PERGAMON INTERNATIONAL LIBRARY
of Science, Technology, Engineering and Social Studies

*The 1000-volume original paperback library in aid of education,
industrial training and the enjoyment of leisure*

Publisher: Robert Maxwell, M.C.

Perspectives in Abnormal Behavior

PGPS-37

PERGAMON GENERAL PSYCHOLOGY SERIES

Editor: Arnold P. Goldstein, *Syracuse University*
Leonard Krasner, *SUNY, Stony Brook*

TITLES IN THE PERGAMON GENERAL PSYCHOLOGY SERIES
(Added Titles in Back of Volume)

The terms of our inspection copy service apply to all the above books. A complete catalogue of all books in the Pergamon International Library is available on request.

The Publisher will be pleased to receive suggestions for revised editions and new titles.

Perspectives in Abnormal Behavior

Edited by

RICHARD J. MORRIS

Department of Psychology
Syracuse University

PERGAMON PRESS INC.

New York / Toronto / Oxford / Sydney / Braunschweig / Paris

Pergamon Press Offices:

U. S. A.	Pergamon Press Inc., Maxwell House, Fairview Park, Elmsford, New York 10523, U.S.A.
U. K.	Pergamon Press Ltd., Headington Hill Hall, Oxford OX3 0BW, England
C A N A D A	Pergamon of Canada, Ltd., 207 Queen's Quay West, Toronto 1, Canada
A U S T R A L I A	Pergamon Press (Aust.) Pty. Ltd., 19a Boundary Street, Rushcutters Bay, N.S.W. 2011, Australia
F R A N C E	Pergamon Press SARL, 24 rue des Ecoles, 75240 Paris, Cedex 05, France
W E S T G E R M A N Y	Pergamon Press GMbH, 3300 Braunschweig, Postfach 2923, Burgplatz 1, West Germany

Library of Congress Cataloging in Publication Data

Morris, Richard J   comp.
    Perspectives in abnormal behavior.

    (Pergamon general psychology series, PGPS-37)
    Includes bibliographies.
    1.   Psychiatry--Addresses, essays, lectures.
I.   Title.   [DNLM: 1.   Psychopathology--Collected
works.   WM100 M877p   1974]
RC458.M63 1974   616.8'9   73-7975
ISBN 0-08-017738-7
ISBN 0-08-017739-5   (pbk.)

Reprinted 1975

Printed in the United States of America

To my mother and in memory of my father

Contents

Preface

There have been many changes in the field of abnormal psychology over the past 20 years. Changes in treatment have ranged from a general disenchantment with insight oriented psychotherapy to treatment techniques based on learning theory, and to encounter groups. Changes with respect to *when* treatment should be initiated have also occurred, giving rise to the community mental health movement with its emphasis on prevention and the handling of everyday "problems in living." In addition, there have been changes in terms of the focus of therapy. Instead of treating the individual *in vacuo*, many therapists have begun to modify the individual's environment as well as his maladaptive behavior within that environment.

Moreover, the recent emphasis in abnormal psychology on the role of social, environmental, cultural, genetic, and biochemical factors as contributing variables to the development and maintenance of maladaptive behavior has led many professionals into disciplines with which they were previously little concerned. Thus, within the last 20 years we find a movement in the field of abnormal psychology away from the strict psychological theorizing of the pre-1950s and toward an interdisciplinary approach to the understanding and treatment of maladaptive behavior.

This is not to say that mental health professionals have totally abandoned such psychological theorizing as psychoanalysis to understand their fellow man, but that within the last decade or so they have begun to realize that there are factors other than the individual's psyche that are contributing to the development and maintenance of his maladaptive behavior.

Just as Freud's position in the early 1900s was considered to be revolutionary, so must the developments in abnormal psychology since 1950. One cannot deny the research findings that have consistently demonstrated the effects of non-psychological variables as contributors to the development, maintenance, and treatment of maladaptive behavior. Nor can one overlook the importance of the exponentially increasing research that has evolved from the learning theories of Hull and Skinner as well as Pavlov and social-learning theory. This research, with little exception, has shown that behavior can be modified by its consequences.

Before 1950, most psychotherapists viewed insight oriented psychotherapy as the method of choice for the treatment of various behavior disorders, the emphasis being on the medical model. However, over the last 20 years, the literature has shown that techniques derived from other models are as effective and perhaps more efficient in the treatment of many of the same maladaptive behaviors.

There have been changes in abnormal psychology in addition to those concerned with etiology, treatment, and prevention. Particularly noteworthy over the last decade has been the development among clinicians of a feeling of disillusionment with psychiatric labels and diagnoses—reflecting the growing body of research which has demonstrated the questionable reliability of psychiatric diagnoses. Intimately tied to this development is the concern by most professionals with the stigma attached to those people who have been labeled mentally ill. This concern is reflected in the number of articles that appeared recently, in the professional literature on the consequences of being labeled mentally ill.

It was because of these various changes in the area of abnormal psychology that a decision was made to compile a book of readings which would communicate these changes to students. In order to present this material in a balanced manner, articles were chosen which reflected the major perspectives now subscribed to in abnormal psychology.

Two main criteria were used in the selection of material. First, the article had to be readable, wihout a technical orientation, and had to maintain the tenets of scientific rigor. Second, the article had to reflect the present direction(s) of the particular area covered and suggest further avenues of investigation. The intent was to present a compelling compilation of challenging and informative articles from various perspectives in the area of abnormal psychology.

As is the case with any book, but especially with a book of readings, many people deserve acknowledgment and thanks. I would like to thank the authors and publishers who permitted their material to be reprinted, and many of my students who were interested enough to discuss critically the issues covered in the book. A number of people worked behind the scenes to ready this book for publication. Among them, appreciation is notably due Donna Petta and Ellen Kasher, Catherine LaPlante, Michael Dolker, and Kenneth Suckerman for their assistance in the preparation of the manuscript. I also thank my colleague and friend, Dr. Mark Sherman, for reviewing the manuscript and offering comments. The major typing of the manuscript and the letters of permission was expertly done by Vera Richardson who donated a significant amount of her time to this project. I thank her very much.

I also wish to express my gratitude to Dr. Arnold P. Goldstein, consulting editor at Pergamon Press, for his support and many helpful suggestions concerning the manuscript. Finally, special thanks are due my wife, Vinnie, for her editorial assistance as well as her everpresent encouragement and support from the formulation to the completion of this book.

RICHARD J. MORRIS
Syracuse, New York

About the Author

Richard J. Morris (Ph.D., Arizona State University) is presently Associate Professor of Psychology, Syracuse University, and a member of the Clinical Faculty, Department of Pediatrics, State University of New York, Upstate Medical Center. He has also taught at Arizona State University. Dr. Morris is a member of several professional associations and serves as a Consulting Editor for *Rehabilitation Psychology* and as a Consultant for the Veterans Administration Hospitals. His published works and papers are in the areas of behavior therapy and experimental personality.

UNIT I

Issues in Identifying Abnormal Behavior

INTRODUCTION

The assumption that has been made traditionally by most clinicians is that it is necessary to diagnose and classify a person's abnormal behavior before treatment can take place. This assumption is based on the procedure followed in medicine regarding when people with physical illnesses are treated. Mental health professionals who use this approach generally believe that once the basic cause, or underlying malady, has been diagnosed from a patient's symptoms (maladaptive behaviors), then the best possible treatment procedure can be prescribed. They further point out that since a patient's symptoms are signs of an underlying psychological disorder or neurological defect direct treatment of these symptoms would not be appropriate. Rather, they feel that the underlying disorder should be the focus of treatment. The use of this approach in the diagnosis and treatment of abnormal behavior is known as the *medical model.*

According to this model, before techniques can be developed to successfully treat various abnormal behaviors, a system must be developed whereby these behaviors can be identified and classified. One of the first systematic attempts to classify abnormal behavior was performed by Emil Kraepelin in the last half of the nineteenth century. He defined two major categories of mental illness—manic-depressive psychosis and dementia praecox (later called schizophrenia). These categories were used, with some modification, by mental health professionals until the classification system was completely revised in the early 1950s by a committee of the American Psychiatric Association. This revision resulted in the publication in 1952 of a new and more elaborate classification system called the *Diagnostic and Statistical Manual of Mental Disorders* (DSM-I). In 1968, this manual was revised by a similar committee of the American Psychiatric Association resulting in the publication of the new classification system, also called the *Diagnostic and Statistical Manual of Mental Disorders* (DSM-II). This revised system is the one currently in use in psychiatric settings.

In recent years the validity of the medical model approach has been questioned by an increasing number of professionals in the field of mental health (e.g., Ullmann & Krasner, 1965). They point out that because there may be an underlying basis to the symptoms of a patient with a particular physical illness, it does not

1

necessarily follow that there must also be an underlying cause for the symptoms of a patient with a mental health problem. They further maintain that the maladaptive behaviors (symptoms) a patient shows *are*, in fact, his psychological disorder, that is, there is no underlying cause to these behaviors. This view implies that the clinician should direct his efforts toward the treatment of maladaptive behaviors and not the treatment of a presumed underlying cause. For example, if a patient has a fear of driving over bridges, a fear of flying, a fear of elevators, and a fear of becoming interpersonally close to another person, the psychologist or psychiatrist should consider these maladaptive behaviors as the patient's disorder and treat these problems directly (either separately or all at one time), instead of trying to find the underlying problem causing each of these behaviors.

One prominent person who has questioned the appropriateness of the medical model is Thomas S. Szasz, author of Article 1. He views mental illness as a myth; that is, he feels that there are no underlying neurological causes to mental illness. He points out that the construct "mental illness" has led mental health professionals away from the very problems they should be treating, namely, the patient's maladaptive behaviors. Thus, this construct should either be redefined in terms of maladaptive behaviors that can be observed or be removed from the language of the mental health professions. Szasz also suggests that the symptoms that clinicians observe in patients represent nothing more than "problems in living," or deviations from the social norm, and he reiterates his point that such deviations are what constitute the mental illness.

A similar position is taken by Thomas J. Scheff, author of Article 2, who directs his discussion to that diagnostic category called schizophrenia, the diagnosis given to the majority of individuals who are hospitalized for psychiatric problems. Making use of labeling theory, he states that schizophrenia is a label applied by people in our society (and by societies who share our values) to those individuals who break the established social rules of acceptable conduct. Since behaviors that deviate from the social customs of a society are not usually tolerated by members of that society, and since these unacceptable modes of behavior do not fit into conventional categories such as crime, drunkenness, prostitution, etc., members of the society utilize a socially acceptable approach in dealing with people who show these unacceptable modes of behavior. Specifically, the society makes use of a residual category that involves labeling these people as mentally ill (e.g., as schizophrenic) and thus enables society to maintain what Scheff refers to as the "public order."

In addition to questioning the validity of the medical model, some researchers have taken a critical look at the reliability of the diagnostic classification system used in the mental health field. They are particularly interested in discovering the extent to which clinicians agree on the diagnosis given to a person in a psychiatric setting. The general findings of this research, based on a large number of studies published since 1950, have shown that the reliability of specific psychiatric diagnoses is not impressive. Article 3, by Edward Zigler and Leslie Phillips, is addressed to the issue of the reliability of psychiatric diagnoses, and discusses the advantages and disadvantages of these diagnoses. Zigler and Phillips' review of the diagnostic system shows that the degree of agreement among professionals regarding such general and inclusive psychiatric categories as psychosis, neurosis, or character disorders is at an acceptable level; however, as the classification system narrows to specific diagnoses within these general categories (e.g., anxiety state neurosis or paranoid schizophrenia), the level of agreement decreases. The authors also discuss reasons why many professionals have questioned the utility of psychiatric diagnoses—for example, one reason relates to the lack of clarity regarding which symptoms are associated with each diagnostic category. They conclude that there is merit in the use of psychiatric diagnoses providing that their use is solely descriptive, that they are based on empirically derived behavior correlates, and that they are not used for purposes of inferring cause.

Article 4 by Frederick H. Kanfer and George Saslow, extends the discussion of psychiatric diagnoses an additional step. The authors reject the use of the behavioral correlate approach to diagnoses since they feel that this approach is not reliable, is of limited prognostic value, and does not differentially determine which type of treatment a particular patient should receive. They feel that the clinician should use a classification system that will help him in the planning of a treatment approach for his particular patient. As an alternative to the current diagnostic practice, these authors suggest that the clinician should undertake a behavior analysis of each patient. Such an analysis would include an extensive interview with the patient, as well as the gathering of information about the patient from various people with whom he interacts, the observation of his interactions with others, and a review of the results of his psychological tests. This differs from traditional diagnostic approaches, but the authors feel that once all the information from this behavior analysis is processed and organized the therapist will be in a position to determine the best treatment procedure for the patient. This approach to diagnosis follows quite closely from Kanfer and Saslow's theoretical position concerning the conduct of therapy. Commonly called behavior modification, or behavior therapy, their position utilizes techniques based on various theories of learning. It also rejects the use of labels to summarize a patient's behavior and favors the clinician's detailed description of the patient's behavior.

References

American Psychiatric Association. *Diagnostic and statistical manual of mental disorders.* Washington, D.C.: American Psychiatric Association, 1952.

American Psychiatric Association. *Diagnostic and statistical manual of mental disorders.* (2nd ed.) Washington, D.C.: American Psychiatric Association, 1968.

Ullman, L., & Krasner, L. *Case studies in behavior modification.* New York: Holt, Rinehart & Winston, 1965.

1

The Myth of Mental Illness*

THOMAS S. SZASZ

My aim in this essay is to raise the question "Is there such a thing as mental illness?" and to argue that there is not. Since the notion of mental illness is extremely widely used nowadays, inquiry into the ways in which this term is employed would seem to be especially indicated. Mental illness, of course, is not literally a "thing"—or physical object—and hence it can "exist" only in the same sort of way in which other theoretical concepts exist. Yet, familiar theories are in the habit of posing, sooner or later—at least to those who come to believe in them—as "objective truths" (or "facts"). During certain historical periods, explanatory conceptions such as deities, witches, and microorganisms appeared not only as theories but as self-evident *causes* of a vast number of events. I submit that today mental illness is widely regarded in a somewhat similar fashion, that is, as the cause of innumerable diverse happenings. As an antidote to the complacent use of the notion of mental illness—whether as a self-evident phenomenon, theory, or cause—let us ask this question: What is meant when it is asserted that someone is mentally ill?

In what follows I shall describe briefly the main uses to which the concept of mental illness has been put. I shall argue that this notion has outlived whatever usefulness it might have had and that it now functions merely as a convenient myth.

MENTAL ILLNESS AS A SIGN OF BRAIN DISEASE

The notion of mental illness derives its main support from such phenomena as syphilis of the brain or delirious conditions—intoxications, for instance—in which persons are known to manifest various peculiarities or disorders of thinking and behavior. Correctly speaking, however, these are diseases of the brain, not of the mind. According to one school of thought, *all* so-called mental illness is of this type. The assumption is made that some neurological defect, perhaps a very subtle one, will ultimately be found for all the disorders of thinking and behavior. Many contemporary psychiatrists, physicians, and other scientists hold this view. This position implies that people *cannot* have troubles—expressed in what are *now called* "mental illnesses"—because of differences in personal needs, opinions, social aspirations, values, and so on. *All problems in living* are attributed to physicochemical processes which in due time will be discovered by medical research.

"Mental illnesses" are thus regarded as basically no different than all other diseases (that is, of the body). The only difference, in this view, between mental and bodily diseases is that the former, affecting the brain, manifest themselves by means of mental symptoms; whereas the latter, affecting other organ systems (for example, the skin, liver, etc.), mani-

*From Szasz, T. S., "The myth of mental illness," *American Psychologist*, 1960, **15**, 113–118. Copyright © 1960 by the American Psychological Association, and reproduced by permission.

4

fest themselves by means of symptoms referable to those parts of the body. This view rests on and expresses what are, in my opinion, two fundamental errors.

In the first place, what central nervous system symptoms would correspond to a skin eruption or a fracture? It would *not* be some emotion or complex bit of behavior. Rather, it would be blindness or a paralysis of some part of the body. The crux of the matter is that a disease of the brain, analogous to a disease of the skin or bone, is a neurological defect, and not a problem in living. For example, a *defect* in a person's visual field may be satisfactorily explained by correlating it with certain definite lesions in the nervous system. On the other hand, a person's *belief*—whether this be a belief in Christianity, in Communism, or in the idea that his internal organs are "rotting" and that his body is, in fact, already "dead"—cannot be explained by a defect or disease of the nervous system. Explanations of this sort of occurrence—assuming that one is interested in the belief itself and does not regard it simply as a "symptom" or expression of something else that is *more interesting*—must be sought along different lines.

The second error in regarding complex psychosocial behavior, consisting of communications about ourselves and the world about us, as mere symptoms of neurological functioning is *epistemological*. In other words, it is an error pertaining not to any mistakes in observation or reasoning, as such, but rather to the way in which we organize and express our knowledge. In the present case, the error lies in making a symmetrical dualism between mental and physical (or bodily) symptoms, a dualism which is merely a habit of speech and to which no known observations can be found to correspond. Let us see if this is so. In medical practice, when we speak of physical disturbances, we mean either signs (for example, a fever) or symptoms (for example, pain). We speak of mental symptoms, on the other hand, when we refer to a patient's *communications about himself, others, and the world about him.* He might state that he is Napoleon or that he is being persecuted by the Communists. These would be considered mental symptoms *only* if the observer believed that the patient was *not* Napoleon or that he was *not* being persecuted by the Communists. This makes it apparent that the statement that "*X* is a mental symptom" involves rendering a judgment. The judgment entails, moreover, a covert comparison or matching of the patient's ideas, concepts, or beliefs with those of the observer and the society in which they live. The notion of mental symptom is therefore inextricably tied to the *social* (including *ethical*) *context* in which it is made in much the same way as the notion of bodily symptom is tied to an *anatomical* and *genetic context* (Szasz, 1957a, 1957b).

To sum up what has been said thus far: I have tried to show that for those who regard mental symptoms as signs of brain disease, the concept of mental illness is unnecessary and misleading. For what they mean is that people so labeled suffer from diseases of the brain; and, if that is what they mean, it would seem better for the sake of clarity to say that and not something else.

MENTAL ILLNESS AS A NAME FOR PROBLEMS IN LIVING

The term "mental illness" is widely used to describe something which is very different than a disease of the brain. Many people today take it for granted that living is an arduous process. Its hardship for modern man, moreover, derives not so much from a struggle for biological survival as from the stresses and strains inherent in the social intercourse of complex human personalities. In this context, the notion of mental illness is used to identify or describe some feature of an individual's so-called personality. Mental illness—as a deformity of the personality, so to speak—is then regarded as the *cause* of the human disharmony. It is implicit in this view that social intercourse between people is regarded as something *inherently harmonious,* its disturbance being due solely to the presence of "mental illness" in many people. This is obviously fallacious reasoning, for it makes the abstraction "mental illness" into a *cause,* even though this abstraction was created in the first place to serve only as a shorthand expression for certain types of human behavior. It now becomes necessary to ask: "What kinds of behavior are regarded as indicative of mental illness, and by whom?"

The concept of illness, whether bodily or mental, implies *deviation from some clearly defined norm.* In the case of physical illness, the norm is the structural and functional integrity of the human body. Thus, although the desirability of physical health, as such, is an ethical value, what health *is* can be stated in anatomical and physiological terms. What is the norm, deviation from which is regarded as mental illness? This question cannot be easily answered. But whatever this norm might be, we can be certain of only one thing: namely, that it is a norm that must be stated in terms of *psychosocial, ethical,* and *legal* concepts. For example, notions such as "excessive repression" or "acting out an unconscious impulse" illustrate the use of psychological concepts for judging (so-called) mental health and illness. The idea that chronic hostility, vengefulness, or divorce are indicative of mental illness would be illustrations of the use of ethical norms (that is, the desirability of love, kindness, and a stable marriage relationship). Finally, the widespread psychiatric opinion that only a mentally ill person would commit homicide illustrates the use of a legal concept as a norm of mental health. The norm from which deviation is measured whenever one speaks of a mental illness is a psychosocial and ethical one. Yet, the remedy is sought in terms of *medical* measures which—it is hoped and assumed—are free from wide differences of ethical value. The definition of the disorder and the terms in which its remedy are sought are therefore at serious odds with one another. The practical significance of this covert conflict between the alleged nature of the defect and the remedy can hardly be exaggerated.

Having identified the norms used to measure deviations in cases of mental illness, we will now turn to the question: "Who defines the norms and hence the deviation?" Two basic answers may be offered: (a) It may be the person himself (that is, the patient) who decides that he deviates from a norm. For example, an artist may believe that he suffers from a work inhibition; and he may implement this conclusion by seeking help *for* himself from a psychotherapist. (b) It may be someone other than the patient who decides that the latter is deviant (for example, relatives, physicians, legal authorities, society generally, etc.). In such a case a psychiatrist may be hired by others to do something *to* the patient in order to correct the deviation.

These considerations underscore the importance of asking the question "Whose agent is the psychiatrist?" and of giving a candid answer to it (Szasz, 1956, 1958). The psychiatrist (psychologist or nonmedical psychotherapist), it now develops, may be the agent of the patient, of the relatives, of the school, of the military services, of a business organization, of a court of law, and so forth. In speaking of the psychiatrist as the agent of these persons or organizations, it is not implied that his values concerning norms, or his ideas and aims concerning the proper nature of remedial action, need to coincide exactly with those of his employer. For example, a patient in individual psychotherapy may believe that his salvation lies in a new marriage; his psychotherapist need not share this hypothesis. As the patient's agent, however, he must abstain from bringing social or legal force to bear on the patient which would prevent him from putting his beliefs into action. If his *contract* is with the patient, the psychiatrist (psychotherapist) may disagree with him or stop his treatment; but he cannot engage others to obstruct the patient's aspirations. Similarly, if a psychiatrist is engaged by a court to determine the sanity of a criminal, he need not fully share the legal authorities' values and intentions in regard to the criminal and the means available for dealing with him. But the psychiatrist is expressly barred from stating, for example, that it is not the criminal who is "insane" but the men who wrote the law on the basis of which the very actions that are being judged are regarded as "criminal." Such an opinion could be voiced, of course, but not in a courtroom, and not by a psychiatrist who makes it his practice to assist the court in performing its daily work.

To recapitulate: In actual contemporary social usage, the finding of a mental illness is made by establishing a deviance in behavior from certain psychosocial, ethical, or legal norms. The judgment may be made, as in medicine, by the patient, the physician (psychiatrist), or others. Remedial action, finally, tends to be sought in a therapeutic—or covertly medical—framework, thus creating a situation in which *psychosocial, ethical,* and/or *legal deviations* are claimed to be correctable by (so-called) *medical action.* Since medical action is designed to correct only medical deviations, it seems logically absurd to expect that it will help solve problems whose very existence had been defined and established on nonmedical grounds. I think that these considerations may be fruitfully applied to the present use of tranquilizers and, more generally, to what might be expected of drugs of whatever type in regard to the amelioration or solution of problems in human living.

THE ROLE OF ETHICS IN PSYCHIATRY

Anything that people *do*—in contrast to things that *happen* to them (Peters, 1958)—takes place in a context of value. In this broad sense, no human activity is devoid of ethical implications. When the values underlying certain activities are widely shared, those who participate in their pursuit may lose sight of them altogether. The discipline of medicine, both as a pure science (for example, research) and as a technology (for example, therapy), contains many ethical considerations and judgments. Unfortunately, these are often denied, minimized, or merely kept out of focus; for the ideal of the medical profession as well as of the people whom it serves seems to be having a system of medicine (allegedly) free of ethical value. This sentimental notion is expressed by such things as the doctor's willingness to treat and help patients irrespective of their religious or political beliefs, whether they are rich or poor, etc. While there may be some grounds for this belief—albeit it is a view that is not impressively true even in these regards—the fact remains that ethical considerations encompass a vast range of human affairs. By making the practice of medicine neutral in regard to some specific issues of value need not, and cannot, mean that it can be kept free from all such values. The practice of medicine is intimately tied to ethics; and the first thing that we must do, it seems to me, is to try to make this clear and explicit. I shall let this matter rest here, for it does not concern us specifically in this essay. Lest there be any vagueness, however, about how or where ethics and medicine meet, let me remind the reader of such issues as birth control, abortion, suicide, and euthanasia as only a few of the major areas of current ethicomedical controversy.

Psychiatry, I submit, is very much more intimately tied to problems of ethics than is medicine. I use the word "psychiatry" here to refer to that contemporary discipline which is concerned with *problems in living* (and not with diseases of the brain, which are problems for neurology). Problems in human relations can be analyzed, interpreted, and given meaning only within given social and ethical contexts. Accordingly, it *does* make a difference—arguments to the contrary notwithstanding—what the psychiatrist's socio-ethical orientations happen to be; for these will influence his ideas on what is wrong with the patient, what deserves comment or interpretation, in what possible directions change might be desirable, and so forth. Even in medicine proper, these factors play a role, as for instance, in the divergent orientations which physicians, depending on their religious affiliations, have toward such things as birth control and therapeutic abortion. Can anyone really believe that a psychotherapist's ideas concerning religious belief, slavery, or other similar issues play no role in his practical work? If they do make a difference, what are we to infer from it? Does it not seem reasonable that we ought to have different psychiatric therapies—each expressly recognized for the ethical positions which they embody—for, say, Catholics and Jews, religious persons and agnostics, Democrats and Communists, white supremacists and Negroes, and so on? Indeed, if we look at how psychiatry is actually practiced today (especially in the United States), we find that people do seek psychiatric help in accordance with their social status and ethical beliefs (Hollingshead & Redlich, 1958). This should really not surprise us more than being told that practicing Catholics rarely frequent birth control clinics.

The foregoing position which holds that contemporary psychotherapists deal with problems in living, rather than with mental illnesses and their cures, stands in opposition to a currently prevalent claim, according to which mental illness is just as "real" and "objective" as bodily illness. This is a confusing claim since it is never known exactly what is meant by such words as "real" and "objective." I suspect, however, that what is intended by the proponents of this view is to create the idea in the popular mind that mental illness is some sort of disease entity, like an infection or a malignancy. If this were true, one could *catch* or *get* a "mental illness," one might *have* or *harbor* it, one might *transmit* it to others, and finally one could get *rid* of it. In my opinion, there is not a shred of evidence to support this idea. To the contrary, all the evidence is the other way and supports the view that what people now call mental illnesses are for the most part *communications* expressing unacceptable ideas, often framed, moreover, in an unusual idiom. The scope of this essay allows me to do no more than mention this alternative theoretical approach to this problem (Szasz, 1957c).

This is not the place to consider in detail the similarities and differences between bodily and mental illnesses. It shall suffice for us here to emphasize only one important difference between them: namely, that whereas bodily disease refers to public, physicochemical occurrences, the notion of mental illness is used to codify relatively more private, socio-psychological happenings of which the observer (diagnostician) forms a part. In other words, the psychiatrist does not stand *apart* from what he observes, but is, in Harry Stack Sullivan's apt words, a "participant observer." This means that he is *committed* to some picture of what he considers reality—and to what he thinks society considers reality—and he observes and judges the patient's behavior in the light of these considerations. This touches on our earlier observation that the notion of mental symptom itself implies a comparison between observer and observed, psychiatrist and patient. This is so obvious that I may be charged with belaboring trivialities. Let me therefore say once more that my aim in presenting this argument was expressly to criticize and counter a prevailing contemporary tendency to deny the moral aspects of psychiatry (and psychotherapy) and to substitute for them allegedly value-free medical considerations. Psychotherapy, for example, is being widely practiced as though it entailed nothing other than restoring the patient from a state of mental sickness to one of mental health. While it is generally accepted that mental illness has something to do with man's social (or interpersonal) relations, it is paradoxically maintained that problems of values (that is, of ethics) do not arise in this process.[1] Yet, in one sense, much of psychotherapy may revolve around nothing other than the elucidation and weighing of goals and values—many of which may be mutually contradictory—and the means whereby they might best be harmonized, realized, or relinquished.

The diversity of human values and the methods by means of which they may be realized [are] so vast, and many of them remain so unacknowledged, that they cannot fail but lead to conflicts in human relations. Indeed, to say that human relations at all levels—from mother to child, through husband and wife, to nation and nation—are fraught with stress, strain, and disharmony is, once again, making the obvious explicit. Yet, what may be obvious may be also poorly understood. This I think is the case here. For it seems to me that—at least in our scientific theories of behavior—we have failed to *accept* the simple fact that human relations are inherently fraught with difficulties and that to make them even relatively harmonious requires much patience and hard work. I submit that the idea of mental illness is now being put to work to obscure certain difficulties which at present may be inherent—not that they need be unmodifiable—in the social intercourse of persons. If this is true, the concept functions as a disguise; for instead of calling attention to conflicting human needs, aspirations, and values, the notion of mental illness provides an amoral and impersonal "thing" (an "illness") as an explanation for *problems in living* (Szasz, 1959). We may recall in this connection that not so long ago it was devils and witches who were held responsible for men's problems in social living. The belief in mental illness, as something other than man's trouble in getting along with his fellow man, is the proper heir to the belief in demonology and witchcraft. Mental illness exists or is "real" in exactly the same sense in which witches existed or were "real."

CHOICE, RESPONSIBILITY, AND PSYCHIATRY

While I have argued that mental illnesses do not exist, I obviously did not imply that the social and psychological occurrences to which this label is currently being attached also do not exist. Like the personal and social troubles which people had in the Middle Ages, they are real enough. It is the labels we give them that concerns us and, having labeled them, what we do about them. While I cannot go into the ramified implications of this problem here, it is worth noting that a demonologic conception of problems in living gave rise to therapy along theological lines. Today, a belief in mental illness implies—nay, requires—therapy along medical or psychotherapeutic lines.

What is implied in the line of thought set forth here is something quite different. I do not intend to offer a new conception of "psychiatric illness" nor a new form of "therapy." My aim is more modest and yet also more ambitious. It is to suggest that the phenomena now called mental illnesses be looked at afresh and more simply, that they be removed from the category of illnesses, and that they be regarded as the expressions of man's struggle with the problem of *how* he should live. The last mentioned problem is obviously a vast one, its

---

[1] Freud went so far as to say that: "I consider ethics to be taken for granted. Actually I have never done a mean thing" (Jones, 1957, p. 247). This surely is a strange thing to say for someone who has studied man as a social being as closely as did Freud. I mention it here to show how the notion of "illness" (in the case of psychoanalysis, "psychopathology," or "mental illness") was used by Freud—and by most of his followers—as a means for classifying certain forms of human behavior as falling within the scope of medicine, and hence (by *fiat*) outside that of ethics!

enormity reflecting not only man's inability to cope with his environment, but even more his increasing self-reflectiveness.

By problems in living, then, I refer to that truly explosive chain reaction which began with man's fall from divine grace by partaking of the fruit of the tree of knowledge. Man's awareness of himself and of the world about him seems to be a steadily expanding one, bringing in its wake an ever larger *burden of understanding* (an expression borrowed from Susanne Langer, 1953). *This burden*, then, *is to be expected and must not be misinterpreted.* Our only *rational* means for lightening it is *more understanding*, and appropriate *action* based on such understanding. The main alternative lies in acting as though the burden were not what in fact we perceive it to be and taking refuge in an outmoded theological view of man. In the latter view, man does not fashion his life and much of his world about him, but merely lives out his fate in a world created by superior beings. This may logically lead to pleading nonresponsibility in the face of seemingly unfathomable problems and difficulties. Yet, if man fails to take increasing responsibility for his actions, individually as well as collectively, it seems unlikely that some higher power or being would assume this task and carry this burden for him. Moreover, this seems hardly the proper time in human history for obscuring the issue of man's responsibility for his actions by hiding it behind the skirt of an all-explaining conception of mental illness.

CONCLUSIONS

I have tried to show that the notion of mental illness has outlived whatever usefulness it might have had and that it now functions merely as a convenient myth. As such, it is a true heir to religious myths in general, and to the belief in witchcraft in particular; the role of all these belief-systems was to act as *social tranquilizers*, thus encouraging the hope that mastery of certain specific problems may be achieved by means of substitutive (symbolic-magical) operations. The notion of mental illness thus serves mainly to obscure the everyday fact that life for most people is a continuous struggle, not for biological survival, but for a "place in the sun," "peace of mind," or some other human value. For man aware of himself and of the world about him, once the needs for preserving the body (and perhaps the race) are more or less satisfied, the problem arises as to what he should do with himself. Sustained adherence to the myth of mental illness allows people to avoid facing this problem, believing that mental health, conceived as the absence of mental illness, automatically insures the making of right and safe choices in one's conduct of life. But the facts are all the other way. It is the making of good choices in life that others regard, retrospectively, as good mental health!

The myth of mental illness encourages us, moreover, to believe in its logical corollary: that social intercourse would be harmonious, satisfying, and the secure basis of a "good life" were it not for the disrupting influences of mental illness or "psychopathology." The potentiality for universal human happiness, in this form at least, seems to me but another example of the I-wish-it-were-true type of fantasy. I do believe that human happiness or well-being on a hitherto unimaginably large scale, and not just for a select few, is possible. This goal could be achieved, however, only at the cost of many men, and not just a few being willing and able to tackle their personal, social, and ethical conflicts. This means having the courage and integrity to forego waging battles on false fronts, finding solutions for substitute problems—for instance, fighting the battle of stomach acid and chronic fatigue instead of facing up to a marital conflict.

Our adversaries are not demons, witches, fate, or mental illness. We have no enemy whom we can fight, exorcise, or dispel by "cure." What we do have are *problems in living*—whether these be biologic, economic, political, or sociopsychological. In this essay I was concerned only with problems belonging in the last mentioned category, and within this group mainly with those pertaining to moral values. The field to which modern psychiatry addresses itself is vast, and I made no effort to encompass it all. My argument was limited to the proposition that mental illness is a myth, whose function it is to disguise and thus render more palatable the bitter pill of moral conflicts in human relations.

REFERENCES

Hollingshead, A. B., & Redlich, F. C. *Social class and mental illness.* New York: Wiley, 1958.

Jones, E. *The life and work of Sigmund Freud.* Vol. III. New York: Basic Books, 1957.

Langer, S. K. *Philosophy in a new key.* New York: Mentor Books, 1953.

Peters, R. S. *The concept of motivation.* London: Routledge & Kegan Paul, 1958.

Szasz, T. S. Malingering: "Diagnosis" or social condemnation? *AMA Arch.-Neurol. Psychiat.,* 1956, **76,** 432–443.

Szasz, T. S. *Pain and pleasure: A study of bodily feelings.* New York: Basic Books, 1957. (a)

Szasz, T. S. The problem of psychiatric nosology: A contribution to a situational analysis of psychiatric operations. *Amer. J. Psychiat.,* 1957, **114,** 405–413. (b)

Szasz, T. S. On the theory of psychoanalytic treatment. *Int. J. Psycho-Anal.,* 1957, **38,** 166–182. (c)

Szasz, T. S. Psychiatry, ethics and the criminal law. *Columbia law Rev.,* 1958, **58,** 183–198.

Szasz, T. S. Moral conflict and psychiatry, *Yale Rev.,* 1960, **49,** 555–566.

2

Schizophrenia as Ideology*

THOMAS J. SCHEFF

In lieu of beginning this paper with a (necessarily) abstract discussion of a concept, *the public order*, I shall invite the reader to consider a *gedanken* experiment that will illustrate its meaning. Suppose in your next conversation with a stranger, instead of looking at his eyes or mouth, you scrutinize his ear. Although the deviation from ordinary behavior is slight (involving only a shifting of the direction of gaze a few degrees, from the eyes to an ear), its effects are explosive. The conversation is disrupted almost instantaneously. In some cases, the subject of this experiment will seek to save the situation by rotating to bring his eyes into your line of gaze; if you continue to gaze at his ear, he may rotate through a full 360 degrees. Most often, however, the conversation is irretrievably damaged. Shock, anger, and vertigo are experienced not only by the "victim" but, oddly enough, by the experimenter himself. It is virtually impossible for either party to sustain the conversation, or even to think coherently, as long as the experiment continues.

The point of this experiment is to suggest the presence of a public order that is all-pervasive, yet taken almost completely for granted. During the simplest kinds of public encounter, there are myriad understandings about comportment that govern the participants' behavior—understandings governing posture, facial expression, and gestures, as well as the content and form of the language used. In speech itself, the types of conformity are extremely diverse and include pronunciation; grammar and syntax; loudness, pitch, and phrasing; and aspiration. Almost all of these elements are so taken for granted that they "go without saying" and are more or less invisible, not only to the speakers but to society at large. These understandings constitute part of our society's assumptive world, the world that is thought of as normal, decent, and possible.

The probability that these understandings are, for the most part, arbitrary to a particular historical culture (is shaking hands or rubbing noses a better form of greeting?) is immaterial to the individual member of society whose attitude of everyday life is, *whatever is, is right.* There is a social, cultural, and interpersonal status quo whose existence is felt only when abrogated. Since violations occur infrequently, and since the culture provides no very adequate vocabulary for talking about either the presence or abuse of its invisible understandings, such deviations are considered disruptive and disturbing. The society member's loyalty to his culture's unstated conventions is unthinking but extremely intense.

The sociologist Mannheim referred to such intense and unconscious loyalty to the status quo as *ideological.* Ideology, in this sense, refers not only to the defense of explicit political or economic interests but, much more broadly, to a whole world view or perspective on what reality is. As a contrast to the ideological view, Mannheim cited the *utopian* outlook,

---

*From Scheff, T. J., *Schizophrenia Bulletin*, 1970, **2**, 15–19. Reprinted by permission of the National Institute of Mental Health Services and Mental Health Administration, U.S. Department of Health, Education, and Welfare, and Dr. Scheff.

which tends "to shatter, either partially or wholly, the order of things prevailing at the time"[7]. The attitude of everyday life, which is ideological, is transfixed by the past and the present; the possibility of a radically different scheme of things, or revolutionary changes in custom and outlook, is thereby rejected. The utopian perspective, by contrast, is fixed on the future; it rejects the status quo with abrupt finality. *Social change* arises out of the clash of the ideological and utopian perspectives.

RESIDUAL RULE VIOLATIONS

It is the thesis of this paper that the concepts of mental illness in general—and schizophrenia in particular—are not neutral, value-free, scientifically precise terms but, for the most part, the leading edge of an ideology embedded in the historical and cultural present of the white middle class of Western societies. The concept of illness and its associated vocabulary—symptoms, therapies, patients, and physicians—reify and legitimate the prevailing public order at the expense of other possible worlds. The medical model of disease refers to culture-free processes that are independent of the public order; a case of pneumonia or syphilis is pretty much the same in New York or New Caledonia. (For criticism of the medical model from psychiatric, psychological, and sociological perspectives, see [3, 4, 6, 8, 11, and 13].)

Most of the "symptoms" of mental illness, however, are of an entirely different nature. Far from being culture-free, such "symptoms" are themselves offenses against implicit understandings of particular cultures. Every society provides its members with a set of explicit norms—understandings governing conduct with regard to such central institutions as the state, the family, and private property. Offenses against these norms have conventional names; for example, an offense against property is called "theft," and an offense against sexual propriety is called "perversion." As we have seen above, however, the public order also is made up of countless unnamed understandings. "Everyone knows," for example, that during a conversation one looks at the other's eyes or mouth, but not at his ear. For the convenience of the society, offenses against these unnamed residual understandings are usually lumped together in a miscellaneous, catchall category. If people reacting to an offense exhaust the conventional categories that might define it (e.g., theft, prostitution, and drunkenness), yet are certain that an offense has been committed, they may resort to this residual category. In earlier societies, the residual category was witchcraft, spirit possession, or possession by the devil; today, it is mental illness. The symptoms of mental illness are, therefore, violations of residual rules.

To be sure, some residual-rule violations are expressions of underlying physiological processes: the hallucinations of the toxic psychoses and the delusions associated with general paresis, for example. Perhaps future research will identify further physiological processes that lead to violations of residual rules. For the present, however, the key attributes of the medical model have yet to be established and verified for the major mental illnesses. There has been no scientific verification of the cause, course, site of pathology, uniform and invariant signs and symptoms, and treatment of choice for almost all of the conventional, "functional" diagnostic categories. Psychiatric knowledge in these matters rests almost entirely on unsystematic clinical impressions and professional lore. It is quite possible, therefore, that many psychiatrists' and other mental-health workers' "absolute certainty" about the cause, site, course, symptoms, and treatment of mental illness represents an ideological reflex, a spirited defense of the present social order.

RESIDUE OF RESIDUES

Viewed as offenses against the public order, the symptoms of schizophrenia are particularly interesting. Of all the major diagnostic categories, the concept of schizophrenia (although widely used by psychiatrists in the United States and in those countries influenced by American psychiatric nomenclature) is the vaguest and least clearly defined. Such categories as obsession, depression, and mania at least have a vernacular meaning. Schizophrenia, however, is a broad gloss; it involves, in no very clear relationship, ideas such as "inappropriateness of affect," "impoverishment of thought," "inability to be involved in meaningful human relationships," "bizarre behavior" (e.g., delusions and hallucinations), "disorder of speech and communication," and "withdrawal."

These very broadly-defined symptoms can be redefined as offenses against implicit social understandings. The appropriateness of emotional expression is, after all, a cultural judgment. Grief is deemed appropriate in our society at a funeral, but not at a party. In other cultures, however, such judgments of propriety may be reversed. With regard to thought disorder, cultural anthropologists have long been at pains to point out that ways of thought are fundamentally different in different societies. What constitutes a meaningful human relationship, anthropologists also report, is basically different in other times and places. Likewise, behavior that is bizarre in one culture is deemed tolerable or even necessary in another. Disorders of speech and communication, again, can be seen as offenses against culturally prescribed rules of language and expression. Finally, the notion of "withdrawal" assumes a cultural standard concerning the degree of involvement and the amount of distance between the individual and those around him.

The broadness and vagueness of the concept of schizophrenia suggest that it may serve as the residue of residues. As diagnostic categories such as hysteria and depression have become conventionalized names for residual rule breaking, a need seems to have developed for a still more generalized, miscellaneous diagnostic category. If this is true, the schizophrenic explores not only "inner space" (Ronald Laing's phrase) but also the normative boundaries of his society.

These remarks should not be taken to suggest that there is no internal experience associated with "symptomatic" behavior; the individual with symptoms *does* experience distress and suffering, or under some conditions, exhilaration and freedom. The point is, however, that public, consensual "knowledge" of mental illness is based, by and large, on knowledge not of these internal states but of their overt manifestations. When a person goes running down the street naked and screaming, lay and professional diagnosticians alike assume the existence of mental illness within that person—even though they have not investigated his internal state. Mental-health procedure and the conceptual apparatus of the medical model posit internal states, but the events actually observed are external.

LABELING THEORY

A point of view which is an alternative to the medical model, and which acknowledges the culture-bound nature of mental illness, is afforded by labeling theory in sociology. (For a general statement of this theory, see [2].) Like the evidence supporting the medical model, which is uneven and in large measure unreliable, the body of knowledge in support of the labeling theory of mental illness is by no means weighty or complete enough to prove its correctness. (Useful supporting material can be found in [1, 5, 6, 9, and 10].) But even though labeling theory is hypothetical, its use may afford perspective—if only because it offers a viewpoint that, along a number of different dimensions, is diametrically opposed to the medical model.

The labeling theory of deviance, when applied to mental illness, may be presented as a series of nine hypotheses:

1. Residual rule breaking arises from fundamentally diverse sources (i.e., organic, psychological, situations of stress, volitional acts of innovation or defiance).

2. Relative to the rate of treated mental illness the rate of unrecorded residual rule breaking is extremely high.

3. Most residual rule breaking is "denied" and is of transitory significance.

4. Stereotyped imagery of mental disorder is learned in early childhood.

5. The stereotypes of insanity are continually reaffirmed, inadvertently, in ordinary social interaction.

6. Labeled deviants may be rewarded for playing the stereotyped deviant role.

7. Labeled deviants are punished when they attempt the return to conventional roles.

8. In the crisis occurring when a residual rule breaker is publicly labeled, the deviant is highly suggestible and may accept the label.

9. Among residual rule breakers, labeling is the single most important cause of careers of residual deviance.

The evidence relevant to these hypotheses is reviewed in the author's *Being Mentally Ill* [8].

According to labeling theory, the societal reaction is the key process that determines outcome in most cases of residual rule breaking. That reaction may be either denial (the most frequent reaction) or labeling. Denial is to "normalize" the rule breaking by ignoring or rationalizing it ("boys will be boys"). The key hypothesis in labeling theory is that, when residual rule breaking is denied, the rule breaking will generally be transitory (as when the stress causing rule breaking is removed; e.g., the cessation of sleep deprivation), compensated for, or channeled into some socially acceptable form. If, however, labeling occurs (i.e., the rule breaker is segregated as a stigmatized deviant), the rule breaking which would otherwise have been terminated, compensated for, or channeled may be stabilized; thus, the offender, through the agency of labeling, is launched on a career of "chronic mental illness." Crucial to the production of chronicity, therefore, are the contingencies (often external to the deviants) that give rise to labeling rather than denial; e.g., the visibility of the rule breaking, the power of the rule breaker relative to persons reacting to his behavior, the tolerance level of the community, and the availability in the culture of alternative channels of response other than labeling (among Indian tribes, for example, involuntary trance states may be seen as a qualification for a desirable position in the society, such as that of shaman).

"SCHIZOPHRENIA"—A LABEL

On the basis of the foregoing discussion, it would seem likely that labeling theory would prove particularly strategic for facilitating the investigation of schizophrenia. Schizophrenia is the single most widely used diagnosis for mental illness in the United States, yet the cause, site, course, and treatment of choice are unknown, or the subject of heated and voluminous controversy. Moreover, there is some evidence that the reliability of diagnosis of schizophrenia is quite low. Finally, there is little agreement on whether a disease entity of schizophrenia even exists, what constitutes schizophrenia's basic signs and symptoms if it *does* exist, and how these symptoms are to be reliably and positively identified in the diagnostic process. Because of the all but overwhelming uncertainties and ambiguities inherent in its definition, "schizophrenia" is an appellation, or "label," which may be easily applied to those residual rule breakers whose deviant behavior is difficult to classify.

In this connection, it is interesting to note the perfectly enormous anomaly of classification procedures in most schizophrenia research. The hypothetical cause of schizophrenia, the independent variable in the research design—whether it is a physiological, biochemical, or psychological attribute—is measured with considerable attention to reliability, validity, and precision. I have seen reports of biochemical research in which the independent variable is measured to two decimal places. Yet the measurement of the dependent variable, the diagnosis of schizophrenia, is virtually ignored. The precision of the measurement, obviously, is virtually nil, since it represents at best an ordinal scale, or, much more likely, a nominal scale. In most studies, the reliability and validity of the diagnosis receives no attention at all: An experimental group is assembled by virtue of hospital diagnoses—leaving the measurement of the dependent variable to the mercy of the obscure vagaries of the process of psychiatric screening and diagnosis. Labeling theory should serve at least to make this anomaly visible to researchers in the field of schizophrenia.

More broadly, the clash between labeling theory and the medical and psychological models of mental illness may serve to alert researchers to some of the fundamental assumptions that they may be making in setting up their research. Particular reference should be made to the question of whether they are unknowingly aligning themselves with the social status quo; for example, by accepting unexamined the diagnosis of schizophrenia, they may be inadvertently providing the legitimacy of science to what is basically a social value judgment. For the remainder of this paper, I wish to pursue this point—the part that medical science may be playing in legitimating the status quo.

As was earlier indicated, there is a public order which is continually reaffirmed in social interaction. Each time a member of the society conforms to the stated or unstated cultural expectations of that society, as when he gazes at the eyes of the person with whom he is in conversation, he is helping to maintain the social status quo. Any deviation from these expectations, however small and regardless of its motivation, may be a threat to the status quo, since most social change occurs through the gradual erosion of custom.

Since all social orders are, as far as we know, basically arbitrary, a threat to society's fundamental customs impels its conforming members to look to extrasocial sources of legitimacy for the status quo. In societies completely under the sway of a single, monolithic religion, the source of legitimacy is always supernatural. Thus, during the Middle Ages, the legitimacy of the social order was maintained by reference to God's commands, as found in the Bible and interpreted by the Catholic Church. The Pope was God's deputy, the kings ruled by divine right, the particular cultural form that the family happened to take at the time—the patrilocal, monogamous, nuclear family—was sanctified by the church, and so on.

In modern societies, however, it is increasingly difficult to base legitimacy upon appeals to supernatural sources. As complete, unquestioning religious faith has weakened, one very important new source of legitimacy has emerged: In the eyes of laymen, modern science offers the kind of absolute certainty once provided by the church. The institution of medicine is in a particularly strategic position in this regard, since the physician is the only representative of science with whom the average man associates. To the extent that medical science lends its name to the labeling of nonconformity as mental illness, it is giving legitimacy to the social status quo. The mental-health researcher may protest that he is interested not in the preservation of the status quo but in a scientific question: "What are the causes of mental illness?" According to the argument given here, however, his question is loaded—like, "When did you stop beating your wife?" or, more to the point, "What are the causes of witchcraft?" (For a comparison of the treatment of witches and the mentally ill, see [12].) Thus, a question about causality may also be ideological, in Mannheim's sense, in that it reaffirms current social beliefs, if only inadvertently.

REFERENCES

1. Balint, M. *The doctor, the patient, and the illness.* New York: International Universities Press, 1957.
2. Becker, H. *Outsiders.* New York: Free Press, 1963.
3. Goffman, E. *Asylums.* New York: Doubleday-Anchor Books, 1961.
4. Laing, R. *The politics of experience.* New York: Pantheon Books, 1967.
5. Laing, R., & Esterson, A. *Sanity, madness and the family.* London: Tavistock, 1964.
6. Lemert, E. M. *Social pathology.* New York: McGraw-Hill, 1951.
7. Mannheim, K. *Ideology and utopia.* London: Routledge & Kegan Paul, 1936.
8. Scheff, T. J. *Being mentally ill: A sociological theory.* Chicago: Aldine, 1966.
9. Scheff, T. J. *Mental illness and social processes.* New York: Harper & Row, 1967.
10. Spitzer, S. P., & Denzin, N. K. *The mental patient: Studies in the sociology of deviance.* New York: McGraw-Hill, 1968.
11. Szasz, T. S. *The myth of mental illness.* New York: Hoeber-Harper, 1961.
12. Szasz, T. S. *The manufacture of madness.* New York: Harper & Row, 1970.
13. Ullman, L. P., & Krasner, L. *A psychological approach to abnormal behavior.* Englewood Cliffs, N.J.: Prentice-Hall, 1969.

3

Psychiatric Diagnosis: A Critique*[1]

EDWARD ZIGLER and LESLIE PHILLIPS

The inadequacies of conventional psychiatric diagnosis have frequently been noted (Ash, 1949; Cattell, 1957; Eysenck, 1952; Foulds, 1955; Harrower, 1950; Hoch & Zubin, 1953; Jellinek, 1939; King, 1954; Leary & Coffey, 1955; Mehlman, 1952; Menninger, 1955; Noyes, 1953; Phillips & Rabinovitch, 1958; Roe, 1949; Rogers, 1951; Rotter, 1954; Scott, 1958; Thorne, 1953; Wittenborn & Weiss, 1952; Wittman & Sheldon, 1948). The responses to this rather imposing body of criticism have ranged from the position that the present classificatory system is in need of further refinement (Caveny, Wittson, Hunt, & Herman, 1955; Foulds, 1955), through steps toward major revisions (Cattell, 1957; Eysenck, 1952; Leary & Coffey, 1955; Phillips & Rabinovitch, 1958; Thorne, 1953; Wittman & Sheldon, 1948), to a plea for the abolishment of all "labeling" (Menninger, 1955; Noyes, 1953; Rogers, 1951). As other investigators have noted (Caveny et al., 1955; Jellinek, 1939), this last position suggests that the classificatory enterprise is valueless. This reaction against classification has gained considerable popularity in clinical circles. The alacrity with which many clinicians have accepted this view seems to represent more than a disillusionment with the specific current form of psychiatric diagnosis. These negative attitudes appear to reflect a belief that diagnostic classification is inherently antithetical to such clinically favored concepts as "dynamic," "idiographic," etc. Thus, a question is raised as to whether any diagnostic schema can be of value. Let us initially direct our attention to this question.

ON CLASSIFICATION

The growth among clinicians of sentiment against categorization has coincided with a period of critical reappraisal within the behavioral sciences generally (Beach, 1950; Brower, 1949; Cronbach, 1957; Guthrie, 1950; Harlow, 1953; Koch, 1951; MacKinnon, 1953; Marquis, 1948; Rapaport, 1947; Roby, 1959; Scott, 1955; Tolman, 1953; Tyler, 1959). This parallel development is more than coincidental. The reaction against "labeling" can be viewed as an extreme outgrowth of this critical self-evaluation, i.e., that psychology's conceptual schemata are artificial in their construction, sterile in terms of their practical predictions, and lead only to greater and greater precision about matters which are more and more irrelevant. It is little wonder that in this atmosphere, conceptualization has itself become

*From Zigler, E., and Phillips, L., "Psychiatric diagnosis: A critique," *Journal of Abnormal and Social Psychology*, 1961, 3, 607–618. Copyright © 1961 by the American Psychological Association, and reproduced by permission.

[1]This investigation was supported by the Dementia Praecox Research Project, Worcester State Hospital, and a research grant (M-896) from the National Institute of Mental Health, United States Public Health Service.

suspect nor that Maslow's (1948) exposition of the possible dangers of labeling or naming has been extended (Rotter, 1954) as a blanket indictment of the categorizing process.

The error in this extension is the failure to realize that what has been criticized is not the conceptual process but only certain of its products. The criticisms mentioned above have not been in favor of the abolishment of conceptualization, but have rather been directed at the prematurity and rarifications of many of our conceptual schemata and our slavish adherence to them. Indeed, many of these criticisms have been accompanied by pleas for lower-order conceptualization based more firmly on observational data (Koch, 1951; Mac-Kinnon, 1953; Tolman, 1953).

In the clinical area, the sentiment against classification has become sufficiently serious that several investigators (Cattell, 1957; Caveny *et al.*, 1955; Eysenck, 1952; Jellinek, 1939) have felt the need to champion the merits of psychiatric categorization. They have pointed out that diagnosis is a basic scientific classificatory enterprise to be viewed as essentially the practice of taxonomy, which is characteristic of all science. Eysenck (1952) puts the matter quite succinctly in his statement, "Measurement is essential to science, but before we can measure, we must know what it is we want to measure. Qualitative or taxonomic discovery must precede quantitative measurement" (p. 34).

Reduced to its essentials, diagnostic classification involves the establishment of categories to which phenomena can be ordered. The number of class systems that potentially may be constructed is limited only by man's ability to abstract from his experience. The principles employed to construct such classes may be inductive, deductive, or a combination of both, and may vary on a continuum from the closely descriptive to the highly abstract.

Related to the nature of the classificatory principle are the implications to be derived from class membership. Class membership may involve nothing more than descriptive compartmentalization, its only utility being greater ease in the handling of data. Obversely, the attributes or correlates of class membership may be widespread and far-reaching in their consequences. The originators of a classificatory schema may assert that specified behavioral correlates accompany class membership. This assertion is open to test. If the hypothesized correlates represent the full heuristic value of the diagnostic schema and class membership is found not to be related to these correlates, then revision or discard is in order. A somewhat different type of problem may also arise. With the passage of time, correlates not originally related to the schema may erroneously be attributed to class membership. Nevertheless, the original taxonomy may still possess a degree of relevance to current objectives in a discipline. In these circumstances, its maintenance may be the rational choice, although a clarification and purification of categories is called for. The relationship of the two problems outlined here to the criticism of contemporary psychiatric diagnosis will be discussed later. What should be noted at this point is that the solution to neither problem implies the abolishment of the attempt at classification.

Another aspect of taxonomy is in need of clarification. When a phenomenon is assigned to a class, certain individual characteristics of that phenomenon are forever lost. No two class members are completely identical. Indeed, a single class member may be viewed as continuously differing from itself over time. It is this loss of uniqueness and an implied unconcern with process that have led many clinicians to reject classification in principle. While classificatory schemata inevitably involve losses of this type, it must be noted that they potentially offer a more than compensatory gain. This gain is represented in the significance of the class attributes and correlates. Class membership conveys information ranging from the descriptive similarity of two phenomena to a knowledge of the common operative processes underlying the phenomena.

A conceptual system minimizes the aforementioned loss to the extent that only irrelevant aspects of a phenomenon are deleted in the classificatory process. The implicit assumption is made that what is not class relevant is inconsequential. The dilemma, of course, lies in our lacking divine revelation as to what constitutes inconsequentiality. It is this issue which lies at the heart of the idiographic versus nomothetic controversy (Allport, 1937, 1946; Beck, 1953; Eysenck, 1954; Falk, 1956; Hunt, 1951a, 1951b; Skaggs, 1945, 1947). The supporters of the idiographic position (Allport, 1937; Beck, 1953) have criticized certain conceptual schemata for treating idiosyncratic aspects of behavior as inconsequential when they are in fact pertinent data which must be utilized if a comprehensive and adequate view of human behavior is to emerge. However, the idiographic position is not a movement toward the abolishment of classification, a fact emphasized by Allport (1937) and Falk (1956). Rather, it represents a plea for broader and more meaningful classificatory schemata.

A conceptually different type of argument against the use of any diagnostic classification has been made by the adherents of nondirective psychotherapy (Patterson, 1948; Rogers, 1946, 1951). This position has advanced the specific contention that differential diagnosis is unnecessary for, and perhaps detrimental to, successful psychotherapy. This attitude of the nondirectivists has been interpreted (Thorne, 1953) as an attack on the entire classificatory enterprise. To argue against diagnosis on the grounds that it affects therapeutic outcome is to confuse diagnosis as an act of scientific classification with the present clinical practice of diagnosis with its use of interviewing, psychological testing, etc. The error here lies in turning one's attention away from diagnosis as an act of classification, a basic scientific enterprise, and attending instead to the immediate and prognostic consequences of some specific diagnostic technique in a specific therapeutic situation, i.e., an applied aspect. To reject the former on the basis of the latter would appear to be an unsound decision.

Although the nondirectivists' opposition to diagnosis seems to be based on a confusion between the basic and applied aspects of classification, implicitly contained within their position is a more fundamental argument against the classificatory effort. Undoubtedly, diagnosis both articulates and restricts the range of assumptions which may be entertained about a client. However, the philosophy of the nondirectivist forces him to reject any theoretical position which violates a belief in the unlimited psychological growth of the client. It would appear that this position represents the rejection, in principle, of the view that any individual can be like another in his essential characteristics, or that any predictable relationship can be established between a client's current level of functioning and the ends which may be achieved. In the setting of this assumption, a transindividual classificatory schema is inappropriate. There is no appeal from such a judgment, but one should be cognizant that it rejects the essence of a scientific discipline. If one insists on operating within the context of a predictive psychology, one argues for the necessity of a classificatory system, even though particular diagnostic schemata may be rejected as irrelevant, futile, or obscure.

Let us now direct our discussion toward some of the specific criticisms of conventional psychiatric diagnosis—that the categories employed lack homogeneity, reliability, and validity.

HOMOGENEITY

A criticism often leveled against the contemporary diagnostic system is that its categories encompass heterogeneous groups of individuals, i.e., individuals varying in respect to symptomatology, test scores, prognosis, etc. (King, 1954; Rotter, 1954; Wittenborn, 1952; Wittenborn & Bailey, 1952; Wittenborn & Weiss, 1952). Contrary to the view of one investigator (Rotter, 1954), a lack of homogeneity does not necessarily imply a lack of reliability. King (1954) has clearly noted the distinction between these two concepts. Reliability refers to the agreement in assigning individuals to different diagnostic categories, whereas homogeneity refers to the diversity of behavior subsumed within categories. While the two concepts may be related, it is not difficult to conceptualize categories which, though quite reliable, subsume diverse phenomena.

King (1954) has argued in favor of constructing a new diagnostic classification having more restrictive and homogeneous categories. He supports his argument by noting his own findings and those of Kantor, Wallner, and Winder (1953), which have indicated that within the schizophrenic group subcategories may be formed which differ in test performance. King found further support for the construction of new and more homogeneous diagnostic categories in a study by Windle and Hamwi (1953). This study indicated that two subgroups could be constructed within a psychotic population which was composed of patients with diverse psychiatric diagnoses. Though matched on the distribution of these diagnostic types, the subgroups differed in the relationship obtained between test performance and prognosis. On the basis of these studies, King suggests that the type of homogeneous categories he would favor involves such classificatory dichotomies as reactive versus process schizophrenics and chronic versus nonchronic psychotics.

An analysis of King's (1954) criticism of the present diagnostic system discloses certain difficulties. The first is that King's heterogeneity criticism does not fully take into consideration certain basic aspects of classification. A common feature of classificatory systems is that they utilize classes which contain subclasses. An example drawn from biology would be a genus embracing a number of species. If schizophrenia is conceptualized as a genus, it cannot be criticized on the grounds that all its members do not share a particular attribute. Such a criticism would involve a confusion between the more specific attributes of the species and the more general attributes of the genus. This is not to assert that schizophrenia does in fact possess the characteristics of a genus. It is, of course, possible that a careful analysis will reveal that it does not, and the class schizophrenia will have to be replaced by an aggregate of entities which does constitute a legitimate genus. However, when a genus is formulated, it cannot be attacked because of its heterogeneous nature since genera are characterized by such heterogeneity.

A more serious difficulty with King's (1954) heterogeneity criticism lies in the inherent ambiguity of a homogeneity-heterogeneity parameter. To criticize a classificatory system because its categories subsume heterogeneous phenomena is to make the error of assuming that homogeneity is a quality which inheres in phenomena when in actuality it is a construction of the observer or classifier. In order to make this point clear, let us return to King's argument. What does it mean to assert that chronic psychosis is an example of an homogeneous class, while schizophrenia is an example of an heterogeneous one? In terms of the descriptively diverse phenomena encompassed, the latter would appear to have the greater homogeneity. The statement only has meaning insofar as a particular correlate—for instance, the relationship of test score to prognosis—is shared by all members of one class but not so shared by the members of the other class. Thus, the meaningfulness of the homogeneity concept is ultimately dependent on the correlates or attributes of class membership or to the classificatory principle related to these correlates or attributes. The intimacy of the relationship between the attributes of classes and the classificatory principle can best be exemplified by the extreme case in which a class has but a single attribute, and that attribute is defined by the classificatory principle, e.g., the classification of plants on the basis of the number of stamens they possess. Therefore, the heterogeneity criticism of a classificatory system is nothing more than a plea for the utilization of a new classificatory principle so that attention may be focused on particular class correlates or attributes not considered in the original schema. While this plea may be a justifiable one, depending on the significance of the new attributes, it has little to do with the homogeneity, in an absolute sense, of phenomena. Indeed, following the formulation of a new classificatory schema, the heterogeneity criticism could well be leveled against it by the adherents of the old system, since the phenomena encompassed by the new categories would probably not be considered homogeneous when evaluated by the older classificatory principle.

Although differing in its formulation, the heterogeneity criticism of present psychiatric classification made by Wittenborn and his colleagues (Wittenborn, 1952; Wittenborn & Bailey, 1952; Wittenborn & Weiss, 1952) suffers from the same difficulties as does King's (1954) criticism. Wittenborn's findings indicated that individuals given a common diagnosis showed differences in their symptom cluster score profiles based on nine symptom clusters isolated earlier by means of factor analytic techniques (Wittenborn, 1951; Wittenborn & Holzberg, 1951). It is upon the existence of these different profiles within a diagnostic category that Wittenborn bases his heterogeneity criticism. Here again the homogeneity-heterogeneity distinction is only meaningful in terms of an independent criterion, a particular symptom cluster score profile. Had it been discovered that all individuals placed into a particular diagnostic category shared a common symptom cluster score profile, then this category would be described as subsuming homogeneous phenomena. But the phenomena—the symptoms mirrored by the symptom profile—are not homogeneous in any absolute sense because the pattern of symptoms may involve the symptoms in descriptively diverse symptom clusters. Thus, the homogeneity ascribed to the category would refer only to the fact that individuals within the category homogeneously exhibited a particular pattern of descriptively diverse behaviors. However, the organization of symptoms mirrored by the symptom cluster profiles is not in any fundamental sense different from that observed in conventional diagnostic syndromes. Both methods of categorization systematize diverse behaviors because of an observed regularity in their concurrent appearance.

The difference between these two approaches, then, lies only in the pattern of deviant behaviors that define the categories. Indeed, Eysenck (1953) has noted that both the clinician and the factor analyst derive syndromes in essentially the same manner, i.e., in terms of the observed intercorrelations of various symptoms. It is the difference in method, purely observational versus statistical, that explains why the final symptom structure may differ. The assumption must not be made that the advantage lies entirely with the factor analytic method. The merit accruing through the greater rigor of factor analysis may be outweighed by the limitations imposed in employing a restricted group of symptoms and a particular sample of patients. Thus, the factor analyst cannot claim that the class-defining symptom pattern he has derived is a standard of homogeneity against which classes within another schema can be evaluated. The plea that symptom cluster scores, derived from factor analytic techniques, substitute for the present method of psychiatric classification has little relevance to the heterogeneity issue.

In the light of this discussion we may conclude that the concept of homogeneity has little utility in evaluating classificatory schemata. Since the heterogeneity criticism invariably involves an implicit preference for one classificatory principle over another, it would perhaps be more fruitful to dispense entirely with the homogeneity-heterogeneity distinction, thus, allowing us to direct our attention to the underlying problem of the relative merits of different classificatory principles.

RELIABILITY AND VALIDITY

A matter of continuing concern has been the degree of reliability of the present diagnostic system. Considerable energy has been expended by both those who criticize the present system for its lack of reliability (Ash, 1949; Boisen, 1938; Eysenck, 1952; Mehlman, 1952; Roe, 1949; Rotter, 1954; Scott, 1958) and those who defend it against this criticism (Foulds, 1955; Hunt, Wittson, & Hunt, 1953; Schmidt & Fonda, 1956; Seeman, 1953). Certain investigators (Foulds, 1955; Schmidt & Fonda, 1956) who have offered evidence that the present system is reliable have also pointed out that the earlier studies emphasizing the unreliability of psychiatric diagnosis have suffered from serious conceptual and methodological difficulties.

In evaluating the body of studies concerned with the reliability of psychiatric diagnosis, one must conclude that so long as diagnosis is confined to broad diagnostic categories, it is reasonably reliable, but the reliability diminishes as one proceeds from broad, inclusive class categories to narrower, more specific ones. As finer discriminations are called for, accuracy in diagnosis becomes increasingly difficult. Since this latter characteristic appears to be common to the classificatory efforts in many areas of knowledge, it would appear to be inappropriate to criticize psychiatric diagnosis on the grounds that it is less than perfectly reliable. This should not lead to an underestimation of the importance of reliability. While certain extraclassificatory factors, e.g., proficiency of the clinicians, biases of the particular clinical settings, etc., may influence it, reliability is primarily related to the precision with which classes of a schema are defined. Since the defining characteristic of most classes in psychiatric diagnosis is the occurrence of symptoms in particular combinations, the reliability of the system mirrors the specificity with which the various combinations of symptoms (syndromes) have been spelled out. It is mandatory for a classificatory schema to be reliable since reliability refers to the definiteness with which phenomena can be ordered to classes. If a system does not allow for such a division of phenomena, it can make no pretense of being a classificatory schema.

While reliability is a prerequisite if the diagnostic system is to have any value, it must not be assumed that if human effort were to make the present system perfectly reliable, it could escape all the difficulties attributed to it. This perfect reliability would only mean that individuals within each class shared a particular commonality in relation to the classificatory principle of symptom manifestation. If one were interested in attributes unrelated or minimally related to the classificatory principle employed, the perfect reliability of the system would offer little cause for rejoicing. Perfect reliability of the present system can only be the goal of those who are interested in nothing more than the present classificatory principle and the particular attributes of the classes constructed on the basis of this principle.

When attention is shifted from characteristics which define a class to the correlates of class membership, this implies a shift in concern from the reliability of a system to its validity. The distinction between the reliability and validity of a classificatory system would appear to involve certain conceptual difficulties. It is perhaps this conceptual difficulty which explains why the rather imposing body of literature concerned with diagnosis has been virtually silent on the question of the validity of the present system of psychiatric diagnosis. Only one group of investigators (Hunt, 1951; Hunt, Wittson, & Barton, 1950a, 1950b; Hunt, Wittson, & Hunt, 1953; Wittson & Hunt, 1951) has specifically been concerned with the predictive efficacy of diagnoses and, thus, to the validity of psychiatric classifications; and even in this work, the distinction between validity and reliability is not clearly drawn.

In order to grasp the distinction between the reliability and the validity of a classificatory schema, one must differentiate the defining characteristics of the classes from the correlates of the classes. In the former case, we are interested in the principles upon which classes are formed; in the latter, in the predictions or valid statements that can be made about phenomena once they are classified. The difficulty lies in the overlap between the classifying principles and the class correlates. If a classificatory system is reliable, it is also valid to the extent that we can predict that the individuals within a class will exhibit certain characteristics, namely, those behaviors or attributes which serve to define the class.

It is the rare class, however, that does not connote correlates beyond its defining characteristics. The predictions associated with class membership may vary from simple extensions of the classificatory principles to correlates which would appear to have little connection with these principles. Let us examine a simple illustration and see what follows from categorizing an individual. Once an individual has been classified as manifesting a manic-depressive reaction, depressed type, on the basis of the symptoms of depression of mood, motor retardation, and stupor (American Psychiatric Association, 1952), the prediction may be made that the individual will spend a great deal of time in bed, which represents an obvious extension of the symptom pattern. One may also hypothesize that the patient will show improvement if electroshock therapy is employed. This is a correlate which has little direct connection with the symptoms themselves. These predictions are open to test, and evidence may or may not be found to support them. Thus, measures of validity may be obtained which are independent of the reliability of the system of classification.

The problem of validity lies at the heart of the confusion which surrounds psychiatric diagnosis. When the present diagnostic schema is assailed, the common complaint is that class membership conveys little information beyond the gross symptomatology of the patient and contributes little to the solution of the pressing problems of etiology, treatment procedures, prognosis, etc. The criticism that class membership does not predict these important aspects of a disorder appears to be a legitimate one. This does not mean the present system has no validity. It simply indicates that the system may be valid in respect to certain correlates but invalid in respect to others. Much confusion would be dispelled if as much care were taken in noting the existing correlates of classes as is taken in noting the classificatory principles. A great deal of effort has gone into the formalization of the defining characteristics of classes (American Psychiatric Association, 1952), but one looks in vain for a formal delineation of the extraclassificatory attributes and correlates of class membership. As a result, the various diagnostic categories have been burdened with correlates not systematically derived from a classificatory principle but which were attributed to the classes because they were the focal points of clinical interest. A major question is just what correlates can justifiably be attributed to the class categories. To answer this question we must turn our attention to the purposes and philosophy underlying contemporary psychiatric diagnosis.

PHILOSOPHY AND PURPOSE OF CONVENTIONAL DIAGNOSIS

The validity of the conventional diagnostic system is least ambiguous and most free from potential criticism as a descriptive schema, a taxonomy of mental disorders analogous to the work of Ray and Linnaeus in biology. In this sense, class membership confirms that the inclusion of an individual within a class guarantees only that he exhibit the defining characteristics of that class. Only a modest extension of this system, in terms of a very limited number of well established correlates, makes for a system of impressive heuristic value, even though it falls considerably short of what would now be considered an optimal classificatory schema. As has been noted (Caveny *et al.*, 1955; Hunt *et al.*, 1953), the present diagnostic system is quite useful when evaluated in terms of its administrative and, to a lesser extent, its preventive implications. Caveny *et al.* (1955) and Wittenborn, Holzberg, and Simon (1953) should be consulted for a comprehensive list of such uses, but examples would include legal determination of insanity, declaration of incompetence, type of ward required for custodial care, census figures and statistical data upon which considerable planning is based, screening devices for the military services or other agencies, etc. In view of the extensive criticism of contemporary diagnosis, the surprising fact is not that so few valid predictions can be derived from class membership, but that so many can.

The value of the present psychiatric classification system would be further enhanced by its explicit divorcement from its Kraepelinian heritage by an emphasis on its descriptive aspect and, through careful empirical investigation, the cataloging of the reliable correlates of its categories. That this catalog of correlates would be an impressive one is expressed in Hoch's (1953) view that the present system is superior to any system which has been evolved to replace it. It is an open question whether the system merits this amount of praise. In general, however, the defense of the present system—or, for that matter, diagnosis in general (Caveny *et al.*, 1955; Eysenck, 1952; Hunt *et al.*, 1953; Jellinek, 1939)—tends to rest on the merits of its descriptive, empirical, and nondynamic aspects.

The present classificatory system, even as a purely descriptive device, is still open to a certain degree of criticism. Its classificatory principle is organized primarily about symptom manifestation. This would be adequate for a descriptive system if this principle were consistently applied to all classes of the schema and if the symptoms associated with each diagnostic category were clearly specified. There is some question, however, whether the system meets these requirements (Phillips & Rabinovitch, 1958; Rotter, 1954). The criticism has been advanced that the present system is based on a number of diverse principles of classification. Most classes are indeed defined by symptom manifestation, but the organic disorders, for example, tend to be identified by etiology, while such other factors as prognosis, social conformity, etc., are also employed as classificatory principles. This does not appear, however, to be an insurmountable problem, for the system could be made a completely consistent one by explicitly defining each category by the symptoms encompassed. The system would appear to be eminently amenable to the unitary application of this descriptive classificatory principle, for there are actually few cases where classes are not so defined. Where reliable relations between the present categories and etiology and prognosis have been established, these also could be incorporated explicitly within the system. Etiology and prognosis would be treated not as inherent attributes of the various classifications, but rather as correlates of the particular classes to which their relationship is known. They would, thus, not be confounded with the classificatory principle of the system.

This course of action would satisfy the requirement of consistency in the application of the classificatory principle. A remaining area of ambiguity would be the lack of agreement in what constitutes a symptom. In physical medicine, a clear distinction has been made between a symptom, which is defined as a subjectively experienced abnormality, and a sign, which is considered an objective indication of abnormality (Holmes, 1946). This differentiation has not, however, been extended to the sphere of mental disorders. A source of difficulty may lie in the definition of what is psychologically abnormal. In psychiatric terminology, symptoms include a wide range of phenomena from the grossest type of behavior deviation, through the complaints of the patient, to events almost completely inferential in nature. One suggestion (Yates, 1958) has been to eliminate the term "symptom" and direct attention to the manifest responses of the individual. This suggestion appears to be embodied in the work of Wittenborn and his colleagues (Wittenborn, 1951, 1952; Wittenborn & Bailey, 1952; Wittenborn & Holzberg, 1951; Wittenborn *et al.*, 1953; Wittenborn & Weiss, 1952). Wittenborn's diagnostic system, in which symptoms are defined as currently discernible behaviors, represents a standard of clarity for purely descriptive systems of psychiatric classification. This clarity was achieved by clearly noting and limiting the group of behaviors which would be employed in the system. But even here a certain amount of ambiguity remains. The number of responses or discernible behaviors which may be considered for inclusion within a diagnostic schema borders on the infinite. The question arises, then, as to how one goes about the selection of those behaviors to be incorporated in the classificatory system. Parsimony demands that only "meaningful" items of behavior be chosen for inclusion, and this selective principle has certainly been at work in the construction of all systems of diagnosis. In this sense, the present method of psychiatric classification is not a purely descriptive one, nor can any classification schema truly meet this criterion of purity. Meaning and utility inevitably appear among the determinants of classificatory systems.

Several investigators (Cameron, 1953; Jellinek, 1939; Magaret, 1952) have stressed the inappropriateness of discussing diagnosis in the abstract, pointing out that such a discussion should center around the question of "diagnosis for what?" Indeed, a diagnostic system cannot be described as "true" or "false," but only as being useful or not useful in attaining prescribed goals. Therefore, when a system is devised, its purposes should be explicitly stated so that the system can be evaluated in terms of its success or failure in attaining these objectives. Furthermore, these goals should be kept explicit throughout the period during which the system is being employed. The present diagnostic schema has not met this requirement. Instead, its goals have been carried along in an implicit manner and have been allowed to become vague. The result has been that some see the purpose of the schema as being an adequate description of mental disorders (Hunt *et al.*, 1953), others view it as being concerned with prognosis (Hoch, 1953), and still others view the schemata goal as the discovery of etiology (Cameron, 1953).

Typically, the present schema has been conceptualized as descriptive in nature, but a brief glance at its history indicates that the original purposes and goals in the construction of this schema went far beyond the desire for a descriptive taxonomy. As Zilboorg and Henry (1941) clearly note, Kraepelin not only studied the individual while hospitalized, but also the patient's premorbid history and posthospital course. His hope was to make our understanding of all mental disorders as precise as our knowledge of the course of general paresis. He insisted on the classification of mental disorders according to regularities in symptoms and course of illness, believing this would lead to a clearer discrimination among the different disease entities. He hoped for the subsequent discovery of a specific somatic malfunction responsible for each disease. For Kraepelin, then, classification was related to etiology, treatment, and prognosis. Had the system worked as envisaged, these variables would have become the extraclassificatory attributes of the schema. When matched against this aspiration, the present system must be considered a failure since the common complaint against it is that a diagnostic label tells us very little about etiology, treatment, or prognosis (Miles, 1953). However, it would be erroneous to conclude that the present system is valueless because its classes are only minimally related to etiology and prognosis.

What should be noted is that etiology and prognosis, though important, are but two of a multitude of variables of interest. The importance of these variables should not obscure the fact that their relationship to a classificatory system is exactly the same as that of any other variables. This relationship may take one of two forms. Etiology and prognosis may be the correlates of the classes of a diagnostic system which employs an independent classificatory principle like symptom manifestation. Optimally, we should prefer a classificatory schema in which the indices of etiology and preferred modes of treatment would be incorporated (Hunt *et al.*, 1953; Pepinsky, 1948). In essence, this was Kraepelin's approach, and it continues to underlie some promising work in the area of psychopathology. Although Kraepelin's disease concept is in disrepute (Hoch & Zubin, 1953; Marzoff, 1947; Rotter, 1954), it is the opinion of several investigators (Eysenck, 1953; Phillips & Rabinovitch, 1958; Wittenborn *et al.*, 1953) that further work employing the descriptive symptomatic approach could well lead to a greater understanding of the etiology underlying abnormal "processes."

Another manner in which etiology, treatment, or prognosis could be related to a classificatory schema is by utilizing each of these variables as the classificatory principle for a new diagnostic system. For instance, we might organize patients into groups which respond differentially to particular forms of treatment like electroshock, drugs, psychotherapy, etc. The new schemata which might be proposed could be of considerable value in respect to certain goals but useless in regard to others. Since we do not possess a diagnostic system based on all the variables of clinical interest, we might have to be satisfied with the construction of a variety of diagnostic systems, each based on a different principle of classification. These classificatory techniques would exist side by side, their use being determined by the specific objectives of the diagnostician.

ETIOLOGY VERSUS DESCRIPTION IN DIAGNOSIS

The classical Kraepelinian classification schema shows two major characteristics a commitment to a detailed description of the manifest symptomatic behaviors of the individual and an underlying assumption that such a descriptive classification would be transitory, eventually leading to and being replaced by a system whose classificatory principle was the etiology of the various mental disorders. Major criticism of this classificatory effort has been directed at the first of these. The reservations are that, in practice, such a descriptive effort allows no place for a process interpretation of psychopathology and that it has not encouraged the development of prevention and treatment programs in the mental disorders.

The authors do not feel that the failure of the Kraepelinian system has demonstrated the futility of employing symptoms as the basis for classification. It does suggest that if one approaches the problem of description with an assumption as to the necessary correlates of such descriptions, then the diagnostic system may well be in error. Kraepelin's empiricism is contaminated in just this way. For example, he refused to accept as cases of dementia praecox those individuals who recovered from the disorder, since he assumed irreversibility as a necessary concomitant of its hypothesized neurophysiological base. Bleuler, on the other hand, who was much less committed to any particular form of causality in this illness, readily recognized the possibility of its favorable outcome. It is not, then, the descriptive approach itself which is open to criticism, but description contaminated by preconception. An unfettered description of those schizophrenics with good prognosis in contrast to those with poor prognosis reveals clear differences in the symptom configuration between these kinds of patients (Farina & Webb, 1956; Phillips, 1953).

Kraepelin's basic concern with the problem of etiology has remained a focus of efforts in the clinical area. Although his postulate of central nervous system disease as the basis of mental disorder is in disrepute, and his systematic classificatory efforts are assailed, one nevertheless finds a striking congruence between Kraepelin's preconceptions and certain current attempts at the solution of the problem of psychopathology. There is an unwavering belief that some simple categorical system will quickly solve the mysteries of etiology. The exponents of these newer classificatory schemata have merely replaced symptoms by other phenomena like test scores (King, 1954), particular patterns of interpersonal relations (Leary & Coffey, 1955), etc. It is the authors' conviction that these new efforts to find short-cut solutions to the question of etiology will similarly remain unsuccessful. The amount of descriptive effort required before etiological factors are likely to be discovered has been underestimated (Kety, 1959a, 1959b), and the pursuit of etiology should represent an end point rather than a beginning for classificatory systems. The process of moving from an empirical orientation to an etiological one is, of necessity, inferential and therefore susceptible to the myriad dangers of premature inference. We propose that the greatest safeguard against such prematurity is not to be found in the scrapping of an empirical descriptive approach, but in an accelerated program of empirical research. What is needed at this time is a systematic, empirical attack on the problem of mental disorders. Inherent in this program is the employment of symptoms, broadly defined as meaningful and discernible behaviors, as the basis of a classificatory system. Rather than an abstract search for etiologies, it would appear more currently fruitful to investigate such empirical correlates of symptomatology as reactions to specific forms of treatment, outcome in the disorders, case history phenomena, etc.

The pervasive concern with etiology may derive from a belief that if this were known, prevention would shortly be forthcoming, thus, making the present complex problems of treatment and prognosis inconsequential. Unfortunately, efforts to short-circuit the drudgery involved in establishing an empirically founded psychiatry has not resulted in any major breakthroughs. Etiology is typically the last characteristic of a disorder to be discovered. Consequently, we would suggest the search for etiology be put aside and attempted only when a greater number of the correlates of symptomatic behaviors have been established.

The authors are impressed by the amount of energy that has been expended in both attacking and defending various contemporary systems of classification. We believe that a classificatory system should include any behavior or phenomenon that appears promising in terms of its significant correlates. At this stage of our investigations, the system employed should be an open and expanding one, not one which is closed and defended on conceptual grounds. Systems of classification must be treated as tools for further discovery, not as bases for polemic disputation.

As stated above, it is possible that a number of systems of classification may be needed to encompass the behaviors presently of clinical interest. It may appear that the espousal of this position, in conjunction with a plea for empirical exploration of the correlates of these behaviors, runs headlong into a desire for conceptual neatness and parsimony. It may be feared that the use of a number of classificatory systems concurrently, each with its own correlates, may lead to the creation of a gigantic actuarial table of unrelated elements. However, the authors do not feel that such a fear is well founded because it assumes that the correlates of these systems have no eventual relation one to the other.

We believe that this latter view is unnecessarily pessimistic. While in principle a multiplicity of classificatory systems might be called for, results from the authors' own research program suggest that a single, relatively restricted and coherent classification system can be derived from an empirical study of the correlates of symptomatic behaviors (Phillips & Rabinovitch, 1958; Zigler & Phillips, 1960). Such a system might serve a number of psychiatrically significant functions, including the optimum selection of patients for specific treatment programs and the prediction of treatment outcomes. In conclusion, a descriptive classificatory system appears far from dead, and if properly employed, it can lead to a fuller as well as a more conceptually based understanding of the psychopathologies.

REFERENCES

Allport, G. *Personality: A psychological interpretation.* New York: Holt, 1937.

Allport, G. Personalistic psychology as science: A reply. *Psychol. Rev.,* 1946, **53**, 132–135.

American Psychiatric Association, Mental Hospital Service, Committee on Nomenclature and Statistics of the American Psychiatric Association. *Diagnostic and statistical manual: Mental disorders.* Washington, D.C.: APA, 1952.

Ash, P. The reliability of psychiatric diagnosis, *J. abnorm. soc. Psychol.,* 1949, **44**, 272–277.

Beach, F. The snark was a boojum. *Amer. Psychologist,* 1950, **5**, 115–214.

Beck, S. The science of personality: Nomothetic or idiographic? *Psychol. Rev.,* 1953, **60**, 353–359.

Boisen, A. Types of dementia praecox: A study in psychiatric classification. *Psychiatry,* 1938, **1**, 233–236.

Brower, D. The problem of quantification in psychological science. *Psychol. Rev.,* 1949, **56**, 325–333.

Cameron, D. A theory of diagnosis. In P. Hoch & J. Zubin (Eds.), *Current problems in psychiatric diagnosis.* New York: Grune & Stratton, 1953. Pp. 33–45.

Cattell, R. *Personality and motivation structure and measurement.* New York: World Books, 1957.

Caveny, E., Wittson, C., Hunt, W., & Herman, R. Psychiatric diagnosis, its nature and function. *J. nerv. ment. Dis.,* 1955, **121**, 367–380.

Cronbach, L. The two disciplines of scientific psychology. *Amer. Psychologist,* 1957, **12**, 671–684.

Eysenck, H. *The scientific study of personality.* London: Routledge & Kegan Paul, 1952.

Eysenck, H. The logical basis of factor analysis. *Amer. Psychologist,* 1953, **8**, 105–113.

Eysenck, H. The science of personality: Nomothetic. *Psychol. Rev.,* 1954, **61**, 339–341.

Falk, J. Issues distinguishing idiographic from nomothetic approaches to personality theory. *Psychol. Rev.,* 1956, **63**, 53–62.

Farina, A., & Webb, W. Premorbid adjustment and subsequent discharge. *J. nerv. ment. Dis.,* 1956, **124**, 612–613.

Foulds, G. The reliability of psychiatric, and the validity of psychological diagnosis. *J. ment. Sci.,* 1955, **101**, 851–862.

Guthrie, E. The status of systematic psychology. *Amer. Psychologist,* 1950, **5**, 97–101.

Harlow, H. Mice, monkeys, men, and motives. *Psychol. Rev.,* 1953, **60**, 23–32.

Harrower, M. (Ed.) *Diagnostic psychological testing.* Springfield, Ill.: Charles C. Thomas, 1950.

Hoch, P. Discussion. In P. Hoch & J. Zubin (Eds.), *Current problems in psychiatric diagnosis.* New York: Grune & Stratton, 1953. Pp. 46–50.

Hoch, P., & Zubin, J. (Eds.) *Current problems in psychiatric diagnosis.* New York: Grune & Stratton, 1953.

Holmes, G. *Introduction to clinical neurology.* Edinburgh: Livingstone, 1946.

Hunt, W. Clinical psychology—science or superstition. *Amer. Psychologist,* 1951, **6**, 683—687. (a)

Hunt, W. An investigation of naval neuropsychiatric screening procedures. In H. Gruetskaw (Ed.), *Groups, leadership, and men.* Pittsburgh, Pa.: Carnegie Press, 1951. Pp. 245–256. (b)

Hunt, W., Wittson, C., & Barton, H. A further validation study of naval neuropsychiatric screening. *J. consult. Psychol.,* 1950, **14**, 485–488. (a)

Hunt, W., Wittson, C., & Barton, H. A validation study of naval neuropsychiatric screening. *J. consult. Psychol.,* 1950, **14**, 35–39. (b)

Hunt, W., Wittson, C., & Hunt, E. A theoretical and practical analysis of the diagnostic process. In P. Hoch & J. Zubin (Eds.), *Current problems in psychiatric diagnosis.* New York: Grune & Stratton, 1953. Pp. 53–65.

Jellinek, E. Some principles of psychiatric classification. *Psychiatry,* 1939, **2**, 161–165.

Kantor, R., Wallner, J., & Winder, C. Process and reactive schizophrenia. *J. consult. Psychol.,* 1953, **17**, 157–162.

Kety, S. Biochemical theories of schizophrenia. Part I. *Science*, 1959, **129**, 1528–1532. (a)

Kety, S. Biochemical theories of schizophrenia. Part II. *Science*, 1959, **129**, 1590–1956. (b)

King, G. Research with neuropsychiatric samples. *J. Psychol.*, 1954, **38**, 383–387.

Koch, S. The current status of motivational psychology. *Psychol. Rev.*, 1951, **58**, 147–154.

Leary, T., & Coffey, H. Interpersonal diagnosis: Some problems of methodology and validation *J. abnorm. soc. Psychol.*, 1955, **50**, 110–126.

MacKinnon, D. Fact and fancy in personality research. *Amer. Psychologist*, 1953, **8**, 138–146.

Magaret, A. Clinical methods: Psychodiagnostics. *Annu. Rev. Psychol.*, 1952, **3**, 283–320.

Marquis, D. Research planning at the frontiers of science. *Amer. Psychologist*, 1948, **3**, 430–438.

Marzoff, S. S. The disease concept in psychology. *Psychol. Rev.*, 1947, **54**, 211–221.

Maslow, A. Cognition of the particular and of the generic. *Psychol. Rev.*, 1948, **55**, 22–40.

Mehlman, B. The reliability of psychiatric diagnosis. *J. abnorm. soc. Psychol.*, 1952, **47**, 577–578.

Menninger, K. The practice of psychiatry. *Dig. Neurol. Psychiat.*, 1955, **23**, 101.

Miles, H. Discussion. In P. Hoch & J. Zubin (Eds.), *Current problems in psychiatric diagnosis*. New York: Grune & Stratton, 1953, Pp. 107–111.

Noyes, A. *Modern clinical psychiatry*. Philadelphia: Saunders, 1953.

Patterson, C. Is psychotherapy dependent on diagnosis? *Amer. Psychologist*, 1948, **3**, 155–159.

Pepinsky, H. B. Diagnostic categories in clinical counseling. *Appl. psychol. Monogr.*, 1948, No. 15.

Phillips, L. Case history data and prognosis in schizophrenia. *J. nerv. ment. Dis.*, 1953, **117**, 515–525.

Phillips, L., & Rabinovitch, M. Social role and patterns of symptomatic behaviors. *J. abnorm. soc. Psychol.*, 1958, **57**, 181–186.

Rapaport, D. The future of research in clinical psychology and psychiatry. *Amer. Psychologist*, 1947, **2**, 167–172.

Roby, T. An opinion on the construction of behavior theory. *Amer. Psychologist*, 1959, **14**, 129–134.

Roe, A. Integration of personality theory and clinical practice. *J. abnorm. soc. Psychol.*, 1949, **44**, 36–41.

Rogers, C. Significant aspects of client-centered therapy. *Amer. Psychologist*, 1946, **1**, 415–422.

Rogers, C. *Client-centered therapy*. Boston: Houghton Mifflin, 1951.

Rotter, J. *Social learning and clinical psychology*. Englewood Cliffs, N.J.: Prentice-Hall, 1954.

Schmidt, H., & Fonda, C. The reliability of psychiatric diagnosis: A new look. *J. abnorm. soc. Psychol.*, 1956, **52**, 262–267.

Scott, J. The place of observation in biological and psychological science. *Amer. Psychologist*, 1955, **10**, 61–63.

Scott, W. Research definitions of mental health and mental illness. *Psychol. Bull.*, 1958, **55**, 1–45.

Seeman, W. Psychiatric diagnosis: An investigation of interperson-reliability after didactic instruction. *J. nerv. ment. Dis.*, 1953, **118**, 541–544.

Skaggs, E. Personalistic psychology as science. *Psychol. Rev.*, 1945, **52**, 234–238.

Skaggs, E. Ten basic postulates of personalistic psychology. *Psychol. Rev.*, 1947, **54**, 255–262.

Thorne, F. Back to fundamentals. *J. clin. Psychol.*, 1953, **9**, 89–91.

Tolman, R. Virtue rewarded and vice punished. *Amer. Psychologist*, 1953, **8**, 721–733.

Tyler, L. Toward a workable psychology of individuality. *Amer. Psychologist*, 1959, **14**, 75–81.

Windle, C., & Hamwi, V. An exploratory study of the prognostic value of the complex reaction time tests in early and chronic psychotics. *J. clin. Psychol.*, 1953, **9**, 156–161.

Wittenborn, J. Symptom patterns in a group of mental hospital patients. *J. consult. Psychol.*, 1951, **15**, 290–302.

Wittenborn, J. The behavioral symptoms for certain organic psychoses. *J. consult. Psychol.*, 1952, **16**, 104–106.

Wittenborn, J., & Bailey, C. The symptoms of involutional psychosis. *J. consult. Psychol.*, 1952, **16**, 13–17.

Wittenborn, J., & Holzberg, J. The generality of psychiatric syndromes. *J. consult. Psychol.*, 1951, **15**, 372–380.

Wittenborn, J., Holzberg, J., & Simon, B. Symptom correlates for descriptive diagnosis. *Genet. psychol. Monogr.*, 1953, **47**, 237–301.

Wittenborn, J., & Weiss, W. Patients diagnosed manic-depressive psychosismanic state. *J. consult. Psychol.*, 1952, **16**, 193–198.

Wittman, P., & Sheldon, W. A proposed classification of psychotic behavior reactions. *Amer. J. Psychiat.*, 1948, **105**, 124–128.

Wittson, C., & Hunt, W. The predictive value of the brief psychiatric interview. *Amer. J. Psychiat.*, 1951, **107**, 582–585.

Yates, A. Symptoms and symptom substitution. *Psychol. Rev.*, 1958, **65**, 371–374.

Zigler, E., & Phillips, L. Social effectiveness and symptomatic behaviors. *J. abnorm. soc. Psychol.*, 1960, **61**, 231–238.

Zilboorg, G., & Henry, G. W. *History of medical psychology.* New York: Norton, 1941.

4

Behavioral Analysis: An Alternative to Diagnostic Classification*[1]

FREDERICK H. KANFER and GEORGE SASLOW

During the past decade attacks on conventional psychiatric diagnosis have been so widespread that many clinicians now use diagnostic labels sparingly and apologetically. The continued adherence to the nosological terms of the traditional classificatory scheme suggests some utility of the present categorization of behavior disorders, despite its apparently low reliability[1, 21]; its limited prognostic value[7, 26]; and its multiple feebly related assumptive supports. In a recent study of this problem, the symptom patterns of carefully diagnosed paranoid schizophrenics were compared. Katz et al.[12] found considerable divergence among patients with the same diagnosis and concluded that "diagnostic systems which are more circumscribed in their intent, for example, based on manifest behavior alone, rather than systems which attempt to comprehend etiology, symptom patterns and prognosis, may be more directly applicable to current problems in psychiatric research" (p. 202).

We propose here to examine some sources of dissatisfaction with the present approach to diagnosis, to describe a framework for a behavioral analysis of individual patients which implies both suggestions for treatment and outcome criteria for the single case, and to indicate the conditions for collecting the data for such an analysis.

I. PROBLEMS IN CURRENT DIAGNOSTIC SYSTEMS

Numerous criticisms deal with the internal consistency, the explicitness, the precision, and the reliability of psychiatric classifications. It seems to us that the more important fault lies in our lack of sufficient knowledge to categorize behavior along those pertinent dimensions which permit prediction of responses to social stresses, life crises, or psychiatric treatment. This limitation obviates anything but a crude and tentative approximation to a taxonomy of effective individual behaviors.

Zigler and Phillips[28], in discussing the requirement for an adequate system of classification, suggest that an etiologically-oriented closed system of diagnosis is premature. Instead, they believe that an empirical attack is needed, using "symptoms broadly defined as meaningful and discernible behaviors, as the basis of the classificatory system" (p. 616). But symptoms as a class of responses are defined after all only by their nuisance value to

*From Kanfer, F., and Saslow, G., Archives of General Psychiatry, 1965, 12, 529–538. Copyright © 1965 by the American Medical Association. Reprinted by permission of the American Medical Association and Drs. Kanfer and Saslow.

[1]This paper was written in conjunction with Research grant MH 06921–03 from the National Institutes of Mental Health, United States Public Health Service.

the patient's social environment or to himself as a social being. They are also notoriously unreliable in predicting the patient's particular etiological history or his response to treatment. An alternate approach lies in an attempt to identify classes of dependent variables in human behavior which would allow inferences about the particular controlling factors, the social stimuli, the physiological stimuli, and the reinforcing stimuli, of which they are a function. In the present early stage of the art of psychological prognostication, it appears most reasonable to develop a program of analysis which is closely related to subsequent treatment. A classification scheme which implies a program for behavioral change is one which has not only utility but the potential for experimental validation.

The task of assessment and prognosis can therefore be reduced to efforts which answer the following three questions: (a) which specific behavior patterns require change in their frequency of occurrence, their intensity, their duration or in the conditions under which they occur? (b) what are the best practical means which can produce the desired changes in this individual (manipulation of the environment, of the behavior, or the self-attitudes of the patient)? and (c) what factors are currently maintaining it and what are the conditions under which this behavior was acquired? The investigation of the history of the problematic behavior is mainly of academic interest, except as it contributes information about the probable efficacy of a specific treatment method.

Expectations of current diagnostic systems In traditional medicine, a diagnostic statement about a patient has often been viewed as an essential prerequisite to treatment because a diagnosis suggests that the physician has some knowledge of the origin and future course of the illness. Further, in medicine, diagnosis frequently brings together the accumulated knowledge about the pathological process which leads to the manifestation of the symptoms, and the experiences which others have had in the past in treating patients with such a disease process. Modern medicine recognizes that any particular disease need not have a single cause or even a small number of antecedent conditions. Nevertheless, the diagnostic label attempts to define at least the necessary conditions which are most relevant in considering a treatment program. Some diagnostic classification system is also invaluable as a basis for many social decisions involving entire populations. For example, planning for treatment facilities, research efforts and educational programs take into account the distribution frequencies of specified syndromes in the general population.

Ledley and Lusted[14] give an excellent conception of the traditional model in medicine by their analysis of the reasoning underlying it. The authors differentiate between a disease complex and a symptom complex. While the former describes known pathological processes and their correlated signs, the latter represents particular signs present in a particular patient. The bridge between disease and symptom complexes is provided by available medical knowledge and the final diagnosis is tantamount to labeling the disease complex. However, the current gaps in medical knowledge necessitate the use of probability statements when relating disease to symptoms, admitting that there is some possibility for error in the diagnosis. Once the diagnosis is established, decisions about treatment still depend on many other factors including social, moral, and economic conditions. Ledley and Lusted[14] thus separate the clinical diagnosis into a two-step process. A statistical procedure is suggested to facilitate the primary or diagnostic labeling process. However, the choice of treatment depends not only on the diagnosis proper. Treatment decisions are also influenced by the moral, ethical, social, and economic conditions of the individual patient, his family and the society in which he lives. The proper assignment of the weight to be given to each of these values must in the last analysis be left to the physician's judgment (Ledley and Lusted[14]).

The Ledley and Lusted model presumes available methods for the observation of relevant behavior (the symptom complex), and some scientific knowledge relating it to known antecedents or correlates (the disease process). Contemporary theories of behavior pathology do not yet provide adequate guidelines for the observer to suggest what is to be observed. In fact, Szasz[25] has expressed the view that the medical model may be totally inadequate because psychiatry should be concerned with problems of living and not with diseases of the brain or other biological organs. Szasz[25] argues that "mental illness is a myth, whose function it is to disguise and thus render more potable the bitter pill of moral conflict in human relations" (p. 118).

The attack against use of the medical model in psychiatry comes from many quarters. Scheflen[23] describes a model of somatic psychiatry which is very similar to the traditional medical model of disease. A pathological process results in onset of an illness; the symptoms are correlated with a pathological state and represent our evidence of "mental disease." Treatment consists of removal of the pathogen, and the state of health is restored. Scheflen suggests that this traditional medical model is used in psychiatry not on the basis of its adequacy but because of its emotional appeal.

The limitations of the somatic model have been discussed even in some areas of medicine for which the model seems most appropriate. For example, in the nomenclature for diagnosis of disease of the heart and blood vessels, the criteria committee of the New York Heart Association[17] suggests the use of multiple criteria for cardiovascular diseases, including a statement of the patient's functional capacity. The committee suggests that the functional capacity be ". . . estimated by appraising the patient's ability to perform physical activity" (p. 80), and decided largely by inference from his history. Further[17], ". . .[it] should not be influenced by the character of the structural lesion or by an opinion as to treatment or prognosis" (p. 81). This approach makes it clear that a comprehensive assessment of a patient, regardless of the physical disease which he suffers, must also take into account his social effectiveness and the particular ways in which physiological, anatomical, and psychological factors interact to produce a particular behavior pattern in an individual patient.

Multiple diagnosis   A widely used practical solution and circumvention of the difficulty inherent in the application of the medical model to psychiatric diagnosis is offered by Noyes and Kolb[18]. They suggest that the clinician construct a diagnostic formulation consisting of three parts: (1) A *genetic* diagnosis incorporating the constitutional, somatic, and historical-traumatic factors representing the primary sources or determinants of the mental illness; (2) a *dynamic* diagnosis which describes the mechanisms and techniques unconsciously used by the individual to manage anxiety, enhance self-esteem, i.e., that traces the psychopathological processes; and (3) a *clinical* diagnosis which conveys useful connotations concerning the reaction syndrome, the probable course of the disorder, and the methods of treatment which will most probably prove beneficial. Noyes' and Kolb's multiple criteria[18] can be arranged along three simpler dimensions of diagnosis which may have some practical value to the clinician: (1) etiological, (2) behavioral, and (3) predictive. The kind of information which is conveyed by each type of diagnostic label is somewhat different and specifically adapted to the purpose for which the diagnosis is used. The triple-label approach attempts to counter the criticism aimed at use of any single classificatory system. Confusion in a single system is due in part to the fact that a diagnostic formulation intended to describe current behavior, for example, may be found useless in an attempt to predict the response to specific treatment, or to postdict the patient's personal history and development, or to permit collection of frequency data on hospital populations.

Classification by etiology   The Kraepelinian system and portions of the 1952 APA classification emphasize etiological factors. They share the assumption that common etiological factors lead to similar symptoms and respond to similar treatment. This dimension of diagnosis is considerably more fruitful when dealing with behavior disorders which are mainly under control of some biological condition. When a patient is known to suffer from excessive intake of alcohol his hallucinatory behavior, lack of motor coordination, poor judgment, and other behavioral evidence of disorganization can often be related directly to some antecedent condition such as the toxic effect of alcohol on the central nervous system, liver, etc. For these cases, classification by etiology also has some implications for prognosis and treatment. Acute hallucinations and other disorganized behavior due to alcohol usually clear up when the alcohol level in the blood stream falls. Similar examples can be drawn from any class of behavior disorders in which a change in behavior is associated primarily or exclusively with a single, *particular* antecedent factor. Under these conditions this factor can be called a pathogen and the situation closely approximates the condition described by the traditional medical model.

Utilization of this dimension as a basis for psychiatric diagnosis, however, has many problems apart from the rarity with which a specified condition can be shown to have a direct "causal" relationship to a pathogen. Among the current areas of ignorance in the fields of psychology and psychiatry, the etiology of most common disturbances probably takes first place. No specific family environment, no dramatic traumatic experience, or known constitutional abnormality has yet been found which results in the same pattern of disordered behavior. While current research efforts have aimed at investigating family patterns of schizophrenic patients, and several studies suggest a relationship between the mother's behavior and a schizophrenic process in the child[10], it is not at all clear why the presence of these same factors in other families fails to yield a similar incidence of schizophrenia. Further, patients may exhibit behavior diagnosed as schizophrenic when there is no evidence of the postulated mother-child relationship.

In a recent paper Meehl[16] postulates schizophrenia as a neurological disease, with learned content and a dispositional basis. With this array of interactive etiological factors, it is clear that the etiological dimension for classification would at best result in an extremely cumbersome system, at worst in a useless one.

Classification by symptoms   A clinical diagnosis often is a summarizing statement about the way in which a person behaves. On the assumption that a variety of behaviors are correlated and consistent in any given individual, it becomes more economical to assign the individual to a class of persons than to list and categorize all of his behaviors. The utility of such a system rests heavily on the availability of empirical evidence concerning correlations among various behaviors (response-response relationships), and the further assumption that the frequency of occurrence of such behaviors is relatively independent of specific stimulus conditions and of specific reinforcement. There are two major limitations to such a system. The first is that diagnosis by symptoms, as we have indicated in an earlier section, is often misleading because it implies common etiological factors. Freedman[7] gives an excellent illustration of the differences both in probable antecedent factors and subsequent treatment response among three cases diagnosed as schizophrenics. Freedman's patients were diagnosed by at least two psychiatrists, and one would expect that the traditional approach should result in whatever treatment of schizophrenia is practiced in the locale where the patients are seen. The first patient eventually gave increasing evidence of an endocrinopathy, and when this was recognized and treated, the psychotic symptoms went into remission. The second case had a definite history of seizures and appropriate anticonvulsant medication was effective in relieving his symptoms. In the third case, treatment directed at an uncovering analysis of the patient's adaptive techniques resulted in considerable improvement in the patient's behavior and subsequent relief from psychotic episodes. Freedman [7] suggests that schizophrenia is not a disease entity in the sense that it has a unique etiology, pathogenesis, etc., but that it represents the evocation of a final common pathway in the same sense as do headache, epilepsy, sore throat, or indeed any other symptom complex. It is further suggested that the term "schizophrenia has outlived its usefulness and should be discarded" (p. 5). Opler [19, 20] has further shown the importance of cultural factors in the divergence of symptoms observed in patients collectively labeled as schizophrenic.

Descriptive classification is not always this deceptive, however. Assessment of intellectual performance sometimes results in a diagnostic statement which has predictive value for the patient's behavior in school or on a job. To date, there seem to be very few general statements about individual characteristics, which have as much predictive utility as the IQ.

A second limitation is that the current approach to diagnosis by symptoms tends to center on a group of behaviors which is often irrelevant with regard to the patient's total life pattern. These behaviors may be of interest only because they are popularly associated with deviancy and disorder. For example, occasional mild delusions interfere little or not at all with the social or occupational effectiveness of many ambulatory patients. Nevertheless, admission of their occurrence is often sufficient for a diagnosis of psychosis. Refinement of such an approach beyond current usage appears possible, as shown for example by Lorr *et al.* [15] but this does not remove the above limitations.

Utilization of a symptom-descriptive approach frequently focuses attention on by-products of larger behavior patterns, and results in attempted treatment of behaviors (symptoms) which may be simple consequences of other important aspects of the patient's life. Emphasis on the patient's subjective complaints, moods, and feelings tends to encourage use of a syndrome-oriented classification. It also results frequently in efforts to change the feelings, anxieties, and moods (or at least the patient's report about them), rather than to investigate the life conditions, interpersonal reactions, and environmental factors which produce and maintain these habitual response patterns.

Classification by prognosis   To date, the least effort has been devoted to construction of a classification system which assigns patients to the same category on the basis of their similar response to specific treatments. The proper question raised for such a classification system consists of the manner in which a patient will react to treatments, regardless of his current behavior, or his past history. The numerous studies attempting to establish prognostic signs from projective personality tests or somatic tests represent efforts to categorize the patients on this dimension.

Windle [26] has called attention to the low degree of predictability afforded by personality (projective) test scores, and has pointed out the difficulties encountered in evaluating research in this area due to the inadequate description of the population sampled and of the improvement criteria. In a later review Fulkerson and Barry [8] came to the similar conclusion that psychological test performance is a poor predictor of outcome in mental illness. They suggest that demographic variables such as severity, duration, acuteness of onset, degree of precipitating stress, etc., appear to have stronger relationships to outcome than test data. The lack of reliable relationships between diagnostic categories, test data, demographic variables, or other measures taken on the patient on the one hand, and duration of illness, response to specific treatment, or degree of recovery, on the other hand, precludes the construction of a simple empiric framework for a diagnostic-prognostic classification system based only on an array of symptoms.

None of the currently used dimensions for diagnosis is directly related to methods of modification of a patient's behavior, attitudes, response patterns, and interpersonal actions. Since the etiological model clearly stresses causative factors, it is much more compatible with a personality theory which strongly emphasizes genetic-developmental factors. The classification by symptoms facilitates social-administrative decisions about patients by providing some basis for judging the degree of deviation from social and ethical norms. Such a classification is compatible with a personality theory founded on the normal curve hypothesis and concerned with characterization by comparison with a fictitious average. The prognostic-predictive approach appears to have the most direct practical applicability. If continued research were to support certain early findings, it would be indeed comforting to be able to predict outcome of mental illness from a patient's premorbid social competence score[28], or from the patient's score on an ego-strength scale[4], or from many of the other signs and single variables which have been shown to have some predictive powers. It is unfortunate that these powers are frequently dissipated in cross validation. As Fulkerson and Barry have indicated[8], single predictors have not yet shown much success.

II. A FUNCTIONAL (BEHAVIORAL-ANALYTIC) APPROACH

The growing literature on behavior modification procedures derived from learning theory[3, 6, 11, 13, 27] suggests that an effective diagnostic procedure would be one in which the eventual therapeutic methods can be directly related to the information obtained from a continuing assessment of the patient's current behaviors and their controlling stimuli. Ferster[6] has said ". . . a functional analysis of behavior has the advantage that it specifies the causes of behavior in the form of explicit environmental events which can be objectively identified and which are potentially manipulable" (p. 3). Such a diagnostic undertaking makes the assumption that a description of the problematic behavior, its controlling factors, and the means by which it can be changed are the most appropriate "explanations." It further makes the assumption that a diagnostic evaluation is never complete. It implies that additional information about the circumstances of the patient's life pattern, relationships among his behaviors, and controlling stimuli in his social milieu and his private experience is obtained continuously until it proves sufficient to effect a noticeable change in the patient's behavior, thus resolving "the problem." In a functional approach it is necessary to continue evaluation of the patient's life pattern and its controlling factors, concurrent with attempted manipulation of these variables by reinforcement, direct intervention, or other means until the resultant change in the patient's behavior permits restoration of more efficient life experiences.

The present approach shares with some psychological theories the assumption that psychotherapy is *not* an effort aimed at removal of intrapsychic conflicts, nor at a change in the personality structure by therapeutic interactions of intense nonverbal nature, (e.g., transference, self-actualization, etc.). We adopt the assumption instead that the job of psychological treatment involves the utilization of a variety of methods to devise a program which controls the patient's environment, his behavior, and the consequences of his behavior in such a way that the presenting problem is resolved. We hypothesize that the essential ingredients of a psychotherapeutic endeavor usually involve two separate stages: (1) a change in the perceptual discriminations of a patient, i.e., in his approach to perceiving, classifying, and organizing sensory events, including perception of himself, and

(2) changes in the response patterns which he has established in relation to social objects and to himself over the years[11]. In addition, the clinician's task may involve direct intervention in the patient's environmental circumstances, modification of the behavior of other people significant in his life, and control of reinforcing stimuli which are available either through self-administration, or by contingency upon the behavior of others. These latter procedures complement the verbal interactions of traditional psychotherapy. They require that the clinician, at the invitation of the patient or his family, participate more fully in planning the total life pattern of the patient outside the clinician's office.

It is necessary to indicate what the theoretical view here presented does *not* espouse in order to understand the differences from other procedures. It does *not* rest upon the assumption that (a) insight is a sine qua non of psychotherapy, (b) changes in thoughts or ideas inevitably lead to ultimate changes in actions, (c) verbal therapeutic sessions serve as replications of and equivalents for actual life situations, and (d) a symptom can be removed only by uprooting its cause or origin. In the absence of these assumptions it becomes unnecessary to conceptualize behavior disorder in etiological terms, in psychodynamic terms, or in terms of a specifiable disease process. While psychotherapy by verbal means may be sufficient in some instances, the combination of behavior modification in life situations as well as in verbal interactions serves to extend the armamentarium of the therapist. Therefore verbal psychotherapy is seen as an *adjunct* in the implementation of therapeutic behavior changes in the patient's total life pattern, not as an end in itself, nor as the sole vehicle for increasing psychological effectiveness.

In embracing this view of behavior modification, there is a further commitment to a constant interplay between assessment and therapeutic strategies. An initial diagnostic formulation seeks to ascertain the major variables which can be directly controlled or modified during treatment. During successive treatment stages additional information is collected about the patient's behavior repertoire, his reinforcement history, the pertinent controlling stimuli in his social and physical environment, and the sociological limitations within which both patient and therapist have to operate. Therefore, the initial formulation will constantly be enlarged or changed, resulting either in confirmation of the previous therapeutic strategy or in its change.

A guide to a functional analysis of individual behavior   In order to help the clinician in the collection and organization of information for a behavioral analysis, we have constructed an outline which aims to provide a working model of the patient's behavior at a relatively low level of abstraction. A series of questions are so organized as to yield immediate implications for treatment. This outline has been found useful both in clinical practice and in teaching. Following is a brief summary of the categories in the outline.

  1. Analysis of a Problem Situation:[2] The patient's major complaints are categorized into classes of behavioral excesses and deficits. For each excess or deficit the dimensions of frequency, intensity, duration, appropriateness of form, and stimulus conditions are described. In content, the

---

[2]For each patient a detailed analysis is required. For example, a list of behavioral excesses may include specific aggressive acts, hallucinatory behaviors, crying, submission to others in social situations, etc. It is recognized that some behaviors can be viewed as excesses or deficits depending on the vantage point from which the imbalance is observed. For instance, excessive withdrawal and deficient social responsiveness, or excessive social autonomy (nonconformity) and deficient self-inhibitory behavior may be complementary. The particular view taken is of consequence because of its impact on a treatment plan. Regarding certain behavior as excessively aggressive, to be reduced by constraints, clearly differs from regarding the same behavior as a deficit in self-control, subject to increase by training and treatment.

response classes represent the major targets of the therapeutic intervention. As an additional in-dispensable feature, the behavioral assets of the patient are listed for utilization in a therapy program.

2. Clarification of the Problem Situation: Here we consider the people and circumstances which tend to maintain the problem behaviors, and the consequences of these behaviors to the patient and to others in his environment. Attention is given also to the consequences of changes in these behaviors which may result from psychiatric intervention.

3. Motivational Analysis: Since reinforcing stimuli are idiosyncratic and depend for their effect on a number of unique parameters for each person, a hierarchy of particular persons, events, and objects which serve as reinforcers is established for each patient. Included in this hierarchy are those reinforcing events which facilitate approach behaviors as well as those which, because of their aversiveness, prompt avoidance responses. This information has as its purpose to lay plans for utilization of various reinforcers in prescription of a specific behavior therapy program for the patient, and to permit utilization of appropriate reinforcing behaviors by the therapist and signifi-cant others in the patient's social environment.

4. Developmental Analysis: Questions are asked about the patient's biological equipment, his sociocultural experiences, and his characteristic behavioral development. They are phrased in such a way as (a) to evoke descriptions of his habitual behavior at various chronological stages of his life, (b) to relate specific new stimulus conditions to noticeable changes from his habitual be-havior, and (c) to relate such altered behavior and other residuals of biological and sociocultural events to the present problem.

5. Analysis of Self-Control: This section examines both the methods and the degree of self-control exercised by the patient in his daily life. Persons, events, or institutions which have successfully reinforced self-controlling behaviors are considered. The deficits or excesses of self-control are evaluated in relation to their importance as therapeutic targets and to their utiliza-tion in a therapeutic program.

6. Analysis of Social Relationships: Examination of the patient's social network is carried out to evaluate the significance of people in the patient's environment who have some influence over the problematic behaviors, or who in turn are influenced by the patient for his own satisfactions. These interpersonal relationships are reviewed in order to plan the potential participation of significant others in a treatment program, based on the principles of behavior modification. The review also helps the therapist to consider the range of actual social relationships in which the patient needs to function.

7. Analysis of the Social-Cultural-Physical Environment: In this section we add to the preced-ing analysis of the patient's behavior as an individual, consideration of the norms in his natural environment. Agreements and discrepancies between the patient's idiosyncratic life patterns and the norms in his environment are defined so that the importance of these factors can be decided in formulating treatment goals which allow as explicitly for the patient's needs as for the pressures of his social environment.

The preceding outline has as its purpose to achieve definition of a patient's problem in a manner which suggests specific treatment operations, or that none are feasible, and specific behaviors as targets for modification. Therefore, the formulation is *action oriented.* It can be used as a guide for the initial collection of information, as a device for organizing avail-able data, or as a design for treatment.

The formulation of a treatment plan follows from this type of analysis because know-ledge of the reinforcing conditions suggests the motivational controls at the disposal of the clinician for the modification of the patient's behavior. The analysis of specific problem be-haviors also provides a series of goals for psychotherapy or other treatment, and for the evaluation of treatment progress. Knowledge of the patient's biological, social, and cultural conditions should help to determine what resources can be used, and what limitations must be considered in a treatment plan.

The various categories attempt to call attention to important variables affecting the patient's *current* behavior. Therefore, they aim to elicit descriptions of low-level abstraction. Answers to these specific questions are best phrased by describing classes of events reported by the patient, observed by others, or by critical incidents described by an informant. The analysis does not exclude description of the patient's habitual verbal-symbolic behaviors. However, in using verbal behaviors as the basis for this analysis, one should be cautious not to "explain" verbal processes in terms of postulated internal mechanisms without adequate supportive evidence, nor should inference be made about nonobserved processes or events without corroborative evidence. The analysis includes many items which are not known or not applicable for a given patient. Lack of information on some items does not necessarily indicate incompleteness of the analysis. These lacks must be noted nevertheless because they often contribute to the better understanding of what the patient needs to learn to become an autonomous person. Just as important is an inventory of his existing socially effective behavioral repertoire which can be put in the service of any treatment procedure.

This analysis is consistent with our earlier formulations of the principles of comprehensive medicine[9, 22] which emphasized the joint operation of biological, social, and psychological factors in psychiatric disorders. The language and orientation of the proposed approach are rooted in contemporary learning theory. The conceptual framework is consonant with the view that the course of psychiatric disorders can be modified by systematic application of scientific principles from the fields of psychology and medicine to the patient's habitual mode of living.

This approach is not a substitute for assignment of the patient to traditional diagnostic categories. Such labeling may be desirable for statistical, administrative, or research purposes. But the current analysis is intended to replace other diagnostic formulations purporting to serve as a basis for making decisions about specific therapeutic interventions.

III. METHODS OF DATA COLLECTION FOR A FUNCTIONAL ANALYSIS

Traditional diagnostic approaches have utilized as the main sources of information the patient's verbal report, his nonverbal behavior during an interview, and his performance on psychological tests. These observations are sufficient if one regards behavior problems only as a property of the patient's particular pattern of associations or his personality structure. A mental disorder would be expected to reveal itself by stylistic characteristics in the patient's behavior repertoire. However if one views behavior disorders as sets of response patterns which are learned under particular conditions and maintained by definable environmental and internal stimuli, an assessment of the patient's behavior output is insufficient unless it also describes the conditions under which it occurs. This view requires an expansion of the clinician's sources of observations to include the stimulation fields in which the patient lives, and the variations of patient behavior as a function of exposure to these various stimulational variables. Therefore, the resourceful clinician need not limit himself to test findings, interview observations in the clinician's office, or referral histories alone in the formulation of the specific case. Nor need he regard himself as hopelessly handicapped when the patient has little observational or communicative skill in verbally reconstructing his life experiences for the clinician. Regardless of the patient's communicative skills the data must consist of a description of the patient's behavior *in relationship* to varying environmental conditions.

A behavioral analysis excludes no data relating to a patient's past or present experiences as irrelevant. However, the relative merit of any information (as, e.g., growing up in a broken home or having had homosexual experiences) lies in its relation to the independent variables which can be identified as controlling the current problematic behavior. The observation that a patient has hallucinated on occasions may be important only if it has bearing on his present problem. If looked upon in isolation, a report about hallucinations may be misleading, resulting in emphasis on classification rather than treatment.

In the *psychiatric interview* a behavioral-analytic approach opposes acceptance of the content of the verbal self-report as equivalent to actual events or experiences. However, verbal reports provide information concerning the patient's verbal construction of his environment and of his person, his recall of past experiences, and his fantasies about them. While these self-descriptions do not represent data about events which actually occur internally, they do represent current behaviors of the patient and indicate the verbal chains and repertoires which the patient has built up. Therefore, the verbal behavior may be useful for description of a patient's thinking processes. To make the most of such an approach, variations on traditional interview procedures may be obtained by such techniques as role playing, discussion, and interpretation of current life events, or controlled free association. Since there is little experimental evidence of specific relationships between the patient's verbal statements and his nonverbal behavioral acts, the verbal report alone remains insufficient for a complete analysis and for prediction of his daily behavior. Further, it is well known that a person responds to environmental conditions and to internal cues which he cannot describe adequately. Therefore, any verbal report may miss or mask the most important aspects of a behavioral analysis, i.e., the description of the relationship between antecedent conditions and subsequent behavior.

In addition to the use of the clinician's own person as a controlled stimulus object in interview situations, *observations of interaction with significant others* can be used for the analysis of variations in frequency of various behaviors as a function of the person with whom the patient interacts. For example, use of prescribed standard roles for nurses and attendants, utilization of members of the patient's family or his friends, may be made to obtain data relevant to the patient's habitual interpersonal response pattern. Such observations are especially useful if in a later interview the patient is asked to describe and discuss the observed sessions. Confrontations with tape recordings for comparisons between the patient's report and the actual session as witnessed by the observer may provide information about the patient's perception of himself and others as well as his habitual behavior toward peers, authority figures, and other significant people in his life.

Except in working with children or family units, insufficient use has been made of material obtained from *other informants* in interviews about the patient. These reports can aid the observer to recognize behavioral domains in which the patient's report deviates from or agrees with the descriptions provided by others. Such information is also useful for contrasting the patient's reports about his presumptive effects on another person with the stated effects by that person. If a patient's interpersonal problems extend to areas in which social contacts are not clearly defined, contributions by informants other than the patient are essential.

It must be noted that verbal reports by other informants may be no more congruent with actual events than the patient's own reports and need to be equally related to the informant's own credibility. If such crucial figures as parents, spouses, employers can be so interviewed, they also provide the clinician with some information about those people with whom the patient must interact repeatedly and with whom interpersonal problems may have developed.

Some observation of the patient's daily *work behavior* represents an excellent source of information, if it can be made available. Observation of the patient by the clinician or his staff may be preferable to descriptions by peers or supervisors. Work observations are especially important for patients whose complaints include difficulties in their daily work activity or who describe work situations as contributing factors to their problem. While freer use of this technique may be hampered by cultural attitudes toward psychiatric treatment in the marginally adjusted, such observations may be freely accessible in hospital situations or in sheltered work situations. With use of behavior rating scales or other simple measurement devices, brief samples of patient behaviors in work situations can be obtained by minimally trained observers.

The patient himself may be asked to provide samples of his own behavior by using tape recorders for the recording of segments of interactions in his family, at work, or in other situations during his everyday life. A television monitoring system for the patient's behavior is an excellent technique from a theoretical viewpoint but it is extremely cumbersome and expensive. Use of recordings for diagnostic and therapeutic purposes has been reported by some investigators[2, 5, 24]. Playback of the recordings and a recording of the patient's reactions to the playback can be used further in interviews to clarify the patient's behavior toward others and his reaction to himself as a social stimulus.

Psychological tests represent problems to be solved under specified interactional conditions. Between the highly standardized intelligence tests and the unstructured and ambiguous projective tests lies a dimension of structure along which more and more responsibility for providing appropriate responses falls on the patient. By comparison with interview procedures, most psychological tests provide a relatively greater standardization of stimulus conditions. But, in addition to the specific answers given on intelligence tests or on projective tests these tests also provide a behavioral sample of the patient's reaction to a problem situation in a relatively stressful interpersonal setting. Therefore, psychological tests can provide not only quantitative scores but they can also be treated as a miniature life experience, yielding information about the patient's interpersonal behavior and variations in his behavior as a function of the nature of the stimulus conditions.

In this section we have mentioned only some of the numerous life situations which can be evaluated in order to provide information about the patient. Criteria for their use lies in economy, accessibility to the clinician, and relevance to the patient's problem. While it is more convenient to gather data from a patient in an office, it may be necessary for the clinician to have first-hand information about the actual conditions under which the patient lives and works. Such familiarity may be obtained either by utilization of informants or by the clinician's entry into the home, the job situation, or the social environment in which the patient lives. Under all these conditions the clinician is effective only if it is possible for him to maintain a nonparticipating, objective, and observational role with no untoward consequences for the patient or the treatment relationship.

The methods of data collecting for a functional analysis described here differ from traditional psychiatric approaches only in that they require inclusion of the physical and social stimulus field in which the patient actually operates. Only a full appraisal of the patient's living and working conditions and his way of life allow a description of the actual problems which the patient faces and the specification of steps to be taken for altering the problematic situation.

SUMMARY

Current psychiatric classification falls short of providing a satisfactory basis for the understanding and treatment of maladaptive behavior. Diagnostic schemas now in use are based on etiology, symptom description, or prognosis. While each of these approaches has a limited utility, no unified schema is available which permits prediction of response to treatment or future course of the disorder from the assignment of the patient to a specific category.

This paper suggests a behavior-analytic approach which is based on contemporary learning theory, as an alternative to assignment of the patient to a conventional diagnostic category. It includes the summary of an outline which can serve as a guide for the collection of information and formulation of the problem, including the biological, social, and behavioral conditions which are determining the patient's behavior. The outline aims toward integration of information about a patient for formulation of an action plan which would modify the patient's problematic behavior. Emphasis is given to the particular variables affecting the *individual* patient rather than determination of the similarity of the patient's history or his symptoms to known pathological groups.

The last section of the paper deals with methods useful for collection of information necessary to complete such a behavior analysis.

REFERENCES

1. Ash, P. Reliability of psychiatric diagnosis. *J. abnorm. soc. Psychol.*, 1949, **44**, 272–277.
2. Bach, G. In Alexander, S. Fight promoter for battle of sexes. *Life*, May 17, 1963, **54**, 102–108.
3. Bandura, A. Psychotherapy as learning process. *Psychol. Bull.*, 1961, **58**, 143–159.
4. Barron, F. Ego-strength scale which predicts response to psychotherapy. *J. consult. Psychol.*, 1953, **17**, 235–241.
5. Cameron, D. E., *et al.* Automation of psychotherapy. *Compr. Psychiat.*, 1964, **5**, 1–14.
6. Ferster, C. B. Classification of behavioral pathology. In L. P. Ullmann & L. Krasner (Eds.), *Behavior modification research.* New York: Holt, Rinehart & Winston, 1965.
7. Freedman, D. A. Various etiologies of schizophrenic syndrome. *Dis. Nerv. Syst.*, 1958, **19**, 1–6.
8. Fulkerson, S. E., & Barry, J. R. Methodology and research on prognostic use of psychological tests. *Psychol. Bull.*, 1961, **58**, 177–204.
9. Guze, S. B., Matarazzo, J. D., & Saslow, G. Formulation of principles of comprehensive medicine with special reference to learning theory. *J. clin. Psychol.*, 1953, **9**, 127–136.
10. Jackson, D. D. A. *Etiology of schizophrenia.* New York: Basic Books, 1960.
11. Kanfer, F. H. Comments on learning in psychotherapy. *Psychol. Rep.*, 1961, **9**, 681–699.
12. Katz, M. M., Cole, J. O., & Lowery, H. A. Nonspecificity of diagnosis of paranoid schizophrenia. *Arch. Gen. Psychiat.*, 1964, **11**, 197–202.
13. Krasner, L. Therapist as social reinforcement machine. In H. Strupp & L. Luborsky (Eds.), *Research in psychotherapy.* Washington, D.C.: American Psychological Association, 1962.
14. Ledley, R. S., & Lusted, L. B. Reasoning foundations of medical diagnosis. *Science*, 1959, **130**, 9–21.
15. Lorr, M., Klett, C. J., & McNair, D. M. *Syndromes of psychosis.* New York: Macmillan, 1963.
16. Meehl, P. E. Schizotaxia, schizotypy, schizophrenia. *Amer. Psychologist*, 1962, **17**, 827–838.
17. New York Heart Association. *Nomenclature and criteria for diagnosis of diseases of the heart and blood vessels.* New York: New York Heart Association, 1953.
18. Noyes, A. P., & Kolb, L. C. *Modern clinical psychiatry.* Philadelphia: Saunders, 1963.
19. Opler, M. K. Schizophrenia and culture. *Sci. Amer.*, 1957, **197**, 103–112.
20. Opler, M. K. Need for new diagnostic categories in psychiatry. *J. Nat. Med. Assoc.*, 1963, **55**, 133–137.
21. Rotter, J. B. *Social learning and clinical psychology.* Englewood Cliffs, N. J.: Prentice-Hall, 1954.
22. Saslow, G. On concept of comprehensive medicine. *Bull. Menninger Clin.*, 1952, **16**, 57–65.
23. Scheflen, A. E. Analysis of thought model which persists in psychiatry. *Psychosom. Med.*, 1958, **20**, 235–241.

24. Slack, C. W. Experimenter-subject psychotherapy—A new method of introducing intensive office treatment for unreachable cases. *Ment. Hyg.*, 1960, **44**, 238–256.
25. Szasz, T. S. Myth of mental illness. *Amer. Psychol.*, 1960, **15**, 113–118.
26. Windle, C. Psychological tests in psychopathological prognosis. *Psychol. Bull.*, 1952, **49**, 451–482.
27. Wolpe, J. *Psychotherapy in reciprocal inhibition.* Stanford, Calif.: Stanford University Press, 1958.
28. Zigler, E., & Phillips, L. Psychiatric diagnosis: Critique. *J. abnorm. soc. Psychol.*, 1961, **63**, 607–618.

Suggested Additional Readings

Adams, H. B. "Mental illness" or interpersonal behavior? *American Psychologist*, 1964, **19**, 191–197.

Alexander, F. G., & Selesnick, S. T. *The history of psychiatry.* New York: Harper & Row, 1961.

American Psychiatric Association. *Diagnostic and statistical manual of mental disorders.* (2nd ed.) Washington, D. C.: American Psychiatric Association, 1968.

Ausubel, D. P. Personality disorder *is* disease. *American Psychologist*, 1961, **16**, 69–74.

Boring, E. G. *A history of experimental psychology.* New York: Appleton-Century-Crofts, 1950.

Laing, R. D. *The politics of experience.* New York: Ballantine Books, 1968.

Mechanic, D. Some factors in identifying and defining mental illness. *Mental Hygiene*, 1962, **46**, 66–74.

Rosenhan, D. L. On being sane in insane places. *Science*, 1973, **179**, 250–258.

Sarbin, T. R. On the futility of the proposition that some people be labeled "mentally ill." *Journal of Consulting Psychology*, 1967, **31**, 447–453.

Scott, W. A. Research definitions of mental health and mental illness. *Psychological Bulletin*, 1958, **55**, 29–45.

Shoben, E. J., Jr. Toward a concept of the normal personality. *American Psychologist*, 1957, **12**, 183–189.

Skinner, B. F. *Science and human behavior.* New York: Macmillan, 1953.

Szasz, T. S. *Ideology and insanity.* New York: Anchor Books, 1970.

Szasz, T. S. *The myth of mental illness.* New York: Harper & Row, 1961.

UNIT II

Perspectives in the Development of Abnormal Behavior

INTRODUCTION

Prior to the nineteenth century, the most popular belief concerning the development of abnormal behavior was related to metaphysical-religious beliefs. Accordingly, people who were considered to be mentally ill were seen as being possessed by demons, evil spirits, or both, or as being punished by God for wrongdoing. Later perspectives regarding the nature of abnormal behavior took a position more congruent with the Hippocratic school. Specifically, this position viewed mental illness as a disease resulting from such natural causes as brain dysfunction. This view accounted for most of the theorizing that took place during the nineteenth century prior to the publication near the turn of the century of Freud's theory of personality development.

Freud's position paralleled the physical disease model, discussed in the previous unit, and soon became the major theoretical position regarding personality development and the etiology of abnormal behavior, although a number of his contemporaries (e.g., Adler, Jung, and Horney) sharply criticized various aspects of his work and published their own theoretical positions regarding the nature of personality and the development of maladaptive behavior.

Nevertheless, for many years Freud's theory was seen as holding great promise for practitioners, theoreticians, and researchers, because it was general enough to be applied to all facets of abnormal psychology. However, its very generality and its emphasis on the gratification of sexual drives and on the unconscious determinants of man's behavior led many mental health professionals to become increasingly disenchanted with it. This discontent became evident in the early and mid-1950s. During this time a number of theoretically oriented articles and texts were published, each of which presented a different explanation of the development and maintenance of maladaptive behavior. For example, Dollard and Miller (1950) published their reinterpretation of Freudian theory in terms of Hull's (1943) learning theory; Rogers (1951) published his phenomenological interpretation of, and treatment approach to, human behavior; Skinner (1953) described his account of human behavior from the learning theory position he had formulated earlier; Sullivan (1953) presented his interpersonal theory of psychiatry; Rotter (1954) discussed his social learning interpretation of personality; and later Wolpe (1958) published his learning theory account of the development and treatment of particular maladaptive behaviors.

These publications, along with a few others (e.g., Mowrer, 1950; Delly, 1955), contributed to the formulation of new theoretical models of maladaptive behavior and the expansion of other models. Sullivan's theory, for example, contributed to the already existing *psychodynamic or medical, model*; Rogers' position contributed to the formulation of the *humanistic model*; and the learning theory orientations helped systematize the *behavioral model*.

Another event of the 1950s that further affected our understanding of maladaptive behavior was the publication of Hollingshead's and Redlich's (1953, 1958) findings regarding the relationship between socioeconomic level and type of mental illness. Psychosis, for example, was found to be significantly more prevalent in the lower than in the higher socioeconomic levels, and the reverse was true for the prevalence of neurosis. These results gave credence to the increasingly held view that factors other than psychological variables contributed to the development of maladaptive behavior.

The present unit samples material showing a number of perspectives concerning the etiology of maladaptive behavior. Specifically, six major areas which have significantly contributed to the understanding of the development of abnormal behavior are considered under five section headings: Psychological Factors, Sociological Factors, Ecological Factors, Anthropological Factors, and Genetic and Biochemical Factors.

Psychological Factors

The first section presents a discussion of some of the psychological variables that have been theorized to contribute to the development of maladaptive behavior. Lewis R. Wolberg presents an overview of Freud's *psychoanalytic theory* and the basis upon which this theory was formulated. Wolberg points out that Freud placed a great deal of emphasis on the repression of certain experiences and desires as a major contributor to the development of mental illness. The article also summarizes Freud's theorized stages of psychosexual development in the child as well as his conceptualization of the various components of the psyche.

Arthur W. Combs presents another view in the next selection. He discusses maladjustment from a *phenomenological* perspective, that is, the way in which an individual perceives himself and his environment. Combs believes that maladaptive behavior is a function of an individual's perception of threat to his concept of self and that this perception produces a state of tension in the person which is characteristic of maladaptation. The concept of self is also viewed as constituting a person's frame of reference and as the guide to his behavior. The implications of this viewpoint as well as its application to therapy are also discussed.

A learning theory explanation of maladaptive behavior, called *social-learning theory*, is discussed in Article 7 by Albert Bandura. According to Bandura, an individual's behavior is not inherently maladaptive; that is, it is not representative of a disease, but is defined as maladaptive according to the social judgments of his behavior made by others and by the person himself. Bandura is basically in agreement with Scheff and Szasz (discussed in Unit I) on this position, and he notes that many factors seem to affect such a judgment—for example, the *appropriateness* of the behavior in a particular situation, *behavioral deficits* in the person, the *intention* others attribute to his behavior, such *personal attributes* as age, sex, race, occupation, and the person's own *self-definition* of his behavior. Bandura further points out that social-learning theory uses principles of learning to explain the occurrence of maladaptive behavior rather than accounting for such behavior on the basis of unconscious factors, the status of the person's psyche, or his self-concept.

Article 8 is by Stephen Fleck and is addressed to a perspective that is not directly psychological, but that has become associated with psychological variables in contributing to the development of maladaptive behavior. Fleck considers the role of *family interactions* in one type of behavior disorder, schizophrenia. From his studies of the families of a group of schizophrenics, he concludes that each of the families was abnormal, and that the type of family setting contributed to the development of schizophrenia in particular family members—for schizophrenia was a means of coping with the family situation. According to Fleck, however, these findings are not sufficient to resolve any questions pertaining to the cause of schizophrenia.

Sociological Factors

The three articles in the next section are primarily addressed to a discussion of the role of sociological factors in the development of maladaptive behavior. Article 9 by August B. Hollingshead and Frederick C. Redlich, summarizes the initial findings of their classic research on the relationship between socioeconomic level and type of psychiatric disorder. It also discusses additional findings on the relationship between socioeconomic level and the type of psychiatric treatment patients received.

Since the publication of Hollingshead's and Redlich's findings, a number of investigators have performed research in this area. These and other studies are critically reviewed in Article 10 by Melvin L. Kohn. He points out various weaknesses in the research, but he still concludes that the findings reported over the years do indicate that there is a concentration in the lower classes of people diagnosed as schizophrenic. Furthermore, he states that these results seem to suggest that social class is causally related to schizophrenia, but adds that other factors related to social class life, such as level of stress, family structure, and reward and opportunity limitations, may also be contributing to the development of schizophrenia. But, since definitive research on the importance of these other factors has not been done, their degree of importance must remain speculative.

Article 11 by Richard H. Seiden summarizes recent findings on the etiology of adolescent suicide. Though not solely directed toward a discussion of sociological variables, this article does discuss various sociological factors that have been theorized and found to be associated with adolescent suicide. After describing the various psychodynamic characteristics related to suicide among youth, and differentiating between attempted and committed suicides, Seiden examines two main types of etiological determinants of suicide—individual and social determinants. His discussion is particularly thought-provoking and comprehensive.

Ecological Factors

The material presented in the third section is concerned with the role of ecological factors (i.e., those factors which affect the relationship between man and his environment) in the development of maladaptation. In Article 12, Omer R. Galle, Walter R. Gove, and J. Miller McPherson, review the findings from animal research on population density and pathology, and discuss the degree to which these findings can be generalized to man. The authors believe that the results of this research seem to indicate that high population density has a serious effect on many animals, producing lower fertility rates, the neglect of the young by mothers, high mortality of the young, disruption of social and sexual behavior, etc. In order to determine the relevance of these findings to humans, Galle, Gove, and McPherson studied the relationship between the prevalence of certain social pathological behaviors and the population density of various community areas in Chicago. Specifically, they were interested in the following indices of social pathology: mortality rate, fertility rate, ineffectual care of the young, juvenile delinquency rate, and rate of admissions to mental hospitals. The results of their study, even after social class and ethnicity were controlled for, suggest that increased population density may seriously affect the social behavior of humans. They further point out that population density should be considered when social scientists (and others) try to explain the occurence of various social pathological behaviors.

Another aspect of ecology, urban-ethnic ecology, and its relationship to the occurrence of psychosis is discussed in Article 13 by Norbett L. Mintz and David T. Schwartz. These authors were particularly interested in studying the effects of the density of an ethnic group in a particular area on the incidence of two forms of psychosis—schizophrenia and manic-depression. They chose as their ethnic sample the Italian population in the greater Boston area. Their findings showed that the density of Italians in the greater Boston area was inversely correlated with the incidence of schizophrenia and manic-depression. No significant correlation was found between socioeconomic status and incidence of psychosis. These findings are discussed in terms of their relationship to the etiology of maladaptive behavior.

Anthropological Factors

The three articles in the fourth section explore the role of cultural factors in maladaptation. Article 14, by E. D. Wittkower and J. Fried, surveys the frequency of, and manifestations associated with, various types of behavior disorders across many cultures. The authors report, for example, that such major behavior disorders as schizophrenia seem to be omnipresent but that the frequency of these disorders does not appear to be distributed evenly across cultures. In addition to discussing their findings, these authors describe some of the problems associated with doing cross-cultural research.

In Article 15, H. B. M. Murphy also reports on the role of cultural factors in the etiology of abnormal behavior, but, unlike Wittkower and Fried, Murphy focuses his discussion on the cultural determinants of schizophrenia. After reviewing the literature, he concludes that culture should not be considered the sole factor in the development of schizophrenia, but as only one of many variables in the history of the individual which may combine to set the stage for maladaption.

Genetic and Biochemical Factors

The two perspectives considered in the last section are related to some of the early physical disease conceptualizations of abnormal behavior that were associated with the Hippocratic school. These perspectives include the role of genetic and of biochemical factors in the etiology of abnormal behavior. In Article 16, David Rosenthal reviews the recent published research on the role of heredity in the development of schizophrenia. Rosenthal suggests that the presently available data does support the position of a genetic basis to schizophrenia. He also discusses some of the implications of genetics for the prevention and treatment of schizophrenia.

The role of chromosome abnormalities in the occurrence of various types of abnormal behavior is summarized by John H. Heller in Article 17. He describes a number of syndromes that have been associated with chromosomal abnormalities and also discusses some of the social and legal implications of the YY syndrome (i.e., the person with an XYY chromosome makeup).

Articles 18 and 19 focus on biochemical factors and their relationship to the development of abnormal behavior. Article 18, by a World Health Organization (WHO) Scientific Group, summarizes recent research on the effect of particular biochemical factors on the development of mental retardation, affective disorders such as manic-depressive reaction, and periodic psychoses like melancholia and paranoia. In Article 19, Seymour S. Kety, on the other hand, addresses himself to the role of biochemical factors in the development of one behavior disorder—schizophrenia. Kety notes that though there are many problems associated with conducting this type of research, work should continue. He discusses several areas that merit further research—for example, the role played by specific protein metabolism dysfunction and the importance of a dysfunction in the transmethylation mechanism in the development of schizophrenia.

REFERENCES

Dollard, J. and Miller, N. E. *Personality and psychotherapy.* New York: McGraw-Hill, 1950.
Hollingshead, A. B., & Redlich, F. C. Social stratification and psychiatric disorders. *American Sociological Review,* 1953, **18**, 163–169.
Hollingshead, A. B., & Redlich, F. C. *Social class and mental illness.* New York: Wiley, 1958.
Hull, C. *Principles of behavior.* New York: Appleton-Century-Crofts, 1943.
Kelly, G. A. *The psychology of personal constructs.* New York: Norton, 1955.
Mowrer, O. H. *Learning theory and personality dynamics.* New York: Ronald Press, 1950.
Rogers, C. R. *Client-centered therapy.* Cambridge, Mass.: Riverside Press, 1951.
Rotter, J. B. *Social learning and clinical psychology.* Englewood Cliffs, N.J.: Prentice-Hall, 1954.
Skinner, B. F. *Science and human behavior.* New York: Macmillan, 1953.
Sullivan, H. S. *The interpersonal theory of psychiatry.* New York: Norton, 1953.
Wolpe, J. *Psychotherapy by reciprocal inhibition.* Stanford, Calif.: Stanford University Press, 1958.

Psychological Factors

5

Freudian Psychoanalytic Theory*

LEWIS R. WOLBERG

In 1880, Joseph Breuer discovered that when an hysterical girl under hypnosis was induced to speak freely, she expressed profound emotion and experienced relief from her symptoms. Under the impression that her hysteria originated in certain painful experiences while caring for her sick father, Breuer enjoined her, while she was in an hypnotic state, to remember and to relive the traumatic scenes. This seemed to produce a cure in her hysteria.

Ten years later, in conjunction with Freud, Breuer continued his research, and, in 1895, the two men published their observations in a book, *Studien Über Hysteria* (1936). Their conclusions were that hysterical symptoms developed as a result of experiences so traumatic to the individual that they were repressed. The mental energy associated with the experiences was blocked off, and not being able to reach consciousness was converted into bodily innervations. The discharge of strangulated emotions (abreaction), through its normal channels during hypnosis, would relieve the necessity of diverting the energy into symptoms. This method was termed "catharsis."

Freud soon found that equally good therapeutic results could be obtained without hypnosis by permitting the patient to talk freely, expressing whatever ideas came to his mind. Freud invented the term "psychoanalysis" for the process of uncovering and permitting the verbal expression of hidden traumatic experiences. Freud found that there were forces that kept memories from invading consciousness, and he discovered that it was necessary to neutralize the repressing forces before recall was possible. An effective way to overcome resistances was to permit the patient to relax and to talk freely about any idea or fantasy that entered his mind no matter how trivial or absurd. Freud could observe in this "free association" a sequential theme that gave clues to the nature of the repressed material.

Mainly through an introspective analysis of his own dreams (1938a) Freud was able to show how dreams were expressions of unconscious wishes and fears, evading the barriers of repression through the assumption of symbolic disguises. He perfected a technique of arriving at the meaning of the unconscious material through translation of symbols.

Freud also observed that when the patient was encouraged to say whatever came to his mind, he verbalized irrational attitudes toward the therapist, such as deep love, fear, hate, overvaluation, expectancy, disappointment and other strivings that were not justified by the reality situation. He noted too that the patient identified the therapist with significant personages in his past, particularly with his parents, and that this identification motivated the transfer over to the therapist of attitudes similar to those he originally had toward his parents. This phenomenon Freud called "transference." For example, a patient with a phobia of being subject to imminent, but indefinable injury might, at a certain phase in his analysis, begin to develop an aversion and dread of the analyst, expressed in fears of being mutilated. At the same time, incestuous wishes for the mother might appear in dreams.

*From Wolberg, L. R., *Techniques of psychotherapy.* Copyright © 1954 by Grune & Stratton, Inc. Reprinted by permission of Grune & Stratton, Inc., publishers, and Dr. Wolberg.

Analysis of the relationship with the analyst (transference) would then possibly reveal an identification of the analyst with the patient's father. It would then become apparent that the patient secretly feared injury by the father for his forbidden wish to possess the mother, and that his phobia was an expression of this fear of mutilation which had been dissociated from awareness by repression. The bringing of the patient's attention to the sources of his fear, and his realization of its irrational nature, would result in an amelioration or cure of his neurosis.

The material uncovered by Freud from his studies of free association, dream interpretation and analysis of the transference, suggested to him that there was a dynamic portion of the psyche, closely associated with the emotional disorder, that did not follow the normal laws of mental functioning. Freud called this aspect of the mind the "unconscious," and he set about to determine the unique laws which dominated the repressed psychic component. In studying the symbols issuing from the unconscious, Freud noted that they were concerned chiefly with sexual material, and he concluded from this that the unconscious was preoccupied for the most part with sexual wishes and fears. Consequently, he assumed that the most important traumatic events which had been repressed were sexual in nature. It was largely on this evidence that he evolved his "theory of instincts" or the "libido theory."

In his theory of instincts, Freud postulated the fact that all energy had its origin in instincts which persistently expressed themselves (repetition compulsion) and were represented mentally as ideas with an emotional charge (cathexis). A fundamental instinct was that of *eros*, the sexual or life instinct, manifesting itself in a force called "libido." Freud hypothesized a permeation of the body by this vital instinctual force, the "libido," which powered the individual's development toward mature sexuality. Libido was, however, subject to many developmental vicissitudes in its destined course to adult genitality. During the first year of life, it concentrated itself around the oral zone, the mouth and lips, the child gaining a kind of erotic pleasure by sucking and later by biting. At the end of the first year, there was a partial shift in libido to the anal zone, and intense pleasures were derived from the retention and expulsion of feces. During this period, the child's interests were more or less concentrated on himself (narcissism), and satisfactions were primarily localized within his own body (auto-erotism). Relationships with people were primitive, being circumscribed to only part of the parent (part-object relationships), like the nipple or breast instead of the entire parent.

Around the age of three, libido was centered around the phallic zone—the penis or clitoris. "Object relationships" were less primitive and were extended to a more complete relatedness with the parent. Yet, fundamentally, the child was ambivalent, responding to his parents and other people with a mixture of love and hate.

This stage of psychosexual growth continued into the Oedipal period, during which the little boy developed toward his mother a profound interest, with strong sexual overtones and desires for exclusive ownership. The little girl, envying men for their possession of a penis, created in part by a desire to repudiate her femininity and to become a male (penis envy), and resenting the fact that she had no penis, accused the mother of responsibility for this deprivation and turned to the father with an intensified sexual interest. In the case of the boy, hostility toward the father, due to a desire to eliminate him as a rival, generated a fear of counter-hostility, and particularly a fear of castration, which inspired such anxiety as to induce him to give up his interest in the mother and to make friends with his father. The intensity of fear became so overwhelming and so unendurable that the boy was forced to yield to his more powerful competitor by renouncing, repudiating and repressing sexual feelings toward the maternal love-object. He was obliged also to repress concomitant hostile impulses toward the father. The little girl similarly resolved her enmity toward her mother, as well as her sexual interest in her father. This drama, known as the Oedipus complex, was to Freud the crucial nuclear conflict in the development of the personality contributing to both character formation and neurotic symptoms.

The incorporation of parental injunctions and prohibitions, and the repudiation of sexual and hostile aims as related to the parents, resulted in the crystallization of an aspect of the psyche which took over the judging, prohibiting and punitive functions hitherto vested in the parents. This aspect became the conscience or super-ego. The adequate resolution of the Oedipus complex was associated with channelization of libido into the genital zone, with capacities for complete, mature, unambivalent, "whole-object" relationships.

Following upon the Oedipal period, there was an era characterized by the neutralization of sexual impulses. This Freud called the "latency period." With the advent of puberty, however, increased libido, due to the heightened activity of the genital glands, reactivated the old Oedipal interests. The person then lived through the revived early Oedipal conflict, and his capacity to solve this anew was determined by the extent of previous vicissitudes and the adequacy with which his conflict had formerly been resolved. In "normal" solutions, the child transferred his or her sexual interest to extra-familial persons of the opposite sex. The little girl renounced her boyish interests and accepted a passive female role.

Under certain conditions, normal psychosexual development was impeded by a "fixation" of libido onto oral, anal and phallic zones. The libido, bound down in this way, was unable to participate in the development of full genitality. Freud believed that both constitutional and experiential factors were responsible for this. Most prominent were excessive gratifications or inordinate frustrations experienced at an early stage of growth. Not only did libidinal fixations interfere with the development of mature sexuality, but they constituted stations to which the individual might return when confronted with overwhelming stress or frustration. Under these circumstances, the libidinal stream was said to undergo "regression" to pregenital fixation points. When this happened, there were revived attitudes and interests characteristic of childhood, with immature sexual strivings, interest in "part-objects" and narcissism. Infantile conflicts and patterns were also revivified in this process. Sexual perversions constituted the positive expression of pregenital libidinal fixations, while neurotic symptoms were a negative or converted expression (Freud, 1938b).

Freud conceived of the mental apparatus as an organ that prevented the damming up of energy. Pain was related to an increase of energy, and pleasure to a decrease. In order to help understand the operations of the mental apparatus, Freud elaborated a topographic structure of the psyche, as involving a reservoir of instinctual energy, the *id*; a supervisory area serving a censoring and sanctioning function, the *super-ego*; and a structure that mediated internal and external adjustments, the *ego*. These sub-divisions, although recognized by Freud as arbitrary, empiric and metapsychologic, were retained by him as a conceptual necessity (Freud, 1930).

Freud classified the id as the original undifferentiated mind, the repository of inherited urges and instinctual energy. It contained the instincts of Eros—the life or sexual instinct, and Thanatos—the death instinct. It provided the individual with dynamic energy (libido), which vitalized every organ and tissue and sought expression in response to a "pleasure principle," along whatever channels were available for it. Through impressions received by the perceptual organs, the id underwent modifications immediately after birth. Differentiation by the child of himself as an entity apart from the world was in keeping with the evolution of the ego, which increasingly assumed the function of an executive organ, harnessing the id to the demands of reality (reality principle). Important impressions, particularly those related to experiences with parents or their surrogates, and frustrations created by prohibitions of pleasure strivings, registered themselves on the child's psyche and stimulated primitive mechanisms of projection and introjection. In projection, aggression was discharged outward and directed toward parents; in introjection, the frustrating parental agencies were "incorporated" within the child's psychic apparatus. Through these mechanisms, rudiments of a super-ego developed which later, with the resolution of the Oedipus complex, crystallized and took over the guiding and prohibitive functions of the parents. One aspect of the super-ego contained constructive ideals toward which the individual felt driven (ego ideal).

Under the lash of the super-ego, the ego created repressions against libidinal strivings and their ideational representatives. Such repressions served to avoid conflict. When, however, for any reason, repression relaxed or proved insufficient, the ego was invaded with some of the content of the repressed. This threat to the individual's security inspired anxiety, a danger signal that indicated a break-through of the repressed material.

As Freud continued his work, he laid less and less stress on strangulated emotions due to early traumatic experiences as the primary cause of neurosis. More and more he became cognizant of the purposeful nature of symptoms, and, in 1926, he revised his theory of neurosis drastically, claiming that symptoms were not only manifestations of repressed instinctive strivings, but also represented defenses against these strivings (Freud, 1936).

Freud contended, however, that the essence of a neurosis was a repression of infantile fears and experiences which continually forced the individual to act in the present as if he were living in the past. The neurotic seemed to be dominated by past anxieties that, split off, operated autonomously and served no further function in reality.

Internal dangers were constantly threatened by the efforts of the id to discharge accumulated tension. Such discharge was opposed by the mental force of the super-ego in the form of repression to prevent the release of tension. Repression was a dynamic force which attempted to seal off internal dangers. However, the maintenance of repression required an enormous expenditure of energy. The ego derived this energy from the id in a subversive manner. Thus, an idea or tendency invested with libido (cathexis) would be stripped of libido and this energy used to oppose the idea or tendency (anti-cathexis).

Subtle mechanisms such as symbolization, condensation, distortion and displacement were employed to evade repressive forces and to provide a substitutive discharge of repressed energy, and a consequent relief of tension. Fantasies, dreams and symptoms were expressions of such mechanisms. Where the substitutive expression was in harmony with social values and super-ego ideals, it provided a suitable means of relief (sublimation). Where it was not in harmony, conflict resulted and repressive mechanisms were again invoked. If repression proved ineffective in mediating tension, a regression to earlier modes of adaptation was possible. This happened particularly where the individual was confronted by experiences similar to, or representative of, those which initiated anxiety in childhood. The ego reacted automatically to these experiences, as if the reality conditionings of later years had had no corrective effect on the original danger situation. It responded with essentially the same defenses of childhood, even though these were now inappropriate.

A retention of a relationship to reality at the expense of an intrapsychic balance produced a psychoneurotic disturbance. The existing conflict here was between the ego and the id. If an intrapsychic balance developed at the expense of reality relationships, the consequence was psychosis. The latter resulted when the ego was overwhelmed by id forces, the conflict being between the ego and the environment.

In addition to the libido theory described above, Freud elaborated the theory of the death instinct to account for phenomena not explicable in terms of libido. He postulated that an instinct existed in the id which prompted aggressive and destructive drives. This instinct manifested itself in a (repetition compulsion) to undo the forward evolutionary development of the organism, and to return it to its primordial inorganic state. The death instinct, though sometimes libidinized (sadism) was totally different from the sexual instinct.…

REFERENCES

Breuer, J., & Freud, S. *Studies in hysteria.* Washington, D.C.: Nervous & Mental Disease Publishing Company, 1936.

Freud, S. The interpretation of dreams. In *Basic writings of Sigmund Freud.* New York: Modern Library, 1938.

Freud, S. Three contributions to the theory of sex. In *Basic writings of Sigmund Freud.* New York: Modern Library, 1938.

Freud, S. *The ego and the id.* London: Hogarth, 1930.

Freud, S. *The problem of anxiety.* New York: Norton, 1936.

6

A Phenomenological Approach to Adjustment
Theory*

ARTHUR W. COMBS

To state that personality theory and the practice of psychotherapy should be closely interwoven seems obvious. Yet, amazingly enough, until recent years we have behaved almost as though this conspicuous relationship did not exist. In the past there has been some justification for this separation. For, on the one hand, traditional normative personality theory contributed little that was very helpful to the psychotherapist in dealing with his unique client. On the other hand, the psychotherapists were so busy developing and comparing methods that they were blind to the importance of sound personality theory. But all this is changing. We seem now to be developing a new group of theorists who are therapists, and therapists who are theorists, which promises much for both theory and practice. We are discovering now that the microcosm of therapy can both stimulate and test the concepts of theory[10]. At the same time we are beginning to understand that effective methods of therapy must find their justification in accurate and consistent personality theory.

In this paper I should like to add what impetus I can to the movement by developing more fully several concepts of personality organization discussed in separate papers by Rogers[10] and by Combs[3] at the 1947 meetings of the American Psychological Association. In particular, I should like to explore the concepts of adjustment and maladjustment as these appear from a phenomenological point of view. The position I have taken grows out of a dual interest in personality theory and the practice of therapy and seems to me to have implications for both fields of psychology. It is based upon a number of concepts and principles already widely held in many areas of psychological thought and represents an attempt to integrate these in a consistent organization.

TWO FRAMES OF REFERENCE FOR OBSERVING BEHAVIOR

There seem to be two possible frames of reference from which we can examine the problem of adjustment. The first we might call the external or objective approach and the second, the *personal or phenomenological* point of view.

1. The *external* or *objective* frame of reference is the traditional method of psychology. In this approach we attempt to observe the behavior of adjusted or maladjusted individuals from the viewpoint of an outside observer. When we make our observations in this way we usually arrive at either of two positions: (a) We describe the individual's behavior in

*From Combs, A. W., "A phenomenological approach to adjustment theory," *Journal of Abnormal and Social Psychology*, 1949, **44**, 29–35. Copyright © 1949 by the American Psychological Association, and reproduced by permission.

normative or statistical terms in which people who conform to social expectancies are described as normal while those who do not are considered to be maladjusted. Or (b), examining behavior more closely, we describe adjustment as a frustration when confronted with a barrier to need satisfaction. Both descriptions have been useful but have also had serious limitations when applied to the practical problems of therapy. The normative position has little to offer the psychotherapist, who must deal with clients just as apt to be the exception as the rule. The frustration concept also does not help us very much, for it describes *all* behavior in these terms and does not help us to understand the unique character of maladjustment in terms of which an adequate therapy must be developed.

2. The second frame of reference from which we may observe the dynamics of adjustment is from the point of view of the individual himself. This approach has been called by Rogers[10], in connection with therapy, "*the client-centered approach,*" and by Snygg and Combs[11], in a more general sense, "*the phenomenological frame of reference.*" In this frame of reference we are concerned with the client's perceptions of himself and his environment rather than the way in which things appear to an outside observer. When we examine adjustment and maladjustment in this way, we arrive at a very different concept of adjustment and one that seems to offer a more adequate guide to the practical problems of therapy. In this paper let us examine the dynamics of adjustment as they seem to appear from the subject's own viewpoint.

MALADJUSTMENT AS A FUNCTION OF PERCEIVED THREAT

The most universally described characteristic of maladjustment from an external point of view is the tension under which "maladjusted" people appear to be operating. In fact, the term "tension-states" is often used almost synonymously with maladjustment. Tension states, however, are mere descriptions of the client's condition and are not adequate for the construction of therapy. Tension, itself, is caused and it is necessary for us to understand how such conditions come about.

When we examine these tensions through the client's own eyes, they appear to be produced by the individual's perception of threat to his self. The presence of threatening perceptions seems to force upon the individual an emergency situation which must be dealt with. His body responds to this emergency by going on what Cannon[2] has called a "war footing" and produces the tension states characteristic of maladjustment. This effect of threatening perceptions is well known to all of us. We can observe it in our own reactions to things which worry or concern us and we can observe it in the reactions of others when they feel afraid or angry. As psychologists, we even make practical use of this principle in our experiments with "lie detection." It would thus appear from a phenomenological point of view that a maladjusted personality is equivalent to a threatened one. Conversely, a well-adjusted personality seems to be one unthreatened by its perceptions.

Describing maladjustment as a function of the perception of threat, however, is not enough. We need to know specifically what it is that is threatened. We have described threat to this point as a threat to self. Yet, when we observe the behavior of individuals from their own point of view, it does not seem to be their physical selves, alone, which they are attempting to preserve. For the most part, threats to our physical selves are seldom of long duration in our society and most of us have learned to deal with them smoothly and effectively. The more serious and long-lasting threats which we experience seem to arise out of social and personal situations that threaten, not our physical selves, but our perceptions of ourselves. Most of our perceptions of threat appear to occur when we are faced with humiliation, the loss of love or prestige, or from a thousand other threats to the way we see ourselves.

THE CONCEPT OF SELF IN ADJUSTMENT

This perceived self Raimy[9] has defined as a complex organization of perceptions about self made up of many perceptions of greater or lesser degree of importance to the individual and defining his relationships to the world as he sees it. Many psychologists have come to feel that the concept of self gives consistency to behavior and lies at the very core of personality[6, 7, 10]. A great deal, if not all, of our behavior appears to be governed by our self-concepts in the myriad life-situations in which we find ourselves. In my own case, for example, when I see myself as a professor, I behave in ways appropriate to my concept of what a professor should be like. At other times I behave in terms of my concept of myself as a parent, as a husband, as a host, as a cigarette smoker, or as a man who enjoys reading "lil Abner," to name but a few of the many concepts I have of myself. Not all of these concepts will be of equal importance in the total organization of my self-concept but all are aspects in terms of which I behave at one time or another.

This principle of the determining effect of the self-concept upon behavior has been demonstrated experimentally in many studies. Piaget[8], for example, has shown how the child's concept of himself selects his perceptions in conformity with the self-concept held. The same phenomenon has been demonstrated by Frenkel-Brunswik[4] with young adults and in a fascinating experiment by Bruner and Goodman[1] showing differences in children's perception of coin sizes.

THE CENTRAL CHARACTER OF THE SELF-CONCEPT
IN THE INDIVIDUAL ECONOMY

In the personal economy of any individual, the concept of self seems to represent the individual's guide to every behavior. Its development is the result of long and arduous experience and stands, at any moment, as the individual's personal frame of reference. Indeed, it is himself from his own point of view. To the individual the concept of self seems a very precious thing to be maintained or enhanced at all costs. As Gardner Murphy[7] has expressed it: "This cherished possession must forever be made more adequate, more worthy; and it must forever be defended against stain and injury whether from the acts of others or of the . . . . organism [itself]." Snygg and Combs[11] have suggested that the need to maintain and enhance the concept of self is, in fact, the basic human need.

In terms of this analysis, it seems to be the self-concept which the individual perceives to be threatened rather than his self as he appears to others. Almost any psychotherapist has among his clients many individuals who from an external point of view seem to be living satisfactory lives. There may even be some who feel a need of therapy themselves, although they are described by other people as "remarkably well adjusted" and may, even, be pointed out to our youth as notable examples, worthy of emulation. Yet these same persons often reveal themselves in the therapy sessions to be deeply threatened and unhappy. It matters very little what things look like to others. The crucial factor is the individual's own perception of threat to his concept of self. Knowing that other people think he is unthreatened does not produce less threat for the individual. It merely proves how little other people really understand him!

SOME IMPLICATIONS OF THE PERCEPTIVE VIEW
OF BEHAVIOR FOR THERAPY

If the client comes to the therapist believing he is being picked on by his boss, this perception of self in relation to his world must be the subject of therapy. Whether the client is *really* being picked on, as others may see it, is unimportant insofar as that individual is concerned.[1] Indeed, it is even possible that, if the therapist makes an investigation and discovers that the objective facts in the case are that the boss is *not* picking on his client, he may end by convincing his client that the therapist has joined the boss in the "picking on" process.

If it is true that human behavior is a function of the individual's perceptions, then it seems necessary to change our concept of therapy. Therapy in the light of this theoretical position becomes a technique for changing perception, rather than a way of changing the client's behavior. Since perceptions lie within the client and are not open to direct manipulation, the therapist cannot change behavior directly. He can only create a situation in which the client can change himself. The task of therapy thus becomes, not so much one of *changing the client's behavior*, as one of *creating a situation in which change in perception is facilitated and encouraged.* This will be true whether we are speaking of individual or environmental treatment, whether we attempt to induce some specific and predetermined change in perception, or whether we are content to let the client choose his own direction of change.

To construct such a therapy it will be necessary for us to understand thoroughly the dynamics of change in perception, and that is a job for personality theory. If we can develop a satisfactory understanding of these dynamics the development of therapeutic techniques for its best implementation should quickly become clear to us. Without such an understanding, it seems likely we shall remain mired in the confusion of methodologies in which we now find ourselves. The fundamental question in the construction of any therapeutic method is, not "what method shall I use?" but, "what are the dynamics of behavior?" If we can answer the latter question, methods should easily follow.

THE CONCEPT OF THE ADEQUATE SELF

Up to this point I have described maladjustment as a function of perceived threat to the self. We have not yet, however, examined why, and under what conditions, the self is perceived as threatened. From our observations of behavior, both in and out of therapy, the experience of threat seems to be at a minimum when the concept of self is perceived as being adequate to deal with the perception of events. For example, the person who sees himself as a successful public speaker feels unthreatened by the necessity for making a speech. Indeed, he may even feel enhanced by an invitation to appear before an audience. Feeling adequate to his task, he can accept his perceptions into his organization and feels unthreatened by them. He operates smoothly and effectively and with a minimum of tension. Rogers[10] has described the results of this feeling of adequacy as follows:

> It would appear that when all of the ways in which the individual perceives himself—all perceptions of the qualities, abilities, impulses and attitudes of the person and all perceptions of himself in relation to others—are accepted into the organized conscious concept of self, then this achievement is accompanied by feelings of comfort and freedom from tension which are experienced as psychological adjustment.

---

[1] It is not unimportant, of course, from a social point of view.

The person with an inadequate self-definition, however, finds himself in a very different position. Feeling inadequate to deal effectively with his perceptions, he is more or less seriously threatened by them. The person who feels himself inadequate or unable to speak in public finds his perception of the necessity for making a speech a threatening and disturbing experience. He feels more and more threatened as the time for action approaches. This is an experience common to many of us who at one time or another have suffered from stage fright. The experience of threat appears to be the result of a self-concept inadequate to cope with the perception. What is more, the threat continues so long as the self is defined as inadequate to cope with the perception or the perception remains in the field.

Since the individual is always under the necessity for maintaining and enhancing the self-concept, perceptions which threaten the self cannot be accepted into the personal organization. Unfortunately, this failure to accept a perception does not eliminate the threat. It continues the threat, for the individual will feel threatened so long as the perception remains in figure and the self is defined in a manner inadequate to cope with it. The mother who feels inadequate to handle her child, for example, remains threatened by the perception of her child whether the youngster is present in the flesh or not. Until either the child is removed or the mother defines herself as adequate to cope with her responsibility she will continue to feel threatened and disturbed.

It follows from this discussion that therapy may attempt to produce change in the perception of self, or the perception of external events, or both. It will often be possible to change the perception of external events by changing the client's environment and may even be possible to induce changes in the concept of self by environmental treatment. But the possibilities of environmental treatment will often be drastically restricted, for there are limits to the degree to which we can change our society for a single individual. More often than not, it will be necessary for us to find ways of aiding threatened individuals to develop more adequate concepts of self. If we could do this well, it is even possible that environmental treatment, in many cases, would be unnecessary.

The development of an adequate concept of self, however, is greatly complicated by the selective effect upon perceptions that any concept of self exerts. We have already observed in the studies of Bruner[1] and others that the concepts of self we hold tend to select perceptions in terms of existing self-definitions. This effect is true of inadequate perceptions of self as well. Seeing himself inadequately, the individual selects his perceptions in terms of his self-definitions and so perpetuates his errors of perception. The child who feels he is rejected is likely to see his parent's slightest reprimand as proof of what he already thinks—that his parents don't love him. In the same way, the housewife who feels inadequate in giving a tea is likely to be far more engrossed with her own social errors than with the fact that the affair was generally successful. An inadequate perception of self tends to select its perceptions in such a way as to conform with its definition and makes new perceptions of self more difficult to achieve.

THE EFFECTS OF THREAT UPON PERCEPTION

To assist clients to the development of a more adequate concept of self it will be necessary for us to discover ways of freeing the client to make new perceptions of self more adequate than those he has previously held. Unfortunately, the very existence of threat in the perceptive field seems to have effects which complicate and obstruct change in perception. For successful therapy, it will be necessary to develop methods by which these effects can be eliminated or reduced.

If the maintenance and enhancement of the self-concept is as important in the dynamics of behavior as Snygg and Combs[11] have suggested, it follows that any threat to this concept must be resisted by the client. A self under threat has no choice but to defend itself. It is a common saying that "nobody ever wins an argument." In fact, the more strongly we are threatened, the more we seem driven to defend ourselves and the positions we have taken. This leaves us with a fine dilemma in therapy. We have theorized that an inadequate self is threatened, and the perception of threat forces the self to maintain its position. Clearly, so long as the individual is under the necessity for defending himself, the self-concept is not likely to change. Yet, therapy, to be successful, must result in change in the concept of self, not in the maintenance of the status quo.

It appears that, in order to break into this vicious circle, it will be necessary somehow to shield the client from threat. This seems to be the major principle upon which nondirective therapy depends in its attempt to create a warm, permissive, accepting atmosphere for the client. The transference phenomenon of psychoanalysis also appears to have this effect at least in part. It also seems to be true of other forms of therapy which shelter the client from threat, such as play therapy, some forms of group therapy, and, in a more limited way, some types of environmental treatment like foster-home placement. By shielding the client from threat in the therapeutic relationship these therapies seem to make it possible for the client to arrive at new self-perceptions. It would appear that absolute respect for the integrity of the client is not only a fine democratic principle but just good business in therapy. If this theoretical position is sound, it also raises grave doubts about the effects of certain types of highly traumatic therapies. If our argument that threat forces the self to defend itself is accurate, it is conceivable that traumatic therapies may even result in driving some clients deeper into their maladjustments.

A second result of threat to the self is its restrictive effect upon the field of perceptions. This is a common phenomenon often observed in work on emotion and has been given the name "tunnel vision." It is also familiar to most of us in our daily lives. When we feel threatened, the field of our perceptions is greatly narrowed to the vicinity of the perceptions which appear threatening to us. For example, in a situation where we are frightened or angry, our perceptions are narrowed to the immediate field of the threatening object and we may be totally unaware of other factors in the situation to which we would normally have attended. It is a common observation in therapy too, that clients who have seriously threatening problems are deeply engrossed in these matters. And no wonder. A threat to self is no laughing matter. It cannot be shrugged off. It must be attended to. In this sense it is understandable that maladjusted persons should be egocentric. This restrictive effect of threat upon perceptions appears to be responsible for much of the perseverative character of maladjusted behavior.

In a restricted perceptive field the number of possibilities for new perceptions is sharply delimited. Yet this restrictive effect of threat upon perception is exactly the opposite of what we desire for therapy. In therapy we want to help our clients to explore freely a wide variety of perceptions from which they may discover better and more satisfying ways of behaving. Anything which prevents such exploration is contrary to the goal of therapy. For effective therapy we must find ways of freeing the individual from threat so that free exploration of the field is possible. To make this possible it will be necessary to understand the dynamics of threat and to discover ways of controlling the effects of threat in the therapeutic process.

In this paper I have attempted to outline some of the dynamics of adjustment and maladjustment as these appear from a phenomenological frame of reference. While this approach represents a considerable departure from traditional concepts of adjustment, it is often true that new frames of reference provide new perspective upon old problems. Parts of this theoretical position have already been corroborated by research. Others remain to be demonstrated. In the final analysis, such hypotheses as I have presented here must stand the test of experimental demonstration, theoretical consistency, and demonstration in the practical test of therapy.

REFERENCES

1. Bruner, J. S., & Goodman, C. C. Value and need as organizing factors in perception. *J. abnorm. soc. Psychol.*, 1947, **42**, 33–44.
2. Cannon, W. B. *The wisdom of the body*. New York: Norton, 1932.
3. Combs, A. W. Phenomenological concepts in non-directive therapy. *J. consult. Psychol.* August 1948.
4. Frenkel-Brunswik, E. Mechanisms of self deception. *J. soc. Psychol.*, 1939, **10**, 409–420.
5. Kelley, E. *Education for what is real*. New York: Harper, 1948.
6. Lecky, L. *Self-consistency*. New York: Island Press, 1945.
7. Murphy, G. *Personality: A biosocial approach to origins and structure*. New York: Harper, 1947.
8. Piaget, J. *The child's conception of the world*. New York: Harcourt, Brace, 1929.
9. Raimy, V. C. The self concept as a factor in counseling and personality organization. Unpublished doctoral thesis, Ohio State University, 1943.
10. Rogers, C. R. The organization of personality. *Amer. Psychologist*, 1947, **2**, 358–368.
11. Snygg, D., & Combs, A. W. *Individual behavior: A new frame of reference for psychology*. New York: Harper, 1949.

7

A Social-Learning Explanation
of Deviant Behavior*

ALBERT BANDURA

The development of principles and procedures of behavioral change is largely determined by the model of causality to which one subscribes. The methods used to modify psychological phenomena therefore cannot be fully understood independently of the personality theory upon which they are based. The major differences between rival theoretical orientations are most strikingly revealed in their interpretations of grossly deviant behavior. Consequently, the systems that have been advanced to explain these perplexing conditions will be considered in some detail here . . . .

The earliest conceptions of psychopathology viewed behavioral anomalies as external manifestations of evil spirits that entered the victim's body and adversely affected his behavior. Treatment accordingly was directed toward exorcising demons by various methods, such as cutting a hole in the victim's skull, performing various magical and religious rituals, or brutally assaulting—physically and socially—the bearer of the pernicious spirits. Hippocrates was influential in supplanting the demonological conceptions of deviant behavior by relabeling it disease rather than demonic manifestations. Wholesome diets, hydrotherapy, bloodletting, and other forms of physical intervention, some benign, others less humane, were increasingly employed as corrective treatments.

Although psychological methods gradually replaced physical procedures in modifying deviant response patterns, the analogy of physical health and disease nevertheless continued to dominate theories of psychopathology. In this conceptualization, behavioral patterns that depart widely from accepted social and ethical norms are considered to be derivatives or symptoms of an underlying disease. Modification of social deviance thus became a medical specialty, with the result that persons exhibiting atypical behavior are labeled "patients" suffering from a "mental illness," and they generally are treated in medically oriented facilities. The disease concepts are likewise indiscriminately applied even to social phenomena, as evidenced by the frequent designation of cultural response patterns as "healthy" or "sick." Had Hippocrates represented behavioral anomalies as products of idiosyncratic social-learning experiences rather than as expressions of a somatic illness, the conceptualization and treatment of divergent response patterns might have taken an entirely different course.

A quasi-disease model is still widely employed in explanations of grossly deviant behavior, but the underlying pathology is generally considered to be psychic rather than neurophysiological in nature. This conceptual scheme became further confused when the appropriateness of the disease analogy to social behavior was increasingly challenged (Szasz, 1961). Most personality theorists eventually discarded the notion that deviant behavior is a manifestation of an underlying mental disease, but they nevertheless unhesitat-

---

ingly label anomalous behaviors as symptoms and caution against the dangers of symptom substitution. In these theories, the conditions supposedly controlling behavior continue to function analogously to toxic substances in producing deviant responses; however, the disturbing agents comprise a host of inimical psychodynamic forces (for example, repressed impulses, energized traits, psychic complexes, latent tendencies, self-dynamisms, and other types of energy systems) somewhat akin to the pernicious spirits of ancient times. Many contemporary theories of psychopathology thus employ a quasi-medical model fashioned from an amalgam of the disease and demonology conceptions, which have in common the belief that deviant behavior is a function of inimical inner forces. Consequently, attention is generally focused, not on the problem behavior itself, but on the presumably influential internal agents that must be exorcised by "catharsis," "abreaction," and acquisition of insight through an extended interpretive process. Indeed, direct modification of so-called symptomatic behavior is considered not only ineffective but actually dangerous, because, it is held, removal of the symptom has no effect upon the underlying disorder, which will manifest itself again in a new, possibly more debilitating symptom.

SOCIAL LABELING OF DEVIANT BEHAVIOR

Although most psychotherapists agree that direct "symptom" removal is inadvisable and few of them would acknowledge engaging in such forms of treatment, remarkably little attention has been devoted to the definition of what constitutes a "symptom." Categorizing a pattern of behavior as symptomatic of an underlying disorder actually involves a complex set of criteria, most of which are quite arbitrary and subjective. Whether specific actions are called normal or symptomatic expressions will depend upon whether certain social judges or the person himself disapproves of the behavior being exhibited. Since symptom labeling primarily reflects the evaluative responses that a given behavior evokes from others, rather than distinguishable qualities of the behavior itself, an identical response pattern may be viewed as a pathological derivative or as wholesome behavior by persons whose judgmental orientations differ. Aggressiveness in children, for example, may be positively reinforced and regarded as a sign of masculinity and healthy social development by some parents, while the same behavior is generally viewed by educational, legal, and other societal agents as a symptom of a personality disorder (Bandura, 1960; Bandura & Walters, 1959).

The designation of behavior as pathological thus involves social judgments that are influenced by, among other factors, the normative standards of persons making the judgments, the social context in which the behavior is exhibited, certain attributes of the behavior, and numerous characteristics of the deviator himself. An adequate theory of deviant behavior must therefore be concerned with the factors determining evaluative judgments. Unfortunately, in spite of widespread use of diagnostic classifications and the potentially serious consequences of labeling persons as mentally disturbed, there has been surprisingly little systematic study of the factors governing such judgmental behavior.

Psychopathology is characteristically inferred from the degree of deviance from the social norms that define how persons are expected to behave at different times and places. Consequently, the *appropriateness* of symbolic, affective, or social responses to given situations constitutes one major criterion in labeling "symptomatic" behavior. Departures from normative standards that do not inconvenience or interfere with the well-being of others are usually tolerated; deviations that produce rewarding consequences for the members of a society, as in the case of technological inventions and intellectual and artistic innovations, may be actively promoted and generously rewarded. On the other hand, deviance that generates aversive consequences for others elicits strong societal disapproval, is promptly labeled abnormal, and generally is met by coercive pressures to eliminate it.

The appropriateness criterion poses serious problems in societies, such as our own, that are differentiated into many subcultures whose members subscribe to divergent behavioral norms and therefore do not agree on what is suitable social behavior. Members of social groups who want rewards that are highly valued in the culture but lack the means of obtaining them in legitimate ways (Cloward & Ohlin, 1960; Merton, 1957) are often forced to resort to socially unacceptable activities. In these instances, antisocial patterns are not only normatively sanctioned, but the social environment provides these persons ample opportunities, through appropriate reinforcement contingencies and role models, to develop and to perfect deviant modes of behavior. According to the prevailing normative structure of these subcultures, skillfully executed antisocial behavior represents emulative rather than sick behavior and is governed by the same types of variables that control the prosocial response patterns displayed by members of the larger society.

Other subgroups are classified as social deviants, and therefore "sick" or "crazy," not because they adhere to culturally disapproved means of gaining highly rated objectives but because they withdraw from the dominant social system and reject the basic cultural goals themselves. The conforming majority within a society may label nonconformist groups, such as "Bohemians," "beatniks," and "hippies," that refuse to strive for the goals highly valued in the culture as exhibiting maladaptive behavior. From the perspective of the deviants, the life style of conforming members is a symptomatic manifestation of an overcommercialized, "sick" society. Thus the same pattern of behavior may be deemed a symptom by one social group but judged healthy and positively reinforced by persons who adhere to a different code of behavior. Similarly, when a society radically alters its social and legal norms, either the presence or absence of the same responses may be judged inappropriate, and, consequently, labeled symptoms of an underlying pathology. Thus, a citizen socialized in other respects who commits a brutal homicide will be diagnosed as suffering from a serious mental disorder, but a military recruit's inability to behave homicidally on the battlefield will likewise be viewed as symptomatic of a "war neurosis." The latter example further illustrates how behavior can come to be thought of as symptomatic because of changes in societal norms rather than because of a psychopathology reflected in the behavior itself.

The discussion thus far has been concerned with the deviant behavior of members of groups, who mutually support and reinforce each other's ideologies and actions. Some individuals display gross behavioral eccentricities that appear totally inexplicable; persons from different subgroups who do not share the same normative systems are apt to view these eccentricities as pathological manifestations. Even in these instances, when the idiosyncratic social-learning history for the behavior is known there is no need to assume an underlying disease process. Lidz, Cornelison, Terry, & Fleck (1958) report a case, for example, in which sibling schizophrenics believed, among other strange things, that "disagreement" meant constipation. This clearly inappropriate conceptual behavior was the result of exposure to bizarre social-learning contingencies and not an expression of a mental illness. Whenever the sons disagreed with their mother, she informed them that they were constipated and required an enema. The boys were then disrobed and given anal enemas, a procedure that dramatically conditioned an unusual meaning to the word "disagreement." The cases cited by Lidz and his associates (Lidz, Fleck, & Cornelison, 1965) provide compelling evidence of development of delusions, suspiciousness, grandiosity, extreme denial of reality, and other forms of "schizophrenic" behavior through direct reinforcement, and of their social transmission by parental modeling of incredibly deviant behavior patterns.

In addition to the influence of normative commitments in determining judgmental responses, certain properties of behavior readily invite one to label an emotional disorder symptomatic. Responses of high magnitude, for instance, often produce unpleasant experiences for others; they are therefore more likely to be considered pathological manifestations than are responses of low or moderate intensities. A youngster who is continually wrestling other children will generally be viewed as exhibiting youthful exuberance; in contrast, a child whose physically aggressive behavior is more forceful and hurtful will in all likelihood be regarded as emotionally disturbed. Although pervasive and intense emotional responses may be reliably categorized, disagreements are apt to arise in the labeling of behavior that falls at less extreme points on the response-intensity continuum. The line separating normality and abnormality may be variously located depending upon the tolerance limits for aversiveness of different judges. Even if a high degree of consensus could be achieved in designating the acceptable limits of amplitude for various behaviors, no evidence exists that emotional responses of high intensity are mediated by psychopathological internal processes, whereas similar responses of lesser strength are governed by nonpathological internal processes.

Behavioral deficits are also frequently interpreted as symptoms of emotional disorder, particularly when the deficits produce hardships and aversiveness for others. Adequately endowed children, for example, who are incontinent and who exhibit marked deficiencies in interpersonal, verbal, and academic skills, and adults who are unable to meet social, marital, and vocational task requirements tend to be labeled as emotionally disturbed. It is generally assumed, moreover, that the greater the deficits, the more extensive the underlying psychopathology. The arbitrary and relativistic nature of the deficit or competence criterion would become readily apparent if one were to vary the minimum standards of competence required in any given situation. If the standards were set at a comparatively low level, practically all members of a society would be judged competent and healthy, whereas the vast majority would suddenly acquire a psychopathology if exceedingly high standards were adopted. In the latter case, therapists and diagnosticians might devote much time to locating the source of pathology within the individuals.

The *intention* attributed to an action will affect its categorization by others as a symptomatic expression. When the variables governing physical and biological phenomena remained unknown, a host of internal forces and deities were invoked as causal agents. As scientific knowledge increased, these fanciful driving forces were replaced by explanatory concepts involving manipulable variables. Similarly, interpretations of psychological phenomena often assume pathological inner agents in cases where deviance appears unintelligible. If a person engages in disapproved behavior to attain generally valued material objects, his activities—being readily understandable—are less likely to be regarded as manifestations of emotional disease than if his deviant behavior has no apparent utilitarian value. Delinquents who strike victims on the head to extract their wallets expediently are generally labeled semiprofessional thieves exhibiting income-producing instrumental aggression. By contrast, delinquents who simply beat up strangers but show no interest in their victims' material possessions are supposedly displaying emotional aggression of a peculiarly disturbed sort. It is evident that in many cases of so-called nonutilitarian aggression, the behavior is highly instrumental in gaining the approval and admiration of peers and in enhancing status in the social hierarchy of the reference group. Peer-group approval is often more powerful than tangible rewards as an incentive for, and reinforcer of, aggressively deviant behavior (Buehler, Patterson, & Furniss, 1966).

The influential role of social reinforcement in regulating dangerous, senseless behavior is clearly revealed in a field study by Yablonsky (1962), who found that the dominant reinforcement contingencies in many delinquent gangs have shifted from utilitarian antisocial activities to destructive assaults executed in a "cool" and apparently indifferent manner on persons and property. The way in which aggression has taken on status-conferring value and in which threat of loss of "rep" may compel a person to engage in a homicidal assault is graphically illustrated in the following excerpt from an interview with one of the boys studied by Yablonsky.

> Momentarily I started to thinking about it inside; I have my mind made up I'm not going to be in no gang. Then I go on inside. Something comes up, then here comes all my friends coming to me. Like I said before, I'm intelligent and so forth. They be coming to me—then they talk to me about what they gonna do. Like, "Man, we'll go out there and kill this cat." I say, "Yeah." They kept on talkin'. I said, "Man, I just gotta go with you." Myself, I don't want to go, but when they start talkin' about what they gonna do, I say, "So, he isn't gonna take over my rep. I ain't gonna let him be known more than me." And I go ahead [p. vii].

External contingencies of reinforcement rather than internal emotional disease also appear to be the major determinants of the behavior of another youth involved in a gang killing: "If I would of got the knife, I would have stabbed him. That would have gave me more of a build-up. People would have respected me for what I've done and things like that. They would say, 'There goes a cold killer' [p. 8]." Similar reinforcement contingencies operated in the practice of a gang apprehended that used attacks upon people without provocation as its main admissions requirement. Each physical assault, which had to be observed by a club member to be valid, was valued at 10 points; and a total of 100 points was required for full-fledged membership (*San Francisco Chronicle*, 1964).

It should be noted in passing that prosocial approval-seeking behavior like athletic achievements or musical accomplishments, which may likewise have no apparent utilitarian value, is seldom labeled as emotionally disturbed behavior. Certain subgroups simply value and reward skillful "stomping" more highly than musical virtuosity.

The instrumental versus emotional dichotomy, therefore, appears primarily to reflect differences in the types of rewards sought, and not basic differences in the purposiveness of the behavior itself, or in the nature of the mediating internal events. Since some members of a society are likely to be brought up under atypical contingencies of social reinforcement, events which are ordinarily neutral or aversive for others may acquire a strong positive valence; consequently, the puzzling behavior exhibited by these individuals may appear to have little or no instrumental value, and thus tend to be explained by reference to internal psychopathological processes.

Certain behavioral requirements are prescribed according to a person's age, sex, social position, occupation, race, ethnic origin, or religion. Therefore *personal attributes* also enter into social judgment of behavior that deviates from role demands. For example, behavior considered to be normal at an early age may be regarded as a symptom of personality disturbance later, as in the case of enuresis. It is very appropriate, in this connection, to repeat Mowrer's (1950) query: "And when does persisting behavior of this kind suddenly cease to be normal and become a symptom [p. 474]?" Or consider the attribute of sex. The differential cultural tolerance for cross-sex behavior displayed by males and females illustrates the role of sex characteristics in the assignment of symptomatic status to deviant behavioral patterns. The wearing of female apparel by males is considered to be indicative of a serious psychological disorder, requiring prompt legal and psychiatric attention. On the other hand, females may adopt masculine garb, hair styles, and a wide range of characteristically masculine response patterns without being labeled as mentally disturbed. Since masculine role behavior occupies a position of relatively high prestige and power in our society and often is more generously rewarded than feminine role behavior, the emulation of masculine tendencies by females is more understandable and, therefore, less likely to be interpreted by reference to disease processes.

There is another side to the influence of personal attributes on judgmental responses. The social-learning background and characteristics of the person making the judgments may significantly affect his designation of particular behaviors as indicative of mental health or psychic pathology. Spohn (1960) found that therapists' social values were related to their mental health judgments of patients' behavior that reflected similar value dimensions: that is, therapists thought the patients more like themselves were the healthier ones.

Although the presence of psychic illness is frequently judged in terms of deviance from particular social norms, in many cases it is primarily based on *self-definition*. As Terwilliger & Fiedler (1958) have shown, persons often label themselves as emotionally disturbed, whereas others may judge them to be functioning satisfactorily within the prevailing social norms. Evaluative discrepancies of this type typically arise when persons impose excessive demands upon themselves and suffer subjective distress as a result of failure to meet self-imposed standards. A comprehensive theory of deviance must take into consideration self-reactions as well as societal reactions to one's behavior.

It is apparent from the foregoing discussion that the categorization of behavior as symptomatic of an underlying pathology depends upon a host of subjective criteria, and as a consequence, the same behavior may be characterized as "healthy" or "sick" by different judges, in different social contexts, and on the basis of performers' social characteristics. It is true, of course, that questions of value and social judgment arise also in the diagnosis of physical disorders. In such cases the symptom-disease model is quite appropriate since internal organic pathologies do in fact exist and can be verified independently of their peripheral manifestations. Brain tumors and dysfunctions involving respiratory, circulatory, or digestive organs are observable events. Where deviant behavior is concerned, analogy with the symptom-disease model is misleading because there are no infected organs or psychic disease entities that can be identified as causal agents. The psychic conditions that are assumed to underlie behavioral malfunctioning are merely abstractions from the behavior. In the disease analogy these abstractions are not only given substance and existence independent of the behavior from which they were inferred, but they are then invoked as the causes of the same behavioral referents. For these reasons, so-called symptomatic behavior can be more adequately explained in terms of social learning and value theory than through inappropriate medical analogizing. An extended account of a social-learning taxonomy of behavioral phenomena generally subsumed under the term "psychopathology" is presented elsewhere (Bandura, 1968). The preceding discussion reviewed some of the principal factors determining the attribution of sickness to deviant behavior. Similar social judgment processes are, of course, involved in the attachment of descriptive labels such as aggression, altruism, dependency, or achievement to particular response patterns.

HYPOTHETICAL INTERNAL DETERMINANTS OF BEHAVIOR

The questions raised concerning the utility and validity of the concept of "symptom" apply equally to the psychopathology presumed to underlie the troublesome behavior. From the focusing of attention on inner agents and forces, many fanciful theories of deviant behavior have emerged. The developmental history of social behavior is rarely known, and its reconstruction from interview material elicited by therapists or diagnosticians is of doubtful validity. In fact, the content of reconstruction is highly influenced by the interviewer's suggestive probing and selective reinforcement of content that is in accord with his theoretical orientation. Heine (1953), for example, found that clients who were treated by client-centered, Adlerian, and psychoanalytic therapists tended to account for changes in their behavior in terms of the explanations favored by their respective interviewers. Even a casual survey of interview protocols would reveal that psychotherapists of different theoretical affiliations tend to find evidence for their own preferred psychodynamic agents rather than those cited by other schools. Thus, Freudians are likely to unearth Oedipus complexes and castration anxieties, Adlerians discover inferiority feelings and compensatory power strivings, Rogerians find compelling evidence for inappropriate self-concepts, and existentialists are likely to diagnose existential crises and anxieties. It is equally true that Skinnerians, predictably, will discern defective conditions of reinforcement as important determinants of deviant behavior. In the latter explanatory scheme, however, the suspected controlling conditions are amenable to systematic variation; consequently the functional relationships between reinforcement contingencies and behavior are readily verifiable.

Theoretical models of dubious validity persist largely because they are not stated in refutable form. The lack of accurate knowledge of the genesis of behavioral deviations further precludes any serious evaluation of suggested determinants that are so involved that they could never be produced under laboratory conditions. When the actual social-learning history of maladaptive behavior is known, principles of learning appear to provide a completely adequate interpretation of psychopathological phenomena, and psychodynamic explanations in terms of symptom-underlying disorder become superfluous. The spuriousness of the supposition that psychodynamic forces produce symptomatic behavior can be best illustrated by cases in which the antecedents of aberrant response patterns are known. Such examples are hard to obtain since they require the production of deviant behavior under controlled conditions. Ayllon, Haughton, & Hughes (1965) furnish a graphic illustration of how a bizarre pattern of behavior—which was developed, maintained, and subsequently eliminated in a schizophrenic woman simply by altering its reinforcing consequences—was interpreted erroneously as a symptomatic manifestation of complex psychodynamic events by diagnosticians who were unaware of the specific conditions of reinforcement regulating the patient's behavior.

Unfortunately, the exact antecedents of deviant behavior are rarely known, and in the absence of powerful techniques that permit adequate control over behavioral phenomena, clinical endeavors have until recently lacked the self-corrective features necessary for eliminating weak or invalid theories of psychopathology. As a consequence, rival interpretations of social behavior have for decades retained a secure status with little risk that any one type of theory might prove more cogent than another.

In recent years there has been a fundamental departure from conventional views regarding the nature, causes, and treatment of behavioral dysfunctions. According to this orientation, behavior that is harmful to the individual or departs widely from accepted social and ethical norms is viewed not as symptomatic of some kind of disease but as a way that the individual has learned to cope with environmental and self-imposed demands. Treatment then becomes mainly a problem in social learning rather than one in the medical domain. In this conceptual scheme the remaining vestiges of the disease-demonic model have been discarded. Response patterns are not viewed as symptoms and their occurrence is not attributed to internal, pernicious forces.

Social learning and psychodynamic theories differ not only in whether they view deviant behavior as a quasi disease or as a by-product of learning, but also in what they regard to be the significant controlling factors, and in the status assigned to internal events....[Also] social-learning approaches treat internal processes as covert events that are manipulable and measurable. These mediating processes are extensively controlled by external stimulus events and in turn regulate overt responsiveness. By contrast, psychodynamic theories tend to regard internal events as relatively autonomous. These hypothetical causal agents generally bear only a tenuous relationship to external stimuli, or even to the "symptoms" that they supposedly produce....

... The major deficiencies of theories that explain behavior primarily in terms of conjectural inner causes would have been readily demonstrated had they been judged, not in terms of their facility in interpreting behavioral phenomena that have already occurred, but rather on the basis of their efficacy in predicting or modifying them. Because the internal determinants propounded by these theories (such as mental structures, Oedipal complexes, collective unconscious) could not be experimentally induced, and rarely possessed unequivocal consequences, psychodynamic formulations enjoyed an immunity to genuine empirical verification. If progress in the understanding of human behavior is to be accelerated, psychological theories must be judged by their predictive power, and by the efficacy of the behavioral modification procedures that they produce....

REFERENCES

Allyon, T., Haughton, E., & Hughes, H. B. Interpretation of symptoms: Fact or fiction. *Behav. Res. & Therapy*, 1965, **3**, 1–7.

Bandura, A. Relationship of family patterns to child behavior disorders. (Progress Report, 1960, Stanford University, Project No. M-1734) United States Public Health Service.

Bandura, A. A social learning interpretation of psychological dysfunctions. In P. London & D. Rosenhan (Eds.), *Foundations of abnormal psychology*. New York: Holt, Rinehart & Winston, 1968. Pp. 293–344.

Bandura, A. & Walters, R. H. *Adolescent aggression*. New York: Ronald Press, 1959.

Buehler, R. E., Patterson, G. R., & Furniss, J. M. The reinforcement of behavior in institutional settings. *Behav. Res. & Therapy*, 1966, **4**, 157–167.

Cloward, R. A., & Ohlin, L. E. *Delinquency and opportunity: A theory of delinquent gangs*. New York: Free Press, 1960.

Heine, R. W. A comparison of patients' reports on psychotherapeutic experience with psychoanalytic, nondirective and Adlerian therapists. *Am. J. Psychother.*, 1953, **7**, 16–23.

Lidz, T., Cornelison, A. R., Terry, D., & Fleck, S. Intrafamilial environment of the schizophrenic patient: VI. The transmission of irrationality. *AMA Arch. Neurol. & Psychiat.*, 1958, **79**, 305–316.

Lidz, T., Fleck, S., & Cornelison, A. R. *Schizophrenia and the family*. New York: International Universities Press, 1965.

Merton, R. K. *Social theory and social structure*. (Rev. ed.) New York: Free Press, 1957.

Mowrer, O. H. *Learning theory and personality dynamics*. New York: Roland Press, 1950.

San Francisco Chronicle, November 26, 1964. P. 3.

Spohn, H. E. The influence of social values upon the clinical judgments of psychotherapists. In J. G. Peatman & E. L. Hartley (Eds.), *Festschrift for Gardner Murphy*. New York: Harper & Row, 1960. Pp. 274–290.

Szasz, T. S. *The myth of mental illness*. New York: Harper & Row, 1961.

Terwilliger, J. S., & Fiedler, F. E. An investigation of determinants inducing individuals to seek personal counseling. *J. consult. psychol.*, 1958, **22**, 288.

Yablonsky, L. *The violent gang*. New York: Macmillan, 1962.

8

Family Dynamics and Origin of Schizophrenia*[1]

STEPHEN FLECK

An intensive study of the families of young upper-class schizophrenic patients initiated by Dr. Theodore Lidz in 1952, is now in the seventh year (not counting the first year's pilot study by Drs. Lidz and Beulah Parker.) The team whose research is reported here consisted of two and occasionally more psychiatrists, a social worker, a psychologist, and research assistants. We selected families in which at least the mother and one sibling were available for the study. In most of our families both parents have been available because the bias in our sample has been intentionally directed toward better organized families than would be provided by a random sample of the families of schizophrenics[31, 54]. By dealing mostly with structurally intact families unencumbered by serious economic problems, we hoped to eliminate some of the more extraneous disorganizing factors that beset so many lower-class families[24].

Contact with some of the families has been maintained through most of the research period and with all at least over many months. Interviews, held weekly in many cases, most commonly have involved the social worker and a family member[9]. Several parents, however, have been seen by one of the psychiatrists for long periods, although usually not at weekly intervals. Also, we often sought out and interviewed other relatives, especially grandparents, friends, and sometimes former servants. Home visits by the social worker have been made at least once in almost every instance. In addition, all available members of each nuclear family have been given a battery of psychological tests[17]. We have found it more useful not to record interviews verbatim but to dictate them as promptly as possible after a session. Even this condensed raw material on some families extends to several volumes of typed material. When satisfied that we had learned as much as we were likely to about a family, or when the patient had been discharged, we summarized the material in 50–100 typewritten pages. We feel that the data for 16 families are at this time reasonably complete.

On one level, the findings can be stated quite simply. No family that functioned or had ever functioned in a way that could be characterized as wholesome or normal or as falling within the usual range of family life has been found. All were severely disturbed, distorted by conflict, and beset by role uncertainties of family members other than the patient. I recognize that such a statement is methodologically not very satisfactory, but the team has been more concerned with describing and delineating the difficulties and disturbances that characterize these families than with an attempt to establish some sort of controlled study.

*From Fleck, S., *Psychosomatic Medicine*, 1960, **22**, 333–343. Copyright © 1960 by Harper & Row, Publishers, Inc. Reprinted by permission of Harper & Row, Publishers, Inc., and Dr. Fleck.

[1]The research reported here has been supported by grants from the National Institute of Mental Health and from the Social Research Foundation.

Presented in part at the program honoring Dr. John C. Whitehorn during the Meeting of the Johns Hopkins Medical and Surgical Association, February 27, 1959, Baltimore, Md.

I shall, however, attempt to spell out some of these differences between the study families and other families later on. We have been encouraged in the pursuit of our approach by the concordant findings of other groups who have studied families of schizophrenics in recent years, such as the National Institute of Mental Health[5, 53], the group under Drs. Don Jackson and Gregory Bateson in Palo Alto[3, 22, 26], and in particular, by similar findings abroad[2, 10]. Notably, Alanen of Finland has made a statement almost identical with the above: All but 16 of 100 mothers of schizophrenic patients he studied suffered from a clear neurosis or more serious psychopathologic disturbance, but each of these 100 families had to be considered severely disturbed[2].

It is not easy, however, to list and delineate the abnormalities in family function that we have discerned manifest in disturbed family interaction and in the personalities of its members. In part, such a list encompasses the titles of previous publications, each only a fragment of the total reconstruction of family histories and the histories of the persons in it. This presentation also can deal only with some segments of the unexpectedly rich and complicated material that we have accumulated so far. Despite a multifaceted approach, we are by no means certain that we have as yet grasped the total picture of all the essentials of interaction in these families that have been studied from months to many years, or for that matter, of family dynamics in general. Our task is further complicated by the absence of a set of concepts (or a communication model for group interaction) that would simultaneously convey both a cross section of transactions at a given time and a longitudinal historical dimension.

The family is a unique type of group and operates under more complicated dynamics than do the synthetic groups usually studied in detail by sociologists or psychologists. Our traditional psychodynamic concepts alone are not suited to the description and analysis of the family-group process over a period of time. We have borrowed from social anthropologists and sociologists[6], especially from Parsons[42, 43], Kluckhohn[28] and group psychologists[44] in an effort to place some of our work in a suitable frame of reference[7, 16, 21, 48, 49]. Without their work and that of many others in allied disciplines, we would have no suitable models to answer our needs at least in part[12, 20]. As I seek to describe some of our findings, it must be emphasized that different methods of abstraction as well as different conceptual approaches have been employed in describing different phases of the disturbed family milieu.

Certain facets of the disturbed family interaction we have observed have been separated out rather artificially, but the respective areas of interaction blend and, in actuality, of course, occur together. For the psychiatrist it is naturally easier to describe individual personal characteristics. In this work, however, impressive as the abnormalities of each family member often are, not to mention those of the patient, we have found that family interaction and the interlocking roles and role shifts appear to have more bearing upon the development of schizophrenia in one member than the characteristics of individual parents or siblings.

PARENTAL PERSONALITIES

At the start it became obvious to us, as it has to others, that many mothers of schizophrenic patients appear severely disturbed, often bordering on the psychotic[1, 2, 23, 34, 40, 45, 46]. Many such personal characteristics of these mothers have been described by others, notably by Dr. Trudi Tietze[51]. We are not yet prepared, however, to amplify these earlier descriptions or to render them more inclusive but should note that none of them applies to all the mothers we have studied. We have found a wider range of disturbances, and no one personality type has emerged. At least half the mothers of our patients were psychotically disturbed. We are in the process of examining the characteristics of mothers in various ways, including the use of a sorting technique employing several hundred items, a modification of a similar study undertaken by Don Jackson and his colleagues[26]. Some of the disturbed interaction patterns and irrational rearing techniques of these mothers will become evident in later sections; here, I note our conclusion that in any analysis of material personalities and in searching for common characteristics, the mothers of schizophrenic sons and of schizophrenic daughters must be considered separately[38].

We realized soon that the intrapsychic disturbances of the mothers were not nearly as relevant to what happened to one or more children in the family (especially to the child who became schizophrenic) as was the fact that these women were paired with husbands who would either acquiesce to their many irrational and bizarre notions of how the family should be run or who would constantly battle with and undermine an already anxious and insecure mother[34, 35]. Furthermore, half the families were dominated by an equally irra-tional, often paranoid father paired with a submissive, acquiescing spouse, or at least by a disturbed husband who clashed with a constantly nagging and depreciating wife. Our first communication therefore concerned the characteristics of some of these fathers[33]. We have noted that while no characteristic type of disturbed father occurred in our series, many were so caught up in their personal problems—very often conscious and unconscious concerns about their masculinity—that they could not function in a parental fashion. Some used the child to gratify their narcissistic needs for admiration or completion of their selves quite as much as has been observed in the mother-child relationships of schizophrenic patients[23, 32]. Still others abdicated parental roles in the face of hostile, chronically nag-ging, and domineering spouses but might possibly have fulfilled parental functions more adequately if they had married supportive, less disturbed women. The reverse can also be said of some mothers, as Lidz and Lidz noted many years ago[31]. As far as the develop-ment of schizophrenia in an offspring is concerned, we now believe that more typical profiles for either parent may emerge if we group them according to the patient's sex[38, 40].

PARENTAL INTERACTION

We have discerned and attempted to describe the disturbed interaction as certain pat-terns seemed to become understandable. These patterns, we believe, have a significant im-pact upon our patients' development and seem pertinent to symptomatology, if not to the basic illness. We have documented these intrafamilial disturbances with detailed examples in a number of papers and in this paper summarize them only briefly.

Schismatic Families

Schismatic families are beset by chronic strife and controversy, primarily between the parents. The friction may focus on specific issues such as religion or the family's social status, and these topics are constantly dragged into family discussion and interaction. Usu-ally, however, such specific contents are only the outward symptom of a basic distrust and often hatred of one spouse for the other[35].

> The Readings were such a family. A paranoid, grandiose, and autocratic father dominated it. After 20 yr. of marriage he had remained emotionally closer to his mother than to his wife. He was very intelligent and productive, but he resisted his wife's burning ambition to rise in the social scale—a source of constant open controversy between them. However, any issue was apt to

produce a fight, and when the older of their two daughters became schizophrenic at 21, the illness, the hospitalization, and the treatment all offered more opportunities for mutual nagging, for undermining the other's plans and hopes, and for holding each other responsible for this disaster. The patient spent most of her time in catatonic muteness, possibly the only way open to her to remove herself from the family battlefield.

The topic of her illness and its relation to the family dynamics will receive further comment in a following section.

The schismatic families in which the parents undermine each other's worth, despising each other as man or woman, depriving each other of much needed support (often a narcissistic need in at least one of the parents), can create insurmountable identity problems for their offspring. To be like one parent incurs the wrath or disparagement of the other, and neither parent may be very self assured about his gender to begin with. We can trace in this way some of the identity problems of schizophrenics and also can appreciate that young people raised in such families break down just at a time when a sense of identity essential to a more independent social role outside the home is expected of them in early adulthood [37, 39].

Skewed Families

Another form of distorted family milieu has been designated as skew. Such families differ from schismatic ones in that the marriage itself may be peaceful and mutually satisfactory because the spouses have overtly or covertly reached a compromise concerning a serious personality defect in one or the other. Usually one partner had given in to the more disturbed and domineering one, but peace between them may be maintained at the expense of the children because the parental alliance also preempts their emotional resources, and then truly parental obligations suffer [35].

Mr. Lamb, for instance, was a very successful business man but a most inadequate parent. As a young adult he had been an outstanding athlete but had to leave his school for disciplinary reasons. Soon after marriage he began to drink heavily, and by the time his wife became pregnant for the first time, he was an alcoholic. From the time of the son's conception on, he made every possible effort to retain all of his wife's attention and affection, and to keep her away from his son, who later was our patient. Mr. Lamb was much less competitive with a subsequent daughter. His wife largely acceded to his demands and wishes although she was aware of her son's unfulfilled needs. Instead of standing up to the father and objecting to his behavior, she tended to look at times to the son for emotional support that the husband could not give her. Moreover, she encouraged the talented son to fulfill her own artistic tendencies. These were entirely lost on her husband, who openly criticized the son as effeminate, weak, and unathletic, after having thwarted the son's earlier efforts to be physically active by sneering at the child's performance in games or sports.

At 20 the son indeed showed all these characteristics. But he had absorbed more from the parental interaction. The father drank, and yet both spouses maintained that he was not an alcoholic. He was unfaithful, and this also remained masked except for one occasion on which it became a community-wide scandal. Cheating and lying caused the patient's removal from school prior to his hospitalization, and prevarication remained a serious handicap in his therapeutic relationship for a long time. During the first year of his hospitalization he also lorded it over the staff, as well as his mother, treating everybody like an underling, as his father had often done at home.

The father had been a sham from the son's point of view. Instead of a father he was a competitor; the lack of integrity in his personal life could not be concealed, despite the parental conspiracy to deny the obvious. The concealment and deceit were reflected in the patient's symptoms and behavior in schizophrenic form.

Knowing the family history thoroughly and from many different vantage points, one is at a loss to find a position at any time to which this youngster could have regressed in order to re-experience some degree of security or satisfaction. Only autistic withdrawal seemed open to him. To live up to his father's "expectations" he had to be weak and passive in one sense, and an athlete in another; to please his mother he had to be artistic; but to assume a male role in any area carried the threat of incestuous closeness to his mother and indeed constituted a threat to his father's shaky masculinity. Thus, in this type of family also we can observe that the patient in his personality development is confronted with irreconcilable identity prototypes.

As far as these identity problems in young schizophrenics are concerned, we find that equivalent phenomena have been pointed out in a more general way by Erickson in his writings on identity crisis[11, 37]. We shall return to this topic later in connection with sexual problems.

The skew in the family can exist in another form: The dominant emotional dyad may be one parent and one offspring[39]. In these latter families the assignment to either group becomes somewhat arbitrary. Not only may a parental schism lead to hostile pairings or camps in the family, but one of these couplings may preempt the family's emotional resources just as importantly as the parental coalition illustrated above.

THE IRRATIONALITY OF THE FAMILY MILIEU AND SYMPTOM FORMATION

Another skewed family may illustrate this important process observed in many of our families—the transmission of irrationality or, one might almost say, the learning of symptoms[8, 14, 36].

Young Dollfuss came to us from another hospital, to which he had been admitted following a serious suicide attempt. Although relatively compliant and cooperative at first, he soon became increasingly resistant to hospital routines, spoke less and less with anybody, neglected his appearance, grew a beard, and would not allow his hair to be cut, so that long locks soon framed his shoulders. Being unusually tall, he not only looked like the Messiah but was indeed preoccupied with strange mystical religions—seemingly of his own invention. As if this appearance were not bizarre enough in the setting of an unbelievably messy room in which he hoarded food, a typical daily scene showed him almost naked, sitting on his toilet, studying stock quotations in the *Wall Street Journal*. It may be noted in passing that he showed a typically schizophrenic phenomenon, exhibiting severe psychotic and delusional behavior, unable to have any comfortable human contact, while still able to select a stock portfolio for his therapist that he predicted correctly would increase 40 per cent on the market in a year's time—a coexistence of abnormal and normal high-order mentation never encountered in any known organic brain disorder.

As we began to learn about the family background, it became clear that the patient conducted his hospital life in the same autocratic, pompous, and captious manner in which the father had governed the parental household. Mr. Dollfuss was an ingenious and successful foreign-born manufacturer, but at home he ruled his roost like an Eastern potentate, a role for which he also claimed divine sanction and inspiration via a special mystical cult that he shared only with a very few select friends. The patient would permit only a chosen few of the staff into his sanctum, just as the father had secluded himself in his bedroom during most of the time that he spent at home, with only his wife and the children's governess permitted to enter and attend to his needs. Mr. Dollfuss, successful inventor and merchant, would sit there in his underclothes reading religious books by the hour. The entire household participated in the religious rites, the mother sharing his beliefs completely and continuing to do so even after his death, which according to the cult meant continuing life in a different form; the widow did not dare to disavow his teachings, because she believed he would know of it.

More than imitation and caricaturization of the father's behavior was involved. Both the patient and his only sister were emotionally deprived children who were isolated from the parents *and* from the surrounding community because the family milieu was so aberrant. Thus, when not mute, the patient often consented to communicate only in foreign languages, as if to emphasize his and the family's estrangement from the surroundings. He "communicated" his sense of deprivation by hoarding food, and during one stage of his illness by devising a complicated airline system designed exclusively for transporting and distributing food supplies in such a way that his needs would be gratified from all over the world.

This case provides a striking example of the irrationality of the parental relationship that came to pervade the entire household and of the aberrant patterns that the child had to cope with and ultimately learn himself, in order to live within the family. To question the bizarre family milieu, as he became aware that people outside did live and perceive the world differently, might have endangered his place as a child, leading to further distance from the parents or others in the household, all of whom shared or seemed to share the abnormal mode of life. To live outside this family the child had to learn other ways of living, if he could—and our patient could not.

VIOLATION OF GENERATION BOUNDARIES

We were further impressed that in both skewed and schismatic families, one child might perceive that in reality he was more important to one or the other parent than was the spouse. In schismatic families, loyalty to one parent, often seductively engendered by that parent, might invite hostility and derogation from the other, just as the spouse to whom the child was close was despised by the partner. In addition to the obvious difficulties this created for the child who sought or needed to identify with one parent, such disregard of the familial generation boundaries had important bearing on the sexual confusions and panics from which practically all schizophrenics suffer[15]. Finally, by being all-important to one parent, or to both as a pawn of battle, the patient became predisposed to symptoms of grandiosity.

The skew in some families, as already described, might consist of a close, erotically colored continuing relationship between one parent and a child. Typically this kind of bond was highly charged with anxiety, since the two individuals never could find a comfortable distance or closeness in their interaction[53]. Therefore, the catatonic issue, "If I make one move, something terrible is going to happen—somebody will be harmed if I initiate a move," was a reality chronically confronting patients who grew up in such families.

We have discovered—especially in connection with the issue of institutionalization itself—that some parents were truly incapable of living without the child and could not tolerate the separation imposed by hospitalization[13]; this conclusion confirms earlier reports by the Lidzes[32], Hill[23], and others[5, 18], based on findings in individual therapy that the so-called symbiotic tie between patient and parent may be more essential to the parent's existence than to that of the patient. When a mother a thousand miles away awakens every morning at 6 a.m. because this is 7 a.m. Eastern time and the moment when her schizophrenic son receives his insulin injection and continues to experience the insulin injection vicariously through the morning over all this distance, day after day, we can appreciate that she cannot leave her son long in the hands of his therapists. We can also understand why the son is right in claiming that every move he makes is of world-shaking consequence because, indeed, it is so to his mother, whose anxiety he in turn heightened by letting her know in detail "how the insulin softened his brain."

We have described in another communication a skewed family containing twins, one of whom became our patient[39]. The birth of these twins was the mother's longed-for triumph over her own nonidentical twin sister, and the twins became the center of her life as well as the masters of the family's existence. Shortly after their birth the father was evicted from his wife's bed and bath rooms and, together with the older son, was relegated literally to inferior roles in the house, being permitted, for example, to use only the basement lavatory. One day when the mother, who was given to temper tantrums, received a spanking from one of the twins, the father tried to intercede, but the mother forbade him to interfere. Most of the violations of the generation boundaries we have noted are somewhat less bizarre and drastic, but not necessarily less damaging to a child's need to find a child's role and position in the family, on the basis of which further personality development and socially adaptive growth can proceed[15, 37, 42, 43].

SEXUAL PROBLEMS

In connection with the Lamb case we have referred to the serious impediments such a family situation can represent to the development in a child of a sense of identity, and also how difficult it may be for an offspring to find in two warring parents suitable prototypes for identification. Whether fighting with each other or supporting each other at the expense of adequate reality presentation to their offspring, most of our parents were usually also very insecure about their own sexuality.

> During visiting hours one of our patients, Dora Nussbaum, suddenly ran from her room in greater panic than observed ever before during several months of hospitalization. On investigation it was learned that she suddenly panicked while sitting on her bed with her father. We knew already that the patient had often fallen asleep in her father's arms. The mother had told us of her disgust over these intimacies between father and daughter, which bothered Mrs. Nussbaum all the more because of the absence of any physical intimacies between herself and her husband. This was a schismatic family in which the parents had become irreconcilably estranged because of a feud between their respective primary families, to whom both spouses were still very much attached. Dora's older brother and the mother had a workable if not close relationship, but Dora was disliked by the mother and preferred by the father, a condition that resulted in a rather incestuous bond between them. In adolescence, Dora began to object to his habit of frequently sleeping on her bed, out of fear that she would become pregnant (we have no evidence of actual incestuous behavior). However, frequent close physical contact was resumed during Dora's psychosis at times when the father tried to calm her. One of Dora's early psychotic manifestations was fear that she would be raped while at the same time she behaved promiscuously with strangers. The father claimed to be impotent but tried to make his wife and daughter believe that he had a mistress. Whether true or not, it bespeaks his insecure masculinity, also expressed in other effeminate, narcissistic tendencies.

Thus one can discern the roots of a schizophrenic patient's sexual and incestuous problems and their close relationship to panic states, symptoms which become understandable through scrutiny of the family background and dynamics[15, 37].

Another father, who never achieved satisfactory sexual relations with his wife, promoted both homosexual and incestuous tendencies in his schizophrenic son. He often spoke to him about arranging dates for him, specifically mentioning an actress who, he pointed out, resembled his mother very strongly. The father also arranged for a friend whom he knew to be homosexual to share the boy's bedroom, besides taking showers himself with the son, comparing the size of their genitals or rubbing each other's backs. During therapy it was learned that one of the patient's tenacious symptoms—a magical need to repeat certain figures—was specifically related to conscious efforts to keep incestuous ideas in abeyance.

In the Reading family, which was split into two camps (page 75), the patient was also aware of the incestuous potential. Her suspicious, cantankerous father, who preferred her over the sister—not to mention his wife, whom he blamed for the illness—also was highly critical of the hospital, as well as suspicious that we were giving him "a run for his money." Realistically, she made no progress, possibly at least in part because of the father's disapproval of our efforts, a parallel to his undermining the mother's social and educational ambitions for her daughters. There were many threats to remove the patient from the hospital, and this he finally did. Once he proposed the following therapeutic solution: the family should split up, the mother and the patient's sister, who formed one faction, would live together, and he would live with and look after the patient himself. When the patient learned of this plan, she made one of her few excursions into reality from her state of catatonic muteness and stated, "I'll do anything for my father, but he can't have me that way."

We have spelled out in more detail in two other communications the nature of the many areas of family dysfunction that we have observed and their possible specific implications for the development of conscious incestuous and homosexual conflicts on the part of patients [15, 39]. The entire family interaction may promote such conscious preoccupations rather than further repression in offspring and parents alike. The continuation of incestuous impulses may be an index of family disorganization, a view supported by Parsons' psychosocial formulations [42, 43]. We found that Parsons' essential prerequisites of family life, which must exist if a child is to de-eroticize his parental attachments, acquire a sexual identity, and prepare for sociocultural adaptation, are often absent in the families we have studied [11, 16, 43]. Among the prerequisites that most, if not all, of our parents failed to observe were the maintenance of generation boundaries, a personal sense of security in each as to sexual, parental, and social roles, a certain degree of marital harmony, the ability to share or compromise on cultural values, and a capacity for role reciprocity [37, 49].

SOCIOCULTURAL ISOLATION

We have illustrated how some of our families do not maintain differential roles in the sense of parents who nurture and lead as against children who are dependent and learn; that sexuality in these families is not limited to parental activity; that the parents, although often competent in their jobs or professions, are rigid, inflexible, and uncompromising in their intrafamilial behavior, and that many provide a home life quite deviant from the surrounding culture. The social life of these families often appears very limited, except that some families are still anchored in the patient's grandparental families or in one of the parent's collateral sibling families. There is failure to form a nuclear family of their own. This we found in six of our schismatic families; in a sense, this failure also constitutes another form of violating generation boundaries—at least in modern America.

Individual parental pathologic traits and role deficiencies aside, it is therefore the irrational and idiosyncratic environment that these families create which seems most important and which has led us to speak of *"folie à famille"* in situations like that of the Dollfusses [14]. Furthermore, not only does the transmission of aberrant percepts seem specifically related to the later development of schizophrenic manifestations, but the feedback between the children and parents creates a self-perpetuating, irrational, and ambivalence-laden atmosphere. The interaction circuit may be one of axe-grinding between parents, or of a parent and child alternating between avoiding anxiety-arousing closeness—incestuous closeness—and efforts to overcome icy distance, but whichever it is, all family members must adapt to it in different roles.

Even if these family environments were not as deviant from the surrounding culture as many are, one gets the impression that intrafamilial life of the kinds described may absorb so much energy that but little emotional investment seems possible for learning and socializing tasks outside the home. Moreover, in many of these families the tools, especially the communication tools essential to the establishment of meaningful relationships outside the family, are simply not furnished[14, 38]. Thus, a vicious cycle exists because the aberrant family environment is self-perpetuating unless corrected from the outside. But the isolating nature of the pathological forces within the family deprives its members of meaningful contacts with the outside world, and therewith, of the potential corrective impact of intimate interaction with people outside the family circle. For instance, the incest issue may arouse enough guilt feelings in one or the other member to render difficult any other friendships; but in the absence of cathected relationships outside the family, those within become all the more intense and conflictful. The child caught in the special bind with a parent is most crucially affected. Seeking friends outside the bond endangers the very essential tie to the parent, and the absence of other ties renders the bond to that parent more intense and more ambivalent.

GENERAL COMMENT

Although the evidence is impressive, even from the fraction of our material presented, that the families discussed are unusually disturbed, we cannot state with certainty the extent to which the families are distinctive in structure and *modi operandi*. The nature of the abnormalities and the distortions of family life that we have observed fall into behavioral categories such as personal, interpersonal, group dynamics, and psychology, and their specific relevance to the development of schizophrenia remains to be documented in detail by further search and study.

We do not intend to promulgate an environmental interpersonal approach as against a genetic or biochemical path to the etiology of schizophrenia. Our material is not suited to settle questions of causation, as we are not searching for a particular cause but have been exploring essentially uncharted territory. This material, pertinent to schizophrenia, may also help us to understand better the mode of transmission from generation to generation of the highest cerebral functions, in particular all those specifically human functions concerned with interpersonal communication through complicated, abstract, verbal and nonverbal symbols, whether normal or schizophrenic. Thus, the study of schizophrenia leads us to the problems of personality development in the human and to the broad question of how meaning and logic and a sense of identity are acquired.

We have previously stated that schizophrenia can be viewed as one possible outcome of personality development, or as Sullivan phrased it, a "way of life"[50]. This view does not exclude organic determinants, as genetic and nongenetic physiochemical influences obviously underlie and impinge upon the learning processes through which every individual must pass to acquire an identity and to develop his intellectual and sociocultural adaptive capacities. The physiological aspects of learning processes are only partially understood, but the development and the integration of symbolic processes and behavior occur after birth, whereas only simple reflexlike response patterns can be acquired prenatally [25, 30]. It seems fruitful, therefore, to scrutinize postnatal interactional phenomena, and such studies indeed render a great deal of this learning or transmission of behavior and attitudes, whether schizophrenic or not, more understandable, even if done retrospectively. This was expressed by Adolf Meyer 50 years ago: "We are, I believe, justified in directing our attention to the factors which we see at work in the life history of so-called dementia praecox. We are justified in emphasizing the process of crowding-out of normal reactions, of a substitution of inferior reactions some of which determine a cleavage along distinctly psychological lines incompatible with reintegration" [41]. I am not citing these words because they may be truer or more appealing than other statements, but rather because if one rereads Bleuler [4], Kraepelin [29], Jung [27], Meyer [41], Freud [19], and others who worked in this field half a century or more ago, recent studies of others and our own data seem to bear out Meyer's admonition above all others.

To explain bizarre behavior such as that of our Christ-like patient who sat in his bathroom with the *Wall Street Journal*, we neither have to fall back on or search for obscure pathological tissue processes on the one hand, nor do we have to speculate about all the possible symbolic meanings of such an activity, which is not to say that either consideration is irrelevant. Nor must we inject some psychotomimetic drug or postulate some sudden regressive break in the personality make-up to find explicable some of the other symptoms we described. To understand how items of behavior developed, however, is not necessarily to understand causality—certainly not the causality of as complicated a condition or process, whichever it may be, as schizophrenia. As long as there is no physical or chemical indicator for schizophrenia, we are left essentially with a conglomerate of clinical manifestations in making a diagnosis and are no better off today in this respect than was Bleuler half a century ago [4], when he stressed that diagnosis rests on the psychological manifestations. In our day we prefer a still less limited area of diagnostic criteria by considering the patient's interpersonal behavior.

How can we be certain that the family interactions we have observed are pathological? Can we or anybody undertake "control studies?" If so, what variables should be controlled? We have designedly put this problem aside. It has taken months and years to arrive at reasonably plausible and congruous reconstructions of fewer than 20 families in terms of the personalities involved and their interaction patterns. Our data in themselves and even for the same family differ in reliability in that we have direct evidence about some phenomena from several sources and only plausible conjectures concerning other observations. Obviously, to duplicate such a study in detail would be an enormous task and open to question from the beginning if done by a different team because of the different personalities involved. We have undertaken recently to study also families of upper-class delinquents—not to compare variables, but to see how, if at all, these families differ, in the hope that we can sharpen our conceptualizations [38].

Another question is: How are the phenomena described related to schizophrenia? Obviously we have not explained or made understandable all possible schizophrenic manifestations, nor is it likely that all of them are rooted in family interaction. Our data indicate, however, that the study of these families sheds much light on many schizophrenic manifestations, and that aspects of the parental personalities and of intrafamilial behavior of all members determine much of what we consider characteristic or pathognomonic of schizophrenia when we, as diagnosticians, approach a patient.

Another question that seemed formidable at first concerned the presence of "normal" and schizophrenic siblings in the same family. We have been working on this problem recently and have found it to be much less difficult. The patients' siblings are not unaffected by the abnormal environment. But when the entire family situation is known and the respective roles are understood, the development of the siblings' personalities, whether more nearly schizophrenic or more nearly normal, also fits into the total family pattern [2a, 38].

SUMMARY

In summary, some of the characteristic forms of family dysfunction related to schizophrenic manifestations that we observed are: (1) failure to form a nuclear family in that one or both parents remain primarily attached to one of his or her parents or siblings; (2) family schisms due to parental strife and lack of role reciprocity; (3) family skews when one dyadic relationship within it dominates family life at the expense of the needs of other members; (4) blurring of generation lines in the family, e.g., (a) when one parent competes with children in skewed families, (b) when one parent establishes a special bond with a child giving substance to the schizophrenic's claim that he or she is more important to a parent than the spouse, and (c) when continued erotization of a parent-child relationship occurs; (5) pervasion of the entire family atmosphere with irrational, usually paranoid, ideation; (6) persistence of conscious incestuous preoccupation and behavior within the group; (7) sociocultural isolation of the family as a concomitant of the six preceding conditions; (8) failure to educate toward and facilitate emancipation of the offspring from the family, a further consequence of points 1–5; (9) handicapping of a child in achieving sexual identity and maturity by the parents' uncertainty over their own sex roles; and (10) presentation to a child of prototypes for identification that are irreconcilable in the necessary process of consolidating his own personality.

Intensive work with these families has therapeutic implications which transcend our research plans as such and therewith the scope of this presentation. Other investigators of family dynamics have focused more on this aspect of the schizophrenia problem. The further development of rational psychotherapy, whether with the patient alone or with the family group, will depend upon better understanding and clarification of the complex interrelatedness of family dynamics, ego development, and identity formation. Thus, the study of schizophrenia and the quest for its origins leads us to the question of human development, and better understanding of the latter may illuminate the nature of schizophrenia as well as facilitate the treatment of schizophrenic patients.

REFERENCES

1. Abrahams, J., & Varon, E. J. *Maternal Dependency and Schizophrenia: Mother and Daughter in a Therapeutic Group.* New York: International Universities Press, 1953.
2. Alanen, Y. O. The mothers of schizophrenic patients. *Acta psychiat. et neurol. scandinav.* Suppl. 124, 1958.
2a. Alanen, Y. O. Work in progress.
3. Bateson, G., Jackson, D. D., Halfy, J., & Weakland, J. Towards the theory of schizophrenia. *Behavioral Sc.,* 1956, **1,** 251.
4. Bleuler, E. Dementia Praecox oder Gruppe der Schizophrenien. In G. Aschaffenburg (Ed.), *Handbuch der Psychiatrie.* Leipzig & Wien, 1911.
5. Bowen, M. Family relationships in schizophrenia. Presented at Hawaiian Divisional Meeting of American Psychiatric Association, May, 1958.
6. Bott, E. *Family and Social Network.* London: Tavistock Publications, 1957.

7. Buell, B., *et al. Classification of Disorganized Families for Use in Family Oriented Diagnosis and Treatment.* New York, New York: Community Research Associates, 1953.
8. Cameron, N. The paranoid pseudo-community revisited. *Amer. J. Sociol.*, 1959, **65**, 52.
9. Cornelison, A. Casework interviewing as a research technique in a study of families of schizophrenic patients. *Ment. Hyg.*, 1960, **44**, 551–559.
10. Delay, J., Deniker, P., & Green, A. Le milieu familial des schizophrenics. *Encéphale*, 1957, **46**, 189.
11. Erickson, E. The problem of ego identity. *J. Amer. Psychoanalyt. A.*, 1956, **4**, 56.
12. Fisher, S., & Mendell, D. The communication of neurotic patterns over two and three generations. *Psychiatry*, 1956, **19**, 41.
13. Fleck, S., *et al.* The intrafamilial environment of the schizophrenic patient. III. Interaction between hospital staff and families. *Psychiatry*, 1957, **20**, 343.
14. Fleck, S., *et al.* The intrafamilial environment of the schizophrenic patient. V. The understanding of symptomatology through the study of family interaction. Presented at meeting of the American Psychiatric Association, May 15, 1957.
15. Fleck, S., *et al.* The intrafamilial environment of the schizophrenic patient. Incestuous and homosexual problems. In J. H. Masserman (Ed.), *Science and Psychoanalysis: Individual and Familial Dynamics.* New York: Grune, 1959, Vol. II.
16. Flugel, J. C. *Man, Morals and Society: A Psychoanalytic Study.* New York: International Universities Press, 1955.
17. Frazee, H. E. Children who later become schizophrenics. *Smith Coll. Studies in Social Work*, 1953, **23**, 125.
18. Fromm-Reichmann, F. Notes on the mother role in the family group. *Bull. Menninger Clin.*, 1940, **4**, 132.
19. Freud, S. Neurose and Psychose (1924). In *Gesammte Werke.* London: Imago, 1940. Vol. XIII.
20. Gerard, D. L., & Siegel, J. The family background of schizophrenia. *Psychiat. Quart.*, 1950, **24**, 47.
21. Goldberg, E. M. Experiences with families of young men with duodenal ulcer and "normal" control families: Some problems of approach and method. *Brit. J. M. Psychol.*, 1953, **26**, 204.
22. Haley, J. The family of the schizophrenic: A model system. *J. nerv. & ment. Dis.*, 1959, **129**, 357–374.
23. Hill, L. *Psychotherapeutic Interaction in Schizophrenics.* Chicago: University Chicago Press, 1955.
24. Hollingshead, A. B., & Redlich, F. *Social Class and Mental Illness.* New York: Wiley, 1958.
25. Hooker, D. Unpublished address to medical sociology seminar, Yale University, 1958.
26. Jackson, D. D. The question of family homeostasis. *Psychiat. Quart.*, 1957, Suppl. **31**, 79.
27. Jung, G. *The Psychology of Dementia Praecox.* New York: Nerv. & Ment. Dis. Publ. Co., 1936.
28. Kluckhohn, F. *Variants in Value Orientations.* Evanston, Ill.: Row Peterson, 1957.
29. Kraepelin, E. Zur Diagnose und Prognose der Dementia Praecox. *Allg. Ztschr. Psychiatrie*, 1899, **56**, 254.
30. Langworthy, O. R. *Development of Behavior Patterns and Myelinization of the Nervous System in the Human Fetus. Contributions to Embryology No. 124.* Washington, D.C.: Carnegie Institute, 1933.
31. Lidz, R. W., & Lidz, T. The family environment of schizophrenic patients. *Amer. J. Psychiat.*, 1949, **106**, 332.
32. Lidz, R. W., & Lidz, T. Therapeutic considerations arising from the intense symbiotic needs of schizophrenic patients. In G. Brady and F. Redlich (Eds.), *Psychotherapy with Schizophrenics.* New York: International Universities Press, 1952.
33. Lidz, T., *et al.* The intrafamilial environment of the schizophrenic patient. I. The father. *Psychiatry*, 1957, **20**, 329.
34. Lidz, T., *et al.* The intrafamilial environment of the schizophrenic patient. IV. Parental personalities and family interaction. *Amer. J. Orthopsychiat.*, 1958, **28**, 764.
35. Lidz, T., *et al.* The intrafamilial environment of schizophrenic patients. II. Marital schism and marital skew. *Amer. J. Psychiat.*, 1957, **114**, 241.
36. Lidz, T., *et al.* The intrafamilial environment of the schizophrenic patient. VI. The transmission of irrationality. *AMA Arch. Neurol. & Psychiat.*, 1958, **79**, 305.

37. Lidz, T., & Fleck, S. Schizophrenia, human integration and the role of the family. In *The Etiology of Schizophrenia.* New York: Basic Books, 1960. P. 323.
38. Lidz, T., & Fleck, S. Studies in progress.
39. Lidz, T., *et al.* The intrafamilial environment of the schizophrenic patient: VII. The differentiation of personalities and symptoms in identical twins. Unpublished.
40. Mark, J. D. The attitudes of mothers of male schizophrenics towards child behavior. *J. abnorm. soc. Psychol.,* 1953, **48**, 185.
41. Meyer, A. The dynamic interpretation of dementia praecox. *Amer. J. Psychol.,* 1910, **21**, 385.
42. Parson, T. The incest taboo in relation to social structure and the socialization of the child. *Brit. J. Sociology,* 1954, **5**, 101.
43. Parsons, T. Social Structure and the Development of Personality. *Psychiatry,* 1958, **21**, 321.
44. Parsons, T., *et al. Family. Socialization and Interaction.* Glencoe, Ill.: Free Press. 1955.
45. Prout, C. T., & White, M. A. A controlled study of personality relationships in mothers of schizophrenic male patients. *Amer. J. Psychiat,* 1951, **107**, 251.
46. Reichard, S., & Tillman, C. Patterns of parent-child relationships in schizophrenia. *Psychiatry,* 1950, **13**, 247.
47. Sohler, D. T., *et al.* The prediction of family interaction from a battery of projective tests. *J. Proj. Tech.,* 1957, **21**, 199.
48. Spiegel, J. P. The resolution of role conflict with the family. *Psychiatry,* 1957, **20**, 1.
49. Spiegel, J., *et al. Integration and Conflict in Family Behavior. Report 27.* Topeka, Kan., Group for the Advancement of Psychiatry, 1954.
50. Sullivan, H. S. *The Interpersonal Theory of Psychiatry (Part III).* Edited by H. S. Perz and M. L. Gavel, New York: Norton, 1953.
51. Tietze, T. A study of mothers of schizophrenic patients. *Psychiatry,* 1949, **12**, 55.
52. Wahl., C. W. Antecedent factors in family histories of 392 schizophrenics. *Amer. J. Psychiat.,* 1954, **110**, 668.
53. Wynne, L. C., *et al.* Pseudo-mutuality in the family relations of schizophrenics. *Psychiatry,* 1958, **21**, 205.

Suggested Additional Readings

Bandura, A., & Walters, R. H. *Social learning and personality development*. New York: Holt, Rinehart & Winston, 1963.

Eysenck, H. J. (Ed.) *Behavior therapy and the neuroses*. New York: Pergamon Press, 1960.

Frankl, V. E. Dynamics, existence and values. *Journal of Existential Psychology*, 1961, **2**, 5–16.

Fromm, E. Individual and social origins of neurosis. *American Sociological Review*, 1944, **9**, 380–384.

Hall, C. S. & Lindzey, G. *Theories of personality*. (2nd ed.) New York: Wiley, 1968.

Horney, K. Culture and neurosis. *American Sociological Review*, 1936, **1**, 221–230.

Jones, E. (Ed.) *Collected papers of Sigmund Freud*. New York: Basic Books, 1959.

Jung, C. G. On the psychogenesis of schizophrenia. *Journal of Mental Science*, 1939, **85**, 993–1011.

Jackson, D. D. (Ed.) *The etiology of schizophrenia*. New York: Basic Books, 1960.

Lidz, T., Fleck, S., & Cornelison, A. R. *Schizophrenia and the family*. New York: International Universities Press, 1965.

Maslow, A. H. *Motivation and personality*. New York: Harper & Row, 1954.

Mowrer, O. H. *Learning theory and behavior*. New York: Wiley, 1960.

Skinner, B. F. Critique of psychoanalytic concepts and theories. *Scientific Monthly*, 1954, **79**, 300–305.

Ullman, L., & Krasner, L. *Case studies in behavior modification*. New York: Holt, Rinehart & Winston, 1965. Pp. 1–67.

Vetter, H. J., & Smith, B. D. (Eds.) *Personality theory: A source book*. New York: Appleton-Century-Crofts, 1971.

Watson, J. B., & Rayner, R. Conditioned emotional reaction. *Journal of Experimental Psychology*, 1920, **3**, 1–4.

Sociological Factors

9

Social Stratification and Psychiatric Disorders*

AUGUST B. HOLLINGSHEAD and FREDERICK C. REDLICH†

The research reported here grew out of the work of a number of men, who, during the last half century, have demonstrated that the social environment in which individuals live is connected in some way, as yet not fully explained, to the development of mental illness.[1] Medical men have approached this problem largely from the viewpoint of epidemiology.[2] Sociologists, on the other hand, have analyzed the question in terms of ecology,[3] and of social disorganization.[4] Neither psychiatrists nor sociologists have carried on extensive research into the specific question we are concerned with, namely, interrelations between the class structure and the development of mental illness. However, a few sociologists and psychiatrists have written speculative and research papers in this area.[5]

---

*From Hollingshead, A. B., and Redlich, F. C., *American Sociological Review*, 1953, **18**, 163–169. Copyright © 1953 by the American Sociological Association. Reprinted by permission of the American Sociological Association, and Dr. Hollingshead.

†Paper read at the annual meeting of the American Sociological Society, September 3–5, 1952. The research reported here is supported by a grant from the National Institute of Mental Health of the United States Public Health Service to Yale University under the direction of Dr. F. C. Redlich, Chairman, Department of Psychiatry, and Professor August B. Hollingshead, Department of Sociology.

[1]For example, see, A. J. Rosanoff, *Report of a Survey of Mental Disorders in Nassau County, New York*, New York: National Committee for Mental Hygiene, 1916; Ludwig Stern, *Kulturkreis und Form der Geistigen Erkrankung*, (Sammlung zwangloser Abhandlungen aus dem Gebiete der Nerven-und-Geisteskrankheiten), X, No. 2, Halle a. S:C. Marhold, 1913, pp. 1–62; J. F. Sutherland, "Geographical Distribution of Lunacy in Scotland," *British Association for Advancement of Science*, Glasgow, Sept. 1901; William A. White, "Geographical Distribution of Insanity in the United States," *Journal of Nervous and Mental Disease*, XXX (1903), pp. 257–279.

[2]For example, see: Trygve Braatoy, "Is it Probable that the Sociological Situation is a Factor in Schizophrenia?" *Psychiatrica et Neurologica*, XII (1937), pp. 109–138; Donald L. Gerard and Joseph Siegel, "The Family Background of Schizophrenia," *The Psychiatric Quarterly*, 24 (January, 1950), pp. 47–73; Robert W. Hyde and Lowell V. Kingsley, "Studies in Medical Sociology, I: The Relation of Mental Disorders to the Community Socio-economic Level," *The New England Journal of Medicine*, 231, No. 16 (October 19, 1944), pp. 543–548; Robert W. Hyde Lowell V. Kingsley, "Studies in Medical Sociology, II: The Relation of Mental Disorders to Population Density," *The New England Journal of Medicine*, 231, No. 17 (October 26, 1944), pp. 571–577; Robert M. Hyde and Roderick M. Chisholm, "Studies in Medical Sociology, III: The Relation of Mental Disorders to Race and Nationality," *The New England Journal of Medicine*, 231, No. 18 (November 2, 1944), pp. 612–618; William Malamud and Irene Malamud, "A Socio-Psychiatric Investigation of Schizophrenia Occurring in the Armed Forces," *Psychosomatic Medicine*, 5 (October, 1943), pp. 364–375; B. Malzberg, *Social and Biological Aspects of Mental Disease*, Utica N.Y.: State Hospital Press, 1940; William F. Roth and Frank H. Luton, "The Mental Health Program in Tennessee: Statistical Report of a Psychiatric Survey in a Rural County," *American Journal of Psychiatry*, 99 (March, 1943), pp. 662–675; J. Ruesch and Others, *Chronic Disease and Psychological Invalidism*, New York: American Society for Research in Psychosomatic Problems, 1946; J. Ruesch and others, *Duodenal Ulcer: A Socio-psychological Study*

The present research, therefore, was designed to discover whether a relationship does or does not exist between the class system of our society and mental illnesses. Five general hypotheses were formulated in our research plan to test some dimension of an assumed relationship between the two. These hypotheses were stated positively; they could just as easily have been expressed either negatively or conditionally. They were phrased as follows:

I. The *expectancy* of a psychiatric disorder is related significantly to an individual's position in the class structure of his society.
II. The *types* of psychiatric disorders are connected significantly to the class structure.
III. The type of *psychiatric treatment* administered is associated with patient's positions in the class structure.
IV. The *psycho-dynamics* of psychiatric disorders are correlative to an individual's position in the class structure.
V. *Mobility* in the class structure is neurotogenic.

Each hypothesis is linked to the others, and all are subsumed under the theoretical assumption of a functional relationship between stratification in society and the prevalence of particular types of mental disorders among given social classes or strata in a specified population. Although our research was planned around these hypotheses, we have been forced by the nature of the problem of mental illness to study *diagnosed* prevalence of psychiatric disorders, rather than *true* or *total* prevalence.

---

of Naval Enlisted Personnel and Civilians, Berkeley and Los Angeles: University of California Press, 1948; Jurgen Ruesch, Annemarie Jacobson, and Martin B. Loeb, "Acculturation and Illness," *Psychological Monographs: General and Applied*, Vol. 62, No. 5, Whole No. 292, 1948 (American Psychological Association, 1515 Massachusetts Ave., N.W., Washington 5, D.C.); C. Tietze, Paul Lemkau and M. Cooper, "A Survey of Statistical Studies on the Prevalence and Incidence of Mental Disorders in Sample Populations," *Public Health Reports*, 1909–27, 58 (December 31, 1943); C. Tietze, P. Lemkau and Marcia Cooper, "Schizophrenia, Manic Depressive Psychosis and Social-Economic Status," *American Journal of Sociology*, XLVII (September, 1941), pp. 167–175.

[3]Robert E. L. Faris, and H. Warren Dunham, *Mental Disorders in Urban Areas*, Chicago: University of Chicago Press, 1939; H. Warren Dunham, "Current Status of Ecological Research in Mental Disorder," *Social Forces*, 25 (March, 1947), pp. 321–326; R. H. Felix and R. V. Bowers, "Mental Hygiene and Socio-Environmental Factors," *The Milbank Memorial Fund Quarterly*, XXVI (April, 1948), pp. 125–147; H. W. Green, *Persons Admitted to the Cleveland State Hospital, 1928–1937*, Cleveland Health Council, 1939.

[4]R. E. L. Faris, "Cultural Isolation and the Schizophrenic Personality," *American Journal of Sociology*, XXXIX (September, 1934), pp. 155–169; R. E. L. Faris, "Reflections of Social Disorganization in the Behavior of a Schizophrenic Patient," *American Journal of Sociology*, L (September, 1944), pp. 134–141.

[5]For example, see: Robert E. Clark, "Psychoses, Income, and Occupational Prestige," *American Journal of Sociology*, 44 (March, 1949), pp. 433–440; Robert E. Clark, "The Relationship of Schizophrenia to Occupational Income and Occupational Prestige," *American Sociological Review*, 13 (June, 1948), pp. 325–330; Kingsley Davis, "Mental Hygiene and the Class Structure," *Psychiatry*, I (February, 1938), pp. 55–56; Talcott Parsons, "Psychoanalysis and the Social Structure," *The Psychoanalytical Quarterly*, XIX, No. 3 (1950), pp. 371–384; John Dollard and Neal Miller, *Personality and Psychotherapy*, New York: McGraw-Hill, 1950; Jurgen Ruesch, "Social Technique, Social Status, and Social Change in Illness," Clyde Kluckholn and Henry A. Murray (editors), in *Personality in Nature, Society, and Culture*, New York: Alfred A. Knopf, 1949, pp. 117–130; W. L. Warner, "The Society, the Individual and his Mental Disorders," *American Journal of Psychiatry*, 94, No. 2 (September, 1937), pp. 275–284.

METHODOLOGICAL PROCEDURE

The research is being done by a team of four psychiatrists,[6] two sociologists,[7] and a clinical psychologist.[8] The data are being assembled in the New Haven urban community, which consists of the city of New Haven and surrounding towns of East Haven, North Haven, West Haven, and Hamden. This community had a population of some 250,000 persons in 1950.[9] The New Haven community was selected because the community's structure has been studied intensively by sociologists over a long period. In addition, it is served by a private psychiatric hospital, three psychiatric clinics, and 27 practicing psychiatrists, as well as the state and Veterans Administration facilities.

Four basic technical operations had to be completed before the hypotheses could be tested. These were: the delineation of the class structure of the community, selection of a cross-sectional control of the community's population, the determination of who was receiving psychiatric care, and the stratification of both the control sample and the psychiatric patients.

August B. Hollingshead and Jerome K. Myers took over the task of delineating the class system. Fortunately, Maurice R. Davie and his students had studied the social structure of the New Haven community in great detail over a long time span.[10] Thus, we had a large body of data we could draw upon to aid us in blocking out the community's social structure.

The community's social structure is differentiated *vertically* along racial, ethnic, and religious lines; each of these vertical cleavages, in turn, is differentiated *horizontally* by a series of strata or classes. Around the socio-biological axis of race two social worlds have evolved: A Negro world and a white world. The white world is divided by ethnic origin and religion into Catholic, Protestant, and Jewish contingents. Within these divisions there are numerous ethnic groups. The Irish hold aloof from the Italians, and the Italians move in different circles from the Poles. The Jews maintain a religious and social life separate from the gentiles. The *horizontal* strata that transect each of these vertical divisions are based upon the social values that are attached to occupation, education, place of residence in the community, and associations.

The vertically differentiating factors of race, religion and ethnic origin, when combined with the horizontally differentiating ones of occupation, education, place of residence and so on, produce a social structure that is highly compartmentalized. The integrating factors in this complex are twofold. First, each stratum of each vertical division is similar in its cultural characteristics to the corresponding stratum in the other divisions. Second, the cultural pattern for each stratum or class was set by the "Old Yankee" core group. This core group provided the master cultural mold that has shaped the status system of each

---

[6]F. C. Redlich, B. H. Roberts, L. Z. Freedman, and Leslie Schaffer.

[7]August B. Hollingshead and J. K. Myers.

[8]Harvey A. Robinson.

[9]The population of each component was as follows: New Haven, 164,443; East Haven, 12,212; North Haven, 9,444; West Haven, 32,010; Hamden, 29,715; and Woodbridge, 2,822.

[10]Maurice R. Davie, "The Pattern of Urban Growth," G. P. Murdock (editor), in *Studies in the Science of Society*, New Haven: 1937, pp. 133–162; Ruby J. R. Kennedy, "Single or Triple Melting-Pot: Intermarriage Trends in New Haven, 1870–1940," *American Journal of Sociology*, 39 (January, 1944), pp. 331–339; John W. McConnell, *The Influence of Occupation Upon Social Stratification*, Unpublished Ph.D. thesis, Sterling Memorial Library, Yale University, 1937; Jerome K. Myers, "Assimilation to the Ecological and Social Systems of a Community," *American Sociological Review*, 15 (June, 1950), pp. 367–372; Mhyra Minnis, "The Relationship of Women's Organizations to the Social Structure of a City," Unpublished Ph.D. thesis, Sterling Memorial Library, Yale University, 1951.

sub-group in the community. In short, the social structure of the New Haven community is a parallel class structure within the limits of race ethnic origin, and religion.

This fact enabled us to stratify the community, for our purposes, with an *Index of Social Position*.[11] This *Index* utilizes three scaled factors to determine an individual's class position within the community's stratificational system: ecological area of residence, occupation, and education. Ecological area of residence is measured by a six point scale; occupation and education are each measured by a seven point scale. To obtain a social class score on an individual we must therefore know his address, his occupation, and the number of years of school he has completed. Each of these factors is given a scale score, and the scale score is multiplied by a factor weight determined by a standard regression equation. The factor weights are as follows: Ecological area of residence, 5; occupation, 8; and education, 6. The three factor scores are summed, and the resultant score is taken as an index of this individual's position in the community's social class system.

This *Index* enabled us to delineate five main social class strata within the horizontal dimension of the social structure. These principal strata or classes may be characterized as follows:

Class I.   This stratum is composed of wealthy families whose wealth is often inherited and whose heads are leaders in the community's business and professional pursuits. Its members live in those areas of the community generally regarded as "the best;" the adults are college graduates, usually from famous private institutions, and almost all gentile families are listed in the New Haven *Social Directory*, but few Jewish families are listed. In brief, these people occupy positions of high social prestige.

Class II.   Adults in this stratum are almost all college graduates; the males occupy high managerial positions, many are engaged in the lesser ranking professions. These families are well-to-do, but there is no substantial inherited or acquired wealth. Its members live in the "better" residential areas; about one-half of these families belong to lesser ranking private clubs, but only 5 per cent of Class II families are listed in the New Haven *Social Directory*.

Class III.   This stratum includes the vast majority of small proprietors, white-collar office and sales workers, and a considerable number of skilled manual workers. Adults are predominately high school graduates, but a considerable percentage have attended business schools and small colleges for a year or two. They live in "good" residential areas; less than 5 per cent belong to private clubs, but they are not included in the *Social Directory*. Their social life tends to be concentrated in the family, the church, and the lodge.

Class IV.   This stratum consists predominately of semi-skilled factory workers. Its adult members have finished the elementary grades, but the older people have not completed high school. However, adults under thirty-five have generally graduated from high school. Its members comprise almost one-half of the community; and their residences are scattered over wide areas. Social life is centered in the family, the neighborhood, the labor union, and public places.

Class V.   Occupationally, class V adults are overwhelmingly semi-skilled factory hands and unskilled laborers. Educationally most adults have not completed the elementary grades. The families are concentrated in the "tenement" and "cold-water flat" areas of New Haven. Only a small minority belong to organized community institutions. Their social life takes place in the family flat, on the street, or in neighborhood social agencies.

The second major technical operation in this research was the enumeration of psychiatric patients. A Psychiatric Census was taken to discover the number and kinds of

---

[11]A detailed statement of the procedures used to develop and validate this *Index* will be described in a forthcoming monograph on this research tentatively titled *Psychiatry and Social Class* by August B. Hollingshead and Fredrick C. Redlich.

psychiatric patients in the community. Enumeration was limited to residents of the community who were patients of a psychiatrist or a psychiatric clinic, or were in a psychiatric institution on December 1, 1950. To make reasonably certain that all patients were included in the enumeration, the research team gathered data from all public and private psychiatric institutions and clinics in Connecticut and nearby states, and all private practitioners in Connecticut and the metropolitan New York area. It received the cooperation of all clinics and institutions, and of all practitioners except a small number in New York City. It can be reasonably assumed that we have data comprising at least 98 per cent of all individuals who were receiving psychiatric care on December 1, 1950.

Forty-four pertinent items of information were gathered on each patient and placed on a schedule. The psychiatrists gathered material regarding symptomatology and diagnosis, onset of illness and duration, referral to the practitioner and the institution, and the nature and intensity of treatment. The sociologists obtained information on age, sex, occupation, education, religion, race and ethnicity, family history, marital experiences, and so on.

The third technical research operation was the selection of a control sample from the normal population of the community. The sociologists drew a 5 per cent random sample of households in the community from the 1951, New Haven *City Directory*. This directory covers the entire communal area. The names and addresses in it were compiled in October and November, 1950—a period very close to the date of the Psychiatric Census. Therefore there was comparability of residence and date of registry between the two population groups. Each household drawn in the sample was interviewed, and data on the age, sex, occupation, education, religion, and income of family members, as well as other items necessary for our purposes were placed on a schedule. This sample is our Control Population.

Our fourth basic operation was the stratification of the psychiatric patients and of the control population with the *Index of Social Position.* As soon as these tasks were completed, the schedules from the Psychiatric Census and the 5 per cent Control Sample were edited and coded, and their data were placed on Hollerith cards. The analysis of these data is in process.

SELECTED FINDINGS

Before we discuss our findings relative to Hypothesis I, we want to reemphasize that our study is concerned with *diagnosed* or *treated* prevalence rather than *true* or *total* prevalence. Our Psychiatric Census included only psychiatric cases under treatment, diagnostic study, or care. It did not include individuals with psychiatric disorders who were not being treated on December 1, 1950, by a psychiatrist. There are undoubtedly many individuals in the community with psychiatric problems who escaped our net. If we had *true* prevalence figures, many findings from our present study would be more meaningful, perhaps some of our interpretations would be changed, but at present we must limit ourselves to the data we have.

Hypothesis I, as revised by the nature of the problem, stated: *The diagnosed prevalence of psychiatric disorders is related significantly to an individual's position* in the class structure. A test of this hypothesis involves a comparison of the normal population with the psychiatric population If no significant difference between the distribution of the normal population and the psychiatric patient population by social class is found, Hypothesis I may be abandoned as unproved. However, if a significant difference is found between the two populations by class, Hypothesis I should be entertained until more conclusive data are assembled. Pertinent data for a limited test of Hypothesis I are presented in Table 9-1. The data included show the number of individuals in the normal population and the psychiatric population, by class level. What we are concerned with in this test is how these two populations are distributed by class.

Table 9-1 Distribution of Normal and Psychiatric Population by Social Class.

Social Class	Normal Population*		Psychiatric Population	
	Number	Per cent	Number	Per cent
I	358	3.1	19	1.0
II	926	8.1	131	6.7
III	2500	22.0	260	13.2
IV	5256	46.0	758	38.6
V	2037	17.8	723	36.8
Unknown†	345	3.0	72	3.7
Total	11,422	100.0	1,963	100.0

Chi square = 408.16, P less than 0.001.
*These figures are preliminary. They do not include Yale students, transients, institutionalized persons, and refusals.
†The unknown cases were not used in the calculation of chi square. They are individuals drawn in the sample, and psychiatric cases whose class level could not be determined because of paucity of data.

When we tested the reliability of these population distributions by the use of the chi square method, we found a *very significant* relation between social class and treated prevalence of psychiatric disorders in the New Haven community. A comparison of the percentage distribution of each population by class readily indicates the direction of the class concentration of psychiatric cases. For example, Class I contains 3.1 per cent of the community's population but only 1.0 per cent of the psychiatric cases. Class V, on the other hand, includes 17.8 per cent of the community's population, but contributed 36.8 per cent of the psychiatric patients. On the basis of our data Hypothesis I clearly should be accepted as tenable.

Hypothesis II postulated a significant connection between the *type* of psychiatric disorder and social class. This hypothesis involves a test of the idea that there may be a functional relationship between an individual's position in the class system and the type of psychiatric disorder that he may present. This hypothesis depends, in part, on the question of diagnosis. Our psychiatrists based their diagnoses on the classificatory system developed by the Veterans Administration.[12] For the purposes of this paper, all cases are

---

[12]*Psychiatric Disorders and Reactions*, Washington: Veterans Administration, Technical Bulletin 10A-78, October, 1947.

grouped into two categories: the neuroses and the psychoses. The results of this grouping by social class are given in Table 9-2.

Table 9-2   Distribution of Neuroses and Psychoses by Social Class.

Social Class	Neuroses		Psychoses	
	Number	Per cent	Number	Per cent
I	10	52.6	9	47.4
II	88	67.2	43	32.8
III	115	44.2	145	55.8
IV	175	23.1	583	76.9
V	61	8.4	662	91.6
Total	449		1,442	

Chi square = 296.45, P less than 0.001.

A study of Table 9-2 will show that the neuroses are concentrated at the higher levels and the psychoses at the lower end of the class structure. Our team advanced a number of theories to explain the sharp differences between the neuroses and psychoses by social class. One suggestion was that the low percentage of neurotics in the lower classes was a direct reaction to the cost of psychiatric treatment. But as we accumulated a series of case studies, for tests of Hypotheses IV and V, we became skeptical of this simple interpretation. Our detailed case records indicate that the social distance between psychiatrist and patient may be more potent than economic considerations in determining the character of psychiatric intervention. This question therefore requires further research.

The high concentration of psychotics in the lower strata is probably the product of a very unequal distribution of psychotics in the total population. To test this idea, Hollingshead selected schizophrenics for special study. Because of the severity of this disease it is probable that very few schizophrenics fail to receive some kind of psychiatric care. This diagnostic group comprises 44.2 per cent of all patients, and 58.7 per cent of the psychotics, in our study. Ninety-seven and six-tenths per cent of these schizophrenic patients had been hospitalized at one time or another, and 94 per cent were hospitalized at the time of our census. When we classify these patients by social class we find that there is a very significant inverse relationship between social class and schizophrenia.

Hollingshead decided to determine, on the basis of these data, what the probability of the prevalence of schizophrenia by social class might be in the general population. To do this he used a proportional index to learn whether or not there were differentials in the distribution of the general population, as represented in our control sample, and the distribution of schizophrenics by social class. If a social class exhibits the same proportion of schizophrenia as it comprises of the general population, the index for that class is 100. If schizophrenia is disproportionately prevalent in a social class the index is above 100; if schizophrenia is disproportionately low in a social class the index is below 100. The index for each social class appears in the last column of Table 9-3.

The fact that the Index of Prevalence in class I is only one-fifth as great as it would be if schizophrenia were proportionately distributed in this class, and that it is two and one-half

Table 9-3   Comparison of the Distribution of the Normal Population with Schizophrenics by Class, with Index of Probable Prevalence.

Social Class	Normal Population		Schizophrenics		Index of Prevalence
	No.	Per cent	No.	Per cent	
I	358	3.2	6	0.7	22
II	926	8.4	23	2.7	33
III	2,500	22.6	83	9.8	43
IV	5,256	47.4	352	41.6	88
V	2,037	18.4	383	45.2	246
Total	11,077	100.0	847	100.0	

times as high in class V as we might expect on the basis of proportional distribution, gives further support to Hypothesis II. The fact that the Index of Prevalence is 11.2 times as great in class V as in class I is particularly impressive.

Hypothesis III stipulated that the type of psychiatric treatment a patient receives is associated with his position in the class structure. A test of this hypothesis involves a comparison of the different types of therapy being used by psychiatrists on patients in the different social classes. We encountered many forms of therapy but they may be grouped under three main types; psychotherapy, organic therapy, and custodial care. The patient population, from the viewpoint of the principal type of therapy received, was divided roughly into three categories: 32.0 per cent received some type of psychotherapy; 31.7 per cent received organic treatments of one kind or another; and 36.3 per cent received custodial care without treatment. The percentage of persons who received no treatment care was greatest in the lower classes. The same finding applies to organic treatment. Psychotherapy, on the other hand, was concentrated in the higher classes. Within the psychotherapy category there were sharp differences between the types of psychotherapy administered to the several classes. For example, psychoanalysis was limited to classes I and II. Patients in class V who received any psychotherapy were treated by group methods in the state hospitals. The number and percentage of patients who received each type of therapy is given in Table 9-4. The data clearly support Hypothesis III.

At the moment we do not have data available for a test of Hypotheses IV and V. These will be put to a test as soon as we complete work on a series of cases now under close study. Preliminary materials give us the impression that they too will be confirmed.

Table 9-4   Distribution of the Principal Types of Therapy by Social Class.

Social Class	Psychotherapy		Organic Therapy		No Treatment	
	Number	Per cent	Number	Per cent	Number	Per cent
I	14	73.7	2	10.5	3	15.8
II	107	81.7	15	11.4	9	6.9
III	136	52.7	74	28.7	48	18.6
IV	237	31.1	288	37.1	242	31.8
V	115	16.1	234	32.7	367	51.2

Chi square = 336.58, P less than 0.001.

CONCLUSIONS AND INTERPRETATIONS

This study was designed to throw new light upon the question of how mental illness is related to social environment. It approached this problem from the perspective of social class to determine if an individual's position in the social system was associated significantly with the development of psychiatric disorders. It proceeded on the theoretical assumption that if mental illnesses were distributed randomly in the population, the hypotheses designed to test the idea that psychiatric disorders are connected in some functional way to the class system would not be found to be statistically significant.

The data we have assembled demonstrate conclusively that mental illness, as measured by diagnosed prevalence, is not distributed randomly in the population of the New Haven community. On the contrary, psychiatric difficulties of so serious a nature that they reach the attention of a psychiatrist are unequally distributed among the five social classes. In addition, types of psychiatric disorders, and the ways patients are treated, are strongly associated with social class position.

The statistical tests of our hypotheses indicate that there are definite connections between particular types of social environments in which people live, as measured by the social class concept, and the emergence of particular kinds of psychiatric disorders, as measured by psychiatric diagnosis. They do not tell us what these connections are, nor how they are functionally related to a particular type of mental illness in a given individual. The next step, we believe, is to turn from the strictly statistical approach to an intensive study of the social environments associated with particular social classes, on the one hand, and of individuals in these environments who do or do not develop mental illnesses, on the other hand. Currently the research team is engaged in this next step but is not yet ready to make a formal report of its findings.

REFERENCES

Braatoy, T. Is it probable that the sociological situation is a factor in schizophrenia? *Psychiatrica et Neurologica*, 1937, **12**, 109–138.

Clark, R. E. The relationship of schizophrenia to occupational income and occupational prestige. *Amer. Sociol. Rev.*, 1948, **13**, 325–330.

Clark, R.E. Psychoses, income, and occupational prestige. *Amer. J. Sociol.*, 1949, **44**, 433–440.

Davie, M. R. The pattern of urban growth. In G. P. Murdock (Ed.), *Studies in the science of society.* New Haven, 1937. Pp. 133–162.

Davis, K. Mental hygiene and the class structure. *Psychiatry*, 1938, **1**, 55–56.

Dollard, J., & Miller, N. *Personality and psychotherapy.* New York: McGraw-Hill, 1950.

Dunham, H. W. Current status of ecological research in mental disorder. *Social Forces*, 1947, **25**, 321–326.

Faris, R. E. L. Cultural isolation and the schizophrenic personality. *Amer. J. Sociol.*, 1934, **39**, 155–169.

Faris, R. E. L. Reflections of social disorganization in the behavior of a schizophrenic patient. *Amer. J. Sociol.*, 1944, **50**, 134–141.

Faris, R. E. L., & Dunham, H. W. Mental disorders in urban areas. Chicago: University of Chicago Press, 1939.

Felix, R. H., & Bowers, R. V. Mental hygiene and socio-environmental factors. *The Milbank Memorial Fund Quarterly*, 1948, **26**, 125–147.

Gerard, D. L., & Siegel, J. The family background of schizophrenia. *Psychiat. Quart.*, 1950, **24**, 47–73.

Green, H. W. Persons admitted to the Cleveland State Hospital, 1928–1937. Cleveland Health Council, 1939.

Hyde, R. W., & Kingsley, L. V. Studies in medical sociology. I. The relation of mental disorders to the community socio-economic level. *New Eng. J. Med.*, 1944, **231**(16), 543–548. (a)

Hyde, R. W., & Kingsley, L. V. Studies in medical sociology. II. The relation of mental disorders to population density. *New Eng. J. Med.*, 1944, **231**(17), 571–577. (b)

Hyde, R.W., & Chisholm, R. M. Studies in medical sociology. III. The relation of mental disorders to race and nationality. *New Eng. J. Med.*, 1944, **231**(18), 612–618.

Kennedy, R. J. R. Single or triple melting-pot: Intermarriage trends in New Haven, 1870–1940. *Amer. J. Sociol.*, 1944, **39**, 331–339.

Malamud, W., & Malamud, I. A socio-psychiatric investigation of schizophrenia occurring in the armed forces. *Psychosom. Med.*, 1943, **5**, 364–375.

Malzberg, B. *Social and biological aspects of mental disease.* Utica, N.Y.: State Hospital Press, 1940.

McConnell, J. W. The influence of occupation upon social stratification. Unpublished doctoral thesis, Sterling Memorial Library, Yale University, 1937.

Minnis, M. The relationship of women's organizations to the social structure of a city. Unpublished doctoral thesis, Sterling Memorial Library, Yale University, 1951.

Myers, J. K. Assimilation to the ecological and social systems of a community. *Amer. Sociol. Rev.*, 1950, **15**, 367–372.

Parsons, T. Psychoanalysis and the social structure. *Psychoanalytical Quarterly*, 1950, **19**(3), 371–384.

Psychiatric disorders and reactions. (Tech. Bull. No. 10A-78) Washington, D. C.: Veterans Administration, 1947.

Rosanoff, A. J. *Report of a survey of mental disorders in Nassau County, New York.* New York: National Committee for Mental Hygiene, 1916.

Roth, W. F., & Luton, F. H. The mental health program in Tennessee: Statistical report of a psychiatric survey in a rural county. *Amer. J. Psychiat.*, 1943, **99**, 662–675.

Ruesch, J. Social technique, social status, and social change in illness. In C. Kluckhohn & H. A. Murray (Eds.), *Personality in nature, society, and culture.* New York: Knopf, 1949. Pp. 117–130.

Ruesch, J., *et al.* Chronic disease and psychological invalidism. New York: American Society for Research in Psychosomatic Problems, 1946.

Ruesch, J., *et al. Duodenal ulcer: A socio-psychological study of Naval enlisted personnel and civilians.* Berkeley and Los Angeles: University of California Press, 1948.

Ruesch, J., Jacobson, A., & Loeb, M. B. Acculturation and illness. *Psychological Monographs: General and Applied*, 1948, **62**(5, Whole No. 292).

Stern, L. *Kulturkreis und Form der Geistigen Erkrankung* (Sammlung zwangloser Abhandlungen aus dem Gebiete der Nerven-und-Geisteskrankheiten). Vol. X, No. 2. Halle. C. Marhold, 1913. Pp. 1–62.

Sutherland, J. F. Geographical distribution of lunacy in Scotland. *British Association for Advancement of Science*, September, 1901.

Tietze, C., Lemkau, P., & Cooper, M. Schizophrenia, manic depressive psychosis and social-economic status. *Amer. J. Sociol.*, 1941, **47**, 167–175.

Tietze, C., Lemkau, P., & Cooper, M. A survey of statistical studies on the prevalence and incidence of mental disorders in sample populations. *Public Health Reports*, 1909–27, **58**, December 31, 1943.

Warner, W. L. The society, the individual and his mental disorders. *Amer. J. Psychiat.*, 1937, **94**, 275–284.

White, W. A. Geographical distribution of insanity in the United States. *J. nerv. & ment. Dis.*, 1903, **30**, 257–279.

10

Social Class and Schizophrenia:
A Critical Review*

MELVIN L. KOHN

My intent in this paper is to review a rather large and all-too-inexact body of research on the relationship of social class to schizophrenia, to see what it adds up to and what implications it has for etiology.[1] Instead of reviewing the studies one by one, I shall talk to general issues and bring in whatever studies are most relevant. It hardly need be stressed that my way of selecting these issues and my evaluation of the studies represent only one person's view of the field and would not necessarily be agreed to by others.

Before I get to the main issues, I should like to make five prefatory comments:

1. When I speak of schizophrenia, I shall generally be using that term in the broad sense in which it is usually employed in the United States, rather than the more limited sense used in much of Europe. I follow American rather than European usage, not because I think it superior, but because it is the usage that has been employed in so much of the relevant research. Any comparative discussion must necessarily employ the more inclusive, even if the cruder, term.

2. I shall generally not be able to distinguish among various types of schizophrenia, for the data rarely enable one to do so. This is most unfortunate; one should certainly want to consider "process" and "reactive" types of disturbance separately, to distinguish between paranoid and non-paranoid, and to take account of several other possibly critical distinctions.

Worse yet, I shall at times have to rely on data about an even broader and vaguer category than schizophrenia—severe mental illness in general, excluding only the demonstrably organic. The excuse for this is that since the epidemiological findings for severe mental illness seem to parallel those for schizophrenia alone, it would be a shame to ignore

---

*Reprinted with permission from *The transmission of schizophrenia*, edited by D. Rosenthal and S. S. Kety (1968), Pergamon Press, Ltd., and Dr. Kohn.

[1]The *raison d'etre* of this review, aside from its being momentarily current, is in its effort to organize the evidence around certain central issues and to make use of all studies relevant to those issues. There are no definitive studies in this field, but most of them contribute something to our knowledge when placed in perspective of all the others. For an alternative approach, deliberately limited to those few studies that meet the reviewers' standards of adequacy, see Mishler (1963). Dunham has recently argued for a more radical alternative; he disputes the legitimacy of using epidemiological data to make the types of social psychological inference I attempt here and insists that epidemiological studies are relevant only to the study of how social systems function. This seems to me to be altogether arbitrary. But see Dunham (1965, 1966). Some other useful reviews and discussions of issues in this field are: Dunham (1947); Felix & Bowers (1948); Dunham (1948); Clausen (1956, 1957, 1959); Hollingshead (1961); Dunham (1963); and Sanua (1963). This present review leans heavily on my earlier paper (Kohn, 1966), but is more complete in its coverage and represents—for all its similarities to the earlier paper—a thorough re-assessment of the field.

the several important studies that have been addressed to the larger category. I shall, however, rely on these studies as sparingly as possible and stress studies that focus on schizophrenia.

3. Social classes will be defined as aggregates of individuals who occupy broadly similar positions in the hierarchy of power, privilege and prestige (Williams, 1951, p. 89). In dealing with the research literature, I shall treat occupational position (or occupational position as weighted somewhat by education) as a serviceable index of social class for urban society. I shall not make any distinction, since the data hardly permit my doing so, between the concepts "social class" and "socio-economic status." And I shall not hesitate to rely on less than fully adequate indices of class when relevant investigations have employed them.

4. I want to mention only in passing the broadly comparitive studies designed to examine the idea that mental disorder in general, and schizophrenia in particular, are products of civilization, or of urban life, or of highly complex social structure. There have been a number of important studies of presumably less complex societies that all seem to indicate that the magnitude of mental disorder in these societies is of roughly the same order as that in highly urbanized, Western societies....

These data are hardly precise enough to be definitive, but they lead one to turn his attention away from the general hypothesis that there are sizeable differences in rates of mental disorder between simpler and more complex social structures, to look instead at differences within particular social structures, where the evidence is far more intriguing. I do not argue that there are no differences in rates of schizophrenia among societies, only that the data in hand are not sufficient to demonstrate them.[2] We have more abundant data on intra-societal variations.

5. One final prefatory note. Much of what I shall do in this paper will be to raise doubts and come to highly tentative conclusions from inadequate evidence. This is worth doing because we know so little and the problem is so pressing. Genetics does not seem to provide a sufficient explanation,[3] and ... biochemical and physiological hypotheses have thus far failed to stand the test of careful experimentation (Kety, 1960). Of all the social variables that have been studied, those related to social class have yielded the most provocative results. Thus, inadequate as the following data are, they must be taken seriously.

It must be emphasized, however, that there are exceedingly difficult problems in interpreting the data that I am about to review. The indices are suspect, the direction of causality is debatable, the possibility that one or another alternative interpretation makes more sense than the one I should like to draw is very real indeed. These problems will all be taken up shortly; first, though, I should like to lay out the positive evidence for a meaningful relationship between class and schizophrenia.

EVIDENCE ON THE POSSIBLE RELATIONSHIP OF SOCIAL CLASS TO RATES OF SCHIZOPHRENIA

Most of the important epidemiological studies of schizophrenia can be viewed as attempts to resolve problems of interpretation posed by the pioneer studies, Faris and

---

[2]For further documentation of this point, see also Mishler & Scotch (1963); Dunham (1965); and Demerath (1955).

[3]Some of the principal recent studies that bear on this point are: Rosenthal (1962); Tienari (1963); and Kringlen (1964a, 1964b, 1966).

Dunham's (1939) ecological study of rates of schizophrenia for the various areas of Chicago and Clark's (1949) study of rates of schizophrenia at various occupational levels in that same city. Their findings were essentially as follows:

Faris and Dunham   The highest rates of first hospital admission for schizophrenia are in the central city areas of lowest socio-economic status, with diminishing rates as one moves toward higher-status peripheral areas.[4]

Clark   The highest rates of schizophrenia are for the lowest status occupations, with diminishing rates as one goes to higher status occupations.

The concentration of high rates of mental disorder, particularly of schizophrenia, in the central city areas[5] of lowest socio-economic status has been confirmed in a number of American cities—Providence, Rhode Island (Faris & Dunham, 1939); Peoria, Illinois (Schroeder, 1942); Kansas City, Missouri (Schroeder, 1942); St. Louis, Missouri (Dee, 1939; Schroeder, 1942; Queen, 1940); Milwaukee, Wisconsin (Schroeder, 1942); Omaha, Nebraska (Schroeder, 1942); Worcester, Massachusetts (Gerard & Houston, 1953); Rochester, New York (Gardner & Babigian, 1966); and Baltimore, Maryland (Klee, Spiro, Bahn, & Gorwitz, 1967). The two ecological studies done in European cities—Sundby and Nyhus's (1963) study of Oslo, Norway and Hare's (1956a) of Bristol, England—are in substantial agreement, too.

The concentration of high rates of mental disorder, particularly of schizophrenia, in the lowest status occupations has been confirmed again and again. The studies conducted by Hollingshead and Redlich (1957) in New Haven, Connecticut, and by Srole and his associates in midtown, New York City (Srole, Langer, Michael, Opler, & Rennie, 1962), are well-known examples; a multitude of other investigations in the United States have come to the same conclusion.[6] Moreover, Svalastoga's (1965, pp. 100–101) re-analysis of Strömgren's data for northern Denmark is consistent, as are the Leightons' data for "Stirling County," Nova Scotia (Leighton, Harding, Macklin, MacMillan, & Leighton, 1963, pp. 279–294), Ødegaard's (1957) for Norway, Brooke's for England and Wales (as reported in Morris, 1959), Stein's (1957) for two sections of London, Lin's (1953, 1966) for Taiwan, and Stenbäck and Achté's (1966) for Helsinki.

But there are some exceptions. Clausen and I happened across the first, when we discovered that for Hagerstown, Maryland, there was no discernible relationship between

---

[4]The pattern is most marked for paranoid schizophrenia, least so for catatonic, which tends to concentrate in the foreign-born slum communities (Faris & Dunham, 1939, pp. 82–108). Unfortunately, subsequent studies in smaller cities dealt with too few cases to examine the distribution of separable types of schizophrenia as carefully as did Faris & Dunham.

[5]There are some especially difficult problems in interpreting the ecological findings, which I shall not discuss here because most of the later and crucial evidence comes from other modes of research. The problems inherent in interpreting ecological studies are discussed in Robinson (1950) and in Clausen and Kohn (1954).

[6]See, for example, Locke, Kramer, Timberlake, Pasamanick, & Smeltzer (1958); Frumkin (1955); Dunham (1965); Lemkau, Tietze, & Cooper (1942); Fuson (1943); Turner & Wagonfeld (1967). Relevant, too, are some early studies whose full significance was not appreciated until later. See, for example, Nolan (1917); Ødegaard (1932, esp. pp. 182–184); and Green (1939). One puzzling partial-exception comes from Jaco's study of Texas. He finds the highest incidence of schizophrenia among the unemployed, but otherwise a strange, perhaps curvilinear relationship of occupational status to incidence. Perhaps it is only that so many of his patients were classified as unemployed (rather than according to their pre-illness occupational status) that the overall picture is distorted. See Jaco (1957, 1960).

either occupation or the social status of the area and rates of schizophrenia.[7] On a re-examination of past studies, we discovered a curious thing: the larger the city, the stronger the correlation between rates of schizophrenia and these indices of social class. In the metropolis of Chicago, the correlation is large, and the relationship is linear: the lower the social status, the higher the rates. In cities of 100,000 to 500,000 (or perhaps more), the correlation is smaller and not so linear: it is more a matter of a concentration of cases in the lowest socio-economic strata, with not so much variation among higher strata. When you get down to a city as small as Hagerstown—36,000—the correlation disappears.

Subsequent studies in a number of different places have confirmed our generalization. Sundby and Nyhus (1963), for example, showed that Oslo, Norwar, manifests the typical pattern for cities of its half-million size: a high concentration in the lowest social stratum, little variation above. Hollingshead and Redlich's (1957) data on new admissions for schizophrenia from New Haven, Connecticut, show that pattern, too.

There is substantial evidence, too, for our conclusion that socio-economic differentials disappear in areas of small population. The Leightons found that although rates of mental disorder do correlate with socio-economic status for "Stirling County," Nova Scotia, as a whole, they do not for the small (population 3000) community of "Bristol" (Leighton, Harding, Macklin, Hughes, & Leighton, 1963; Leighton, Harding, Macklin, MacMillan, & Leighton, 1963). Similarly, Buck, Wanklin, and Hobbs (1955), in an ecological analysis of Western Ontario, found a high rank correlation between median wage and county first admission rates for mental disorder for counties of 10,000 or more population, but a much smaller correlation for counties of smaller population. And Hagnell (1966) found no relationship between his admittedly inexact measures of socio-economic status and rates of mental disorder for the largely rural area of south-western Sweden that he investigated.

I think one must conclude that the relationship of socio-economic status to schizophrenia has been demonstrated only for urban populations. Even for urban populations, a linear relationship of socio-economic status to rates of schizophrenia has been demonstrated only for the largest metropolises. The evidence, though, that there is an unusually high rate of schizophrenia in the lowest socio-economic strata of urban communities seems to me to be nothing less than overwhelming. The proper interpretation why this is so, however, is not so unequivocal.

THE DIRECTION OF CAUSALITY

One major issue in interpretating the Faris and Dunham, the Clark, and all subsequent investigations concerns the direction of causality. Rates of schizophrenia in the lowest

---

[7]Clausen & Kohn (1959). In that paper, the data on occupational rates were incompletely reported. Although we divided the population into four occupational classes, based on U.S. Census categories, we presented the actual rates for only the highest and lowest classes, leading some readers to conclude, erroneously, that we had divided the population into only two occupational classes. In fact, the average annual rates of first hospital admission for schizophrenia, per 100,000 population aged 15–64, were:

(a) professional, technical, managerial, officials and proprietors: 21.3
(b) clerical and sales personnel: 23.8
(c) craftsmen, foremen, and kindred workers: 10.7
(d) operatives, service workers, and laborers: 21.7

Our measures of occupational mobility, to be discussed later, were based on movement among the same four categories.

socio-economic strata could be disproportionately high either because conditions of life in those strata are somehow conducive to the development of schizophrenia, or because people from higher social strata who become schizophrenic suffer a decline in status. Or, of course, it could be some of both. Discussions of this issue have conventionally gone under the rubric of the "drift hypothesis," although far more is involved.

The drift hypothesis was first raised as an attempt to explain away the Faris and Dunham findings. The argument was that in the course of their developing illness, schizophrenics tend to "drift" into lower status areas of the city. It is not that more cases of schizophrenia are "produced" in these areas, but that schizophrenics who are produced elsewhere end up at the bottom of the heap by the time they are hospitalized, and thus are counted as having come from the bottom of the heap.

When the Clark study appeared, the hypothesis was easily enlarged to include "drift" from higher to lower-status occupations. In its broadest formulation, the drift hypothesis asserts that high rates of schizophrenia in the lowest social strata come about because people from higher classes who become schizophrenic suffer a decline in social position as a consequence of their illness. In some versions of the hypothesis, it is further suggested that schizophrenics from smaller locales tend to migrate to the lowest status areas and occupations of large metropolises; this would result in an exaggeration of rates there and a corresponding underestimation of rates for the place and class from which they come.

Incidentally, the drift hypothesis is but one variant of a more general hypothesis that any differences in rates of schizophrenia are the result of social selection—that various social categories show high rates because people already predisposed to schizophrenia gravitate into those categories. This has long been argued by Ødegaard (1932, 1957, 1962) but with data that are equally amenable to social selection and social causation interpretations. Dunham (1965) has recently made the same point, but I think his data argue more convincingly for social causation than for social selection. Intriguing though the issue is, it is presently unresolvable; so it would be better to focus on the more specific question, whether or not the high concentration of schizophrenia in the lowest socio-economic strata is the result of downward drift.

One approach to this problem has been to study the histories of social mobility of schizophrenics. Unfortunately, the evidence is inconsistent. Three studies indicate that schizophrenics have been downwardly mobile in occupational status,[8] three others that they have not been.[9] Some of these studies do not compare the experiences of the schizophrenics to those of normal persons from comparable social backgrounds. Those that do are nevertheless inconclusive—either because the comparison group was not well chosen, or because the city in which the study was done does not have a concentration of

---

[8]Evidence that schizophrenics have been downwardly mobile in *occupational* status has been presented in Schwartz (1946); Lystad (1957); Turner & Wagonfeld (1967). In addition, there has been some debatable evidence that the ecological concentration of schizophrenia has resulted from the migration of unattached men into the high-rate areas of the city. See Gerard & Houston (1956); Dunham (1965). (Dunham's data, however, show that when rates are properly computed, rate-differentials between high- and low-rate areas of Detroit are just as great for the stable population as for in-migrants.)

[9]Evidence that schizophrenics have not been downwardly mobile in occupational status is presented in Hollingshead & Redlich (1954, 1957, pp. 244–248); Clausen & Kohn (1959); and Dunham (1964, 1965). Evidence that the ecological concentration of schizophrenia has not resulted from in-migration or downward drift is presented in Lapouse, Monk, & Terris (1956); Hollingshead & Redlich (1954); and, as noted in the preceding note, Dunham (1965).

schizophrenia in the lowest social class. Since no study is definitive, any assessment must be based on a subjective weighing of the strengths and weaknesses of them all. My assessment is that the weight of this evidence clearly indicates either that schizophrenics have been no more downwardly mobile (in fact, no less upwardly mobile) than other people from the same social backgrounds, or at minimum, that the degree of downward mobility is insufficient to explain the high concentration of schizophrenia in the lowest socio-economic strata.

There is another and more direct way of looking at the question, however, and from this perspective the question is still unresolved. The reformulated question focuses on the social class origins of schizophrenics; it asks whether the occupations of fathers of schizophrenics are concentrated in the lowest social strata. If they are, that is clear evidence in favor of the hypothesis that lower-class status is conducive to schizophrenia. If they are not, class might still matter for schizophrenia—it might be a matter of stress experienced by lower-class adults, rather than of the experience of being born and raised in the lower class—but certainly the explanation that would require the fewest assumptions would be the drift hypothesis.

The first major study to evaluate the evidence from this perspective argued strongly in favor of lower-class origins being conducive to mental disorder, although perhaps not to schizophrenia in particular. Srole and his associates (1962) found, in their study of midtown New York, that rates of mental disorder correlate nearly as well with their parents' socio-economic status as with the subjects' own socio-economic status. But then Goldberg and Morrison (1963) found that although the occupations of male schizophrenic patients admitted to hospitals in England and Wales show the usual concentration of cases on the lowest social class, their fathers' occupations do not. Since this study dealt with schizophrenia, the new evidence seemed more directly in point. One might quarrel with some aspects of this study—the index of social class is debatable, for example, and data are lacking for 25% of the originally drawn sample—but this is much too good a study to be taken lightly. Nor can one conclude that the situation in England and Wales is different from that in the United States, for Dunham reports that two segments of Detroit show a similar picture (Dunham, 1964; Dunham, Phillips, & Srinivasan, 1966; see also Rinehart, 1966).

There is yet one more study to be considered, however, and this the most important one of all, for it offers the most complete data about class origins, mobility, and the eventual class position of schizophrenics. Turner and Wagonfeld (1967) in a study of Monroe County (Rochester), New York, discovered a remarkable pattern: rates of first treatment for schizophrenia are disproportionately high, both for patients of lowest occupational status and for patients whose fathers had lowest occupational status, but these are by and large not the same patients. Some of those whose fathers were in the lowest occupational class had themselves moved up and some of those ending up in the lowest occupational class had come from higher class origins. Thus, there is evidence both for the proposition that lower-class origins are conducive to schizophrenia and for the proposition that most lower-class schizophrenics come from higher socio-economic origins. No wonder partial studies have been inconsistent!

The next question one would want to ask, of course, is how the schizophrenics' histories of occupational mobility compare to those of normal people of comparable social class origins. Turner and Wagonfeld have not the data to answer this definitively, for they lack an appropriate control group. They are able, however, to compare the mobility experiences of their schizophrenics to those of a cross-section of the population, and from this they learn two important things. More schizophrenics than normals have been downwardly mobile. This downward mobility did not come about because of a loss of occupational position that had once been achieved, but reflected their failure ever to have achieved as high an occupational level as do most men of their social class origins.

This argues strongly against a simple drift hypothesis—it is not, as some have argued, that we have erroneously rated men at lower than their usual class status because we have classified them according to their occupations at time of hospitalization, after they have suffered a decline in occupational position. It is more likely that a more sophisticated drift hypothesis applies—that some people genetically or constitutionally or otherwise predisposed to schizophrenia show some effects of developing illness at least as early as the time of their first jobs, for they are never able to achieve the occupational levels that might be expected of them. If so, the possibilities of some interaction between genetic predisposition and early social circumstances are very real indeed.

One direction that further research must take is well pointed out by the Turner and Wagonfeld study. The question now must be the degree to which the correlation of class and schizophrenia results from a higher incidence of schizophrenia among people born into lower-class families, the degree to which it results from schizophrenics of higher class origins never achieving as high an occupational level as might have been expected of them—and why.

For the present, I think it can be tentatively concluded that despite what Goldberg and Morrison found for England and Wales, the weight of evidence lies against the drift hypothesis being a sufficient explanation. In all probability, lower-class families produce a disproportionate number of schizophrenics, although perhaps by not so large a margin as one would conclude from studies that rely on the patients' own occupational attainments.

Parenthetically, there is another important question involved here, the effects of social mobility itself. Ever since Ødegaard's (1963; see also Astrup, Christian, & Ødegaard, 1960) classic study of rates of mental disorder among Norwegian migrants to the United States, we have known that geographic mobility is a matter of considerable consequence for mental illness (see Tietze, Lemkau, & Cooper, 1942; Leacock, 1957; Mishler & Scotch, 1963), and the same may be true for social mobility (Kleiner & Parker, 1963, see also Myers & Roberts, 1959; Parker & Kleiner, 1966). But we have not known how and why mobility matters—whether it is a question of what types of people are mobile or of the stresses of mobility—and unfortunately later research has failed to resolve the issue.

THE ADEQUACY OF INDICES

The adequacy of indices is another major issue in interpreting the Faris and Dunham, the Clark, and all subsequent investigations. Most of these studies are based on hospital admission rates, which may not give a valid picture of the true incidence of schizophrenia. Studies that do not rely on hospital rates encounter other and perhaps even more serious difficulties, with which we shall presently deal.

The difficulty with using admission rates as the basis for computing rates of schizophrenia is that lower-class psychotics may be more likely to be hospitalized, and if hospitalized to be diagnosed as schizophrenic, especially in public hospitals. Faris and Dunham tried to solve this problem by including patients admitted to private as well as to public mental hospitals. This was insufficient because, as later studies have shown, some people who suffer serious mental disorder never enter a mental hospital. [10]

---

[10] See, for example, Kaplan, Reed, & Richardson (1956); see also all of the major community studies of mental illness.

Subsequent studies have attempted to do better by including more and more social agencies in their search for cases; Hollingshead and Redlich (1957) in New Haven, and Jaco (1960) in Texas, for example, have extended their coverage to include everyone who enters any sort of treatment facility—Jaco going so far as to question all the physicians in Texas. This is better, but clearly the same objections hold in principle. Furthermore, Srole and his associates (1962, esp. pp. 240–251) have demonstrated that there are considerable social differences between people who have been treated, somewhere, for mental illness, and severely impaired people, some large proportion of them schizophrenic, who have never been to any sort of treatment facility. So we must conclude that using treatment—any sort of treatment—as an index of mental disorder is suspect.

The alternative is to go out into the community and examine everyone—or a representative sample of everyone—yourself. This has been done by a number of investigators, for example Essen-Möller in Sweden (Essen-Möller, 1956, 1961; Hagnell, 1966), Srole and his associates (1962) in New York, the Leightons in Nova Scotia (Leighton, Harding, Macklin, MacMillan, & Leighton, 1963). They have solved one problem, but have run into three others.

1. The first is that most of these investigators have found it impossible to classify schizophrenia reliably, and have had to resort to larger and vaguer categories—severe mental illness, functional psychosis, and such. For some purposes, this may be justified. For our immediate purposes, it is exceedingly unfortunate.

2. Second, even if you settle for such a concept as "mental illness," it is difficult to establish criteria that can be applied reliably and validly in community studies (see Dohrenwend & Dohrenwend, 1965). For all its inadequacies, hospitalization is at least an unambiguous index, and you can be fairly certain that the people who are hospitalized are really ill. But how does one interpret the Leightons' estimate that about a third of their population suffer significant psychiatric impairment (Leighton, Harding, Macklin, Hughes, & Leighton, 1963, p. 1026), or Srole's that almost a quarter of his are impaired (Srole *et al.*, 1962, p. 138)?

Personal examination by a single psychiatrist using presumably consistent standards is one potential solution, but usable only in relatively small investigations. Another possible solution is the further development of objective rating scales, such as the Neuropsychiatric Screening Adjunct first developed by social scientists in the Research Branch of the U.S. Army in World War II (Star, 1950) and later incorporated into both the Leightons' and Srole's investigations, but not developed to anything like its full potential in either study. The limitation here is that such scales may be less relevant to the measurement of psychosis than of neurosis.

To make significant further advances, we shall have to break free of traditional methods of measurement. Epidemiological studies still largely rely on a single, undifferentiated overall assessment. Even when such an assessment can be demonstrated to be reliable within the confines of a single study, it has only limited use for comparative studies and is questionable for repeated application in studies designed to ascertain how many new cases arise in some given period of time. At minimum, we must begin to make use of our developing capacities of multivariate analysis. One obvious approach is to try to differentiate the several judgments that go into clinical diagnoses, develop reliable measures of each, and examine their interrelationship. At the same time, it would be well to develop reliable measures of matters conventionally given only secondary attention in epidemiological research—for example, the degree of disability the individual has sustained in each of several major social roles (see Clausen's incisive analysis, 1966). A third path we might try is the further development of objective measures of dimensions of subjective state (such as anxiety, alienation, and self-abasement) thought to be indicative of pathology. All these and others can be measured as separate dimensions, and then empirically related to each other and to clinical assessments.

Whether or not these particular suggestions have merit, I think the general conclusion that it is time for considerable methodological experimentation is indisputable.

3. The third problem in community studies is that it is so difficult to secure data on the incidence of mental disturbance that most studies settle for prevalence data (see Kramer, 1957). That is, instead of ascertaining the number of new cases arising in various population groups during some period of time, they count the number of people currently ill at the time of the study. This latter measure—prevalence—is inadequate because it reflects not only incidence but also duration of illness. As Hollingshead and Redlich (1957) have shown duration of illness—in so far as it incapacitates—is highly correlated with social class.

Various approximations to incidence have been tried, and various new—and often some-what fantastic—statistical devices invented to get around this problem, but without any real success. Clearly, what is needed is repeated studies of the population, to pick up new cases as they arise and thus to establish true incidence figures. (This is what Hagnell did, and it was a very brave effort indeed.) The crucial problem, of course, is to develop reliable measures of mental disorder, for without that our repeated surveys will measure nothing but the errors of our instruments. Meantime, we have to recognize that prevalence studies use an inappropriate measure that exaggerates the relationship of socio-economic status to mental disorder.

So, taken all together, the results of the studies of class and schizophrenia are hardly definitive. They may even all wash out—one more example of inadequate methods leading to premature, false conclusions. I cannot prove otherwise. Yet I think the most reasonable interpretation of all these findings is that they point to something real. Granted that there isn't a single definitive study in the lot, the weaknesses of one are compensated for by the strengths of some other, and the total edifice is probably much stronger than you would conclude from knowing only how frail are its component parts. A large number of complementary studies all seem to point to the same conclusion: that rates of mental disorder, particularly of schizophrenia, are highest at the lowest socio-economic levels, at least in moderately large cities, and this probably isn't just a matter of drift or inadequate indices or some other artifact of the methods we use. In all probability, more schizophrenia is actually produced at the lowest socio-economic levels. At any rate, let us take that as a working hypothesis and explore the question further. Assuming that more schizophrenia occurs at lower socio-economic levels—Why?

ALTERNATIVE INTERPRETATIONS

Is it really socio-economic status, or is it some correlated variable that is operative here? Faris and Dunham did not take socio-economic status very seriously in their interpretation of their data. From among the host of variables characteristic of the high-rate areas of Chicago, they focused on such things as high rates of population turnover and ethnic mix-tures and hypothesized that the really critical thing about the high-rate areas was the degree of social isolation they engendered. Two subsequent studies, one by Jaco (1954) in Texas, the other by Hare (1956a) in Bristol, England, are consistent in that they, too, show a correlation of rates of schizophrenia to various ecological indices of social isolation. The only study that directly examines the role of social isolation in the lives of schizophrenics, however, seems to demonstrate that while social isolation may be symptomatic of developing illness, it does not play an important role in etiology (Kohn & Clausen, 1955; see also Clausen & Kohn, 1954).

Several other interpretations of the epidemiological evidence have been suggested, some supported by intriguing, if inconclusive, evidence. One is that it is not socio-economic status as such that is principally at issue, but social integration. The Leightons have produced plausible evidence for this interpretation (Leighton, Harding, Macklin, MacMillan & Leighton, 1963). The problems of defining and indexing "social integration" make a definite demonstration exceedingly difficult, however, even for the predominantly rural populations with which they have worked.

Another possibility is that the high rates of schizpohrenia found in lower-class populations are a consequence of especially high rates for lower-class members of some "ethnic" groups who happen to be living in areas where other ethnic groups predominate. In their recent study in Boston, for example, Schwartz and Mintz (1963a) showed that Italian-Americans living in predominantly non-Italian neighborhoods have very high rates of schizophrenia, while those living in predominantly Italian neighborhoods do not (see also their more extended discussion, 1963b). The former group contribute disproportionately to the rates for lower-class neighborhoods. (The authors suggest that this may explain why small cities do not show a concentration of lower-class cases: these cities do not have the ethnic mixtures that produce such a phenomenon.)

Wechsler and Pugh (1966) extended this interpretive model to suggest that rates should be higher for any persons living in a community where they and persons of similar social attributes are in a minority. Their analysis of Massachusetts towns provides some surprisingly supportive data.

Other possibilities deal more directly with the occupational component of socio-economic status. Ødegaard (1956) long ago showed that rates of schizophrenia are higher for some occupations that are losing members and lower for some that are expanding. His observation was correct, but it explained only a small part of the occupational rate differences. Others have focused on alleged discrepancies between schizophrenics' occupational aspirations and achievements (Kleiner & Parker, 1963; Myers & Roberts, 1959), arguing that the pivotal fact is not that schizophrenics have achieved so little but that they had wanted so much more. The evidence is limited.

One could argue—and I see no reason to take the argument lightly—that genetics provides a quite sufficient explanation. If there is a moderately strong genetic component in schizophrenia, then one would expect a higher than usual rate of schizophrenia among the fathers and grandfathers of schizophrenics. Since schizophrenia is a debilitating disturbance, this would be reflected in grandparents' and parents' occupations and places of residence. In other words, it could be a rather complex version of drift hypothesis. The only argument against this interpretation is that there is no really compelling evidence in favor of it; one can accept it on faith, or one can keep it in mind while continuing to explore alternatives. Prudence suggests the latter course of action.

There are other possibilities we might examine, but since there is no very strong evidence for any of them, that course does not seem especially profitable. One must allow the possibility that some correlated variable might prove critical for explaining the findings; it might not be social class, after all, that is operative here. Until that is demonstrated, however, the wisest course would seem to be to take the findings at face value and see what there might be about social class that would help us to understand schizophrenia.

CLASS AND ETIOLOGY

What is there about the dynamics of social class that might affect the probability of people becoming schizophrenic? How does social class operate here; what are the intervening processes?

The possibilities are numerous, almost too numerous. Social class indexes...[are] correlated with so many phenomena that might be relevant to the etiology of schizophrenia. Since it measures status, it implies a great deal about how the individual is treated by others—with respect or perhaps degradingly; since it is measured by occupational rank, it suggests much about the conditions that make up the individual's daily work, how closely supervised he is, whether he works primarily with things, with data, or with people; since it reflects the individual's educational level, it connotes a great deal about his style of thinking, his use or non-use of abstractions, even his perceptions of physical reality and certainly of social reality; furthermore, the individual's class position influences his social values and colors his evaluations of the world about him; it affects the family experiences he is likely to have had as a child and the ways he is likely to raise his own children; and it certainly matters greatly for the type and amount of stress he is likely to encounter in a lifetime. In short, social class pervades so much of life that it is difficult to guess which of its correlates are most relevant for understanding schizophrenia. Moreover, none of these phenomena is so highly correlated with class (nor class so highly correlated with schizophrenia) that any one of these facets is obviously more promising than the others.

This being the case, investigators have tended to pursue those avenues that have met their theoretical predilections and to ignore the others. In practice, this has meant that the interrelationship of class, family, and schizophrenia has been explored, and more recently the relationship of class, stress, and schizophrenia, but the other possibilities remain largely unexamined. Given the inherent relevance of some of them—class differences in patterns of thinking, for example, have such obvious relevance to schizophrenia—this is a bit surprising.

But let me review what has been done. The hypothesis that stress is what is really at issue in the class–schizophrenia relationship is in some respects especially appealing, in part because it is so direct. We have not only our own observations as human beings with some compassion for less fortunate people, but an increasingly impressive body of scientific evidence. (Dohrenwend & Dohrenwend, 1970), to show that life is rougher and rougher the lower one's social class position. The stress explanation seems especially plausible for the very lowest socio-economic levels, where the rates of schizophrenia are highest.

There have to my knowledge been only two empirical investigations of the relationship of social class to stress to mental disorder. The first was done by Langner and Michael (1963) in New York as part of the "Midtown" study. This study, as all the others we have been considering, has its methodological defects—it is a prevalence study, and many of the indices it uses are at best questionable—but it tackles the major issues head-on, and with very impressive and very intriguing results. It finds a strong linear relationship between stress and mental disturbance, specifically, the more sources of stress, the higher the probability of mental disturbance. It also finds the expected relationship between social class and stress. So the stress hypothesis has merit. But stress is not all that is involved in the relationship of social class to mental disorder. No matter how high the level of stress, social class continues to be correlated with the probability of mental disturbance; in fact, the more stress, the higher the correlation.[11] Thus, it seems that the effect of social class on the rate of mental disorder is not only, or even principally, a function of different amounts of stress at different class levels.

In a more recent study in San Juan, Puerto Rico, Rogler and Hollingshead (1965) ascribe a more important role to stress. Theirs was an intensive investigation of the life histories of a sample of lower-class schizophrenics, along with comparable studies of a well-matched sample of non-schizophrenics. Rogler and Hollingshead found only insubstantial differences in the early life experiences of lower-class schizophrenics and controls; they did find, however, that in the period of a year or so before the onset of symptoms, the schizophrenics were subjected to an unbearable onslaught of stress. In effect, all lower-class slum dwellers in San Juan suffer continual, dreadful stress; in addition to this "normal" level of stress, however, the schizophrenics were hit with further intolerable stress which incapacitated them in one or another central role, leading to incapacitation in other roles, too.

The picture that Rogler and Hollingshead draw is plausible and impressive. It is not possible, however—at least not yet—to generalize as far from their data as one might like. Their sample is limited to schizophrenics who are married or in stable consensual unions. These one would assume to be predominantly "reactive" type schizophrenics—precisely the group whom one would expect, from past studies, to have had normal childhood social experiences, good social adjustment, and extreme precipitating circumstances. So their findings may apply to "reactive" schizophrenia, but perhaps not to "process" schizophrenia. In addition, for all the impressiveness of the argument, the data are not so unequivocal. Their inquiry was not so exhaustive as to rule out the possibility that the schizophrenics might have had different family experiences from those of the controls. Furthermore, the evidence that the schizophrenics were subjected to significantly greater stress is not so thoroughly compelling as one might want. Thus, the case is not proved. Nevertheless, Rogler and Hollingshead have demonstrated that the possibility that stress plays an important role in the genesis of schizophrenia is to be taken very seriously indeed. Certainly this study makes it imperative that we investigate the relationship of class to stress to schizophrenia far more intensively.

At the same time, we should investigate some closely related possibilities that have not to my knowledge been studied empirically. Not only stress, but also reward and opportunity, are differentially distributed among the social classes. The more fortunately situated not only are less beaten about, but may be better able to withstand the stresses they do encounter because they have many more rewarding experiences to give them strength. And many more alternative courses of action are open to them when they run into trouble. Might this offer an added clue to the effects of class for schizophrenia?

More generally, what is there about the conditions of life of the lowest social strata that might make it more difficult for their members to cope with stress? One can think of intriguing possibilities. Their occupational conditions and their limited education gear their thinking processes to the concrete and the habitual; their inexperience in dealing with the abstract may ill-equip them to cope with ambiguity, uncertainty, and unpredictability; their

---

[11]The latter finding is in part an artifact of the peculiar indices used in this study, and reflects differences not in the incidence of illness but in type and severity of illness in different social classes at various levels of stress. At higher stress levels, lower-class people tend to develop incapacitating psychoses and middle-class people less incapacitating neuroses.

mental processes are apt to be too gross and rigid when flexibility and subtlety are most required. Or, a related hypothesis, the lower- and working-class valuation of conformity to external authority, and disvaluation of self-direction, might cripple a man faced with the necessity of suddenly having to rely on himself in an uncertain situation where others cannot be relied on for guidance.

These hypotheses, unfortunately, have not been investigated; perhaps it is time that they were. The one hypothesis that has been studied, and that one only partially, is that lower- and working-class patterns of parent-child relationships somehow do not adequately prepare children for dealing with the hazards of life. Now we enter what is perhaps the most complicated area of research we have touched on so far, and certainly the least adequately studied field of all.

There has been a huge volume of research literature about family relationships and schizophrenia (see the references in Kohn & Clausen, 1956; Clausen & Kohn, 1960; and Sanua, 1961); most of it inadequately designed. One has to dismiss the majority of studies because of one or another incapacitating deficiency. In many, the patients selected for study were a group from which you could not possibly generalize to schizophrenics at large. Either the samples were comprised of chronic patients, where one would expect the longest and most difficult onset of illness with the greatest strain in family relationships, or the samples were peculiarly selected, not to test a hypothesis, but to load the dice in favor of a hypothesis. In other studies, there have been inadequate control groups or no control group at all. One of the most serious defects of method has been the comparison of patterns of family relationship of lower- and working-class patients to middle- and upper-middle-class normal controls—which completely confounds the complex picture we wish to disentangle. In still other studies, even where the methods of sample and control-selection have been adequate, the method of data-collection has seriously biased the results. This is true, for example, in those studies that have placed patients and their families in stressful situations bound to exaggerate any flaws in their interpersonal processes, especially for people of lesser education and verbal skill who would be least equipped to deal with the new and perplexing situation in which they found themselves (for a more complete discussion, see Clausen & Kohn, 1960, pp. 309–316).

Still, some recent studies have suggested respects in which the family relationships of schizophrenics seem unusual, and unusual in theoretically interesting ways—that is, in ways that might be important in the dynamics of schizophrenic personality development. Work by Bateson and Jackson on communication processes in families of schizophrenics (Bateson, Jackson, Haley, & Weakland, 1956; see also Mishler & Waxler, 1965) and that by Wynne and his associates on cognitive and emotional processes in such families (Wynne, Ryckoff, Day, & Hirsch, 1955; Ryckoff, Day, & Wynne, 1959; see also Mishler & Waxler, 1965), for example, are altogether intriguing.

But—and here I must once again bring social class into the picture—there has not been a single well-controlled study that demonstrates any substantial difference between the family relationships of schizophrenics and those of normal persons from lower- and working-class backgrounds. Now, it may be that the well-controlled studies simply have not dealt with the particular variables that do differentiate the families of schizophrenics from those of normal lower- and working-class families. The two studies that best control for social class—Clausen's and my study in Hagerstown, Maryland (Kohn & Clausen, 1956) and Rogler and Hollingshead's (1965) in San Juan—deal with but a few aspects of family relationship, notably not including the very processes that recent clinical studies have emphasized as perhaps the most important of all. It may be that investigations yet to come will show clear and convincing evidence that some important aspects of family relationships are definitely different for schizophrenia-producing families and normal families of this social background.

If they do not, that still does not mean that family relationships are not important for schizophrenia, or that it is not through the family that social class exerts one of its principal effects. Another way of putting the same facts is to say that there is increasing evidence of remarkable parallels between the dynamics of families that produce schizophrenia and family dynamics in the lower classes generally (Kohn, 1963; Pearlin & Kohn, 1966). This may indicate that the family patterns of the lower classes are in some way broadly conducive to schizophrenic personality development.

Clearly these patterns do not provide a sufficient explanation of schizophrenia. We still need a missing X, or set of X's, to tell us the necessary and sufficient conditions for schizophrenia to occur. Perhaps that X is some other aspect of family relationships. Perhaps lower-class patterns of family relationships are conducive to schizophrenia for persons genetically predisposed, but not for others. Or perhaps they are generally conducive to schizophrenia, but schizophrenia will not actually occur unless the individual is subjected to certain types or amounts of stress. We do not know. But these speculative considerations do suggest that it may be about time to bring all these variables—social class, early family relationships, genetics, stress—into the same investigations, so that we can examine their interactive effects. Meantime, I must sadly conclude that we have not yet unravelled the relationship of social class and schizophrenia, nor learned what it might tell us about the etiology of the disorder.

CONCLUSION

Perhaps, after so broad a sweep, an overall assessment is in order. There is a truly remarkable volume of research literature demonstrating an especially high rate of schizophrenia (variously indexed) in the lowest social class or classes (variously indexed) of moderately large to large cities throughout much of the Western world. It is not altogether clear what is the direction of causality in this relationship—whether the conditions of life of the lowest social classes are conducive to the development of schizophrenia, or schizophrenia leads to a decline in social class position—but present evidence would make it seem probable that some substantial part of the phenomenon results from lower-class conditions of life being conducive to schizophrenia. It is not even certain that the indices of schizophrenia used in these studies can be relied on, although there is some minor comfort in that studies using several different indices all point to the same conclusion. Perhaps it is only an act of faith that permits me to conclude that the relationship of class to schizophrenia is probably real, an act of faith only barely disguised by calling it a working hypothesis.

This working hypothesis must be weighed against a number of alternative interpretations of the data. Many of them are plausible, several are supported by attractive nuggets of data, but none is more compelling than the most obvious interpretation of all: that social class seems to matter for schizophrenia because, in fact, it does.

When one goes on to see what this might imply for the etiology of schizophrenia, one finds many more intriguing possibilities than rigorous studies. There is some evidence that the greater stress suffered by lower-class people is relevant, and perhaps that lower- and working-class patterns of family relationships are broadly conducive to schizophrenia—although the latter is more a surmise than a conclusion.

Finally, it is clear that we must bring genetic predisposition and class, with all its attendant experiences, into the same investigations. That, however, is not the only sort of investigation that calls for attention. We have reviewed a large number of hypotheses, several major conflicts of interpretation, and many leads and hunches that all cry out to be investigated. The most hopeful sign in this confusing area is that several of the recent studies have gone far beyond seeing whether the usual stereotyped set of demographic characteristics correlate with rates of schizophrenia, to explore some of these very exciting issues.

REFERENCES

Astrup, C., & Ødegaard, Ø. Internal migration and disease in Norway. *Psychiatr. Quart.*, 1960, **34**, (Suppl.)116–130.

Bateson, G., with Jackson, D., Haley, J., & Weakland, J. Toward a theory of schizophrenia. *Behav. Sci.*, 1956, **1**, 251–264.

Buck, C., with Wanklin, F. M., & Hobbs, G. E. An analysis of regional differences in mental illness. *J. nerv. & ment. Dis.*, 1955, **122**, 73–79.

Clark, R. E. The relationship of schizophrenia to occupational income and occupational prestige. *Amer. Sociol. Rev.*, 1948 **13**, 325–330.

Clark, R. E. Psychoses, income, and occupational prestige. *Amer. J. Sociol.*, 1949, **54**, 433–440.

Clausen, J. A. *Sociology and the field of mental health.* New York: Russell Sage Foundation, 1956.

Clausen, J. A. The ecology of mental illness. *Symposium on Social and Preventive Psychiatry*, Walter Reed Army Medical Center, Washington, D.C., 1957.

Clausen, J. A. The sociology of mental illness. In R. K. Merton *et al.* (Eds.), *Sociology today, problems and prospects.* New York: Basic Books, 1959.

Clausen, J. A. Values, norms, and the health called "mental": Purposes and feasibility of assessment. Paper presented to the Symposium on Definition and Measurement of Mental Health, Washington, D.C., May 16, 1966. Mimeographed.

Clausen, J. A., & Kohn, M. L. The ecological approach in social psychiatry. *Amer. J. Sociol.*, 1954, **60**, 140–151.

Clausen, J. A., & Kohn, M. L. Relation of schizophrenia to the social structure of a small city. In B. Pasamanick (Ed.), *Epidemiology of mental disorder.* Washington, D.C.: American Association for the Advancement of Science, 1959.

Clausen, J. A., & Kohn, M. L. Social relations and schizophrenia: A research report and a perspective. In D. D. Jackson (Ed.), *The etiology of schizophrenia.* New York: Basic Books, 1960.

Dee, W. L. J. An ecological study of mental disorders in metropolitan St. Lousis. Unpublished masters thesis, Washington University, 1939.

Demerath, N. J. Schizophrenia among primitives. In A. M. Rose (Ed.), *Mental health and mental disorder.* New York: Norton, 1955.

Dohrenwend, B. P., & Dohrenwend, B. S. The problem of validity in field studies of psychological disorder. *J. abnorm. Psychol.*, 1965, **70**, 52–69.

Dohrenwend, B. S., & Dohrenwend, B. P. Class and race as status-related sources of stress. In S. Levine & N. A. Scotch (Eds.), *The study of stress.* Chicago: Aldine, 1970.

Dunham, H. W. Current status of ecological research in mental disorder. *Social Forces*, 1947, **25**, 321–326.

Dunham, H. W. Social psychiatry. *Amer. Sociol. Rev.*, 1948, **13**, 183–197.

Dunham, H. W. Some persistent problems in the epidemiology of mental disorders. *Amer. J. Psychiat.*, 1963, **109**, 567–575.

Dunham, H. W. Social class and schizophrenia. *Amer. J. Orthopsychiat.*, 1964, **34**, 634–642.

Dunham, H. W. *Community and schizophrenia: An epidemiological analysis.* Detroit: Wayne State University Press, 1965.

Dunham, H. W. Epidemiology of psychiatric disorders as a contribution to medical ecology. *Arch. Gen. Psychiat.*, 1966, **14**, 1–19.

Dunham, H. W., Phillips, P., & Srinivasan, B. A research note on diagnosed mental illness and social class. *Amer. Sociol. Rev.,* 1966, **31,** 223–227.

Essen-Möller, E. Individual traits and morbidity in a Swedish rural population. *Acta psychiat. neurol. scand.,* 1956, **100,** (Suppl.) 1–160.

Essen-Möller, E. A current field study in the mental disorders in Sweden. In P. H. Hoch & J. Zubin (Eds.), *Comparative epidemiology of the mental disorders.* New York: Grune & Stratton, 1961.

Faris, R. E. L., & Dunham, H. W. *Mental disorders in urban areas: An ecological study of schizophrenia and other psychoses.* Chicago: University of Chicago Press, 1939.

Felix, R. H., & Bowers, R. V. Mental hygiene and socio-environmental factors. *The Milbank Memorial Fund Quarterly,* 1948, **26,** 125–147.

Frumkin, R. M. Occupation and major mental disorders. In A. M. Rose (Ed.), *Mental health and mental disorder.* New York: Norton, 1955.

Fuson, W. M. Research note: Occupations of functional psychotics. *Amer. J. of Sociol.,* 1943, **48,** 612–613.

Gardner, E. A., & Babigian, H. M. A longitudinal comparison of psychiatric service to selected socio-economic areas of Monroe County, New York. *Amer. J. Orthopsychiat.,* 1966, **36,** 818–828.

Gerard, D. L., & Houston, L. G. Family setting and the social ecology of schizophrenia. *Psychiat. Quart.,* 1953, **27,** 90–101.

Goldberg, E. M., & Morrison, S. L. Schizophrenia and social class. *Brit. J. Psychiat.,* 1963, **109,** 785–802.

Green, H. W. Persons admitted to the Cleveland State hospital, 1928–1937. Cleveland Health Council, 1939.

Hagnell, O. *A prospective study of the incidence of mental disorder.* Stockholm: Svenska Bokförlaget, 1966.

Hare, E. H. Mental illness and social conditions in Bristol. *J. ment. Sci.,* 1956, **102,** 349–357. (a)

Hare, E. H. Family setting and the urban distribution of schizophrenia. *J. ment. Sci.,* 1956, **102,** 753–760. (b)

Hollingshead, A. B. Some issues in the epidemiology of schizophrenia. *Amer. Sociol. Rev.,* 1961, **26,** 5–13.

Hollingshead, A. B., & Redlich, R. C. Social stratification and schizophrenia. *Amer. Sociol. Rev.,* 1954, **19,** 302–306.

Hollingshead, A. B., & Redlich, R. C. *Social class and mental illness.* New York: Wiley, 1957.

Jaco, E. G. The social isolation hypothesis and schizophrenia. *Amer. Sociol. Rev.,* 1934, **19,** 567–577.

Jaco, E. G. Incidence of psychoses in Texas. *Texas State Journal of Medicine,* 1957, **53,** 1–6.

Jaco, E. G. *The social epidemiology of mental disorders.* New York: Russell Sage Foundation, 1960.

Kaplan, B., with Reed, R. B., & Richardson, W. A comparison of the incidence of hospitalized and non-hospitalized cases of psychosis in two communities. *Amer. Sociol. Rev.,* 1956, **21,** 472–479.

Kety, S. S. Recent biochemical theories of schizophrenia. In D. D. Jackson (Ed.), *The etiology of schizophrenia.* New York: Basic Books, 1960.

Klee, G. D., with Spiro, E., Bahn, A. K., & Gorwitz, K. An ecological analysis of diagnosed mental illness in Baltimore. In R. R. Monroe *et al.* (Eds.), *Psychiatric epidemiology and mental health planning.* (Psychiatric Research Report No. 22) American Psychiatric Association, April, 1967.

Kleiner, R. J., & Parker, S. Goal-striving, social status, and mental disorder: A research review. *Amer. Sociol. Rev.,* 1963, **28,** 189–203.

Kohn, M. L. Social class and parent-child relationships: An interpretation. *Amer. J. Sociol.,* 1963, **68,** 471–480.

Kohn, M. L. On the social epidemiology of schizophrenia. *Acta Sociol.,* 1966, **9,** 209–221.

Kohn, M. L., & Clausen, J. A. Social isolation and schizophrenia. *Amer. Sociol. Rev.,* 1955, **20,** 265–273.

Kohn, M. L., & Clausen, J. A. Parental authority behavior and schizophrenia. *Amer. J. Orthopsychiat.,* 1956, **26,** 297–313.

Kramer, M. A discussion of the concepts of incidence and prevalence as related to epidemiologic studies of mental disorders. *Amer. J. Pub. Hlth,* 1947, **47,** 826–840.

Kringlen, E. Discordance with respect to schizophrenia in monozygotic twins: Some genetic aspects. *J. nerv. & ment. Dis.*, 1964, **138**, 26–31. (a)

Kringlen, E. *Schizophrenia in male monozygotic twins.* Oslo: Universitetsforlaget, 1964. (b)

Kringlen, E. Schizophrenia in twins: An epidemiological-clinical study. *Psychiatry*, 1966, **29**, 172–184.

Langner, T. S., & Michael, S. T. *Life stress and mental health.* New York: Free Press, 1963.

Lapouse, R., with Monk, M., & Terris, M. The drift hypothesis and socioeconomic differentials in schizophrenia. *Amer. J. Pub. Hlth*, 1956, **46**, 978–986.

Leacock, E. Three social variables and the occurrence of mental disorder. In A. H. Leighton, J. A. Clausen, & R. N. Wilson (Eds.), *Explorations in social psychiatry.* New York: Basic Books, 1957.

Leighton, D. C., with Harding, J. S., Macklin, D. B., Hughes, C. C., & Leighton, A. H. Psychiatric findings of the Stirling County study. *Amer. J. Psychiat.*, 1963, **119**, 1021–1026.

Leighton, D. C., with Harding, J. S., Macklin, D. B., MacMillan, A. M., & Leighton, A. H. *The character of danger: Psychiatric symptoms in selected communities.* New York: Basic Books, 1963.

Lemkau, P., with Tietze, C., & Cooper, M. Mental hygiene problems in an urban district. Second paper. *Ment. Hyg.*, 1942, **26**, 1–20.

Lin, T. A study of the incidence if mental disorder in Chinese and other cultures. *Psychiatry*, 1953, **16**, 313–336.

Lin, T. Mental disorders in Taiwan, fifteen years later: A preliminary report. Paper presented to the Conference on Mental Health in Asia and the Pacific, Honolulu, March, 1966.

Locke, B. Z., with Kramer, M., Timberlake, C. E., Pasamanick, B., & Smeltzer, D. Problems of interpretation of patterns of first admissions to Ohio State public mental hospitals for patients with schizophrenic reactions. In B. Pasamanick & P. H. Knapp (Eds.), *Social aspects of psychiatry.* (Psychiatric Research Report No. 10) American Psychiatric Association, 1958.

Lystad, M. H. Social mobility among selected groups of schizophrenic patients. *Amer. Sociol. Rev.*, 1957, **22**, 288–292.

Mishler, E. G., & Scotch, N. A. Sociocultural factors in the epidemiology of schizophrenia: A review. *Psychiatry*, 1963, **26**, 315–351.

Mishler, E. G., & Waxler, N. E. Family interaction processes and schizophrenia: A review of current theories. *Merrill-Palmer Quarterly of Behavioral Development*, 1965, **11**, 269–315.

Morris, J. N. Health and social class. *Lancet*, 1959, **7**, 303–305.

Myers, J. K., & Roberts, B. H. *Family and class dynamics in mental illness.* New York: Wiley, 1959.

Nolan, W. J. Occupation and *dementia praecox.* (New York) *State Hospitals Quarterly*, 1917, **3**, 127–154.

Ødegaard, Ø. Emigration and insanity: A study of mental disease among the Norwegian born population of Minnesota. *Acta psychiatr. Neurol.* 1932, (Suppl. 4).

Ødegaard, Ø. Emigration and mental health. *Ment. Hyg.*, 1936, **20**, 546–553.

Ødegaard, Ø. The incidence of psychoses in various occupations. *Internat. J. Soc. Psychiat.*, 1956, **2**, 85–104.

Ødegaard, Ø. Occupational incidence of mental disease in single women. *Living Conditions and Health*, 1957, **1**, 169–180.

Ødegaard, Ø. Psychiatric epidemiology. *Proceedings of the Royal Society of Medicine*, 1962, **55**, 831–837.

Parker, S., & Kleiner, R. J. *Mental illness in the urban Negro community.* New York: Free Press, 1966.

Pearlin, L. I., & Kohn, M. L. Social class, occupation, and parental values: A cross-national study. *Amer. Sociol. Rev.*, 1966, **31**, 466–479.

Queen, S. A. The ecological study of mental disorders. *Amer. Sociol. Rev.*, 1940, **5**, 201–209.

Rinehart, J. W. Communication. *Amer. Sociol. Rev.*, 1966, **31**, 545–546.

Robinson, W. S. Ecological correlations and the behavior of individuals. *Amer. Sociol. Rev.*, 1950, **15**, 351–357.

Rogler, L. H., & Hollingshead, A. B. *Trapped: Families and schizophrenia.* New York: Wiley, 1965.

Rosenthal, D. Problems of sampling and diagnosis in the major twin studies of schizophrenia. *J. Psychiat. Res.*, 1962, **1**, 116–134.

Ryckoff, I., with Day, J., & Wynne, L. C. Maintenance of stereotyped roles in the families of schizophrenics. *AMA Arch. Psychiat.*, 1959, **1**, 93–98.

Sanua, V. D. Sociocultural factors in families of schizophrenia: A review of the literature. *Psychiatry*, 1961, **24**, 246–265.

Sanua, V. D. The etiology and epidemiology of mental illness and problems of methodology: With special emphasis on schizophrenia. *Men. Hyg.*, 1963, **47**, 607–621.

Schroeder, C. W. Mental disorders in cities. *Amer. J. Sociol.*, 1942, **48**, 40–48.

Schwartz, M. S. The economic and spatial mobility of paranoid schizophrenics and manic depressives. Unpublished masters thesis, University of Chicago, 1946.

Schwartz, D. T., & Mintz, N. L. Ecology and psychosis among Italians in 27 Boston comunities. *Social Problems*, 1963, **10**, 371–374.

Schwartz, D. T., & Mintz, N. L. Urban ecology and psychosis: Community factors in the incidence of schizophrenia and manic-depression among Italians in Greater Boston. 1963. Mimeographed.

Srole, L., with Langner, T. S., Michael, S. T., Opler, M. K., & Rennie, T. A. C. *Mental health in the metropolis: The midtown Manhattan study.* New York: McGraw-Hill, 1962. Vol. I.

Star, S. A. The screening of psychoneurotics in the army. In S. A. Stouffer with L. Guttman, E. A. Suchman, P. F. Lazarsfeld, S. A. Star, & J. A. Clausen (Eds.), *Measurement and prediction.* Princeton, N.J.: Princeton University Press, 1950.

Stein, L. 'Social class' gradient in schizophrenia. *Brit. J. Prevent. & Soc. Med.*, 1957, **11**, 181–195.

Stenbäck, A., & Achté, K. A. Hospital first admissions and social class. *Acta Psychiat. Scand.*, 1966, **42**, 113–124.

Sundby, P., & Nyhus, P. Major and minor psychiatric disorders in males in Oslo: An epidemiological study. *Acta Psychiat. Scand.*, 1963, **39**, 519–547.

Svalastoga, K. *Social differentiation.* New York: David McKay, 1965.

Tienari, P. Psychiatric illnesses in identical twins. *Acta Psychiat. Scand.*, 1963, **39** (Suppl. 171).

Tietze, C., with Lemkau, P., & Cooper, M. Personality disorder and spatial mobility. *Amer. J. Sociol.*, 1942, **48**, 29–39.

Turner, R. J., & Wagonfeld, M. O. Occupational mobility and schizophrenia, an assessment of the social causation and social selection hypotheses. *Amer. Sociol. Rev.*, 1967, **32**, 104–113.

Wechsler, H., & Pugh, T. F. Fit of individual and community characteristics and rates of psychiatric hospitalization. Paper presented to the Sixth World Congress of Sociology, Evian, September, 1966.

Williams, R. M., Jr. *American society: A sociological interpretation.* New York: Knopf, 1951.

Wynne, L. C., with Ryckoff, I. M., Day, J., & Hirsch, S. I. Pseudo-mutuality in the family relations of schizophrenics. *Psychiatry*, 1958, **22**, 205–220.

11

Studies of Adolescent Suicidal
Behavior: Etiology*

RICHARD H. SEIDEN

. . .[This article presents a discussion of the etiological factors found to be related to adolescent suicidal behavior. Numerous problems arose in the arrangement and presentation of this material.] These problems were exacerbated by two major considerations: first, the methodological defects and non-comparability of many of the studies, and secondly, the sheer weight of the literature written upon this subject. . . . Many studies contained imprecise definitions or conclusions that frequently went far beyond their data. Particularly common was the failure to distinguish between attempted, committed, threatened, "partial" and "probable" suicides. Various kinds of self-destructive behaviors were frequently combined without due respect for the important differences which exist between them. In some cases the results from a study based upon one group, such as attempted suicides, were over-generalized to other categories of suicidal behavior as well. In other cases the authors drew conclusions which were not evident from their data but which seemed to have been applied "wholesale" from previous studies. Yet another obstacle to neat, synoptic organization was introduced by the great number of factors which had been elicited in the various studies. For example, a prodigious number of psychodynamic characteristics have been causally linked to adolescent suicide, including, among others:

> *Chronic depression* (Lawler, Nakielny, & Wright, 1963; Cerny & Cerna, 1962),
>
> *Hallucinations, delusions, schizophrenic reactions* (Lawler, *et al.*, 1963; Toolan, 1962),
>
> *Feelings of rage and desire for revenge* (Bender & Schilder, 1937; Moss & Hamilton, 1956),
>
> *Guilt*—self-blame for parent's suicide (Cain & Fast, 1966); over sexual freedom (Jensen, 1955); anxiety and guilt over sexual impulses (Mohr & Despres, 1958); arousing guilt as a means of hurting others (Block & Christiansen, 1966); remorse (Bakwin, 1964); shame about failure and reactions of others (Iga, 1961),
>
> *Fear*—of punishment (Bakwin, 1964; MacDonald, 1906–7; Zumpe, 1959); failure in school, especially college (Jensen, 1955; Rook, 1959),
>
> *Feelings of powerlessness* (Parot, Collet, Girard, Jean & Coudert, 1965),
>
> *Desire to control environment* (Mohr & Despres, 1958); need to force attention and love from others (Bender & Schilder, 1937; Bergstrand & Otto, 1962; Faigel, 1966; Gould, 1965); manipulativeness (Toolan, 1962); blackmail (Launay, 1964; Ringel, Spiel & Stepan, 1955),
>
> *Feelings of worthlessness* (Hendin, 1964); of inadequacy (Iga, 1961; Lyman, 1961); severely reduced self-esteem (Munter, 1966); sense of failure (Gunther, 1967),
>
> *Loneliness and creation of unreal world* (Bergsma, 1966; Maycock, 1966); withdrawal (Morrison & Smith, 1967); isolation (Jacobs & Teicher, 1967; Jan-Tausch, n.d.); fantasy life (Lawler, *et al.*, 1963),

---

*From Seiden, R. H., *Suicide among youth*, Washington, D.C.: U.S. Government Printing Office, 1969. Reprinted by permission of the National Institute of Mental Health, Health Services and Mental Health Administration, U.S. Department of Health, Education, and Welfare, and Dr. Seiden. (Emphasized comments have been omitted and tables have been renumbered.)

Feelings of helplessness—dependency needs, insecurity (Iga, 1966); when dependency removed (Lourie, 1966); lack of love and protection (Zumpe, 1959),

Impulsivity (Geisler, 1953; Gould, 1965); ineffective self-control (Iga, 1966); crisis in control of aggressive urges; hypersensitivity, suggestibility, magical thinking (Schneer, Kay & Brozovsky, 1961),

Identification—wish for reunion with dead parent (Keeler, 1954; Launay, 1964; Mohr & Despres, 1958; Moss & Hamilton, 1956); follow example of parent's suicidal behavior (Lourie, 1966),

Feelings of hopelessness—futility; last resort (Jacobs & Teicher, 1967; Tuckman, Youngman, & Leifer, 1966),

Desire for escape from unbearable situation (Bender, 1953); tired of poor treatment (Faigel, 1966); feels unloved (Mohr & Despres, 1958; Peck, 1967a),

Loss of love object, concept of death, puberty (Alexander & Alderstein, 1958; Nagy, 1959). [*Italics* added.]

Our major task was to bring some order into the literature on this subject. We have attempted to evaluate the key studies, and from the numerous papers to select those whose findings had sufficient correspondence to warrant their presentation as a body of consensual knowledge. That is, our criterion was to select the research that was substantially relevant and could be generalized to the study of adolescent suicide.

ATTEMPTED VS. COMMITTED SUICIDE

The most striking defect in many of the studies of adolescent suicides was their frequent failure to distinguish between various self-destructive behaviors, particularly between the general categories of attempted and committed suicides. The only logical way to combine these categories is to assume that cases of attempted and committed suicide come from the same population or are characteristic of the same kinds of persons. This assumption infers that all degrees of self-destructive behavior are essentially attempts at suicide which differ only with respect to how "successful" they are. In other words, the suicidal behavior is regarded as continuous, and fatal attempts simply mark its terminal phase. The unsoundness of this assumption is indicated by a wide body of evidence that persons who attempt suicide do not come from the same population as those who commit suicide. Mintz (1964) conducted the only prevalence study of suicide attempts to be found in the literature. His results indicated that suicide attempters were younger (model age range 14–24) than completed suicides and the sex ratio for attempts was the reverse (females 3:1 over males) of the sex ratio associated with completed suicides. Shneidman and Farberow (1961) summarized the demographic distinctions between attempters and committers in Table 11-1.

On the basis of their investigation they concluded that attempted and committed suicides cannot be combined without masking some extremely important differences. Stengel (1964) also insists that data on attempters and committers should be clearly separated. He points

Table 11-1   Characteristics of Attempted and Committed Suicides.

Variables	Modal Attempter	Modal Committer
Sex	F	M
Age	20–30	40 plus
Method	barbiturates	gunshot
Reasons	marital or depression	ill health, marital or depression

Source: Adapted from Shneidman & Farberow, 1961, p. 44.

out that less than 10 percent of persons who attempt suicide later kill themselves and that many of the people who commit suicide do so on their first attempt. An important reason for distinguishing attempters from committers is that the problems of persons who survive attempted suicide offer the greatest challenge and hope for remedial action: First, for the obvious reason that these people have survived despite their suicidal behavior, but also because they outnumber committed suicides, especially in adolescence, by a ratio which has been estimated from 7:1 (Dublin, 1963) to as high as 50:1 (Jacobziner, 1960). The problem of suicide attempts is particularly significant in adolescence since it is reported that 12 percent of all the suicide attempts in this nation were made by adolescents, and that 90 percent of these attempts were made by adolescent girls (Balser & Masterson, 1959).

Some of the recent studies in progress (e.g. Peck & Schrut, 1967) demonstrate an increased awareness of the important differences manifested among varieties of self-destructive behavior and, in fact, are utilizing these distinctions for comparative study. In their current research on college-student suicide Peck & Schrut (1967) have divided their subjects into four groups: attempted, threatened, and committed suicides and a control group of non-suicidal individuals. Their design calls for comparisons among these four groups to determine differences in demographic factors, factual items, and life style.

Unfortunately, many of the studies encompassed in this review did not make such necessary distinctions. Most of the published studies were based upon suicide attempters (about one-fourth of them were based upon cases of committed suicide, a handful on threatened suicide and other forms of suicidal behavior). Nonetheless, of all the etiological factors presented in the following section, there was only one characteristic which was differentially assigned to one type of suicidal activity. That single characteristic was "social isolation." This determinant was generally attributed to cases of completed suicides but apparently was not seen to be as characteristic of suicide attempters or threateners. Except for this single instance, the causative, dynamic factors were applied to the entire range of suicidal behaviors. More often than not widely different suicidal behavior ranging from the "partial" suicide of a diabetic who disregarded medical dietary advice (Mason, 1954) to the suicide of an adolescent who killed himself by highly lethal means on his first attempt, was attributed to similar if not identical dynamics.

THEORIES OF SUICIDE

Another deficiency of most of the studies of adolescent suicide is the absence of a theoretical orientation from which testable hypotheses can be derived and verified. The absence is not surprising because no theories of suicide are directly based upon adolescent cases. With the possible exception of psychoanalytic theory, which does emphasize the importance of renewed libidinal impulses at puberty, the theories of suicide were derived from the study of adult cases. Little attention has been paid to the specific dynamics leading to youthful self-destruction.

In general, the various theoretical writings on suicide can be divided into two major categories: (1) those formulations where individual, psychodynamic determinants are emphasized and, (2) those in which sociocultural factors are accorded a dominant role.

The psychodynamic formulations fall into two main classifications: non-psychoanalytic and psychoanalytic. The non-psychoanalytic theories are widely diversified, ranging from the view that suicide is caused by a failure in adaptation (Crichton-Miller, 1931) to the idea that suicide is affected by climate (Mills, 1934). The psychoanalytic theories stress the importance of libidinal impulses, particularly dynamic, strongly aggressive impulses directed against an introjected object. Schneer and Kay (1962) specifically apply psychoanalytic formulations to describe the particular dynamics of adolescent suicide. They conceive of adolescent suicide as an immature means of coping with extensive Oedipal conflicts through renewal of infantile primary process thought and action.

Sociocultural theories of suicide place greatest emphasis upon dynamic interrelated social forces influencing the suicide rate. The most important of these formulations was developed by Durkheim (1897) who stated as a general rule that the suicide potential of a given society varied inversely to the degree of cohesion existing within that society. According to Durkheim, suicides could be classified into three types reflecting an individual's relationships and attachments within his social context. Three types of suicide he described were: (1) Anomic, where a poorly structured, normless society provided few ties for an individual; (2) Egoistic, wherein an individual was unwilling to accept the doctrine of his society and; (3) Altruistic, where an individual was too strongly identified with the traditions and mores of his social group. Gibbs and Martin (1964) likewise propose a theory based upon the durability and stability of social relationships and the degree to which different social statuses are successfully integrated by an individual. Paralleling Durkheim, they state as their major premise that the suicide rate of any population will vary inversely with the degree of such status integration. Henry and Short (1954) also employ a sociocultural frame of reference in relating suicide and homicide rates to shifts and trends in the economic business cycle.

These examples afford a brief description of the major theoretical orientations. The reader who wishes a discussion and review of the various theories of suicide is referred to the informative articles written by Jackson (1957) and Farberow (Farberow & Shneidman, 1961) on psychodynamic theories; Broom and Selznick (1958) and Sorokin (1947) for the sociocultural viewpoint on suicide.

ETIOLOGY—INDIVIDUAL DETERMINANTS

Genetic and Familial Tendencies

The literature records several references to families with a history of self-destruction (A family of suicides, 1901; Manganaro, 1957; Shapiro, 1935; Swanson, 1960). Since, in these cases, suicide seemed to "run in the family," it was speculated that a tendency to suicide may be inherited. However, this speculation has never been proven and there is no evidence that self-destructive tendencies can be transmitted genetically. The only studies specifically designed to examine the possibility of genetic influence were done by Kallmann (Kallmann & Anastasio, 1946; Kallmann, De Porte, De Porte, & Feingold, 1949). In these investigations, the case-histories of suicides occurring in sets of identical and fraternal twins (11 sets in the first study, 27 in the second) were compared. Kallmann found that suicidal behavior was not consistent among sets of twins even though they might be similar in personality or even when they were handicapped by comparable mental disorders. He concluded that there were no special hereditary traits predisposing a person to suicide. Instead, he reasoned that suicide was "the result of such a complex combination of motivational factors as to render a duplication of this unusual constellation very unlikely even in identical twin partners."

Puberty

There are indications that, at puberty, a sudden significant increase takes place in the number of suicide attempts. Puberty is also the stage of development where characteristic sex-specific differences in suicidal behavior become apparent (a male preponderance for completed suicide, a female preponderance for suicide attempts). This pubertal increase in suicidal activity has generally been linked to the "stress and strain" of adolescence, especially to conflicts over sexuality and dependency. As Gorceix (1963) points out, the adolescent is sexually mature but his environment does not accept this maturity. According to Schneer, *et al.* (1961), suicidal behavior in adolesence (either attempts or threats) may represent a cry for help in dealing with the problems of sexual identification and with associated libidinal and hostile impulses. A crisis in sexual identity is cited by several authors (Bigras, Gauthier, Bouchard, & Tassé, 1966; Schneer & Kay, 1962; Zilboorg, 1937) who propose that a failure in masculine or feminine identity, or concern about possible homosexual tendencies, may lead to serious suicide attempts. In a recent study, Peck (1967b) pointed out that many boys use their fathers' guns (symbolizing masculinity) to commit suicide. He found that if a boy has a father who places a premium on masculinity, commanding his son to "be a man," this directive may frequently have the opposite effect and lead to a weakening of his sense of masculine identity.

Even when sexual identification is adequate, the increased sexual impulses of adolescence, *per se*, may lead to anxiety, guilt, and frustration. Schrut (1967) as well as Winn and Halla (1966), concluded from their studies of adolescent girls that "guilt over sexual acting out" was a major factor precipitating their suicide attempts. Another example of the eroticization of suicide has been described by McClelland (1963) who proposed that there were persons (mostly women) who fantasied death as a lover—"a mysterious, dark figure who seduces and takes them away..." McClelland calls this feeling of excitement and anticipation, of "flirting with death," the "Harlequin complex." As such his findings would help to explain the greater preponderance of female suicide attempts, particularly among adolescent girls dealing with the renaissance of their sexual impulses. Increased sexual impulsivity may also be responsible for one very unusual and highly sexualized type of self-destruction. That is, the death by hanging of adolescent males acting out erotic fantasies. One of the earliest studies which mention this percular kind of death was published by Stearns (1953) who reported several cases of early-adolescent males who had hanged themselves while dressed in female clothing, in some cases with their feet and hands bound up as well. He made no attempt to explain this phenomenon but regarded it as a case of "probable" suicide. Similar cases where young men hanged themselves while engaging in transvestite activity were also mentioned by Ford (1957); Litman, Curphey, Shneidman, Farberow & Tabachnik (1963); Mulcock (1955); Shankel and Carr (1956). All these instances involved young males who died during autoerotic or transvestite activity. Precautions were frequently taken to avoid disfigurement (e.g. a towel placed around the neck to prevent rope burns). The repetitive history of this unusual activity led these investigators to regard such deaths as accidents caused by excessive eroticized "risk-taking" rather than as clear-cut cases of suicide.

Mental Disorder

The two mental disorders most frequently linked to suicide are depressive states and schizophrenic reactions. However, there are no modern writers who contend that mental disorder is either a necessary or sufficient cause of suicide.

Depression In the clinical evaluation of suicide potential, the role of depression has always been considered important. But, recent studies indicate that depression defined by internalized aggression and self-hatred may not be as important a factor in younger age groups as it is in cases of adult suicide.

If a pathological state of depression occurs in a young person it is usually associated with the loss of a love-object either through death or separation. For example, after the death of a parent, impairment of ego-functioning, coupled with a feeling of helplessness, has been observed. This combination of symptoms may lead to a serious suicide attempt as a means of regaining contact with the lost love-object (Faigel, 1966; Schechter, 1957; Toolan, 1962). Paradoxically the critical period for suicidal behavior does not seem to be during the depressive reaction but shortly after the depression lifts. Apparently a patient's mood may improve chiefly because he has resolved his conflict by making definite plans for his own destruction. Some recent studies (Cerny & Cerna, 1962; Lawler, *et al.*, 1963) found depression to be characteristic of half the young people who attempted suicide. Contrary results were reported by Lourie (1966) who stated that younger children making suicide attempts revealed no depression in the usual adult sense. He suggested that it was not until late adolescence that the clinical picture of depression appears as a prime factor. Likewise, Balser and Masterson (1959) concluded that depression was not important among adolescent suicide attempters. They were joined in their dissent by Winn and Halla (1966) who were similarly skeptical as to the importance of depression in children who threatened suicide.

In brief, if depression is simply and circularly defined as normal grief over the loss of significant relationships, then children and adolescents can be considered depressed. On the other hand, if depression is defined as a syndrome characterized by feelings of guilt, worthlessness and pessimism, then such symptoms would not appear to be as characteristic of youthful suicides as they are of adults.

Schizophrenic reactions   Response to auditory hallucinations or commands may sometimes be the cause of serious suicide attempts among young people (Lawler, *et al.*, 1963; Toolan, 1962). The combination of a rich fantasy life coupled with limited environmental interaction has been proposed as the factor which produces these suicidal hallucinations (Lawler, *et al.*, 1963).

Winn and Halla (1966) diagnosed childhood schizophrenia in 70 percent of the threatened or attempted suicides in their study. Fifty percent of the attempters experienced hallucinations telling them to kill themselves; all of the adolescent boys in their study described "command" hallucinations. Balser and Masterson (1959) found that 23 of 37 adolescent suicide attempters had been diagnosed as schizophrenic, with specific pathology which included dissociation, hallucinations, delusional ideas, withdrawal, suspiciousness, and lack of communicability. These investigators concluded that schizophrenic reactions bear a closer relationship to suicidal tendencies in adolescents than does depression. Maria (1962) supports this hypothesis with his observation that in cases of completed suicides, schizophrenia ia diagnosed more frequently in childhood and adolescent cases than it is in adult cases.

Identification, Imitation, Suggestion

Studies of suicide and suicidal behavior have found that children may imitate the actions or follow the suggestions of people close to them who have died, attempted suicide, are preoccupied by suicidal thoughts, or who openly reveal death wishes toward them.

Death may mean to the child a chance for reunion with a loved one, and there are instances where a child has attempted, through suicide, to join a beloved brother, sister, or parent—or even a favorite pet. In his study of children's reaction to the death of a parent, Keeler (1954) reported fantasies of reunion with the dead parent were present in eight of eleven children and that suicidal preoccupations and attempts in six of these children seem to represent an identification with the dead parent and a wish to be reunited.

Lourie (1966) cited identification (or imitation) as an important dynamic factor for the younger children in his study. A suicide or suicide attempt by a family member may lead the young child to copy his example, even insofar as making the same choice of weapon. Bender and Schilder (1937) suggested that a deep attachment to a mother or father with suicidal preoccupations may spur suicidal preoccupations in a child. Schrut (1964) stated that a young child does not clearly differentiate his identity from that of his mother. If the mother harbors feelings of self-hatred and helplessness, the child may also harbor these same feelings. The opposite case, where lack of identification plays a part in suicidal behavior, was reported by Fowler (1949) on the basis of her work with suicidal children. She cited problems in primary family relationships where the parents provided poor models for the child to identify with as important determinants of suicidal activity.

A child's capacity for responding to suggestion may contribute to suicidal tendencies. Children who are openly rejected by a parent, or whose parents are frequently hostile toward them may respond to these "death wishes" with a suicide attempt. In their study of children who had threatened or attempted suicide, Winn and Halla (1966) found that over 50 percent of the children had experienced hallucinations directing them to kill themselves. Lawler, *et al.* (1963) described these auditory hallucinations as "hearing a voice, speaking in a critical manner, telling [the child] to kill himself." Occasionally, epidemics of suicides among school children have been recorded. These, too, seem to be at least partly motivated by suggestion and imitation.

It is doubtful whether any very young (under age 9) children actually intend to die. Because of their incompletely developed concept of death, any type of threat or attempt by children is particularly dangerous. If a child does not fully anticipate that he may indeed kill himself, his choice of method (jumping from a window, leaping into a river, or running in front of a car or train) may not leave him any of the chances for rescue which characterize the suicide attempt made in later adolescence.

Death Concept

Integrally connected to suicide is an individual's conception of death. To understand why a person takes his own life, we must also understand what death means to that person. Suicide in the young is particularly tragic since they frequently do not seem realistically aware of their own mortality. Winn and Halla (1966) found that young children often attach as much significance to stealing from their mother's purse as they do to a threat to kill themselves. Paradoxically, a child may wish to kill himself but not to die. That is, death is simply and tragically equated to running away or escaping from an unbearable situation. Without the realization that death is final, a child measures his own life's value with a defective yardstick. While young children do not lack a conception of death, their death concept is qualitatively different and frequently distorted when compared to that of a mature adult. A more realistic concept of death seems to emerge in a predictable, developmental sequence which corresponds to chronological age.

The earliest empirical investigation of this topic was conducted by Schilder and Wechsler (1934). Their findings indicated that even a child who was preoccupied with fantasies of death and violence did not really believe in the possibility of his own destruction. Similarly, Bender and Schilder (1937) believed that a child conceived of death as reversible and temporary. Supposedly, a child has this concept because of his difficulty in distinguishing between reality and unreality. Geisler (1953) emphasized the ambivalence of childhood fantasies of suicide which might be violent and motivated by aggressive-sadistic impulses, but also by a desire not to cease existing but to return to a more peaceful existence.

Nagy (1959) published a definitive study of the developmental sequence of children's death concepts. On the basis of compositions, drawings, and discussions collected from children (ages 3–10), she was able to formulate three major developmental stages: Stage 1 (under 5 years) is characterized by a denial of death. Death is seen as separation or similar to sleep and as gradual or temporary. Stage 2 (ages 5–9 years) is where the child reifies and personifies death. Death is imagined as a separate person or is identified with those already deceased. The existence of death at this stage is accepted but averted. At Stage 3 (age 9 years and older) a child begins to realize that death means a final cessation of bodily activities. This general developmental sequence was confirmed by Lourie (1966). Moreover, he pointed out that among the school age children he studied a frequent awareness of death was expressed in their thoughts and even in wishes for their own death. This awareness was evident not only among 70 percent of the children with emotional problems but among 54 percent of the normal school-age population. Rochlin (1965) also indicated that children are quite concerned with death. He disagrees with other writers in maintaining that by as early as age 3 or 4 a child is aware of his own morality. It is for this reason, says Rochlin, that a child sees death as temporary or reversible—to defend himself against an overwhelming fear of his own demise. In this regard he agrees with Ackerly (1967) who also sees the childhood belief in the reversibility of death as a defensive maneuver. In a study comparing different age groups, Alexander and Alderstein (1958) measured emotional responses to the idea of death using word-association tasks. They concluded that the concept of death had greatest emotional significance in young children (5–8 years) and adolescents (13–16 years) as compared to the latency age (9–12 years) child. This discrepancy was attributed to the observation that social roles and self-concepts in the latency age child were more well defined than they were in the other two groups. Death attitudes among adolescents were specifically studied by Kastenbaum (1959). He concluded that the adolescent lived in an intense "present" and paid little attention to such distant future concepts as death. When adolescents did regard the remote future they saw it as risky, unpleasant and devoid of significant value. The findings of Alexander and Alderstein and of Kastenbaum seem to indicate that the concept of death achieves a renewed emotional significance in adolescence but that it is handled by displacement or denial in a manner characteristic of much younger children. Denial of death fears by suicidal adolescents has also been cited by Lester (1967) who developed a scale to measure the fear of death. He concluded that suicidal adolescents feared death less than did their non-suicidal adolescent counterparts. These observations are additionally confirmed by the work of Speigel and Neuringer (1963). Through a detailed study of suicide notes they concluded that normal feelings of dreading death were inhibited as a necessary precondition for suicidal activity.

Aggression

All types of suicidal behavior in young children—whether threats, attempts, or completed suicide—have been customarily explained as displacement of frustrated aggression which becomes self-directed (Bender & Schilder, 1937). However, Stengel (1964) argues that aggression directed toward others, not oneself, is more typical of the suicide attempter. He believes that this means of directing aggression is an important difference which distinguishes suicide attempts from cases of completed suicide.

The particular dynamic relationship between aggression and suicide stems from the belief that direct expressions of hostility or rage—usually provoked by disappointments or deprivation of love—are thwarted (Moss & Hamilton, 1956) and are turned inward for several reasons: (1) The motive of spite or revenge is predominant. Faigel (1966) stated that the desire to punish others who will grieve at their death was one of the most frequent motives to suicide in young children. An angry child, powerless to punish or manipulate his parents directly, may take his revenge through an attempt at self-destruction. Zilboorg (1937) found that spite was a frequent motivation to suicide among primitive people. He suggested that it was a typical and universal reaction. (2) A child may become overwhelmed with guilt, fear, or anxiety about his feelings of hostility, and then direct his aggression against himself (Moss & Hamilton, 1956).

Spite, Revenge, or Manipulation

An almost universal fantasy among children is "If I die, then my parents will feel sorry." Hall (1904) suggested that such desires to punish others were a frequent motive to suicide in young children. Research by Lourie (1966), Bender and Schilder (1937) and Faigel (1966) supported this conclusion. They found that revenge or spite toward a parent was one of the most frequent reasons given by young children for their suicidal behavior. In particular, Lourie maintained that the ultimate goal a child hoped to achieve was the love and attention of the parents while Bender and Schilder declared that suicide threats were frequently used by a youngster to assert his independence.

According to Lawler, *et al.* (1963), these manipulative attempts were not likely to result in death except through miscalculation.

Impulsivity

Suicide threats and attempts are often attributed to the greater impulsiveness of youth. As such, this impulsivity is considered to be the necessary component which translates youthful suicidal thoughts into actions.

Winn and Halla (1966) designated impulsivity as a prominent feature in the personality of a child and noted its existence in two-thirds of their cases of children who threatened suicide. Lawler, *et al.* (1963) described the children in their study of attempts as possessing a rich fantasy life leading to little environmental interaction. This combination, they stated, leads to a control by inner impulses sometimes resulting in self-destructive action.

Lourie (1966) concluded from his study of childhood attempters that the vast majority of these children had impulse control problems. Although most of the children had no particular preoccupation with self-destruction, they came from a cultural setting which encouraged or even stimulated general impulsivity. He suggested that the attempts were "mostly based on the pressure of the moment in an individual with relatively poor impulse control." But he also noted that despite their immediate problems of impulsivity, these children had a chronic history of long-standing problems.

Jacobziner (1960) reported that the high incidence of attempts among adolescent girls is "probably due to the greater impulsivity of the young female, who does not premeditate the act . . . it is, in the main, a precipitous impulsive act, a sudden reaction to a stressful situation." In their study of suicide attemps in Sweden, Bergstrand and Otto (1962) likewise concluded that for most adolescent girls, suicidal attempts seem to be impulsive acts connected with small problems.

A strong note of disagreement with these conclusions was reached by Teicher and Jacobs (1966a). They argue with the idea that suicide attempts are impulsive and precipitated by some trivial, isolated problem. Rather, they suggest that a longitudinal view of a person's total life history demonstrates that "the suicide attempt is considered in advance and is . . . from the conscious perspective of the suicide attempter . . . weighed rationally against other alternatives." In other words, the suicide attempt is not really an impulsive, spur-of-the-moment decision but an end-phase to a long history of problems in adjustment.

Drugs

Of all the "psychedelic" drugs currently popular among the youthful generation, LSD has been most frequently linked with suicide. There has been a great deal of heat, particularly by the mass media, but relatively little light, beamed on this subject. According to Cohen (1967), LSD can be related to suicide in the following ways:

Accidental   Where, under the influence of hallucination or delusion, a subject embarks upon an act which leads to his destruction. Examples: the delusion that one has the ability to fly, hallucinations that cars on highways are toys which can be picked up in motion. In this category, there is no true suicidal intent as such.

Exacerbation of suicide proneness   Cases where suicidal thought has taken place before ingestion and the LSD experience intensified such wishes. This condition can lead to:

1. suicide attempts under LSD or;
2. suicide attempts after the "trip."

Intrusion of suicidal ideas   [Occurs] in "normal" individuals, usually as a result of a panic state in an individual who has not previously thought of suicide. Under LSD, dissociation of body or thoughts that a "bad trip" will never end can take place. These ideas might result in suicidal attempts made during a drug-induced state of agitated depression.

Suicide as a result of LSD-induced fantasy   These are miscellaneous cases where a subject may sense his death is necessary for altruistic reasons. This type of suicide is sometimes associated with a person's feelings of guilt and his conviction that he "must die to save the world."

Flashback suicide   These are cases where LSD effects recur without the drug-magnifying or distorting psychopathology or depression. Panic is intensified by a confusion over what brought the episode on and whether or not it can be ended. Attempts at suicide in this state may be marked by the same motivation to escape psychic pain that occurs in the drugged state.

In these LSD-related suicides there does not seem to be any underlying depression, rather, the main precipitant is an overwhelming emotional experience beyond an individual's control; an experience which can be exacerbated by suggestibility factors when the drug is taken in social groupings. At this stage the psychopharmacology is still not clear, but it seems reasonable to conclude that LSD may act to catalyze underlying conflicts and emotions including suicidal predispositions and to disorient a person to such a degree that his self-destructive potential (lethality) is increased.

It is unclear whether these LSD suicides are really intentional. Shneidman (1963) considers such individuals to be what he calls "psyche-experimenters." Their motivation is not to die but to be in a perceptually altered and befogged state. They wish to remain conscious and alive but benumbed and drugged. Accordingly they may experiment with dosages, sometimes with fatal consequences but this type of death is traditionally considered to be accidental.

While there is scanty evidence of a direct causal connection between adolescent drug usage and suicide, there have been some anecdotal speculations concerning the observed association. Trautman (1966) reports a case study in which drug abuse and an attempt at suicide were viewed as complementary means of escaping an "unbearable family situation." Schonfeld (1967) blames our affluent society which emphasizes immediate rewards, not allowing adolescents to become tolerant of frustration. Subsequently, he writes, when faced with difficulties, they become overwhelmed and turn to escapist measures such as drugs, withdrawal and suicide.

ETIOLOGY—SOCIAL DETERMINANTS

Family Relationships

Family relationships are particularly important in the etiology of adolescent suicide. Not only because the family represents the most viable social unit in our society, but because of the significance of family relationships in the life of the young. Hardly any studies have investigated the protective values of a favorable family environment; instead, most studies have emphasized sibling position, family disorganization, loss, and types of destructive parent-child relationships which lead to suicidal behavior.

Sibling order   Kallmann, *et al.* (1949) observed in their studies that the suicide rate of only children did not differ significantly from that of the general population. Several recent investigators, however, have suggested that a child's sibling position may be related to his suicidal behavior. Toolan (1962) found that 49 of 102 adolescent suicide attempters were first-born children. Lester (1966) compared Toolan's statistics on sibling positions with data from the New York City population. He confirmed that the distribution of sibling positions in Toolan's samples—especially the high number of first-borns—differed significantly from the expected distribution.

Another group of investigators (Lawler, *et al.*, 1963) concluded from their study of suicide attempts that a disproportionate number of suicidal children occupy special sibling positions. Fourteen of the 22 children in their study occupied special positions (three only children, seven first-born, four youngest), but the sample was too small for adequately reliable conclusions. Lester recently (1966) re-examined the relationship between sibling position and suicidal behavior. He reasoned that suicide attempts might express an affiliative tendency to communicate with significant others. Noting that such affiliative tendencies are strongest in first-born and only children, Lester predicted an overrepresentation of first-born and only children attempting suicide. His data did not bear out the hypothesized relationship.

Family disorganization   A significant number of young people who commit or attempt to commit suicide have a history of broken or disorganized homes. A correlation between broken homes and suicide has been noted not only in the United States but has been observed throughout the world by investigators in such countries as Canada (Bigras, *et al.*, 1966); Japan (Iga, 1966); Germany (Zumpe, 1959); France (Porot, *et al.*, 1965; Zimbacca, 1965); England (Mulcock, 1955); and Sweden (Bergstrand & Otto, 1962).

But Stengel (1964) injects a note of controversy by pointing out that the definition of "broken home" varies greatly in the discussions of different authors. To some it means lack of at least one parent. Others seem to include all forms of family disorganization, including severe parental discord or extreme family conflict.

However it is generally agreed that the motives for suicide in children cannot be fully understood without carefully considering their family situations. Most young people who

exhibit suicidal behavior seem to come from homes with grossly disturbed family relationships. Frequently these family problems constitute the dominant motivations provoking the
suicidal behavior.)

In study after study, the home lives of suicidal children have been characterized as
disruptive or chaotic. Their histories generally include several of the following indices of
family disruption: (1) Frequent moving from one neighborhood or city to another, with
many changes of school; (2) family estrangement because of quarreling between parents or
between parent(s) and child; (3) great financial difficulties and impoverishment; (4) sibling
conflict; (5) illegitimate children; (6) paternal or maternal absence; (7) conflict with step-
parent(s); (8) cruelty, rejection, or abandonment by parent(s); (9) institutionalization of
adolescent or family member (hospital, jail, reformatory, etc.); (10) suicide attempts by
parents; and (11) alcoholic parents.

Such poor family life has been hypothesized to lead to the following conflicts: A fear or
knowledge of being unloved; fear of harsh punishment; desire to escape from intolerable
conditions; lack of meaningful relationships, creation of guilt; spite; depression; loneliness;
hostility; conflict; anxiety; and other affective states, any of which can predispose a child to
many forms of anti-social behavior. This consequent anti-social behavior may range from
stealing, fire-setting, running away, sexual promiscuity, to other forms of juvenile delinquency or, in some youngsters, to suicide.

Despite the general agreement that broken homes are causally related to youthful
suicide, a critical view is taken by Jacobs and Teicher (1967) who contend that any valid
analysis must place "broken homes" into the context of an adolescent's total life history. In
their study of adolescent suicide attempts, they found that broken homes *per se* were not
distinctively precursive of suicidal behavior. Both their suicidal and non-suicidal control
groups demonstrated similarly high percentages of broken homes. The real distinction was
that the control group had experienced a stable home life *during the preceding five years*
while the suicide attempter group had not.

Loss The loss of a parent or other loved one (through death, divorce, or prolonged separation) seems to have several significant influences affecting suicidal behavior in children.
First, a loss through death may lead to a desire for reunion with the lost loved one. A young
child may therefore attempt suicide in order to rejoin his dead parent, sibling (or even a
favorite cat), yet not intend to die permanently. An older child or adolescent who believes
in the existence of an afterlife may make a serious attempt at suicide in order to rejoin a
parent, sibling, or friend.

The death of significant persons in the child's life can also stimulate suicidal activity in
other ways:

1. Parental suicide may lead a young child to copy his parent's example.
2. A child may blame himself for the death of his parent and be driven by this guilt to
   make a serious suicide attempt.
3. A child may be predisposed to suicide in later life through parental loss in childhood.

Zilboorg (1937) suggested that "when a boy or girl loses a father, brother, or sister at a
time when he or she is at the height of their Oedipus complex, or transition to puberty,
there is . . . a true danger to suicide." Several studies support the conclusion that the death
of a parent early in a child's life may contribute to his later suicide-susceptibility. Dorpat,
Jackson, and Ripley (1965) studied 114 completed suicides and 121 attempted suicides.
They found that the death of a parent was highest for completed suicides, and concluded

from this that unresolved object-loss in childhood leads to an inability to sustain object-loss in later life. Bruhn (1962) compared a group of attempted suicides against a control group without suicidal tendencies. The group of suicide attempters was distinguished by the lack of both parental figures or had experienced the absence or death of a family member. Similar results were reported by Greer (1964) who found that the incidence of parental loss was higher in suicidal than non-suicidal persons. Paffenbarger and Asnes (1966) discovered that death or absence of the father was the major precursor of suicide among college males. Another consequence of paternal loss or absence is that the mother may be cast in the role of chief disciplinarian. According to Henry (1960), this type of family role structure is associated with children's tendencies toward self-blame. And since the turning of blame inwards has been related to suicide, this type of family structure may predispose children toward suicide.

Again an iconoclastic note is sounded by Jacobs and Teicher (1967), who argue against a simple unitary relationship between loss and suicide. Their research compared the life histories of 50 adolescent suicide attempters with those of 32 control adolescents. Both the suicide attempters and control adolescents had high rates of parental loss in childhood. One group attempted suicide; the other did not. Obviously it was not simply parental loss in childhood which predisposed some subjects to depression and suicides in later life. They concluded that:

> loss of love-object is an important aspect of the process, but it must be viewed as part of a process where particular attention is paid to when it occurred and/or recurred, and not merely to its pressence or absence. Furthermore, it seens that it is not the loss of a love-object *per se* that is so distressing but the loss of love.

4. A child who suffers the loss of a love-object may be predisposed to states of depression linked with suicidal tendencies (Lawler, *et al.*, 1963). The common denominator in all youthful depression is considered to be the loss of the love-object. When this loss occurs to young children it can lead to difficulty in forming the object-relationships required for healthy emotional development. When the loss occurs during adolescence it does not block the development of object-relationships since the critical years for this development are passed. On the other hand, it can cause an adolescent to hate the love-object, who he feels has betrayed and deserted him (Toolan, 1962).

5. Adolescent girls, who make up approximately three-fourths or more of all adolescent suicide attempts, may be especially vulnerable to loss of a father. Lack of a father is frequently noted in their histories and some writers hypothesize that paternal deprivation plays a significant part in the suicidal attempt of young girls (Bigras, *et al.*, 1966; Gorceix, 1963; Toolan, 1962; Zimbacca, 1965).

6. Other forms of love-object losses have also appeared to be significant influences leading to youthful suicide. They include:

(a) Loss of close friends through repeated school transfers (Lawler, *et al.*, 1963).

(b) Loss of older siblings through marriage, college, Army, or moving (Teicher & Jacobs, 1966a).

(c) Loss of boy-friend or girl-friend, where this love-object has become a substitute for a dependency upon the parent (Peck, 1967a).

(d) Loss felt by freshmen at college—a kind of homesickness which overcomes the youngster when he finds himself alone and his dependency needs acutely unsatisfied (Peck, 1967a).

Social Isolation

Of all the psychodynamic attributes associated with suicidal behavior, the factor of human isolation and withdrawal appears to be the most effective in distinguishing those who will kill themselves from those who will not. While withdrawal and alienation can be important determinants of many types of suicidal behavior, they seem to characterize cases of completed suicides rather than suicide attempts or threats.

Jan-Tausch (n.d.) studied New Jersey school children and reported that "in every case of suicide, ... the child [had] no close friends with whom he might share confidences or from whom he received psychological support." The critical difference between attempters who "failed" and those who "succeeded" was that those who failed had a relationship with "someone to whom they felt close." Jan-Tausch goes on to suggest:

> the individual has either withdrawn to the point where he can no longer identify with any person or idea, or (he) sees himself as rejected by all about him and is unable to establish a close supportive relationship with any other individual.

Reese (1966) also investigated school-age suicides and found chronic social isolation to be the single most striking feature of this group. He reported that these youngsters had such a marked lack of involvement with other students or teachers that they were literally "unknown" in their own classrooms. Social isolation was also regarded as a major prodromal sign for college suicides many of whom were described as "terribly shy, virtually friendless individuals, alienated from all but the most minimal interactions" (Seiden, 1966).

Various reasons have been assigned to explain this state of isolation. Stengel (1964) maintains that "lack of secure relationship to a parent figure in childhood may have lasting consequences for a person's ability to establish relationships with other people. Such individuals are likely to find themselves socially isolated in adult life, and social isolation is one of the most important causal factors in the causation of suicidal acts." Schrut (1967) states that, for adolescent females, isolation is a gradual process which takes place over a long period. This process of isolation has also been associated with progressive family conflict which becomes increasingly more severe. He reported that the adolescent female suicide attempter in his studies "characteristically saw herself as being subjected to an unjust, demanding, and often irreconcilable isolation with a typical, chronically progressive, diminution of receptive inter-familial communication." After an adolescent becomes estranged from her parents, she relies upon a boy-friend to become the substitute parental image. A fight with the boy-friend is frequently the final blow and becomes the precipitating factor in her suicide attempt. Jacobs and Teicher (1967) concur with this analysis, adding that suicidal adolescents usually have numerous and serious problems which progressively isolate them. These authors describe a similar chain-reaction of conflicts isolating an adolescent from meaningful social relationships and frequently leading to a suicide attempt: A long period of extreme conflict between an adolescent girl and her parent(s) eventually leads to parent-child alienation; the adolescent girl frequently seeks to re-establish a meaningful relationship through a romance with a boy-friend. During this time she alienates all other friends by concentrating all her time and energy on her boy-friend. When the romance fails, she finds herself isolated from all "significant others," and the possibility of a suicide attempt is likely. The importance of an active social life is emphasized in the research of Barter, *et al.* (1968) where peer group relations were considered an important barrier to suicide attempts. They note that even though the nuclear family life might remain quite disorganized, when the adolescent has an active social life the prognosis is favorable. Additional support for the significance of good peer-group relations can be found in the research of Harlow and Harlow (1966) in their continuing studies of affective relationships among lower[primate] animals.

Communication

Closely related to feelings of social isolation are problems in communicating with others—difficulties which are characteristic of many suicidal individuals. In some cases the suicidal act itself is a form of communication, a desperate "cry for help." In other cases, an individual may attempt suicide because of the loneliness and despair growing out of his failure to communicate.

In many cases of attempted or threatened suicide, self-destruction may not be the dominant purpose. That is, some suicidal activities are distinguished by features which are not entirely compatible with the purpose of self-destruction: Some suicide attempters give warning of their intention (allowing for preventive action) or the attempts are carried out in a setting which makes intervention by others possible or probable (allowing for rescue). Stengel (1964) calls these attempts "Janus-faced," because they are directed toward destruction, but at the same time toward human contact and life. He believes they are really alarm signals which should be regarded as appeals for help. They should be treated as highly emotional types of communication which are different in style and content from the usual kinds of communication. A recent study by Darbonne (1967) investigating this point, indicated that the communication style of suicidal individuals was distinctively different from the non-suicidal individuals.

A large portion of the suicidal behavior of adolescent girls seems to fall into the category of communication attempts. Stengel (1964) thinks these young girls use suicidal threats and acts as appeals to the environment more frequently than males, and that females seem inclined to use the suicidal act as an aggressive manipulative device more often than males.

Why do adolescents resort to this dangerous method of gaining attention and response? Lourie (1966) indicates that they drag with them, into adolescence, poor, distorted answers to the problems of earlier development (i.e. what to do with agression, how to get attention, etc.). Peck (1967b) commented:

> We must . . . wonder at the condition of poverty of one's inner resources, when suicidal behavior becomes one's sole means of obtaining that attention.

But he goes on to state that these young people are not to be shrugged off merely as attention-seeking, manipulating youngsters, but should be regarded as unhappy, helpless, hopeless young people who are apparently unable to change things in more constructive ways.

These attempts to communicate through suicidal behavior may have two outcomes: change or further impasse. On a hopeful note Peck reports:

> . . . when the kinds of problems that underlie a suicidal behavior are appropriately confronted . . . suicidal behavior often disappears as a coping mechanism.

Yet a high percentage of these attempts do not result in improved conditions and when they do not they sometimes end in suicide. Peck (1967a) states that if the communications go unheeded, they become louder and more lethal, and the consequences, regardless of how nonlethally intended, may be disastrous. The possibility of tragic consequences is also confirmed by Teicher and Jacobs (1966a) who similarly observed:

> More often than not adolescents who adopt the drastic measure of an attempt as an attention-getting device find that this too fails . . . (and) the adolescent is then convinced . . . that death is the only solution to what appears to him as the chronic problem of living.

Socio-economic Status

The relationship between socio-economic factors and youthful suicide is, in general, similar to that of adult suicides. That is, suicides are highest in times of economic depression and lowest during periods of war. However, social upheavels do not seem to affect the suicide rate of the young as much as the rate of adults. The factors predisposing to youthful suicide appear to be much more related to home, family, and school life. Poverty has been associated with suicide and so has wealth but on balance there is no real evidence to suggest that suicide is more frequent among the rich or the poor. As Shneidman and Farberow (1961) pointed out, the distribution is very "democratic" and represented proportionately among all levels of society. Nevertheless, suicide is most prevalent in the transitional sections of a community, which are usually impoverished and run-down areas. Sainsbury (1955) has reported that low income by itself does not lead to high suicide rates. In his ecological studies, he discovered that it was the poor stability of a neighborhood not its poverty which accounted for the high rate of suicide.

Religion

There is little reliable evidence to relate religion specifically to suicide. Among the three major religions in this country, the suicide rate is highest among Protestants, lowest among Catholics. Durkheim (1897) proposed that the higher rate among Protestants was because Protestantism had less social intergration and consistency than did Catholicism and therefore the Protestant church had a less moderating effect upon suicides of its members. On the other side of the coin, it is possible that Catholic suicides may frequently be concealed because of religious and social pressures. History indicates that religion has both moderated and facilitated suicidal activity. For example, the history of the Jews is replete with instances of mass suicides which occurred as a consequence of persecution and discrimination. There are also cases of individuals caught up in a religious frenzy or motivated to achieve religious martyrdom through self-immolation.

Simplistic attempts to relate suicide to unitary religious dimensions, e.g. Catholic, Protestant and Jewish, are merely exercises in futility. Questions of religious affiliation do not get at the critical variables influencing suicide. The important unanswered questions concerning religion and suicide were delineated by Shneidman (1964):

> What would seem to be needed would be studies relating self-destructive behaviors to the operational features of religious beliefs; including a detailed explication of the subject's present belief system in relation to an omnipotent God, the efficacy of prayer, the existence of an hereafter, the possibility of reunion with departed loved ones, etc.

Education—The Special Case of Student Suicide

The subject of student suicide appears throughout the 20th century literature; however, the first thorough study of suicide on United States campuses dates back only 30 years (Raphael, Power & Berridge, 1937). Stimulated by the fact that suicides accounted for over half the deaths at the University of Michigan, Raphael and his colleagues investigated the role and function of the university mental hygiene unit in dealing with this problem. Later research on college suicide described the suicide problem at Yale (Parrish, 1957), Cornell (Braaten & Darling, 1962), and Harvard (Temby, 1961). The results of these studies indicated that the suicide problem was substantial and implied that the risk of suicide was greater for students than for their non-academic peers. In addition, these authors attempted to identify the factors which predisposed students to suicide and to offer suggestions for its prevention. (These earlier studies were almost entirely descriptive, and while they did provide informative insights they failed to provide control groups for a baseline against which the validity of their findings could be assessed.) This situation was remedied by later studies (Bruyn & Seiden, 1965; Seiden, 1966) which applied the necessary principle of adequate control or comparison groups to answer two basic questions: (1) Are students at greater risk of suicide than non-students? (2) How do suicidal students differ from their non-suicidal classmates?

Students vs. non-students   Studies by Temby (1961) and Parrish (1957) indicated that students were more suicidal than non-students. Temby reported a suicide rate of 15 per 100,000 at Harvard, and Parrish's work indicated a suicide rate of 14 per 100,000 at Yale. Both of these rates are well in excess of the expected suicide rate for this population (7 to 10 per 100,000). A series of studies in English universities also led to the conclusion that students were more suicidal than their non-academic age peers. Parnell (1951) published a detailed analysis of suicides at Oxford University comparing deaths due to suicide among Oxford students to those in the population at large. He found that the suicide rate was approximately 12 times as great for Oxford students (59.4:5.0). Carpenter (1959), after reviewing cases of suicide among Cambridge undergraduates, also concluded that the rate of [male] students was higher than for comparable groups. Two years later Lyman (1961) investigated suicides at Oxford University comparing the incidence at various British schools. Her data are summarized in Table 11.2.

To test whether the same relationship held in American universities, Bruyn and Seiden (1965) investigated the incidence of suicide among college students at the University of California, Berkeley campus (UCB) and contrasted this incidence with the figures for comparable age groups in the California population. During the 10-year period they studied (1952–1961) there were 23 student suicides whereas only 13 suicides would be expected if the general population rates held. They concluded that the suicide rate among students was significantly greater than for a comparable group of age cohorts. In addition, they found that the general mortality experience [deaths due to all causes] was significantly lower for students when contrasted to a comparable group of age peers.

Table 11.2   Suicide Rates of British Universities.

Populations	Annual Suicide Rate per 100,000 Population Ages 20 to 24
England and Wales	4.1
Oxford University	26.4
Cambridge University	21.3
University of London	16.3
Seven unnamed British universities	5.9

Source: Lyman, 1961, p. 219.

There is one study which indicates lower suicide incidence among [male Finnish University] students, when compared to the general population (Idanpann-Hekkila, *et al.*, 1967). Barring this exception, the general rule obtains that students are at greater risk of suicide than their non-student peers.

Suicidal students vs. non-suicidal classmates   This question was investigated by Seiden (1966) who compared students at the University of California, Berkeley (UCB) who committed suicide during the 10-year period, 1952 through 1961, with the entire UCB student body population during this same decade. The main findings of this research were:

> Suicidal students could be significantly differentiated from their classmates on the variables of age, class standing, major subject, nationality, emotional condition, and academic achievement. Compared to the student population at large, the suicidal group was older, contained greater proportions of graduates, language majors, and foreign students, and gave more indications of emotional disturbance. In addition, the undergraduate suicides fared much better than their fellow students in matters of academic achievement.

Another study which distinguished between suicidal and non-suicidal students was published by Paffenbarger and Asnes (1966). Using the college records of 40,000 former students at the Universities of Pennsylvania and Harvard, they examined the records for characteristics precursive of eventual suicide. Early loss of or absence of the father was found to be the dominant distinguishing characteristic in cases of male suicide.

The effects of school success or failure   There is some disagreement about the importance of school success in relation to suicide. This has been a recurrent question over many years. One of the most famous discussions of the Vienna Psychoanalytical Society was held in 1910 to deal with the specific problem of suicide among students. The Teutonic school system was the target of much public criticism and members of the Viennese psychoanalytic group, including Freud, Adler, Stekel, *et al.*, applied the newly developed insights of dynamic psychology and psychoanalysis to this controversy. A ... translation (Friedman, 1967) of this classic symposium provides an extremely interesting historical and theoretical contribution to the literature.

In more recent times Otto (1965) examined 62 cases where public school problems were indicated as a provoking cause of suicidal attempts. He found that the school problems, when compared to other difficulties, were factors of relatively slight importance. However, Reese (1966), studying public-school-age suicides to assess the effects of the school environment, found that half of the subjects were doing failing work at the time of their suicide.

Reese's study was the only research which showed a relationship between low I.Q. and suicide. He found that in 25 percent of those cases where the I.Q. was available, the scores were borderline or below. In contrast, other studies by various authors have indicated that suicidal adolescents have invariably been of average or better than average intelligence. With college students, the factor of intellectual competence has been characteristically greater in the suicidal students than in their non-suicidal classmates (Seiden, 1966). Students who committed suicide had higher grade point averages (3.18 as opposed to 2.50) and a greater proportion of them had won scholastic awards (58 percent as opposed to 5 percent). The transcripts of these students would indicate that they had done splendidly in their academic pursuits. However, reports from family and friends revealed that these students were never secure despite their high grades. Characteristically, they were filled with doubts of their adequacy, dissatisfied with their grades, and despondent over their general academic aptitude. This propensity for some brilliant academic students to feel that they achieved their eminence by specious means was also reported by Munter (1966) who called this syndrome the "Fraud Complex" and indicated that it was a frequent cause of depression among students.

Suicidal students or academic stress?   A pivotal question is whether students are at greater risk of suicide because they are initially more suicidal than non-students or because the school environment makes them more susceptible. Is the higher student rate due to selection procedures? Rook (1959) maintained that it was when he wrote that "higher standards of entry are more likely to lead to selection of the mentally unstable." Or is the elevated rate due to the institutional inflexibility and the stresses of academe? The Conference on Student Stress implied this viewpoint when they met to deal with the question: "How do stresses of students affect their emotional growth and academic performance?" (Shoben, 1966). The answer to this question needs further research to follow up college students and record their later mortality experience. Unfortunately, the standard death certificate does not supply information regarding education of the decedent. Such data would be helpful for a definitive answer to the controversial question of which is more significant, the susceptible student or the academic stress?

Variation by college   There is no evidence directly bearing upon this question. A definite answer would require standardized reporting procedures probably involving a national clearinghouse for information on student suicide. Nonetheless, the data from Lyman's study of English universities (1961) clearly indicated that the Oxbridge schools had a remarkably high rate of suicide compared to the nation in general and to the unnamed "red-brick" British universities in particular. Accordingly, it may be reasonable to hypothesize that the suicide rates at top-ranked American universities, e.g. Harvard, Yale, Cornell, Berkeley, are higher than the suicide rates at schools of lesser academic reputation. The test of this hypothesis is an interesting subject for future research. Other provocative questions which must await future research are the comparison of suicide rates for: Large vs. small schools; public vs. private schools; and co-ed vs. sexually segregated schools.

Mass Media

Youthful suicide has been a subject for novelists and poets throughout the years. Literature is filled with humorous, insightful and sensitive treatments of the conflicts and despair of adolescents (Beerbohm, 1911; Gide, 1926; Goethe, 1774; Hardy, 1923; Ibsen, 1961; Kleinschmidt, 1956; Reid, 1939; Roth, 1963; Shakespeare, 1936; Stevenson, n.d.). Some people believe that the fictional, romanticized treatment of suicide and adolescence acts as a stimulant to self-destruction. Perhaps the most vigorous advocacy of this position came from Mapes (1903) who wrote that:

> Trashy novels and all kinds of unwholesomely sentimental literature are a very important predisposing cause to suicide in this country. They produce a morbid condition of mind which unfits people for realities.

Mapes' outrage was primarily aroused by one of the most celebrated examples of stormy adolescent love—Goethe's novel, *The Sorrows of Young Werther* (1774). This slim volume became a symbol of 18th century *Weltschmerz* and was vastly popular throughout the world. Soon afterwards Goethe and his book were accused of initiating a wave of school-boy suicides which followed its publication. Goethe himself came in for various denunciations, his book was lampooned (Thackeray, 1903) and banned from public sale in some cities. Even [in modern times] . . . one finds castigating references blaming "Wertherism" for adolescent suicides (Becker, 1965).

Despite the condemnation of "trashy" novels and romantic sentimentality there is no evidence that the treatment of suicide by mass media influences the suicide rate. The only study to directly attack this question was done recently by Motto (1967). To determine whether newspaper publicity about suicides influenced the suicide rate, he studied the incidence of self-destruction in cities which had experienced newspaper blackouts due to strikes. No significant changes were noted when the newspaper coverage was suspended. Motto concluded that newspaper publicity was not an instrumental precipitating factor for suicide. The blame for youthful suicide is no longer placed upon literary influences but on the deeper underlying motives which lead children to suicide. Nonetheless, it is of some passing interest and a reflection of the *Zeitgeist* that *The Ode to Billy Joe* (Gentry, 1967) which tells the story of a teenage suicide was, for many weeks, the number one best-selling phonograph record throughout this country.

Despite the inflammatory accusations leveled against the mass media, the educational aspects of a mass media approach have not been overlooked. There have been numerous films, plays and stories designed to educate the public about the general problem of self-destruction. In the specific area of youthful suicide, such a training film has been produced with the cooperation of the Los Angeles Suicide Prevention Center (Peck, 1969). This film is especially geared to help teachers, counselors, parents and others who have frequent contact with adolescents, to recognize, and deal with the clues prodromal to adolescent suicide.

ETIOLOGY—CULTURAL DETERMINANTS

Cultural factors may influence the suicide rate in three basic ways: (1) By the acute psychological stresses and tensions produced in its members; (2) by the degree of acceptability accorded to suicidal behavior; and (3) by the opportunity for alternative behaviors provided by the culture.

Stresses   Instances of the first type, where the built-in stresses of a culture may catalyze and aggravate the suicide potentiality of its members, were discussed by Bakwin (1957). Writing on the "Prussian" attitude toward children, Bakwin related the high suicide rate among Prussian children to their fear of punishment and to their strong guilt feelings about failure. Prussian children were reared in an atmosphere which demanded a rigid conformity; punishment was frequent and severe. Overly-strict attitudes with few excuses accepted for "misbehavior" were the dominant codes at home and in the classroom. A comprehensive study of cultural factors influencing suicide was published by Hendin (1964) who used a psychoanalytic frame of reference to study individuals and their culture. Hendin investigated the reasons for the consistent differences in suicide incidence among the Scandinavian countries of Denmark, Sweden and Norway. From his observations of parent-child relationships, Hendin formulated modal "psycho-social character" structures which typified each of the three Scandinavian nations and which he related to national differences in child-rearing orientations. Sweden, where the suicide rate is relatively high, was characterized by "performance" types of suicide due to high achievement expectations, self-hatred for failure and problems with affectivity resulting from early maternal separation. Denmark, where the suicide rate is also high, was characterized by "dependency" suicides revolving around such conflicts as anxiety about losing dependency relationships, over-sensitivity to abandonment, and difficulty in expressing overt aggression. In contrast, the suicide rate in Norway is quite low. Hendin proposed that this lower rate occurred because Norwegian mothers were more accepting, less concerned with their children's performance, more tolerant of aggression and strivings for independence than were Swedish or Danish mothers. He believed that those suicides which occurred in

Norway were mainly of a "moralistic" type, stemming from guilt feelings precipitated by puritanical aspects of Norwegian culture. Hendin's hypotheses were later tested by Block and Christiansen (1966) who investigated the reported child-rearing practices of Scandinavian mothers. They found general, but somewhat equivocal, support for Hendin's conclusions. In particular, their results were fairly consistent with Hendin's regarding Denmark and Norway; less so with respect to Sweden.

Acceptability. Examples of the second type, where culturally favorable attitudes may affect the suicide rate were presented by Bakwin (1957) who pointed out that countries such as Austria and Germany, where suicide is regarded as an honorable way to die, produce a higher incidence of self-destruction than countries like England or the United States where suicide is looked upon as cowardly or as a sign of mental aberration. The effect of culturally favorable attitudes toward suicide are probably best exemplified by the extreme case of Japan. In past years children of the nobility and military classes were indoctrinated at an early age with the belief that suicide was an acceptable, often highly valued, means for resolving demands of honor or duty, e.g. *kamikaze, seppuku.* Although traditional suicides are no longer as prevalent in Japan, the general attitude toward suicide is still much more tolerant than it is in many other parts of the world. At present, in Japan, suicide incidence has reached the point where it is the number one cause of death below the age of 30. Contrary to the United States pattern where the frequency of suicide increases with advancing age, Japanese suicides reach a peak at the youthful ages of 20–25. During the age range of 15–24, the suicide rates for Japanese youth are 10–20 times the corresponding United States rates (Iga, 1961). Despite the fact that academic competition (Examination hell, 1962); exaggerated dependency and shame or failure (Iga, 1961); poor family relationships (Iga, 1966); and attempts at symbolic communication (Hayakawa, 1957) have all been cited as significant influences, the singularly distinctive characteristic cited in studies of Japanese suicide is the culturally favorable attitude toward self-destruction.

Alternatives Conversely, where the cultural attitudes are condemnatory or repressive, one finds examples of the third type where the culture provides for alternative behaviors that indirectly satisfy the same end of self-destruction. Wolfgang's research (1959) supported the belief that the relatively high homicide and low suicide rates among young American Negro males were influenced by common values shared by members of this sub-cultural group. That is, suicide was perceived as cowardly and effeminate whereas death by homicide was considered to be masculine and courageous. Lowie (1935) recorded a somewhat parallel phenomenon among the Crow Indians. He observed a cultural pattern which was geared toward those men who were no longer interested in living. They were allowed to become a "Crazy-Dog-Wishing-to-Die."

> Above all, these warriors were pledged to foolhardiness and they deliberately courted death, recklessly dashing up to the enemy so as to die within one season.

A similar cultural pattern had also been observed in past years among the Northern Cheyenne Indians. Formerly, when a Cheyenne warrior became depressed or lost face, he could deal with the situation by organizing a small war party. During the ensuing battle, he could resolve his conflict through a feat of bravery which would renew his self-esteem or by engaging in an extremely dangerous and courageous act during which he was killed (Dizmang, 1967). As such, these cultural alternatives bear some similarity to the fictitious Suicide Club described by Robert Louis Stevenson (n.d.). Members of this club could manage to die without actually doing the killing themselves. As one of the characters re-marked, "the trouble with suicide is removed in that way...."

But what happens when a culture comes to a deadend and no longer offers these alterna-tive outlets for its members? Dizmang (1967), writing on the Northern Cheyenne Indians, observed that their traditional ways of acquiring self-esteem were gone, the culturally ap-proved means of expressing aggression (e.g. Sun Dance, buffalo hunt, inter-tribal warfare) had been denied to them and he reasoned that it was these sorts of deprivation which were responsible for a mass epidemic of adolescent suicide attempts. In this case, Dizmang con-cluded, a whole culture had been "denied means for dealing with instinctual feelings ... and the result was a feeling of hopelessness and helplessness," stemming from this cultural deadend....

REFERENCES

A family of suicides. *Medical Record, New York*, 1901, **60** (17); 660–661.

A student suicide. *Boston Medical Surgical Journal*, 1927, **196** (2); 491.

Ackerly, W. C. Latency age children who threaten or attempt to kill themselves. *Journal of the American Academy of Child Psychiatry*, 1967, **6**, 242–261.

Alexander, I. E., & Alderstein, A. M. Affective responses to the concept of death in a population of children and early adolescents. *Journal of Genetic Psychology*, 1958, **93**, 167–177.

Bakwin, H. Suicide in children and adolescents. *Journal of Pediatrics*, 1957, **50** (6), 749–769.

Balkwin, H. Suicide in children and adolescents. *Journal of the American Medical Women's Associa-tion*, 1964, **19** (6), 489–491.

Balser, B. H., & Masterson, J. F. Suicide in adolescents. *American Journal of Psychiatry*, 1959, **116** (5), 400–404.

Barter, J. T., Swaback, D. O., & Todd, D. Adolescent suicide attempts. *Archives of General Psychiatry (Chicago)*, 1968, **19**, 523–527.

Becker, W. Suicide in youth. *Medizinische Klinik (Munich)*, 1965, **60** (6), 226–231.

Beerbohm, M. *Zuleika Dobson*. New York: Dodd, Mead, 1911.

Bender, L. Children preoccupied with suicide. In L. Bender, *Agression, hostility, and anxiety in children*. Springfield, Ill.: Charles C Thomas, 1953. Pp. 66–90.

Bender, L. L., & Schilder, P. Suicidal preoccupations and attempts in children. *American Journal of Orthopsychiatry*, 1937, **7**, 225–243.

Bergsma, J. Suicide and suicide attempts, especially in young people. *Nederlands Tijdschrift voor de Psychologie en Haar Grensgebieden*, 1963, **21** (4), 245–273.

Bergstrand, C. G., & Otto, U. Suicidal attempts in adolescence and childhood. *Acta Paediatrica*, 1962, **51** (1), 17–26.

Bigras, J., Gauthier, Y., Bouchard, C., & Tassé, Y. Suicidal attempts in adolescent girls: A preliminary study. *Canadian Psychiatric Association Journal*, 1966, (Suppl.), 275–282.

Block, J., & Christiansen, B. A test of Hendin's hypotheses relating suicide in Scandinavia to child-rearing orientations. *Scandinavian Journal of Psychology*, 1966, **7** (4), 267–286.

Braaten, L. J., & Darling, C. D. Suicidal tendencies among college students. *Psychiatric Quarterly*, 1962, **36** (4), 665–692.

Broom, L., & Selznick, P. *Sociology* (2nd ed.). Evanston, Ill.: Row, Peterson, 1958. Pp. 20–24.

Bruhn, J. G. Broken homes among attempted suicides and psychiatric outpatients: A comparative study. *Journal of Mental Science*, 1962, **108** (Whole No. 457), 772–779.

Cain, A. C., & Fast, I. Children's disturbed reactions to parent suicide. *American Journal of Orthopsychiatry*, 1966, **36** (5), 873–880.

Cerny, L., & Cerna, M. Depressive syndrome in children and adolescents with regard to suicidal ten-dencies. *Ceskoslovenska Psychiatrie*, 1962, **58** (3), 162–169.

Cohen, A. Y. LSD and the student: Approaches to educational strategies. Unpublished manuscript, University of California Counseling Center, Berkeley, 1967.

Crichton-Miller, H. The psychology of suicide. *British Medical Journal*, 1931, **2**, 239–241.

Darbonne, A. R. *Dissertation Abstracts*, 1967, **27** (7-B), 2504–2505. (Abstract)

Dizmang, L. H. Suicide among the Cheyenne Indians. *Bulletin of Suicidology*, July 1967, 8–11.

Dorpat, T. L., Jackson, J. K., & Ripley, H. S. Broken homes and attempted and committed suicide. *Archives of General Psychiatry*, 1965, **12** (2), 213–216.

Dublin, L. I. *Suicide: A sociological and statistical study*. New York: Ronald Press, 1963.

Durkheim, E. *Suicide*. New York: Free Press. 1951. (Originally published in 1897.)

Examination hell: Japan's student suicides. (London) *Times Educational Supplement*, October 26. 1962, 2475–2533.

Faigel, H. C. Suicide among young persons. A review for its incidence and causes, and methods of its prevention. *Clinical Pediatrics*, 1966, **5**, 187–190.

Ford, R. Death by hanging of adolescent and young adult males. *Journal of Forensic Sciences*, 1957, **2** (2), 171–176.

Fowler, C. Suicide as a symptom of neurotic conflict in children. *Smith College Studies in Social Work*, 1949, **19** (2), 136–137. (Abstract)

Friedman, P. (Ed.) *On suicide*. New York: International Universities Press, 1967.

Geisler, E. Selbstmord und Todessehnsucht im Kindesalter. (Suicide and death-longing in childhood), *Psychiatrie, Neurologie und Medizinische Psycholgie*, 1953, **5**, 210–216.

Gentry, B. *Ode to Billy Joe*. Capitol Records, 1967 (phonograph record).

Gibbs, J. P., & Martin, W. T. *Status integration and suicide*. Eugene, Oregon: Oregon University Press, 1964.

Gide, A. *The counterfeiters*. New York: Modern Library, 1951. (Originally published in 1926.)

Goethe, J. W. v. The sorrows of young Werther. In T. Mann (Ed.), *The permanent Goethe*, New York: Dial Press, 1948. Pp. 361–448. (Originally published in 1774.)

Gorceix, A. Le suicide l'adolescence et le poison. (Suicide, adolescence and poison), *Semaine des Hopitaux de Paris*, 1963, **39** (50), 2371–2374.

Gould, R. E. Suicide problems in children and adolescents. *American Journal of Psychotherapy*, 1965, **19** (2), 228–246.

Greer, S. The relationship between parental loss and attempted suicide: A control study. *British Journal of Psychiatry*, 1964, **110** (468), 698–705.

Gunther, M. Why children commit suicide. *Saturday Evening Post*, June 11, 1967, 86–89.

Hall, G. S. *Adolescence*. Vol. I. New York: Appleton, 1904. Pp. 374–385.

Hardy, T. *Jude the obscure*. New York: Modern Library, 1923.

Harlow, H. F., & Harlow, M. H. Learning to love. *American Scientist*, 1966, **54**, 244–272.

Hayakawa, S. I. Suicide as a communicative act. *Etc.: Review of General Semantics*, 1957, **15** (1), 46–51.

Hendin, H. *Suicide and Scandinavia*. New York: Grune & Stratton, 1964.

Henry, A. F. Family role structure and self-blame. In N. W. Bell & E. F. Vogel (Eds.), *A modern introduction to the family*. New York: Free Press, 1960. Pp. 538–543.

Henry, A. F., & Short, J. F. *Suicide and homicide*. New York: Free Press, 1954.

Idanpann-Hekkila, P., Idanpann-Hekkila, J., & Savonen, K. Suomen Korkeakouluopiskelijoiden Itsemurhat 1955–1964. (Suicides among Finnish University students in 1955–1964), *Duodecim*, 1967, **83**, 412–418.

Iga, M. Cultural factors in suicide of Japanese youth with focus on personality. *Sociology and Social Research*, 1961, **46** (1), 75–90.

Iga, M. Relation of suicide attempt and social structure in Kamakura, Japan. *International Journal of Social Psychiatry*, 1966, **12**, 221–232.

Jackson, D. D. Theories of suicide. In E. S. Shneidman & N. L. Farberow (Eds.), *Clues to suicide*. New York: McGraw-Hill, 1957. Pp. 11–21.

Jacobs, J., & Teicher, J. D. Broken homes and social isolation in attempted suicide of adolescents. *International Journal of Social Psychiatry*, 1967, **13** (2), 139–149.

Jacobziner, H. Attempted suicides in children. *Journal of Pediatrics*, 1960, **56** (4), 519–525.
Jacobziner, H. Attempted suicides in adolescence. *Journal of the American Medical Association*, 1965, **191** (1), 7–11.
Jacobziner, H. Attempted suicides in adolescents by poisonings: Statistical report. *American Journal of Psychotherapy*, 1965, **19** (2), 247–252.
Jan-Tausch, J. *Suidide of children 1960–63: New Jersey public school students*. Trenton, N.J.: State of New Jersey Department of Education (n.d.).
Jensen, V. W. Evaluating the suicide impulse in the university setting. *Journal-Lancet*, 1955, **75**, 441–444.
Kallmann, F. J., & Anastasio, M. M. Twin studies on the psychopathology of suicide. *Journal of Heredity*, 1946, **37**, 171–180.
Kallmann, F. J., De Porte, J., De Porte, E., & Feingold, L. Suicide in twins and only children. *American Journal of Human Genetics*, 1949, **1**, 113–126.
Kastenbaum, R. Time and death in adolescence. In H. Feifel, (Ed.), *The meaning of death*. New York: McGraw-Hill, 1959. Pp. 99–113.
Keeler, W. R. Children's reaction to the death of a parent. In P. H. Hoch & J. Zubin (Eds.), *Depression*. New York: Grune & Stratton, 1954. Pp. 109–120.
Kleinschmidt, H. J. The death of Elpenor: On a distinct type of self-destructive reaction in a rejected youth. *Journal of Hillside Hospital*, 1956, **5** (3–4), 320–327.
Launay, C., & Col, C. Suicide and attempted suicide in children and adolescents. *Revue Pratique de Psychologie de la Vie Sociale et d'Hygiene Mentale*, 1964, **14** (6), 619–626.
Lawler, R. H., Nakielny, W., & Wright, N. A. Suicidal attempts in children. *Canadian Medical Association Journal*, 1963, **89**, 751–754
Lester, D. Fear of death of suicidal persons. *Psychological Reports*, 1967, **20** (3), (Pt. 2), 1077–1078.
Lester, D. Sibling position and suicidal behavior. *Journal of Individual Psychology*, 1966, **22** (2), 204–207.
Litman, R. E., Curphey, T., Shneidman, E. S., Farberow, N. L., & Tabachnik, N. Investigations of equivocal suicides. *Journal of the American Medical Association*, 1963, **184**, 924–929.
Lourie, R. S. Clinical studies of attempted suicide in childhood. *Clinical proceedings of Children's Hospital of the District of Columbia*, 1966, **22**, 163–173.
Lowie, R. H. *The Crow indians*. New York: Holt, Rinehart & Winston, 1935.
Lyman, J. L. Student suicide at Oxford University. *Student Medicine*, 1961, **10** (2), 218–234.
MacDonald, A. Statistics of child suicide. *American Statistical Association Publication*, 1906–1907, **10**, 260–264.
Manganaro, D. A case of familial suicide. *Rivista di Patologia Nervosa e Mentale* (Florence), 1957, **78**, 1078–1081.
Mapes, C C. Suicide in children. *Medical Age*, 1903, **21** (8), 289–295.
Maria, G. Some considerations apropos of the suicide of minors. *Rassegna Internazionale di Clinica e Terapia* (Naples), 1962, **42**, 985–993.
Mason, P. Suicide in adolescents. *Psychoanalytic Review*, 1954, **41**, 48–54.
Maycock, E. Depression, despair and suicide. (London) *Times Educational Supplement, February 11, 1966*, 407.
McClelland, D. The Harlequin complex. In R. W. White (Ed.), *The Study of Lives*. Englewood Cliffs, N.J.: Prentice-Hall, 1963. Pp. 94–119.
Mills, C. A. Suicides and homicides in their relation to weather changes. *American Journal of Psychiatry*, 1934, **91**, 669–677.
Mintz, R. S. A pilot study of the prevalence of persons in the city of Los Angeles who have attempted suicide. Unpublished manuscript (presented in abbreviated form at American Psychiatric Association meetings, Los Angeles, May, 1964), UCLA Neuropsychiatric Institute. Los Angeles, 1964.
Mohr, G. G., & Depres, M. A. *The stormy decade: Adolescence*. New York: Random House, 1958. Pp. 194–208.
Morrison, G. C., & Smith, W. R. Emergencies in child psychiatry: A definition and comparison of two groups. *American Journal of Orthopsychiatry*, 1967, **372**, 412–413.

Moss, L. M., & Hamilton, D. C. The psychotherapy of the suicidal patient. *American Journal of Psychiatry*, 1956, **112**, 814–820.

Motto, J. Suicide and suggestibility—the role of the press. *American Journal of Psychiatry*, 1967, **124** (2), 252–256.

Mulcock, D. Juvenile suicide. A study of suicide and attempted suicide over a 16-year period. *Medical Officer*, 1955, **94**, 155–160.

Munter, P. K. Depression and suicide in college students. In L. McNeer (Ed.), *Proceedings of Conference on Depression and Suicide in Adolescents and Young Adults.* Fairlee, Vermont, June, 1966. Pp. 20–25.

Nagy, M. H. The child's view of death. In H. Feifel (Ed.). *The meaning of death.* New York: McGraw-Hill, 1959. Pp. 79–98.

Otto, U. Changes in the behavior of children and adolescents preceding suicidal attempts. *Acta Psychiatrica Scandinavica*, 1964, **40** (4) 386–400.

Otto, U. Suicidal attempts made by children and adolescents because of school problems. *Acta Paediactrica Scandinavica*, **54** (4), 348–356.

Paffenbarger, R. S., & Asnes, D. P. Chronic disease in former college students. III. Precursors of suicide in early and middle life. *American Journal of Public Health*, 1966, **56**, 1026–1036.

Parrish, H. M. Epidemiology of suicide among college students. *Yale Journal of Biology and Medicine*, 1957, **29**, 585–595.

Peck, M. L. Optimism and despair among suicidal adolescents. Paper read at "Optimism and Suicide" seminar, San Diego, January, 1967. (a)

Peck, M. L. Suicide and Youth. Paper read at "Suicide Intervention" workshop, Fresno, March, 1967. (b)

Peck, M. L. *Rick: An adolescent suicide.* Los Angeles: Suicide Prevention Center, 1969. (film)

Peck, M. L., & Schrut, A. Statistical data on college student suicide: Los Angeles county. Unpublished manuscript, Suicide Prevention Center, Los Angeles, 1967.

Porot, M., Collet, M., Girard, J., Jean, C., & Coudert, A. Suicide of adolescents. *Revue de Neuropsychiatrie Infantile et d'Hygiene Mentale de l'Enfance*, 1965, **13**, 647–650.

Powers, D. Youthful suicide attempts. *Northwest Medicine*, 1954, **53** (10), 1001–1002: Part 2. 1231–1232.

Powers, D. Suicide threats and attempts in the young. *American Practitioner*, 1956, **7** (7), 1140–1143.

Raphael, T., Power, S. H., & Berridge, W. L. The question of suicide as a problem in college mental hygiene. *American Journal of Orthopsychiatry*, 1937, **7** (1), 1–14.

Reese, F. D. School-age suicide: The educational parameters. *Dissertation Abstracts.* 1967, **27** (9-A), 2895–2896.

Reid, F. *Peter Waring.* London: Faber & Faber, 1939.

Ringel, E., Spiel, W., & Stepan, M. Untersuchungen über kindliche Selbstmordversuche. (An investigation of suicide attempts of children), *Praxis der Kinderpsychologie und Kinderpsychiatrie (Göttingen)*, 1955, 4, 161–168.

Rochlin, C. *Griefs and discontents.* Boston: Little Brown, 1965.

Rook, A. Student suicides. *British Medical Journal*, 1959, **5122**, 599–603.

Roth, P. The conversion of the Jews. In P. Roth, *Goodbye Columbus.* New York: Bantam, 1963. Pp. 100–114.

Sainsbury, P. *Suicide in London.* London: Chapman-Hall, 1955.

Schechter, M. D. The recognition and treatment of suicide in children. In E. S. Shneidman & N. L. Farberow (Eds.), *Clues to suicide.* New York: McGraw-Hill, 1957. Pp. 131–142.

Schilder, P., & Wechsler, D. The attitudes of children toward death. *Journal of Genetic Psychology*, 1934, **45**, 406–451.

Schneer, H. I., & Kay, P. The suicidal adolescent. In S. Lorand & H. Schneer (Eds.), *Adolescents.* New York: Paul Hosbar, 1962. Pp. 180–201.

Schneer, H. I., Kay, P., & Brozovsky, M. Events and conscious ideation leading to suicidal behavior in adolescence. *Psychiatric Quarterly*, 1961, **35** (3), 507–515.

Schonfeld, W. A. Socioeconomic influence as a factor. *New York State Journal of Medicine*, 1967, **67** (14), 1981–1990.

Schrut, A. Suicidal adolescents and children. *Journal of the American Medical Association*, 1964, **188** (13), 1103–1107.

Schrut, A. Some typical patterns in the behavior and background of female adolescents who attempt suicide. Paper read at American Psychiatric Association meetings, Detroit, May, 1967.

Seiden, R. H. Campus tragedy: A study of student suicide. *Journal of Abnormal, Psychology*, 1966, **71** (6), 389–399.

Shakespeare, W. Romeo and Juliet. In G. L. Kittredge (Ed.), *The complete works of Shakespeare*. Boston: Ginn, 1936. Pp. 1005–1044.

Shankel, L. W., & Carr, A. C. Transvestism and hanging episodes in a male adolescent. *Psychiatric Quartertly*, 1956, **30** (1), 478–493.

Shapiro, L. B. Suicide: Psychology and family tendency. *Journal of Nervous and Mental Disease*, 1935, **81**, 547–553.

Shaw, C. R., & Schelkun, R. F. Suicidal behavior in children. *Psychiatry*, 1965, **28** (2), 157–168.

Shneidman, E. S. Orientations toward death. In R. W. White (Ed.), *The study of lives*. Englewood Cliffs, N.J.: Prentice-Hall, 1963. Pp. 201–227.

Shneidman, E. S. Suicide, sleep, and death. *Journal of Consulting Psychology*, 1964, **28** (2), 95–106.

Shneidman, E. S. Suicide among adolescents, *California School Health*, 1966, **2** (3), 1–4. (a)

Shneidman, E. S. Suicide of children and adolescents: A national problem. In L. McNeer (Ed.), *Proceedings of Conference on Depression and Suicide in Adolescents and Young Adults*. Fairlee, Vermont, June, 1966. Pp. 5–8. (b)

Shneidman, E. S., Farberow, N. L., & Leonard, C. V. *Some facts about suicide*. (P.H.S. Publ. No. 852, Health Info. Series No. 101) Washington, D.C.: United States Government Printing Office, 1961.

Shneidman, E. S., & Farberow, N. L. Statistical comparisons between attempted and committed suicides. In N. L. Farberow & E. S. Shneidman (Eds.), *The cry for help*. New York: McGraw-Hill, 1961. Pp. 19–47.

Shneidman, E. S., & Mandelkorn, P. *How to prevent suicide*. (Public Affairs pamphlets no. 406) New York: Public Affairs Committee, 1967.

Sorokin, P. A. *Society, culture and personality*. New York: Harper, 1947. Pp. 6–18.

Speigel, D., & Neuriager, C. Role of dread in suicidal behavior. *Journal of Abnormal and Social Psychology*, 1963, **66**, 507–511.

Stearns, A. W. Cases of probable suicide in young persons without obvious motivation. *Journal of the Maine Medical Association*, 1953, **44** (1), 16–23.

Stengel, E. *Suicide and attempted suicide*. Baltimore: Penguin, 1964.

Stevenson, R. L. The suicide club. In R. L. Stevenson, *New Arabian nights*. London: Thomas Nelson (n.d.). Pp. 9–106.

Swanson, D. W. Suicide in identical twins. *American Journal of Psychiatry*, 1960, **116** (1), 934–935.

Teicher, J. D., & Jacobs, J. Adolescents who attempt suicide: Preliminary findings. *American Journal of Psychiatry*, 1966, **122** (11), 1248–1257. (a)

Teicher, J. D., & Jacobs, J. The physician and the adolescent suicide attempter. *Journal of School Health*, 1966, **36** (9), 406–415. (b)

Temby, W. D. Suicide. In G. B. Blaine & C. C. McArthur (Eds.), *Emotional problems of the student*. New York: Appleton-Century-Crofts, 1961. Pp. 133–152.

Thackeray, W. M. A legend of the Rhine. In W. M. Thackeray, *Burlesques*. London: Macmillan, 1903. Pp. 3–67.

Toolan, J. M. Suicide and suicidal attempts in children and adolescents. *American Journal of Psychiatry*, 1962, **118** (8), 719–724.

Toolan, J. M. Suicide in children. In L. McNeer (Ed.), *Proceedings of Conference on Depression and Suicide in Adolescents and Young Children*. Fairlee, Vermont, June, 1966. Pp. 9–13.

Trautman, E. Drug abuse and suicide attempt of an adolescent girl. *Adolescence*, 1966, **1** (4), 381–392.

Tuckman, J., Youngman, W. F., & Leifer, B. Suicide and family disorganization. *International Journal of Social Psychiatry*, 1966, **12** (3), 187–191.

United States Department of Health, Education and Welfare, Public Health Service, National Office of Vital Statistics. Death rates by age, race and sex, United States, 1900–1953: Suicide *Vital Statistics Special Report*, August 22, 1956, **43** (30), 463–477.

WHO Epidemiological and vital statistics report. *Mortality from Suicide*, 1956, **9**, 243.

Winn, D., & Halla, R. Observations of children who threaten to kill themselves. *Canadian Psychiatric Association Journal*, 1966, **11** (Suppl.), 283–294.

Wolfgang, M. E. Suicide by means of victim-precipitated homicide. *Journal of Clinical and Experimental Psychopathology*, 1959, **20**, 335–349.

Zilboorg, G. Considerations of suicide with particular reference to that of the young. *American Journal of Orthopsychiatry*, 1937, **7**, 15–31.

Zimbacca, N. Suicide in adolescents. *Concours Medical.* 1965, **87**, 4991–4997.

Zumpe, L. Selbstmordversuche von kindern und jugendlichen. (Suicide attempts in children and adolescents.) *Zeitschrift für Psychotherapie und Medizinische Psychologie (Stuttgart)*, 1959, **9**, 223–243.

Suggested Additional Readings

Derogatis, L. R., Covi, L., Lipman, R. S., Davis, D. M., & Rickels, K. Social class and race as mediator variables in neurotic symptomatology. *Archives of General Psychiatry*, 1971, **25**, 31–40.

Goffman, E. *Asylums*. New York: Doubleday, 1961.

Kleiner, R. J., Tuckman, J., & Lavell, M. Mental disorder and status based on race. *Psychiatry*, 1960, **23**, 271–274.

Mishler, E. G., & Scotch, N. A. Sociocultural factors in the epidemiology of schizophrenia. *Psychiatry*, 1963, **26**, 315–351.

Petras, J. W., & Curtis, J. E. The current literature on social class and mental disease in America: Critique and bibliography. *Behavioral Science*, 1968, **13**, 382–398.

Redlich, F. C., Hollingshead, A. B., Roberts, B. H., Robinson, H. A., Freedman, L. Z., & Myers, J. K. Social structure and psychiatric disorders. *American Journal of Psychiatry*, 1953, **109**, 729–734.

Scheff, T. J. The role of the mentally ill and the dynamics of mental disorder. *Sociometry*, 1963, **26**, 436–453.

Schein, E. Reaction patterns to severe, chronic stress in American army prisoners of war of the Chinese. *Journal of Social Issues*, 1957, **13**, 21–30.

Wechsler, H., Solomon, L., & Kramer, B. M. *Social psychology and mental health*. New York: Holt, Rinehart & Winston, 1970.

Wold, C. I. Characteristics of 26,000 suicide prevention center patients. *Bulletin of Suicidology*, 1970, No. 6, 24–28.

Ecological Factors

12

Population density and Pathology:
What Are the Relations for Man?*†

OMER R. GALLE, WALTER R. GOVE and J. MILLER McPHERSON

Studies of various animal populations suggest that high levels of population density frequently produce "pathological" behavior. The results of these studies, coupled with an increased concern about high rates of growth in the human population, have led to speculations about the implications of high levels of density for human populations. We begin this article with a review of some of these studies, noting the implications of possible animal-human similarities, and then take the animal studies as a serious model for human populations and devise a test case.

In 1962, Calhoun published an article detailing the ways in which overcrowding affects the behavior of rats. In his experiment, he gave the rats sufficient food and water, but the density of the population was substantially higher than it is in the rats' natural habitat. Calhoun observed the following "pathological behaviors" under these conditions: increased mortality, especially among the very young; lowered fertility rates; neglect of the young by their mothers; overly aggressive and conflict-oriented behavior; almost total withdrawal from the community (the "somnambulists"); and sexual aberrations and other "psychotic" behavior[1]. It should be noted that these aberrations were much more common in the central pens, where the rats *voluntarily* congregated.

In recent years it has become clear that rats are not alone in being adversely affected by high density[2, 3]. A study by Susiyama[4] of wild monkeys indicated that high density led to a general breakdown in the monkeys' social order and resulted in extremely aggressive behavior, hypersexuality, the killing of young, and so on. High density appears to cause death in hares[5] and shrews[6]. Morris[7] has found that high density causes homosexuality in fish. Probably the most frequently demonstrated effect of density is in the area of natality. For example, under conditions of high density the clutch size of the great tit decreases[8], as does the number of young carried by shrews[6]. It appears likely that high density reduces the fertility of elephants[9]. Female house mice abort if they smell a strange male mouse[10], as do shrews[11].

In sum, high population density appears to have a serious inhibiting effect on many animals. It must be noted, however, that the effect of density is not uniform among different species; different species react to density in different ways. It is probably inevitable that increasing knowledge of the effect of density on animal behavior leads to concern about the effect density may have on human behavior. By now, the idea that density has, or at least may have, serious consequences for man appears to have fairly wide acceptance. Such

*From Galle, O. R., Gove, W. R., and McPherson, J. M., *Science*, 1972, **176**, 23–30. Copyright © 1972 by the American Association for the Advancement of Science. Reprinted by permission of the American Association for the Advancement of Science, and Dr. Galle.

†Evidence from one city suggests that high population density may be linked to "pathological" behavior.

acceptance is obvious in much popular writing[12] as well as in work specifically aimed at behavioral scientists[13].

DENSITY AND PATHOLOGY IN HUMAN POPULATIONS

Although many people have written about the effect overcrowding has on human behavior, there is a paucity of good research. A detailed and careful review of the existing literature by Schorr led him to believe that the effect of poor housing (overcrowding) has been understated. Schorr concluded that poor housing (overcrowding) had the following effects[14, pp. 31–32].

> A perception of one's self that leads to pessimism and passivity, stress to which the individual cannot adapt, poor health, and a state of dissatisfaction; pleasure in company but not in solitude, cynicism about people and organizations, a high degree of sexual stimulation without legitimate outlet, and difficulty in household management and child rearing....

Other authors interpret the existing data differently and feel that such relations have not, in general, been clearly established[15].

The evidence on the relations of pathological behavior and high population density is ambiguous; before the issue is decided, a number of studies of different populations in different settings will have to be undertaken. If, as Hall[3] has suggested, different cultures and different ethnic groups have different spatial requirements, the issue becomes quite complex. A recent and important interview study in Hong Kong suggested that within that culture and in that settling, where virtually everyone lives in an overcrowded environment, variations in crowding are not related to severe emotional strain, but are related to a lack of control over children[16].

We will look at the relation between population density and a variety of pathological behaviors as they vary over the community areas of Chicago[17]. Even if we use the animal studies as a guide, it is not obvious what effects we should look for in humans because, as noted before, density appears to affect different species in different ways. Our analysis will thus, of necessity, be exploratory. Since Calhoun's study has received more attention than others, we use his results as a starting point. There are several practical reasons for doing so. First, he covers a wider range of "pathologies" than do most other researchers. Second, there are a number of indices in the Chicago data that will serve as surrogate measures of Calhoun's "pathologies." In particular, there are indices of (i) fertility, (ii) mortality, (iii) ineffectual care of the young, (iv) asocial, aggressive behavior, and (v) psychiatric disorder. The following are operational definitions of the measures that we use in the statistical analysis.

For each of the 75 community areas of Chicago, the *Local Community Fact Book for Chicago* [18] provides information on the number of persons residing in that area. This, combined with the size of the land area included in each community area[19], gives a measure of population density—the number of persons per acre.

The first two measures we use for indices of "social" pathology are distinctly biological in nature—mortality and fertility. The immediate cause of mortality will generally be specific diseases, although mortality rates will also be affected by such variables as malnutrition, accidents, and suicide. Variations in fertility are due to differences in conception, gestation, parturition, and the factors involved in these processes. However, as Calhoun noted, the factors involved in determining variations in mortality and fertility are largely social in nature. Thus, although mortality is largely the consequence of disease, we are interested in variations in mortality as social phenomena because such variations appear to be indirectly caused by, and certainly are associated with, such variables as social class, ethnicity, and, possibly, population density. The same may be said for the factors involved in the determination of variations in fertility. Let us define, then, the first measure of social pathology as the "standardized mortality ratio." This measure is the age-adjusted death rate of a given community area, express as a ratio to the death rate for the total population of Chicago in 1960. Our second measure of social pathology will be the "general fertility rate," which is simply the number of births in a community area per 1000 women ages 15 to 44 in the same area.

As a measure of ineffectual parental care of the young, we will use the number of recipients of public assistance under 18 years old in May 1962 per 100 persons under 18 years old in April 1960. Although this is not an ideal measure of ineffectual parental care, families receiving such assistance are typically disrupted, having only one parent in residence, and the family is not providing for the children in the normal societal manner. We shall call this the "public assistance rate," but it should be remembered that the rate refers only to the *young* persons of the community area. Our measure of asocial, aggressive behavior will be the "number of male individuals brought before the Family Court of Cook County on delinquency petitions during the years 1958–1961 per 100 male population 12–16 years of age in 1960"[18]. We refer to the measure simply as the "juvenile delinquency rate." Finally, as an indication of withdrawal and other psychotic behavior, the fact book reports age-adjusted rates of admissions to mental hospitals for 1960–1961 per 100,000 persons in the community area in 1960. This we shall call the rate of "admission to mental hospitals"[20].

Variations in the five social pathologies we have just defined are normally explained by social structure factors, such as social class and ethnic (or racial) status. For example, it is assumed that variations in the mortality rate arise from such factors as exposure to disease, access to medical assistance, and knowledge about effective preventive measures and that such factors are mediated by one's social class and ethnic status. Similar arguments are made regarding the other pathologies. The precise explanations of the way in which class and ethnicity relate to each pathology would probably differ—in fact, there may be more than one explanation of how class and ethnicity relate to a particular pathology. Nevertheless, most sociologists see these social structure variables as the primary factors determining the variations in the rates of these pathologies. The case for the population density argument will be substantially strengthened if we can demonstrate not only that variations in population density make a significant contribution to the amount of variance explained in selected social pathologies, but that this contribution remains significant even after taking into account (or controlling for) the traditional sociological variables, social class and ethnic status.

We have chosen three measures as indicators of social class: the percentage of employed males in the community area who have white-collar occupations; the median number of years of school completed by all persons 25 years of age and older in a community area; and the median family income for all families residing in that community area. We have combined these measures into an index of social class[21]. This index was developed in a blatantly post hoc fashion in which we maximized the degree to which class is associated with variations in the different pathologies. Our index of ethnicity is also based on three measures: the percentage of Negroes in the community area, the percentage of Puerto Ricans in the community area, and the percentage of foreign-born in the community area. Again, this index was developed in a post hoc fashion, in which we maximized the degree to which ethnicity is associated with variations in the different pathologies[22].

PRELIMINARY RESULTS

Table 12.1 exhibits, for each of the measures of social pathology, four different correlation coefficients. The relation between population density and social pathology is given, as is the more traditional problem of the relation between social structure and social pathology.

The causal model implicit in an argument like Calhoun's is simply

$$u$$
$$\downarrow$$
Density $\longrightarrow$ Pathology

(The u in this model indicates unmeasured variables not taken into account that impinge on pathological behavior.) For this model, a relevant measure is the set of zero-order correlations between density and each of the five pathologies[23]. These are presented in Table 12.1. For each social pathology, the relation with density is significantly different from zero, but it is relatively small. Furthermore, one of the five coefficients, though significant, is in the wrong direction. That is, the animal studies consistently indicate that the higher the population density, the lower the level of fertility. Here, the relationship is positive: the higher the density, the higher the fertility. However, some investigators might argue that high rates of fertility are pathological for urban populations[24]. Thus, one might conclude that population density has a small but significant effect on social pathology: the higher the density, the higher the pathology.

Table 12.1   Zero-order, Multiple, and Partial Correlation, Coefficients for Social Pathology, Population Density, Ethnicity, and Social Class (Chicago, 1960).

	Social pathologies				
Parameter	Standard Mortality Ratio	General Fertility Rate	Public Assistance Rate	Juvenile Delinquency Rate	Admissions to Mental Hospitals
Population Density and Social Pathology					
Zero-order correlation coefficient of each pathology with population density*	0.283	0.373	0.337	0.492	0.349
Partial correlation coefficient of each pathology with population density, controlling for social class and ethnicity	−0.177†	−0.023†	−0.118†	0.227†	0.142†
Social Class, Ethnicity, and Social Pathology					
Multiple correlation coefficient of each pathology with social class and ethnicity	0.828	0.853	0.885	0.927	0.546
Multiple-partial correlation coefficient of each pathology with ethnicity and social class, controlling for population density	0.817	0.827	0.871	0.907	0.466

*The measure of density, persons per acre is transformed into natural logarithms.
†Not significantly different from zero at $P = 0.05$.

We know, however, that the lower one's social class and ethnic status, the more likely one is to live in areas with a high population density. Thus, it may be that class and ethnicity account for the variations both in population density and in pathology, and that there is no *causal* relation between density and pathology. Alternatively, class and ethnicity may affect density, and density may, in turn, affect the pathologies. In this case, density partially "interprets" the way in which class and ethnicity relate to the pathologies. We assume that, in this latter instance, class and ethnicity also affect the pathologies in ways unrelated to density. These two possibilities are presented in Fig. 12.1.

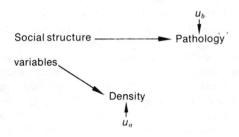

Density as a spurious relation

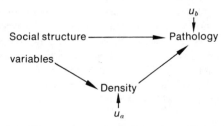

Density as an intervening variable

Fig. 12.1   Models of density as a spurious relation and as an intervening variable; u_a and u_b represent all the unmeasured variables impinging on density and pathology that are not taken into account in the models.

If the relation between density and pathology is spurious, then when we control for class and ethnicity, the partial correlation between density and pathology should approach zero. In contrast, if density is an intervening variable that only partially mediates the effects of class and ethnicity, the partial correlation between density and pathology will not go to zero when class and ethnicity are used as controls, although it may be reduced. Furthermore, if density is a major intervening variable, the partial correlation between the social structure variables and the pathologies would be noticeably reduced when density is used as a control.

As is apparent from Table 12.1, when class and ethnicity are used as controls, the correlations between density and the pathologies are not signficantly different from zero. Furthermore, Table 12.1 shows that controlling for density has virtually no effect on the correlation between the social structure variables and the pathologies. One may assert that these data indicate that the relation between density and the pathologies is spurious[25]. These results are similar to those of Winsborough, who used 1950 data for Chicago[26].

DIMENSIONS OF POPULATION DENSITY

However, before we accept such a conclusion, a reappraisal of our measure of density (persons per acre) may be in order. When the animal ecologists refer to overpopulation of a particular species, they generally indicate the number of animals per some unit of area, such as an acre. However, in the case of human populations, the situation is substantially more complex, especially in an urban setting. On the one hand, there is what might be called overcrowding at the personal, or individual, level. That is, is it possible for an individual to have privacy in the particular housing unit in which he resides, or is he constantly in contact with others? We refer to this type of overcrowding as "interpersonal press." As we have developed the concept, interpersonal press is composed of two distinct factors: the number of persons per room and the number of rooms per housing unit[27].

Population density may also be affected by more "structural" factors. In the urban setting there is considerable variation in the kinds of structures persons live in and in the spacing of these structures. If each individual housing unit is a single, detached structure, then there must be many individual structures per acre to achieve a high level of population density. Alternatively, if there are many high-rise apartment buildings in the area, then the number of housing units per structure will increase dramatically, while another measure, the number of residential structures per acre, may stay relatively low.

A given level of population density in a community area can be achieved by different combinations of four components of density: (i) the number of persons per room; (ii) the number of rooms per housing unit: (iii) the number of housing units per structure; and (iv) the number of residential structures per acre.

Table 12.2 shows the interrelations of the various components of population density for Chicago[28]. The first row shows the zero-order correlations between the overall measure of population density (persons per acre) and each of the four components of this overall level. The next row shows the results of a multiple regression analysis of each of the four components of population density on the general measure of population density (persons per acre). Both rows indicate that it is the structural measures of density (housing units per structure and structures per acre) which account for most of the variance in persons per

Table 12.2   The Interrelations Among the Components of Population Density (Chicago, 1960). (All measures of density are transformed into natural logarithms. For this reason, the multiple regression analysis of the four components of density on persons per acre yields a multiple r of 1.00, and the unstandardized regression coefficients are also 1.00.)

Measures of the Interrelations	Components of Population Density			
	Persons per Room	Rooms per Housing Unit	Housing Units per Structure	Structures per Acre
Zero-order correlations with persons per acre	0.146	−0.560	0.741	0.717
Standardized regression coefficients from a multiple regression analysis of the four components of population density on persons per acre	0.226	0.242	0.811	0.699

acre, while the measures of interpersonal press (persons per room and rooms per housing unit) have only a modest relation to persons per acre.

These data thus suggest that the preceding analysis of the relation between density and pathology may have yielded misleading conclusions. This is particularly obvious if the effect of density on pathology is primarily a consequence of interpersonal press. Therefore we reanalyzed the relation between density and pathology by breaking down population density into its four component parts.

We are still essentially testing the two models outlined in Fig. 12.1, with the one difference that, as density has been broken down into four components, our measure of density is now represented by multiple components; the relation between density and each pathology will therefore be represented by a multiple correlation coefficient. As before, if the relation between the components of density and the pathologies is spurious, the multiple-partial correlation between density and the pathologies should approach zero when we control for class and ethnicity; if density is an intervening variable, the multiple-partial correlation should not go to zero although it may be reduced [29]. The importance of density as an intervening variable should be directly related to the reduction of the multiple-partial correlation between the social structure variables and the pathologies when density is used as a control.

As is shown in Table 12.3, the results of the analysis when population density is broken down into its four components are strikingly different from the results of the original

Table 12.3 Social Pathology, Density, Ethnicity, and Social Class Reexamined.

| | Social Pathologies | | | | |
Parameter	Standard Mortality Ratio	General Fertility Rate	Public Assistance Rate	Juvenile Delinquency Rate	Admissions to Mental Hospitals
Population Densities and Social Pathology					
Multiple correlation coefficients of the four components of density* on each of the social pathologies	0.867	0.856	0.887	0.917	0.689
Multiple-partial correlation coefficient of each pathology with the four components of density, controlling for ethnicity and social class	0.476	0.371	0.584	0.498	0.508
Social Class, Ethnicity, and Social Pathology					
Multiple correlation coefficient of each pathology with social class and ethnicity	0.828	0.853	0.885	0.927	0.546
Multiple-parital correlation coefficient of each pathology with ethnicity and social class, controlling for the four components of population density*	0.143†	0.351	0.574	0.574	0.086†

*All measures of density are transformed into natural logarithms.
†Not significantly different from zero at $P = 0.05$.

analysis shown in Table 12.1. Density is now related to each of the pathologies, and in each case a significant relation between the components of density and the pathologies remains when class and ethnicity are used as controls. Furthermore, the relation between the social structure variables and the pathologies is markedly reduced when the components of density are used as a control. From this revised analysis it appears that at least some of the components intervene between class and ethnicity and the various pathologies, thereby partially interpreting that relationship. We will assume that this is correct, although we emphasize that we have not proved it. For example, we are simply assuming that class and ethnicity "cause" density and thereby ignore the possibility that density (through selective migration) "causes" class and ethnicity.

With the posited model in mind, let us attempt to evaluate the contributions made by class, ethnicity, and the four components of density. Following Duncan[30], we can do this in two different ways. First, we can work back from effect to cause. In this case, the multiple correlation between the components of density and pathology represents the total "effect" of density, including both its "unique" contribution to the variance of the pathology in question and the contribution it "transmits" from the social structure variables (class and ethnicity). The increment added by class and ethnicity that is not "routed" through density can be calculated by subtracting the variance explained by density from the variance explained by density, ethnicity, and class. Alternatively, we can go from earliest cause to effect. In this case, the multiple correlation of ethnicity and class with the pathologies represents the total effect of these social structure variables, including the effect routed through density. We can then calculate the independent effect of density (the effect that is unrelated to ethnicity and class) by subtracting the variance explained by ethnicity and class from the variance explained by density, ethnicity, and class.

The results of these analyses are presented in Table 12.4. If we work back from effect to cause, density appears to "account" for most of the variance, with the social structure variables having relatively little effect on the pathologies except through their effect on the

Table 12.4   The Proportion of Variance Explained by the Four Components of Density and by Class and Ethnicity.

Manner of Partitioning the Explained Variance Between the Major Variables	Social Pathologies				
	Standard Mortality Ratio	General Fertility Rate	Public Assistance Rate	Juvenile Delinquency Rate	Admissions to Mental Hospitals
Working Backward from Effect to Cause					
Total "effect" of the four components of density	75.2	73.3	78.7	84.1	47.5
Increment added by class and ethnicity	0.4	3.2	7.0	5.3	0.4
Total variance explained	75.6	76.5	85.7	89.4	47.9
Working Forward from Prior Cause to Effect					
Total "effect" of class and ethnicity	68.5	72.8	78.3	85.9	29.8
Increment added by the components of density	7.1	3.7	7.4	3.5	18.1
Total variance explained	75.6	76.5	85.7	89.4	47.9

components of density. On the other hand, if we go from earliest cause to effect, we see that class and ethnicity do, at least indirectly, account for most of the variance of the pathologies. It is noteworthy that in most cases the independent increment of explained variance added by either the social structure variables or by the components of density is fairly small. These findings are consistent with the second model proposed in Fig. 12.1; that is, the results are compatible with the assumption that the components of density interpret the relation between the social structure variables and the pathologies.

As a step toward identifying the relative importance of each of the four components of population density, a multiple regression analysis was run for each of the five social pathologies. In four of the five cases, the standardized regression coefficients indicated that the number of persons per room is the most important determinant of the effect of density on pathology. The exception is admissions to mental hospitals, in which case the most important component of density is the other measure of interpersonal press—rooms per housing unit. Next, we found that in four of the five cases the second most important component is housing units per structure. when an analysis such as that outlined in Table 12.4 is performed on a comparison between the effect of persons per room and rooms per housing unit when class and ethnicity are taken into account, the results are strikingly similar. That is, the values differ only slightly from those in Table 12.4, in which all four components of density are considered.

Table 12.5 presents a similar analysis, but with only one component of density considered—persons per room. Because we already suspected that persons per room is not strongly related to admission to mental hospitals, we first focused our attention on the other four pathologies. For these pathologies, the total amount of explained variance dropped relatively slightly. As we move from effect to cause, we find that persons per room accounts for most of the explained variance, although the relation is not as strong as when we used all four components of density. However, compared to our earlier analysis, there is a

Table 12.5 The Proportion of Variance Explained by Persons per Room and by Class and Ethnicity.

Manner of Partitioning the Explained Variance Between the Major Variables	Social Pathologies				
	Standard Mortality Ratio	General Fertility Rate	Public Assistance Rate	Juvenile Delinquency Rate	Admissions to Mental Hospitals*
Working Forward from Prior Cause to Effect					
Total "effect" of persons per room	60.5	65.4	73.3	61.5	15.8(46.8)
Increment added by class and ethnicity	9.8	9.5	10.1	24.4	15.6(0.2)
Total variance explained	70.3	74.9	83.4	85.9	31.4(47.0)
Working Forward from Prior Cause to Effect					
Total "effect" of class and ethnicity	68.5	72.8	78.3	85.9	29.8(29.8)
Increment added by persons per room	1.8	2.1	5.1	0.0	1.6(17.2)
Total variance explained	70.3	74.9	83.4	85.9	31.4(47.0)

*The numbers in parentheses indicate the values that occur when rooms per housing unit are used instead of persons per room.

noticeable increase in the independent increment added by class and ethnicity. Most of this increase can be attributed to the fact that housing units per structure are no longer treated as part of density.

This analysis suggests that, for mortality, fertility, public assistance, and juvenile delinquency, the most important component of density is persons per room. Next, but considerably less important, is the number of housing units per structure. For these four pathologies, the other two components of density—rooms per housing unit and structures per acre—appear to be relatively unimportant.

The pattern is quite different for admissions to mental hospitals. When Table 12.5 is compared with Table 12.4 one can easily see the marked decline in the total amount of variance explained, when the only component of density considered is persons per room. This is not surprising, since the standardized regression cofficients indicate that rooms per housing unit is the most important component of density as a predictor of admissions to mental hospitals. In Table 12.5 we have put in parentheses the variance associated with rooms per housing unit. In comparing these with those obtained when the four components of density are used, it is apparent that rooms per housing unit can account for virtually all of the variance in hospital admissions associated with density.

If our assumptions are correct, these data indicate that density—particularly persons per room (except in the case of admissions to mental hospitals)—may be an important factor in the development of various pathologies.

HOW DENSITY MAY RELATE TO PATHOLOGY

Before considering each pathology separately, let us make some general observations. First, as the number of persons in a dwelling increases, so will the number of social obligations, as well as the need to inhibit individual desires. This escalation of both social demands and the need to inhibit desires would become particularly problematic when people are crowded together in a dwelling with a high ratio of persons per room. Second, crowding will bring with it a marked increase in stimuli that are difficult to ignore. Third, if human beings, like many animals, have a need for territory or privacy, then overcrowding may, in fact, conflict with a basic (biological?) characteristic of man[31].

It would seem reasonable to expect that people would react to the incessant demands, stimulation, and lack of privacy resulting from overcrowding with irritability, weariness, and withdrawal. Furthermore, people are likely to be so completely involved in reacting to their environment that it becomes extremely difficult for them to step back, look at themselves, and plan ahead[32]. It would certainly seem that in an overcrowded situation it would be difficult for them to follow through on their plans. Thus, we might expect the behavior of human beings in an overcrowded environment to be primarily a response to their immediate situation and to reflect relatively little regard for the long-range consequences of their acts.

It seems from the above discussion that the most important component of density, as far as the pathologies are concerned, would be persons per room. This, of course, is the component that our analysis has indicated to be most important. Furthermore, it would seem that, to the degree persons in different dwelling units are involved with each other because of spatial arrangements (that is, could hear arguments, television, and so on), many of the reactions that occur on the interpersonal level (such as irritation and withdrawal) might also occur at this interunit level of interaction. Probably the most significant indicator of overcrowding at the interunit level of interaction is housing units per structure—and this, in our analysis, was the second most important component of density.

We now turn to a brief discussion of the possible effect of density (overcrowding) on each of the five pathologies under consideration.

Mortality

There are at least four possible ways in which overcrowding may be related to mortality. First, increased contact with others increases one's chances of contracting various infectious diseases. Such contact would presumably be related to both the number of persons per room and the number of housing units per structure. Second, if persons do become tired and run-down because of overcrowding[33], overcrowding would increase their susceptibility to disease. Third, sick persons in an overcrowded situation are likely to be constantly disturbed by the activity of others and thus will often not get the rest and relaxation that is important to treatment. And fourth, if overcrowding is associated with irritability, withdrawal, and ineffectual behavior, the treatment the sick person receives (from family members) will not be as effective in an overcrowded situation. Regarding the above points, we would note that investigations of overcrowding do indicate that it is related to poor health[34] and that controlled studies confirm that improved housing reduces the incidence of illness and death[35].

Fertility

Animal studies indicate that overcrowding leads to a drop in natality. However, we found the exact opposite—namely, the greater the density, the greater the fertility. If we are to consider the animal studies as being relevant to human beings, we must reconcile this difference. We reiterate that, although density has a significant impact on many animals, both the effects of density and the mechanisms involved differ widely from species to species. Second, we note that a frequent effect of overcrowding among animals is the development of hypersexuality[1, 4]. Among human beings, an increase in sexual intercourse is likely to lead to increased natality, for women are receptive and able to conceive for 12 months of the year. In contrast, most female animals are receptive and able to conceive during a very specific and limited period of time, and at this time they typically have sexual intercourse. Therefore there is no reason to believe that increased rates of sexual intercourse among animals would typically lead to increased natality, whereas it would among human beings. Third, we note that many factors that would appear to limit natality in animals, such as lack of territory[36] or intense social competition[37], do not appear to be major factors in human populations. Fourth, because overcrowding appears to make it difficult to step back, look at one's situation, and plan ahead, it may be that persons in overcrowded situations are less likely to perceive the long-range consequences of having more children and are thus less likely to want to use birth-control techniques. And finally, because overcrowding makes it difficult to follow through on plans, birth control, even if desired, may be ineffectually practiced.

Ineffectual Parental Care (Public Assistance)

Overcrowding may lead to tensions and irritations in the home. Potentially, this could cause the breakup of the family, which might also mean the loss of financial support. Even if the family does not break up, children may receive less effective care in the home because overcrowding leads to ineffectual performance and withdrawal on the part of the parents. Furthermore, in overcrowded situations parents may be less likely to support their children in the usual manner, through gainful employment, because of weariness, poor health, and ineffectual ways of behaving that affect their performance in the larger community.

Juvenile Delinquency

As noted above, in an overcrowded environment parents are likely to be irritable, weary, harassed, inefficient. Children, in turn, are apt to find the home a relatively unattractive place, full of constant noise and irritation, with no privacy, no place to study, and so on. They are thus inclined to seek relief by getting out of the home. In fact, their disappearance may be partially welcomed by the parents, for it removes, temporarily, a source of irritation. Studies of low-income (overcrowded) families indicate, as our analysis would suggest, a strikingly early cutoff point in parental will and ability to contain children [38].

An important factor in the development of delinquent gangs appears to be a high degree of autonomy. We have suggested that such autonomy is probably greater in dwellings with a high persons-per-room ratio. It may also be that autonomy is greater where there are a large number of housing units per structure, which, as we have already argued, may lead to a decrease in communication between persons in different dwelling units. At any rate, the Chicago data indicate that housing units per structure has more "impact" on delinquency than it does on the other pathologies.

Psychiatric Disorder

From the above discussion, it would seem reasonable to anticipate a fairly strong relation between persons per room and admissions to mental hospitals. However, persons per room has a much weaker relation to admissions to mental hospitals than it does upon the other pathologies. In fact, the density component with by far the strongest relation to admissions to mental hospitals is rooms per housing unit, a finding that does not fit readily into our framework.

Admissions to mental hospitals is highly correlated with the percentage of persons living alone ($r = 0.72$)[39]. It may be that isolation is a contributing factor in the development of mental illness (that is, too little interaction instead of too much). Furthermore, disturbed persons living by themselves are more likely to require hospitalization when they can no longer care for themselves than are persons living with and assisted by others. We suspect, however, that the correlation between rooms per housing unit (or persons living alone) involves primarily a self-selection factor. That is, people who have a history of difficulty in getting along with others are likely to move to small apartments where they live by themselves, and these are the persons who are most likely to be admitted to mental hospitals. If this is the case, then it is the kind of housing that has drawn disturbed persons into particular community areas. This would involve a process that falls completely outside the posited model. It may, of course, be that overcrowding played a role in the creation of the person's initial disorders, which in turn led to his living alone, but these data, while not denying that possibility, do not support it.

CONCLUSION

Our study suggests that overcrowding may have a serious impact on human behavior and that social scientists should consider overcrowding when attempting to explain a wide range of pathological behaviors. Having made this point, we end on a note of caution. We have been using cross-sectional ecological data. Thus, not only have we not proved that there is a causal relation between density and the various pathologies, but the relations that appear at the ecological level may not appear at the individual level. We would also note that, although social structure variables and density are analytically very distinct, they are so highly intercorrelated, at least for these data, that it is difficult to accurately identify their independent effects. Even assuming that the data on Chicago do reflect the importance of density, more research is needed. At the moment, we may speculate about how overcrowding relates to various pathologies, but specific knowledge about casual links, if there are any, is lacking.

REFERENCES AND NOTES

1. J. Calhoun, *Sci. Amer.*, **206**, 139 (February 1962).
2. For a more extensive review of the literature see R. Snyder, in *Progress in Physiological Psychology*, E. Stellar and J. Sprague, Eds. (Academic Press, New York, 1968), pp. 119–160; V. Wynne-Edwards, *Animal Dispersion in Relation to Social Behavior* (Oliver & Boyd, London, 1962).
3. E. Hall, *The Hidden Dimension* (Doubleday, New York, 1966).
4. Y. Susiyama, in *Social Communication among Primates*, S. Altmann, Ed. (Univ. of Chicago Press, Chicago, 1967); pp. 221–236.
5. J. Christian, *J. Mammalogy*, **31**, 247 (1950).
6. J. Christian & D. Davis, *Science* **146**, 1550 (1964).
7. D. Morris, *Behavior*, **4**, 233 (1952).
8. D. Perrins, *J. Anim. Ecol.*, **34**, 601 (1965).
9. R. Laws and I. Parker, in *Symposium of the Zoological Society* (Academic Press, London, 1968) vol. 21, pp. 319–359.
10. R. Chipman, J. A. Holt, K. A. Fox, *Nature* **210**, 653 (1966).
11. F. Clulow and J. Clarke, *ibid.*, **219**, 511 (1968).
12. R. Ardrey, *African Genesis* (Dell, New York, 1961); *The Territorial Imperative* (Dell, New York, 1966); *The Social Contract* (Atheneum, New York, 1970); D. Morris, *The Naked Ape* (Dell, New York, 1967).
13. J. Calhoun, *J. Soc. Issues*, **22**, 46 (1966); R. Sommer, *ibid.*, p. 59; L. Duhl, Ed. *The Union Condition* (Basic Books, New York, 1963); D. Heer, Ed., *Readings on Population* (Prentice-Hall, Englewood Cliffs, N.J., 1968).
14. A. Schorr, *Slums and Social Insecurity* (Government Printing Office, Washington, D.C., 1963). See also S. Riemer, *Amer. Sociol. Rev.*, **8**, 272 (1943).
15. D. Wilner & W. Baer, "Sociocultural factors in residential space," mimeographed, prepared for the Environmental Control Administration of the Department of Health, Education, and Welfare and the American Public Health Association (1970); I. de Groot, R. L. Carroll, R. M. Whitman, "Human health and the spatial environment," mimeographed, prepared for the Environmental Control Administration of the Department of Health, Education, and Welfare and the American Public Health Association (1970); R. Mitchell, "Personal, family and social consequences arising from high density housing in Hong Kong and other major cities in Southeast Asia," mimeographed, prepared for the Environmental Control Administration of the Department of Health, Education, and Welfare and the American Public Health Association (1970).
16. R. Mitchell, *Amer. Sociol. Rev.*, **36**, 18 (1971). As Mitchell notes, 170 square feet (1 square foot = 0.09 square meter) of floor space per person is held to be the lower limit in Europe, and in 1950 the American Public Health Service set the desirable standard at twice this figure. In Mitchell's study the highest category for floor space per person was 67 or more square feet (shown in two tables) and 100 or more square feet (shown in one table).
17. These are ecological data, and relationships that occur at this level of analysis do not necessarily occur at the individual level. However, it seems to us that ecological measures are appropriate and

meaningful when dealing with phenomena such as density. That is, characteristics of areal units may have a significant effect on rates of human behavior.

18. E. Kitagawa & K. Taeuber, Eds., *Local Community Fact Book for Chicago Metropolitan Area, 1960* (Chicago Community Inventory, Chicago, 1963).

19. P. Hauser and E. Kitagawa, *Local Community Fact Book for Chicago, 1950* (Chicago Community Inventory, Chicago, 1953).

20. As noted, there are 75 community areas in Chicago. However, the central business district (community area 32—known as the Loop) is a unique area with regard to various social, economic, and other kinds of indicators. In our case, the measures of pathology are dramatically changed if the central business district is included. Perhaps the most marked case is the rate of admissions to mental hospitals. The city-wide rate is 297.6; the rate for the Loop is 3757.2, and the next highest rate is 851.1. While the elimination of the Loop does not transform the distribution of admissions to mental hospitals into a normal distribution, it does substantially reduce its deviation from this ideal: skewness is reduced from 7.56 to 2.88, and kurtosis is reduced from 62.32 to 15.14 [for a discussion of skewness and kurtosis, see J. Freund, *Modern Elementary Statistics* (Prentice-Hall, Englewood Cliffs, N.J., 1960), pp. 99–105]. Other measures, especially the standardized mortality ratio, are affected in similar, although somewhat less drastic, fashion. For this reason our analysis is based on 74 rather than 75 community areas in Chicago around 1960.

21. A regression analysis of income, education, and occupation was run on each of the pathologies. These five regression equations were then used as a basis for constructing the weighted sum of the three measures as a general index. The equation for the index of social class is as follows: index of social class $= 0.1 \times$ (median family income) $+ 10.0 \times$ (median years of school completed) $+$ (percentage of employed males in white-collar occupations) $- 550.0$. Median family income is by far the most important component of the social class index.

22. A regression analysis of percentage of Negroes, percentage of Puerto Ricans, and percentage of foreign-born was run on each of the pathologies. As with social class, these five regression equations were then used as a basis for constructing the weighted sum of the three measures as a general index. The equation for the index of ethnicity is as follows: index of ethnicity $= 25.0 \times$ (percentage of Negroes) $+ 10 \times$ (percentage of Puerto Ricans) $+ 0.1 \times$ (percentage of foreign-born). The percentage of Negroes is by far the most important component of the ethnicity index.

23. As Blalock notes, grouping by proximity may partially control for independent variables associated with "error" in the dependent variable. Thus to some extent, the size of the correlation between density and the pathologies, and between the social structure variables and the pathologies may be determined by the fact that the community areas, like all ecological variables, involved data grouped by proximity [H. Blalock, *Casual Inferences in Nonexperimental Research* (*Univ. of North Carolina Press, Chapel Hill*, 1974), pp. 102–114].

24. In a subsequent section of this article we will discuss the possibility that in human populations high rates of fertility might be a consequence of population density.

25. The same conclusion is reached if one uses regression coefficients. We would note that there are advantages and disadvantages to using either regression coefficients or partial correlations. Although multiple partial correlations are not strict estimates of the parameters of the causal model, we consider them to be sufficient for our purpose, and using them simplifies the analysis in the second part of the article.

26. H. Winsborough, in *Social Demography*, T. Ford and G. De Jong, Eds. (Prentice-Hall, Englewood Cliffs, N.J., 1970), pp. 84–90.

27. Holding the number of persons per room constant, it is probable that an increase in the number of rooms will increase the likelihood that a person will be able, at least occasionally, to be alone in a room.

28. The number of persons in each community area is reported directly in the *Local Community Fact Book*, as is the number of housing units. The number of rooms per community area and the number of residential structures per community area are, however, based on estimates from openended interval data. The fact book reports the number of housing units with 1, 2, 3, 4, 5, 6, 7, and 8 or more rooms in them. To get an estimate of the number of rooms per community area, we

multiplied the number of housing units at each level by the appropriate number of rooms. The highest interval was multiplied by 8, even though it was an openended interval. The fact book reports the number of housing units in 1-unit structures, 2-unit structures, 3- and 4-unit structures, 5- to 9-unit structures, and 10- or more unit structures. Data from the 1940 fact book suggest that, for that year, slightly over half of the housing units located in the over 10 category were in the over 20 category. To estimate the number of residential structures in the area, we set the midinterval points for these data at 1, 2, 3, 5, 7, and 20. We divided the number of housing units in each category by these midinterval points and added the resulting figures to get the estimate of the number of residential structures for the community area. The four measures of density were then calculated by division: number of persons divided by the number of rooms, the number of rooms divided by the number of housing units, and so on.

29. The cogency of the multiple-partial correlation coefficient as an estimate of the relation is based upon the assumption that all indicators are related to the pathologies in the predicted direction. This assumption is, in general, supported by an examination of a table of the partial regression coefficients relating the four dimensions of density to each of the pathologies, although the general fertility rate increases with density. This table is available from the authors upon request.

30. O. Duncan, in *Sociological Methodology*, E. Borgatta and G. Bohrnstedt, Eds. (Jossey-Bass, San Francisco, 1970). pp. 38–47.

31. R. Sommer, *Personal Space: The Behavioral Basis of Design* (Prentice-Hall, Englewood Cliffs, N.J., 1969).

32. J. Plant, *Amer. J. Psychiat.*, **9**, 849 (1930); in *Modern Introduction to the Family*, N. Bell and E. Vogel, Eds. (Free Press, New York, 1960), pp. 510–520.

33. A. Davis, in *Industry and Society*, W. F. Whyte, Ed, (McGraw-Hill, New York, 1946) pp. 84–106.

34. A. Pond, *Marriage Fam. Living*, **19**, 154 (1957); D. Wilner, R. P. Walkley, M. Tayback, *Amer. J. Public Health*, **46**, 736 (1956).

35. D. Wilner, R. P. Walkley, T. Pinkerton, M. Tayback, *The Housing Environment and Family Life: A Longitudinal Study of the Effects of Housing on Morbidity and Mental Health* (Johns Hopkins Univ. Press, Baltimore, 1962).

36. A. Watson, *Nature*, **215**, 1274 (1967).

37. L. Mech, *The Wolf: The Ecology and Behavior of an Endangered Species* (Natural History Press, Garden City, N.J., 1970).

38. H Lewis, "Child rearing practices among low income families in the District of Columbia," mimeographed, presented at the National Conference on Social Welfare, Minneapolis (1961); S. Riemer, *Amer. Sociol. Rev.* **8**, 272 (1943); R. Mitchell, *ibid.*, **36**, 18 (1971).

39. The relation between the percentage of persons living alone and admissions to mental hospitals remains fairly strong, even after class and ethnicity are used as controls ($r = 0.59$). The percentage of persons living alone also has a high negative correlation with rooms per housing unit $r = -0.91$).

40. The research for this paper was supported in part by the Urban and Regional Development Center, Vanderbilt University. We thank H. Costner, L. Rigsby, A. Gove, and O. D. Duncan for their comments on an earlier draft of this article.

13

Ecological Factors in the Incidence of Schizophrenic and Manic-Depressive Psychoses*

NORBETT L. MINTZ and DAVID T. SCHWARTZ

Numerous studies have suggested that the incidence of mental illness is inversely related to the socioeconomic status of the person's community or the social class of the person himself [25, 37]. The classic study was done by Faris and Dunham [8], who correlated 11 Chicago districts (ranging from high to low socioeconomic stability) with hospital rates of first admission for psychosis. They concluded that the incidence of schizophrenia was inversely related to the socioeconomic stability of a city area, and that the incidence of schizophrenia for racial and for foreign-born groups was higher in areas where these groups were few in number. They stated that the incidence of manic-depressive psychosis showed a *random* pattern with respect both to the stability of an area and to the racial or foreign-born proportions in an area.

CRITIQUE OF EARLIER WORK

While reanalyzing Faris and Dunham's work, we found that their conclusions were not altogether consistent with their data. The stability of an area was inversely related to the incidence of schizophrenia (-0.87), as Faris and Dunham claimed; but it *also* was inversely related to the incidence of manic depression (-0.74). When we reanalyzed their data for racial density in an area, we found, as Faris and Dunham claimed, that racial groups (Negroes and whites), in areas where their numbers were relatively few, had a significantly high incidence of schizophrenia. However, their data showed this inverse relationship *also* to be true for the incidence of manic depression. When we reanalyzed their data for foreign-born density in an area, we found, contrary to Faris and Dunham, that nativity groups (foreign-born and native-born), in areas where they were relatively few, did *not* have a significantly higher incidence of schizophrenia or of manic depression.†

This situation presents an intriguing problem. If Negroes (or whites) living in their "own" areas had generally lower rates for schizophenia and for manic depression than did Negroes (or whites) living in "alien" areas, then why did this reciprocal relation not hold for the native-born and foreign-born? We know of no other study since Faris and Dunham's that has addressed itself to this problem. Dunham was in error [5, pp. 143–145] when he claimed that Dee's findings for St. Louis (reported by Schroeder) supported Faris and Dunham's

*This article originally appeared in *Origins of Abnormal Behavior* (Reading, Mass.: Addison-Wesley, 1971), edited by Corah and Gale. It was supported, in part, by USPHS Grant 5 K01 MH 31,212 from the National Institute of Mental Health. The article contains material that was published previously in *Social Problems*, 1963, **10**, 371–374, and in the *International Journal of Social Psychiatry*, 1964, **10**, 101–118.
†See Mintz and Schwartz for details on these reanalyses [19].

earlier conclusion[8] that persons residing in "alien" areas show high rates of schizophrenia. Dee's study[28] supported this assertion only for whites living in Negro areas. No data were reported for the foreign-born.

RATIONALE

Let us assume that ethnicity and residence does affect the incidence of psychosis. If so, one would expect to find a lower incidence where foreign-born groups live in an area primarily populated by their "own" members. But what constitutes their "own" members, *all* other foreign-born? This seemed to be the assumption of Faris and Dunham, or at least this was the kind of data they had. Our assumption would be that "their own members" only would be the members of *their own ethnic background*. Why should the foreign-born Italian benefit psychologically from living in a foreign-born area which is predominantly Puerto Rican? Since foreign-born areas differ in their distribution of dominant ethnicity, calculating foreign-born rates homogeneously is bound to lead to the inconclusive results found in the data of Faris and Dunham.

A second factor we must consider is how a foreign-born population *experiences* its ethnicity. Foreign-born groups differ in their degree of clannishness, retention of native mores, integration with the dominant culture, language barrier, etc.[21, 30, 31]. Also, different ethnic groups vary in the extent to which the second generation is integrated with, or in conflict with, the immigrant generation. Ethnic groups having a pattern of immigrant-second generation cohesion may experience more of an ethnic community than those with immigrant-second generation disunity or conflict. These factors should influence the degree to which psychosis rates for an ethnic group are affected by the proportion of this group in the community. Unless a separate analysis is done of a single group, inconclusive results again may be found.

We propose that if these various interacting factors were to be untangled, Faris and Dunham's inverse correlations for racial density and incidence (that members of a race have low rates of psychosis in their "own" neighborhoods and high rates in "alien" neighborhoods) would be obtained also for ethnic density and incidence.* If so, then correlations between a community's socioeconomic index and its incidence of psychosis (found for both types of psychosis by our reanalysis of Faris and Dunham's study, and found for schizophrenia in several other studies) may have been brought about by ethnic factors. What follows is the rationale for these assumptions.

In any complex urban area, communities having many foreign-born generally are communities with a low socioeconomic index. There are various reasons for this. Certain indices of community status, such as Faris and Dunham's index of area stability, use a high percentage of foreign-born as one criterion of an area's instability or low status. With such a procedure, there obviously will be an inverse correlation between foreign-born density and socioeconomic status. However, any of several other indices of socioeconomic status (e.g., rental or income) also may place most foreign-born communities on the low end of the scale. Such communities may be immigrant slum areas, consisting of a variety of ethnic populations, and classed by sociologists as socially disintegrating[35]. However, there are

---

*We wish to remind the reader that "incidence of psychosis" or "rate of psychosis" used throughout this article refers to the proportion of individuals from a community admitted for the *first time* to any mental hospital for a psychotic disorder. Such a definition is different from "true prevalence" which would be the proportion of psychotic individuals in a community, whether hospitalized or not.

other foreign-born communities which are not slum areas in the sense of social disintegration. They may consist of one predominant ethnic group, such as Boston's Italian North End[12, 36]. Yet these communities also are low on most socioeconomic scales. Being high in immigrant population, their education is low, in most cases so is their income, and, because their patterns of living lead them to prefer tenement dwellings (economically as well as socially), their rental also is low. (Certain exceptions occur; black ghettos often have higher rentals than economically better, white areas.)

Whatever the specific reasons, communities high in foreign-born generally are low on socioeconomic factors. Since we propose that there is an inverse relation between ethnic density and incidence of psychosis, one then is led to consider that a community's socioeconomic index may not be the causal factor in the inverse relation found between it and incidence of psychosis; it simply may accompany other factors such as ethnic density and distribution. Let us assume the following conditions:

(a) an ethnic group has an average or low incidence of psychosis in its "own" areas but a high incidence in "alien" areas;
(b) a community low on socioeconomic or stability factors is frequently a community with a mixed ethnic population;
(c) in such a mixed community, there are one or two numerically strong groups and several remaining numerically weak groups; and
(d) the numerically strong group in such a community usually consists of a plurality, not a majority.

Given these conditions, the multiethnic community may have *in toto* a relatively high incidence of psychosis. This result can be brought about because:

1. the various smaller ethnic groups have just slightly higher rates of psychosis than does the dominant ethnic group, but because these groups, when combined, outnumber the dominant group, the *average* incidence of psychosis for the area will be weighted with these higher rates;
2. the various smaller groups, even if they do not outnumber the dominant ethnic group, have *disproportionately* higher rates than does the dominant group, again averaging out to a high community incidence; or
3. the smaller ethnic groups outnumber the dominant group, *and* have disproportionately high rates. Such multiethnic communities also have a low socioeconomic index, for reasons given earlier; therefore an inverse correlation will appear between the community's socioeconomic index and its incidence of psychosis. However, this correlation may hold only for the various smaller groups of the low socioeconomic, multiethnic community, *but not necessarily for the dominant members of the community.*

The inverse correlations which have been obtained between a community's socioeconomic index and its incidence of psychosis thus may have reflected only several ethnic groups' minority status in a community and these groups' high rates of psychosis. [For other critiques of the class-incidence relationship, see Refs. 4, 14, 18, 22, 26.]

The above discussion yields two general hypotheses. When a *single* ethnic group is investigated, and when its *experience* is one of shared patterns of distinctive behavior (common origin, religion, language, customs), then:

1. In areas where the members of this group are relatively numerous, their incidence rates, both for schizophrenia and for manic depression, will be lower than in areas where they are relatively few.

2. In cities where the members of this group are represented widely throughout the city, so that their subgroups, both large and small, are scattered among communities sometimes high in socioeconomic status and sometimes low, then for this group *no* correlation will be found between the incidence of schizophrenia or manic depression and community socioeconomic status.

The essence of this second hypothesis is that if the numerical density of an ethnic group either were constant for communities of varying socioeconomic status, or else varied randomly among them, then no correlation for this group would be found between psychosis rates and community socioeconomic status. (This assumes that the class-incidence relationship is an artifact of ethnic density.) Since random variation is easier to obtain than is constancy, the hypothesis was stated in that form. Of course, strict randomness is not obtained either. There usually is some negative correlation between the number of foreign-born in a community and its socioeconomic status, for reasons stated earlier. This may be eliminated by statistical manipulation, as we show later.

PROCEDURES

To test these two propositions, we chose to study the Italian population of Greater Boston. This group, which experiences itself as an ethnic community, also is one of the more firmly established groups of the Boston area, and so it is represented over a fairly wide socioeconomic range of communities. Our general procedure was to correlate rates for the incidence of psychosis among Italians from various communities in the Greater Boston area with these communities' "Italian" density and "socioeconomic" indices.

Reports of first admission to all mental hospitals in Massachusetts (public, private, Veterans) for $2\frac{1}{2}$ years (starting July 1, 1956) were obtained for Italian patients from the Massachusetts Department of Mental Health. An "Italian" patient was someone either Italian-born or American-born but of an Italian parent or parents (second-generation). The "Greater Boston" area was defined as any of 24 communities in Boston Corporate City or any of 23 suburbs within 10 miles of Boston's City Hall. Since our data only spanned a $2\frac{1}{2}$-year period, to have included communities with less than 500 Italian-born inhabitants would have led to erratic incidence rates per year, either very high or zero. Therefore, we used only communities with *at least* 500 Italian-born for the 1950 census. This left us with 28 areas, including Boston's West End. This neighborhood was undergoing redevelopment and population relocation. Therefore, we excluded West End patients from our general analysis, leaving a total of 27 communities (see Table 13.1). These 27 communities had 462 Italian patients admitted to mental hospitals for first admission during these $2\frac{1}{2}$ years; 260 of them were diagnosed as having a schizophrenic disorder (SZ) and 202 as having a manic-depressive disorder (MD). Of the 462 patients, 137 were Italian-born, and 325 were American-born but one or both parents were born in Italy.

Using 1950 U.S. census data[33], we calculated the incidence rates for SZ and for MD among Italian-born and second-generation Italians in each of the 27 communities. For the base population of the number of Italians in a community, we used the census figures for the number of Italian-born in each community (see Table 13.1, data column 1) and then multiplied that figure by 3.25. In other words, we assumed a ratio of Italian-born to second-generation of $1:2.25$ for each community, which Weinman found to be fairly constant for Italians in 25 U.S. city areas in 1950[34]. We then divided the number of SZ and MD first admissions for a community by that community's base population, which gave us

Table 13.1 Community Data for Italian Density, Socioeconomic Status, and Incidence of Psychosis*

Location	Ecological Data for Italian-Born			Incidence† data	
	Number	% of Population	Median Monthly Rent	SZ Rate	MD Rate
Corporate Boston:					
Allston	535	1.6	43.80	46	46
Brighton	564	1.6	52.10	112	45
E. Boston & Orient hts.	7,121	14.1	26.00	58	43
Hyde Park	1,342	4.5	35.20	37	73
Jamaica Plain	886	1.6	34.90	167	69
Meeting House Hill	705	2.0	34.80	87	52
N. Dorchester	1,006	2.2	32.80	66	13
North End	4,484	27.9	21.30	33	22
Roslindale	1,020	3.6	38.90	73	97
Rosbury	1,477	2.1	26.90	81	54
S. Boston	1,003	1.8	27.10	61	98
South End	1,073	2.0	27.80	81	58
Suburban areas:					
Arlington	966	2.2	46.30	71	71
Belmont	781	2.9	46.80	102	68
Cambridge	2,509	2.1	36.90	74	74
Chelsea	950	2.4	28.60	166	52
Everett	2,926	6.0	34.10	48	40
Lynn	1,631	1.6	35.30	45	8
Malden	1,578	2.6	37.00	138	11
Medford	3,535	5.3	39.40	52	49
Newton	1,993	2.4	47.30	56	74
Quincy	2,434	2.9	40.60	65	80
Revere	2,375	6.5	34.40	57	26
Somerville	4,890	4.8	34.80	61	33
Waltham	1,432	3.0	38.30	96	47
Watertown	1,666	4.5	43.30	38	98
Woburn	540	2.6	32.40	22	68
Total	51,422	(Av.) 3.6	(Av.) 36.20	(Av.) 62	(Av.) 48

*Per 100,000 population.
†SZ = Schizophrenia.   MD = Manic depression.

admissions rates for $2\frac{1}{2}$ years. These $2\frac{1}{2}$-year rates were divided by 2.5 to give the rates per year, and multiplied by 100,000 to yield the incidence rates per year per 100,000 population (see Table 13.1, data columns 4 and 5).

These incidence rates were to be correlated with Italian community density and community socioeconomic status. For one index of Italian density we used the number of Italian-born in that community as of 1950, that is, the Italian-born base population described above. This index may serve well in communities with a *large* number of Italian-born inhabitants. A second index was the percentage of Italian-born inhabitants among all inhabitants of that community (Table 13.1, data column 2) obtained from the 1950 census. We suspect that this index may be more accurate in areas with relatively *few* Italian-born inhabitants. Having no supposition as to where the line of separation might be, we used both the percentage and the absolute number of Italian-born as indices of the density of the Italian population in each community.

There are many possible indices for community socioeconomic status. None of them appears to have any overall advantage, and all of them have a high correlation with the simple and readily available median monthly rental[13, 27]. For these reasons, median monthly rental (as given in the 1950 census) became our socioeconomic index for the 27 communities (Table 13.1, data column 3).

RESULTS

Pearsonian correlations were run between ecological indices and incidence data. Table 13.2 shows that there were significant inverse correlations for incidence rates and both the absolute number and the percentage of Italian-born; i.e., communities with high Italian densities had low incidence rates of SZ and MD among their Italian members. In contrast. there were *no* significant correlations between community median monthly rental and incidence either of SZ or of MD among the communities' Italian members. However, there was a possible artifact in these data. As can be seen in Table 13.2, the "Italian" density indices themselves were negatively correlated with monthly rental (− 0.41 and − 0.48). We therefore did an analysis of partial correlation. This controls (a) for the influence of monthly rental on the correlation between "Italian" density and the incidence of SZ or MD, and (b) for the influence of "Italian" density on the correlation between rental and the incidence of SZ or MD.

Table 13.2 Correlations Between Ecological Factors and Incidence of Psychosis.*

	Italian-Born		Median Rental
	No.	%	
Schizophrenia	− 0.41	− 0.33	0.01
Manic depression	− 0.39	− 0.39	0.21
Number of Italian-born		0.65	− 0.41
Per cent of population			− 0.48

*Correlations in italics reached at least the 0.05 level of confidence for a one-tailed test of Pearsonian correlation.

Table 13.3 shows that the inverse correlations found between "Italian" density indices and the community's "Italian" incidence of SZ or MD remained significant even after partial correlation. Table 13.3 also shows that, with partial correlation, we still did not uncover any significant inverse correlations between rental and incidence of SZ or MD.

Three other results, not of central relevance to this report, were found:

1. As noted in the Procedures section, Boston's West End was not included in our study because it was undergoing redevelopment. However, we computed its rates for comparison with the rest of our data. The West End was high in Italian-born (10% and 1,668 in number), which would lead one to expect, on the basis of our other results, a low incidence of SZ and

Table 13.3   Partial Correlations Between Ecological Factors and Incidence of Psychosis.*

	Italian-Born		Median Rental
	No.	%	
Schizophrenia (rental controlled)	−0.44	−0.37	
Schizophrenia (with No. Italian-born controlled)			−0.19
Schizophrenia (with % Italian-born controlled)			−0.16
Manic depression (with rental controlled)	−0.34	−0.34	
Manic depression (with No. Italian-born controlled)			0.04
Manic depression (with % Italian-born controlled)			0.03

*Correlations in italics reached at least the 0.05 level of confidence for a one-tailed test of partial correlation.

of MD among the Italian inhabitants. Actually, the West End rates were *unusually high* (132 for SZ and 74 for MD), falling well above the average for our sample of 27 communities (see Table 13.1). Furthermore, the rates for this area were probably *underestimated*. The population base used to calculate them came from the 1950 census, and a fair percentage of the population had been relocated before or during the period of our study. While we must be cautious in any interpretation, since it is a single instance, this finding certainly supports other findings of high psychosis rates in areas of social disorganization[5].

2. Communities with less than 500 Italian-born in 1950 were not included in our study, for reasons stated in our Procedures section. However, we computed the *average* incidence rates for all 11 such communities within Corporate Boston. These communities totaled 1,974 Italian-born as of 1950, an average of 180 Italian-born per community. The average incidence rate for Italian inhabitants for all 11 communities was 98 for SZ and 72 for MD. As can be seen in Table 13.1, these rates were 50% above the average for the 27 communities having more than 500 Italian-born. Thus, the inverse relationship between density and incidence of psychosis also holds at the extreme of low density.

3. As was seen in Table 13.1, the average rate among Italians for SZ and MD was 62 and 48. These rates seem high, especially the one for MD, when they are compared to standard rates for urban areas. But they differ from standard rates in the following ways:

(a) our rates were based on admissions to *all* types of mental hospitals and include hospitals *throughout* the state, rather than just in Greater Boston;
(b) over 30% of the sample included an immigrant population; and
(c) our rates had a population denominator based on the census six to eight years prior to the admission records, so the rates probably were inflated.

Even if these factors were controlled, our rates should be compared with the rates for Boston's general population before concluding that the rates obtained for Italians were unusually high.

DISCUSSION

Incidence of Schizophrenia

Our inverse correlation between density and SZ is analogous to the findings of Faris and Dunham[8] and of Dee[28]: races living in areas populated by their "own" races had lower incidence rates for SZ than they did in areas populated by "others." In addition, it clarifies why similar results were *not* found in our reanalysis of their data for foreign-born density and SZ. Treating the *entire* ethnic population of a community as a single group, not taking into account the fact that in one area they may be dominant and in another not, was shown by our results to be a source of error in the Faris and Dunham study.

Our lack of correlation between community rental and community incidence of SZ contradicts the findings of those epidemiological studies of large cities which found community socioeconomic status to be inversely correlated with incidence of SZ[5, 8, 26, 28]. But it is consistent with Clausen and Kohn's investigation[3] of a small city (Hagerstown, Maryland) which revealed no correlation between socioeconomic status and SZ. Our study may help to explain these contradictions.

We proposed that communities low on a socioeconomic index often have large combined numbers (various nationalities) of foreign-born. While this can result in high rates for the *combined* ethnic population, any single ethnic group may have low rates in those communities where they are relatively numerous. Since we studied a *single* ethnic group, widely represented throughout various socioeconomic communities, we avoided generating an artificial relationship between socioeconomic indices and incidence rates. (The artifact may also be avoided, where the correlation between density of an ethnic group in various communities and the socioeconomic index of these communities is known, by the technique of partial correlation.) Likewise, Clausen and Kohn's study did not generate this artificial relationship because their city was "an old and settled community... relatively stable in recent decades [and] remarkably homogeneous—preponderantly white, Protestant, and native-born"[4; p. 70]. In effect, then, their study paralleled ours in that it had a single cultural population widely represented throughout the various socioeconomic areas of the city.

Incidence of Manic-Depressive Psychosis

We found that ethnic density in a community also was inversely related to the community incidence of MD. This is analogous to the findings for racial density and MD, uncovered when we reanalyzed Faris and Dunham's data. Similar to our findings for incidence of SZ, our own data also showed no effect of community socioeconomic factors on the community incidence of MD, but, unlike the results for SZ, these findings do not greatly clarify the relation between MD and community socioeconomic factors.

Studies of the incidence of SZ have found either no correlation or a negative correlation with community socioeconomic factors[4, 5, 28, 32]. However, studies of the incidence of MD have found both negative as well as positive correlations with community socioeconomic factors, and sometimes no correlation at all[4, 28, 32]. In fact, within a *single* study one can find this inconsistent situation. For example, the reader will remember that when we reanalyzed Faris and Dunham's data for socioeconomic stability of community, we found there was a negative relationship (-0.74) between it and incidence of MD. Their stability index was composed of several factors, one of which was an educational measure for the area. Yet, when they correlated MD incidence with the area's educational measure alone, they found a positive correlation of 0.41[8]. Given such inconsistency, a likely hypothesis is that correlations found by others between community socioeconomic factors and community incidence of MD have *various* causes. A negative correlation, uncovered by our reanalysis of Faris and Dunham's data and in other studies[28, 32], perhaps can be explained in the same manner as we explained the negative correlation between these factors and the incidence of SZ: as an artifact of the nature of the ethnic composition of lower socioeconomic communities. We know that this was likely for the Faris and

Dunham data, since one factor in their community stability index was the percentage of foreign-born in the area.

This does not explain the *positive* relation between community socioeconomic factors and the incidence of MD sometimes found [5, 8], nor why our data did not show one. One artifact operating in these studies may have been the proportion of patients with this diagnosis who came from private hospitals. Faris and Dunham [8] have shown that many more diagnoses of MD, compared to SZ, were contributed by private hospitals than by state hospitals. This may reflect the higher socioeconomic background of these patients, or it may only reflect different diagnostic fashions, which have been shown to exist [4, 25]. If the latter is the case, then contradictory results can be attributed to differences in sample. Since our own study used *all* mental hospitals, and since it came after there has been some recognition of diagnostic fashion, it is possible that this bias did not operate in our data. However, we did not tabulate diagnosis by the type of hospital, so we have no way of checking this point.

Some Qualifications Regarding Community Socioecomic Factors

Our total patient sample was rather small and was limited to a single ethnic group. Possibly there is a correlation between incidence of psychosis and community socioeconomic factors, but it is so weak that a rather large sample would be needed to demonstrate it. For example, after partial correlation, a weak negative correlation between community incidence of SZ and community rental did appear, but it was not statistically reliable (Table 13.3). Perhaps certain ethnic groups may not show this relationship, while others may. Furthermore,

(a) our rates had a 1950 census base, while our cases were from 1956 to 1958;
(b) our rates were based on an estimated second-generation Italian population; and
(c) our city areas were gross subdivisions, in contrast to Faris and Dunham's finer subdivisions.

Any of these factors may have obscured a possible inverse correlation between socioeconomic factors and incidence of psychosis existing independently of ethnic-ecological factors. Finally, our results in no way pertain to whether or not the socioeconomic status of *patients themselves* is inversely related to psychosis, but only to the question of socioeconomic factors in the *community* and the *community's* incidence of psychosis.

In addition, another consideration must be kept in mind. Previous investigators often assumed that "general stress" would lead to an inverse relationship between socioeconomic factors and psychosis [3, 14]. All other things being equal, having more substantial means should lead to an easier life (and presumably lower rates of psychosis) than having less; but when are *all* other things equal? Socioeconomic status *per se* may be overwhelmed by more relevant factors. Birch has commented on this in discussing the relationship between the incidence of schizophrenia and social structure. He pointed out that, especially in large urban communities, occupation plays no more or less important a role in determining lower socioeconomic status than do such factors as ethnicity, generation, and length of community residence [2; p. 89]. Studies of European and Asian cities with little in- or out-migration, and consequently a homogeneous ethnic population, can be helpful here. If such studies show an inverse relation between community socioeconomic status and incidence rates of psychoses, then the ethnic factor will not be implicated. Unfortunately, cross-cultural data on such problems are scarce [17, 22, 26].

One way to conceptualize the general problem is in terms of the "ins" and the "outs" within a community. The relevant dimension for defining "in-ness" will not be the same for all places at all times. In a homogeneous city within a strongly class-stratified society, socioeconomic factors may be the most relevant dimension; but in the urban United States, lower-class community integration achieved by ethnic groups in "urban villages" (such as Little Italy or Chinatown) can relegate socioeconomic status to secondary importance (at least for the problem of incidence rates of psychosis). It is relevant now to recall our findings for Boston's West End. This area, undergoing redevelopment, had extremely high rates of psychosis, supporting the view that community disintegration affects incidence. In a sense, then, socioeconomic factors may be relevant though indirect. Areas low in socioeconomic status are likely to have a large, combined ethnic population, for reasons mentioned earlier. Under conditions of a highly uniform ethnic population, this may lead to a more stable community, while under conditions of many antagonistic groups, this may lead to a very unstable community. In either case, these communities, whether *organized* lower-class communities or *disorganized* slums, are highly vulnerable to redevelopment schemes, which then lead to a highly disintegrated community[9, 10].

If socioeconomic status does play an independent role, we believe that this, as well as any other factors, may best be approached by the study of community organization. Such a complex variable comes closer to requiring the kind of analysis associated with field studies, rather than census and record studies. This probably is the direction that will have to be taken if fuller understanding of these problems is to be found[15, 22].

Incidence and Etiology

Incidence studies on the rate of psychotic breakdown in a community, such as this one, often attempt to understand the effects of sociocultural forces on the psychogenesis of the psychoses. A less dynamic, though plausible, assumption is that studies such as these do not relate to etiology in a *psychological* sense, but only to the *social definition* of psychosis. Obviously, first admission to a mental hospital is only one measure of incidence, and, in this measure, many selective factors operate. For example, a very large percentage of admissions still come about through the police and the courts[11; p. 187]. Therefore, the "outs" in the community may be "easy targets" for admission to mental hospitals, for punitive or other reasons.

We can delineate at least three (not mutually exclusive) ways in which community dynamics may influence the hospital incidence of psychosis [see also 16, 22]:

1. Definition of psychosis Certain ethnic groups may have greater tolerance for deviation among their members than do others[20, 24, 29]. Also, any ethnic group, where its members are in the minority, may be vulnerable to community hostility and to intolerance of even minor deviation. Likewise, if a community is in some way disrupted, stabilized psychotics existing "at peace" in the community may somewhat arbitrarily be defined as "cases" when no longer protected by normal community functioning. The latter is one possible explanation for the high rates found in Boston's West End.

2. Exacerbation of psychosis This also is not etiological in a psychogenetic sense. Community dynamics may precipitate a dormant psychosis, making hospitalization necessary. For example, relocation of families and its attendant stresses may precipitate breakdown in prepsychotic individuals. This is a second possible reason for the high rates in Boston's West End. Living in a neighborhood that suddenly has an influx of a "hostile" ethnic group offers another opportunity for community dynamics to play a role in precipitating breakdown and hospitalization in borderline individuals.

3. Psychogenesis of psychosis   Here one directly implicates community dynamics in the developmental process. Different communities have different styles of life, which affect child-rearing practices, as well as the values and opportunities available to the growing personality[21]. Benedict's discussion of cultural continuity or discontinuity[1] is relevant not only for total cultures, but also within subgroups of a culture and between subgroups and the entire culture. For example, a second-generation Italo-American growing up in an Irish-American community has the discontinuity of his Italian background with both the dominant American culture and also the more immediate Irish subculture. An immigrant Italian going through the process of "acculturation " is likewise going through a microgenetic, developmental process[6, 7]. While the psychogenetic link with the immigrant is not as strong as with the second generation, one can think of community dynamics as providing a slow integrating or disintegrating effect on the personality over time. (If the disintegration does not develop slowly, but rather occurs soon after immigration, we would class it as social exacerbation.)

Ecological studies of urban incidence of psychosis have yet to untangle psychogenesis from "definition" or "exacerbation." While they always will be interdependent, we expect that ethnic community factors will have separate and discernible effects on the *etiology* of psychoses as well as on their manifestation[20, 22]. But to demonstrate these effects, greater specificity in theory must occur. Many studies proceed on a vague notion of "general stress": incidence rates are lower for certain groups in particular areas because their situation is less stressful[3]. With such a lack of articulation, it is difficult to test psychogenetic hypotheses[14, 22].

SUMMARY

Analysis of the Chicago study of Faris and Dunham led to the restudy of urban-ethnic ecology and the incidence of psychosis. The incidence of schizophrenia and of manic depression among Italians was found to be inversely related to the density of Italians in Greater Boston communities. No correlation was found between community incidence of psychosis and community monthly rental. Correlations found by others between community incidence and community socioeconomic factors may have been due to aspects of urban-ethnic ecology. The relevance of these findings to questions of etiology was discussed.

REFERENCES

1. Benedict, R. Continuities and discontinuities in cultural conditioning. In P. Mullahy (Ed.), *A study of interpersonal relations.* New York: Grove Press, 1949. Pp. 297–309.
2. Birch, H. G. Discussion of schizophrenia and social structure. In B. Pasamanick (Ed.), *Epidemiology of mental disorder.* Washington, D.C.: A.A.A.S. Publ. No. 60, 1959. Pp. 86–90.
3. Clausen, J. A., & Kohn, M. L. The ecological approach in social psychiatry. *Amer. J. Sociol.,* 1954, **60,** 140–151.
4. Clausen, J. A., & Kohn, M. L. Relation of schizophrenia to the social structure of a small city. In B. Pasamanick (Ed.), *Epidemiology of mental disorder.* Washington, D.C.: A.A.A.S. Publ. No. 60, 1959. Pp. 69–86.
5. Dunham, H. W. *Sociological theory and mental disorder.* Detroit: Wayne State University, 1959.

6. Erikson, E. H. *Childhood and society.* New York: Norton, 1950. Pp. 213–218, 244–284.
7. Erikson, E. H. Identity and the life cycle. *Psychol. Issues,* 1959, **1,** 18–50, 147–157.
8. Faris, R., & Dunham, H. W. *Mental disorders in urban areas.* Chicago: University of Chicago, 1939.
9. Gans, H. J. *The urban villagers.* Glencoe, Ill.: Free Press, 1962.
10. Higbee, E. C. *The squeeze: Cities without space.* New York:Morrow, 1960.
11. Hollingshead, A. B., & Redlich, F. C. *Social class and mental illness.* New York: Wiley, 1958.
12. Jacobs, J. *Life and death of the great American city.* New York: Random House, 1961.
13. Kahl, J. A., & Davis, J. A. A comparison of indexes of socioeconomic status. *Amer. Sociol. Rev.,* 1955, **20,** 317–326.
14. Kennedy, D. A. Key issues in cross-cultural study of mental disorders. In B. Kaplan (Ed.), *Studying personality cross culturally.* New York: Row, Peterson, 1961. Pp. 405–427.
15. Kennedy, M. C. Is there an ecology of mental illness? *Int. J. Soc. Psychiat.,* 1964, **10,** 119–133.
16. Leighton, A. H. *My name is Legion.* New York: Basic, 1959. Pp. 133–188.
17. Lin, T. A study of the incidence of mental disorders in other cultures. *Psychiatry,* 1953, **16,** 313–336.
18. Miller, S. M., & Mishler, E. G. Social class, mental illness, and American psychiatry, an expository review. *Milbank Med. Fund Quart.,* 1959, **37,** 174–199.
19. Mintz, N. L., & Schwartz, D. T. Urban ecology and psychosis. *Int. J. Soc. Psychiat.,* 1964, **10,** 101–118.
20. Mintz, N. L., & Wylan, L. Ethnic differences in response to psychotic symptoms. MS in preparation, 1969.
21. Opler, M. K. The influence of ethnic and class subcultures on child care. *Soc. Probl.,* 1955, **3,** 12–21.
22. Opler, M. K. *Culture and social psychiatry.* New York: Atherton, 1967.
23. Opler, M. K., & Singer, J. L. Ethnic differences in behavior and psychopathology. *Int. J. Soc. Psychiat.,* 1956, **2,** 11–22.
24. Owens, M. B. Alternative hypotheses for the explanation of Faris and Dunham's results. *Amer. J. Sociol.,* 1941, 47, 48–57.
25. Plunkett, R. J., & Gordon, J. E. *Epidemiology and mental illness.* New York: Basic, 1960. Chapter 3.
26. Rose, A. M., & Stub, H. R. Summary of studies on the incidence of mental disorders. In A. M. Rose (Ed.), *Mental health and mental disorder.* New York: Norton, 1955. Pp. 87–117.
27. Schmid, C. F., MacCannel, E., & Van Arsdoil, M., Jr. The ecology of the American city. *Amer. Soc. Rev.,* 1958, **23,** 392–401.
28. Schroeder, C. W. Mental disorders in cities. *Amer. J. Sociol.,* 1942, **48,** 40–48.
29. Scott, W. A. Research definitions of mental health and mental disorders. *Psychol. Bull.,* 1958, **55,** 29–45.
30. Srole, L., Langner, T., Michael, S., Opler, M. K., & Rennie, T. *Mental health in the metropolis: The midtown Manhattan study,* Vol. I. New York: McGraw-Hill, 1962.
31. Suttles, G. D. *The social order of the slum.* Chicago: University of Chicago, 1969.
32. Tietze, C., Lemkau, P., & Cooper, M. Schizophrenia, manic-depressive psychosis, and socioeconomic status. *Amer. J. Sociol.,* 1941, **47,** 167–175.
33. U.S. Bureau of Census: *Seventeenth U.S. Census.* Washington, D.C.: Government Printing Office, 1952.
34. Weinman, J. (Station WBOS, Boston). Personal communication, 1958.
35. Woods, R. *The city wilderness.* Boston: Houghton Mifflin, 1898.
36. Whyte, W. F. *Street-corner society.* Chicago: University of Chicago, 1955.
37. Zubin, J. *Field studies in the mental disorders.* New York: Grune & Stratton, 1961.

Suggested Additional Readings

Calhoun, J. B. Population density and social pathology. *Scientific American*, 1962, **206**, 139–146.

Calhoun, J. B. Ecological factors in the development of behavioral anomalies. In J. Zubin & H. F. Hunt (Eds.), *Comparative psychopathology: animal and human*. New York: Grune & Stratton, 1967.

Calhoun, J. B. Design for mammalian living. *Architectural Association Quarterly*, 1970, **1**, 1–12.

Clausen, J. A. & Kohn, M. L. The ecological approach in social psychiatry. *American Journal of Sociology*, 1954, **60**, 140–151.

Morris, D. *The naked ape*. New York: Dell, 1961.

Morris, D. *The human zoo*. New York: McGraw-Hill, 1969.

Proshansky, H. M., Ittelson, W. H., & Rivlin, L. G. The influence of the physical environment on behavior: Some basic assumptions. In H. M. Proshansky, W. H. Ittelson, & L. G. Rivlin (Eds.), *Environmental psychology*. New York: Holt, Rinehart & Winston, 1970.

Schwartz, D. C. On the ecology of political violence: "The long hot summer" as a hypothesis. *American Behavioral Scientist*, 1968, **11**, 24–28.

Somner, R. *Personal space: the behavioral basis of design*. Englewood Cliffs, N.J.: Prentice-Hall, 1969.

Wechsler, H. Community growth, depressive disorders, and suicide. *Annual Journal of Sociology*, 1961, **67**, 9–16.

Anthropological Factors

14

A Cross-Cultural Approach to Mental
Health Problems*[1]

EDWARD D. WITTKOWER and JOHN FRIED

Much thought has been given to the definition of the term and to the delineation of the field of *social psychiatry*. According to M. Opler[1], "the impact of social and cultural environment upon the development of personalities is the central concern of social psychiatry." This general description indicates that social psychiatry, in contrast to clinical psychiatry, invariably involves the complicated play of interpersonal relations between sets of individuals, and that it views the behavior of such individuals against the background of, in interaction with, and in response to their sociocultural environment. Such approach implies and presupposes a thorough knowledge on the part of the social psychiatrist of the social system in which patients under his observation live, or, more realistically, a close collaboration between psychiatrists and social scientists.

However, because the field as outlined by M. Opler[1]—ranging as it does from marriage counseling to the effect of culture change on mental health—is so wide that no single person can encompass it, it appears advisable to detach *cultural psychiatry* from social psychiatry and to treat it as a separate entity. As such the term cultural psychiatry denotes a field of research which explores the frequency, etiology and nosology of mental illness and the care and after-care of the mentally ill within the confines of a cultural unit and in relation to the cultural environment concerned. The term "culture" has gradually emerged from the studies of anthropologists to refer to a uniquely expressed mode of social life based upon patterns of thinking and acting that reflect overtly and covertly organized feelings and perceptions which are held in common by all the normal members of the community.

As regards the interplay between culture and personality, the position taken by us can be defined as follows: Certain drives and infantile experiences are common to all human beings though variations in degree and quality occur. Parental values, attitudes, and controls which reflect cultural tradition are, by precept and example, implanted in, and incorporated and absorbed by, the ego of the child and form the core of his conscious and unconscious superego. Consequently culture does not only represent the fabric of the ways of living of the society in which we live but it also has its counterpart in our inner world. In line with this argument culture conflict has its battleground in the inner as well as in the outer world.

A still wider vista unfolds if human behavior (normal and abnormal) and any of the areas named are subjected to comparison in contrasting cultures. Because this approach

---

*Reprinted from *The American Journal of Psychiatry*, Vol. 116, pp. 423–428, 1959. Copyright © 1959, the American Psychiatric Association.

[1]Read at the 115th annual meeting of The American Psychiatric Association, Philadelphia, Pa., April 27–May 1, 1959.

goes beyond the boundaries of one culture, we have called it *transcultural*; its comparative and contrasting aspects have been labeled cross-cultural.

During the last 3 years Dr. Fried and I have been jointly engaged in a transcultural psychiatric study. The aims of this research are to arrive at conclusions regarding which cultural norms make for mental health and which foster the development of mental illness; and by isolating and defining modifiable sociocultural variables, to work toward prevention, or at least reduction, of mental illness.

SOURCES OF DATA

The data summarized in this paper have come predominantly from correspondence with psychiatrists and social scientists abroad, strategically placed and qualified to be able to give authoritative information. This communication network stretches around the world and has involved over 30 countries.[2]

A SURVEY OF CROSS-CULTURAL MENTAL HEALTH PROBLEMS

Four questions concerning this field of interest which have been raised repeatedly will be taken up successively.

1. Are There Any Significant Differences in the Prevalence and Incidence of Mental Disorders in Different Cultures?

Largely based on rates of mental hospital admissions and hence open to objections regarding their general validity such differences have been reported. For instance mental hospital admissions of schizophrenics according to Ratanakorn[2] amount to 72% in Thailand as against 28.8% in the U.S.S.R.[3] on a survey of 193 Soviet Russian mental institutions. According to several observers, the incidence of depressive psychoses is low among African Negroes[5, 6, 7], and among Indonesians[8]. The suicide rate is reported high in Japan, Denmark, Switzerland, and in Whites resident in South Africa. It is low in Ireland[9], in African Negroes[10], and nonexistent in the Bantu. Margetts[11] reporting from Kenya, doubts whether depressions and suicides in Africa are really as rare as is generally believed. According to him "most Africans do not have much of a concept of depression as an illness though they have words for sadness and grief." Rarity of senile psychosis has been noted in Hong Kong[12] and Formosa[13]. Also open to doubt is the alleged very low incidence of psychoneuroses in African Negroes, Chinese, and Indians. It seems conceivable that the scarcity of trained psychiatrists in these countries is such, and the necessity to deal with psychiatric emergencies is so great, that the problem of psychoneurosis, which looms so large in the Western world, is of minor importance. The writers from Ireland[9] and Greece[14], in Europe, and an Indian psychiatrist, M. R. Gaitonde[15] in Bombay, are the only ones who report on conversion hysterics in appreciable numbers. Obsessional neuroses have been reported as rare on Formosa[13], in Kuwait[16], and among African Negroes[10]. The common belief, recently restated by Stainbrook[17] that the high inci-

---

[2]The information thus received was organized in the form of a number of Newsletters (Newsletter–Transcultural Research in Mental Health Problems) sent to our correspondents and available to others interested in the subject.

dence of psychosomatic disorders is one of the doubtful privileges of Western civilization is not borne out by Parhad's[16] observations in Kuwait and by Seguin's[18] and our own observations in Peruvian Indians. Alcoholism is rare on Formosa[13]. It constitutes a particularly serious problem in Peru[19] and in the Union of South Africa[10]. Sexual perversions have been reported as common in Iran[20], and as rare in Russia[21].

2. Are There Any Mental Disorders Common in Some Cultures but Nonexistent in Others?

From what has been said it is evident that the main categories of mental disorders are ubiquitous. Mental disorders confined to certain geographical areas are those due to malnutrition, to malarial and other infections, toxic psychoses, and variants of drug addictions. African specialists have identified what seems to be some mental syndromes indigenous to that continent, e.g. Carother's[4] "frenzied anxiety." Whether this is an organic illness or a functional psychosis is not clear. Only further research on such apparently unique disturbances can prove whether they are cultural variants of known conditions or totally new phenomena.

3. Are There Any Nosological Differences in the Manifestations of Mental Disease on Comparison of Different Cultures?

The example of schizophrenia may be given. Observers with psychiatric experience in the East and in the West[22], have noted that hospitalized schizophrenic patients are less aggressive and less violent in India and in Japan than schizophrenics in Western mental hospitals. Caudill[23] observed that Japanese schizophrenic patients, more than patients in the United States, maintain contact with other human beings.

Schizophrenia in African natives is said to be quieter and less florid—a poor imitation of European forms[24]. Twilight or confusional states, often of short duration, are common. Severe schizophrenics in various stages of deterioration, with marked blunting of affect and poorly organized, autistic thinking, prevail or at least come predominantly under the care of psychiatrists. Most observers agree that the hebephrenic form of schizophrenia is most commonly seen and that the paranoid form is relatively uncommon. Hallucinations, auditory and visual, are systematized and have a predominantly mythological content. Delusions of being bewitched or poisoned are most common.

4. Are There Any Psychiatric Syndromes Specific to Certain Geographical Areas or Cultural Confines?

Such syndromes to mention just a few, have been described under the names of Koro, Latah, Imu, Arctic hysteria, Youngda-Hte, Hsieh-Ping, Susto, and Windigo psychosis.

Patients suffering from *Koro*, a disorder reported from Malaya and Southern China, are suddenly seized by the belief that their penis is shrinking into their abdomen. To forestall such an event which, according to popular belief, would lead to death, elaborate preventive measures are taken, such as clamping the penis into a wooden box or tying a red string around it[12].

Latah has been reported from various parts of the world (among the Malay races, as Imu among the Ainus of North Japan and as Arctic hysteria among Eskimos and Siberian natives). It is usually precipitated by fright, occurs in middle-aged women, and is characterized by a trancelike state with automatic obedience, alternating with motility storms, echolalia, and echopraxia[12].

A trancelike state under the name of *Hsieh-Ping* has been reported from Formosa[13]. The symptoms during seizures, which last from half an hour to many hours, consist of tremor, disorientation, clouding of consciousness and delirium, often accompanied by visual or auditory hallucinatons. An outstanding feature is ancestor identification. Magical and mystical animal transformation states have been reported from Indonesia[8].

Sal y Rosas[25], one of our correspondents from Peru, reports on a condition named *Susto* (magic fright). It is precipitated by a violent fright experience, occurs usually in children and adolescents and is characterized by intense anxiety, hyperexcitability, and a state of depression accompanied by considerable loss of weight. The patients believe that their "soul" has been separated from their body, and has been absorbed and kidnapped by the Earth. The treatment applied consists of magical acts to recover the fugitive or robbed spirit.

To return to the question raised, it appears that the syndromes described constitute, to some extent, clinical entities, though they are less specific nosologically than is frequently believed. Phenomenological overlap between some of the syndromes described under different names in geographically widely separated areas is noticeable. According to local psychiatric observers, most of the syndromes have been regarded as culture-bound variants of hysteria.

SOME PSYCHOCULTURAL AND SOCIOCULTURAL CONSIDERATIONS

Thus far a brief account has been given of observations which have been made. In appraising their significance, psychocultural as well as sociocultural variables have to be taken into account.

PSYCHOCULTURAL VARIABLES

Obsessional Neurosis

The alleged absence of obsessional neuroses in some cultures, e.g. in African Negroes[26] and in Chinese[13] could be attributed: to the disinclination of obsessive-compulsives all over the world to consult psychiatrists; to the mitigating effect of lenient early toilet training on sphincter morality development; to externalization of a threatening superego in the form of popular beliefs and superstitions; and to absorption of obsessional defenses into culture dictated rituals.

Depression

The rarity of depression, if indeed it is rare, in certain cultures, e.g. among African natives, has been accounted for: by a weak superego formation, by predominance of projective mechanisms and by the prophylactic effect of ritual and ceremonial observances following a death. Contrasting the high incidence of confusional excitement, often combined with homicidal behavior, and the rarity of depression, P. K. Benedict and Jacks[27] suggest that in nonliterate cultures hostility of psychotics is channeled *outward*, whereas in Euro-American culture hostility is more often directed *inward*.

Schizophrenia

Divergent views have been expressed regarding the relevance of Oriental cultures to the incidence of schizophrenia. It has been suggested that the Eastern way of life (a) predisposes to schizophrenia[2] (b) conceals it in prizing and rewarding schizoid trends[28] and (c) safeguards against it by providing outlets for introvert tendencies[29, 30].

Beyond this, it is obvious that the content of schizophrenic delusions is conditioned by culturally patterned orientation and that their paucity or richness reflects the modalities of mental and behavioral activities inherent in diverse cultural systems.

SOCIOCULTURAL VARIABLES

As regards sociocultural variables the effects of detribalization, urbanization, culture change, migration, and culture-determined differences in psychotherapy will be briefly dealt with.

1. Observations made in various parts of Africa[31, 7] and in Haiti[32] show that, as rural, backward and tribal native populations enter urban areas, mental disorders increase in frequency and their clinical manifestations approximate those of the European white settlers.

2. There is general agreement that radical culture change is felt by large sections of the affected populations as a stressful experience. A frequent result of stressful experiences of this kind is an increase in antisocial behavior. However, differing responses to similar experiences have been noted in culturally distinct groups. Thus, in Israel[33], Jewish immigrants from Tunisia have a high rate of delinquency and of other forms of antisocial behavior whereas Yemenites have a low rate.

Other apparently culture-bound variants of mental phenomena reported in migrants include a high frequency of bronchial asthma in Iraqui Jews migrated to Israel and of generalized, shifting pains in Indians migrating from the Andes to the coastal cities of Peru[18].

3. Cross-cultural evidence indicates that differences in culturally based attitudes toward the mentally ill and toward mental hospitals may influence rates of commitment and of release. Irrespective of availability of mental hospitals, there is a high tolerance in Oriental and African societies for what in the Western world would be considered seriously disturbed behavior.

Cultural premises influence types of treatment procedures in different cultures. For instance, adherence to traditional systems of values seems to account for the resistance of Japanese psychiatrists to psychoanalysis and their preference for ego-directed forms of psychotherapy founded on established and accepted religious systems. Prominent among these are: Morita-therapy based on Zen Buddhist disciplines and Nishimaru's Confucian based persuasion therapy[34].

Still another aspect of cultural orientation is applied to psychotherapy by Spiegel[35] who showed that the goals of psychotherapy and the therapeutic process as such, are influenced by concordant or discordant cultural values of therapist and patient.

CRITICALLY ASSESSING VALIDITY OF DATA

The general survey given throws into relief the numerous difficulties which beset the student of, and investigator in, the field of transcultural psychiatry, some of which follow.

Variability of the Concepts of Mental Health and Illness

While it is difficult enough to agree on what is "normal," "still normal" or "already abnormal" in one's own culture, these difficulties are multiplied if standards of normality and abnormality established in one culture have to be compared with those in an entirely different culture. Application of Western standards of normality by Western psychiatric observers in dealing with primitive societies may result in grave errors regarding the frequency of mental illness owing to ethnocentric orientation and ethnocentric bias.

Moreover, it has been pointed out that historically and geographically disease detection, disease-naming and disease acceptance are conditioned by the prevailing social and cultural systems of medical behavior[17] i.e. "being sick" is a cultural phenomenon in itself. For instance, a shamanism which would be regarded as pathological by us is regarded as normal in the countries in which it is practiced and sysmenorrhoea becomes an illness only if the social system in which the sufferer lives considers having pain with menstrual periods as an illness. As mentioned before, the same argument applies to the absence or presence of depression in primitive societies.

Variability of Nomenclature

Visitors from the Far East, accustomed as they are to Kraepelinian diagnostic criteria, are usually amazed by the much wider conception of the term in North America. Similarly, the relatively high figure for incidence of the manic form of manic-depressive psychoses in some cultures has been attributed to the tendency of local psychiatrists to diagnose states of excitement as manic rather than as catatonic excitement or schizo-affective state as undoubtedly many psychiatrists would[17, 27].

Variability of Locale of Observations

Data on mental illness in primitives, as far as psychiatrists are concerned, have been predominantly obtained from hospitalized patients. Since in native culture, a majority of the patients suffering from mental illness do not seek medical help or are attended by native practitioners, observations based on hospitalized patients deal with a highly selected population. Comparison of observations made in field studies with hospitalized patients is clearly impossible.

Other difficulties encountered in establishing valid comparisons include inadequate training of anthropological observers in psychiatry and inadequate training of psychiatric observers in anthropology, as well as differences in the quality, training and orientation of the psychiatric observers, in the methods of sampling, in the intensity of the investigation, and in the methods of computation of data.

Last but not least, differences in cooperation of the populations studied have to be taken into account. Partly because they mistake the white doctor as the stereotype of the "official," partly because they fear hospitalization, natives on being interviewed are apt to adopt evasive tactics[36] or to fabricate. Africans are known to be great storytellers[11]. Moreover when an interview with a preliterate or barely literate person has to be conducted through an interpreter, distortions of meaning will inevitably arise.

SUMMARY AND CONCLUSIONS

There are many ways of viewing the etiology of mental disease. It can be understood as being due to heredity, due to fixation at infantile levels of instinctual development and faulty early object relationships, due to biological dysfunctions and due to influences aris-ing from interpersonal relationships within the society or culture in which an individual lives. None of these viewpoints is "wrong" but each represents a segmental view of a multilateral process.

In the foregoing an attempt has been made to survey our present knowledge regarding the relevance of social and cultural factors to the etiology and treatment of mental illness. In this survey which inevitably had to be incomplete many questions have been raised and few have been answered. It has been shown that the major categories of mental disorders occur ubiquitously, that there is some evidence that they are distributed unevenly, that nosological differences exist between different cultural areas and that differences both in frequency and in nature of clinical manifestations can be related to cultural differences. Methodological difficulties especially of comparative quantitative studies but also of qual-itative studies have been pointed out.

REFERENCES

(The letters N.L. refer to the 5 issues of the Newsletter on Transcultural Research in Mental Health Problems produced and circularized by the Section of Transcultural Psychiatric Studies, McGill Uni-versity.)

1. Opler, M. K. *Culture, psychiatry and human values.* Springfield, Ill.: Charles C Thomas, 1956.
2. Ratanakorn, P. N.L. 3, pp. 4, 20.
3. Brandt, M. Reports of the Osteuropa Institute of the Free University Berlin–Number 31, Medical Series: New Research in Soviet Psychiatry, Berlin. p. 11, 1957.
4. Carothers, J. C. *Psychiatry*, 1948, **11**, 47.
5. Carothers, J. C. *The African mind in health and disease.* Geneva: World Health Organization Monograph No. 17, 1953.
6. Laubscher, B. J. F. *Sex, custom and Psychopathology.* London: Routledge and Sons, 1937.
7. Tooth, G. *Studies in mental illness in the Gold Coast.* London. H.M.S.O. Colonial Research Publi-cations No. 6, 1950.
8. Khing, Kho Tjok. N.L. 4, p. 21.
9. McGrath, S. D. N.L. 1, p. 30.
10. Berman, S. N.L. 4, p. 56.
11. Margetts, E. Personal communication.
12. Yap, P. M. *J. Ment. Science*, 1951, **97**, 313. N.L. 1, p. 23.
13. Lin, Tsung-yi. *Psychiatry*, **16**, 313.
14. Philippopoulos, G. S. N.L. 2, p. 10.
15. Gaitonde, M. R. Cross cultural study of the psychiatric syndromes in outpatient clinics in Bombay, India, and Topeka, Kansas. Paper presented at the 114th annual meeting of the American Psychiatric Association, San Francisco, 1958.
16. Parhad, L. N.L.3, p. 5.
17. Stainbrook, E. N.L. 3, p. 8.
18. Seguin, C. A. *Psychosomatic Med.*, 1956, **18**, 404.
19. Caravedo, B. N.L. 3, p. 7.
20. Valentine, M. N.L. 2, p. 11.
21. Kyerbikov, O. V., Ozyeryetskiy, P. I., Popov, E. A., & Sheshnevskiy, A. V. *Uchyebnik Psichiatrii.* (Textbook of Psychiatry), Moscow, Medhiz: State Editorship of Medical Literature, 1958.
22. Mansani, K. R. N.L. 1, p. 25.
23. Caudill, W. N.L. 4, p. 17.
24. Gordon, H. L. *J. Ment. Science*, 1934, **80**, 167.
25. Sal y Rosas, F. N.L. 4, p. 30.
26. Lambo, T. A. *Br. Med. J.*, 1956, **2**, 1388.
27. Benedict, P. K., & Jacks, I. *Psychiatry*, 1954, **17**, 377.

28. DuBois, C. *Psychoanal. Rev.*, 1937, **24**, 246.
29. Horney, K. *The neurotic personality of our time.* New York: Norton, 1937.
30. Klineberg, O. *Social psychology.* New York: Henry Holt, 1940.
31. Forster, E. F. B. N.L. 1, p. 17.
32. Mars, L. N.L. 5, p. 51.
33. Weinberg, A. N.L. 1, p. 19.
34. Kato, M. Report on Psychotherapy in Japan. Presented at the International Congress of Psychotherapy, Barcelona, Spain, September 1958.
35. Spiegel, J. P. N.L. 5, p. 14.
36. Sinclair, A. Report of a field and clinical survey of the mental health of the Indigenes of the Territories of Papua and New Guinea, 1957. Unpublished.

15

Cultural Factors in the Genesis of Schizophrenia*

H. B. M. MURPHY

Any review of empirical data touching possible sociocultural influences on the genesis of schizophrenia must face serious difficulties, since such influences are overlapping continua, not simple dichotomies of presence or absence, and will almost certainly have interacted elaborately with each other before producing the final result. It is not to be thought, for instance, that the experience of a migrant is the same regardless of the social class he moves in or that patterns of intrafamilial behavior are unaffected by the cultural expectations of the surrounding society. Accordingly, there are a host of concomitant variables which theoretically need to be allowed for when we seek to assess the relevance of any one, and since there is no study which has been able to handle them all the reviewer of such literature has continually to draw inferences from inadequate evidence. It is in some ways much easier to write a theoretical paper in this field, selecting hypotheses and suggesting means of testing them, than to write a descriptive one, when so much of what one would like to describe has never been filled in.

These problems apply to any sociocultural approach to schizophrenia and to most other approaches as well, but one is probably more aware of them when considering specifically cultural influences, since culture interpenetrates all other aspects of social life. Culture, in the sense used in transcultural psychiatry, consists of the values, beliefs, and patterns of behavior which a society teaches to its members, with a view to equipping them better for the task of life. In traditional societies we are accustomed to think of these beliefs and practices as maintaining an existence of their own with very little reasoned relationship to actual living conditions, but they did not start out that way, and beyond a certain point they do not persist in that way either, if they become inappropiate to actual conditions and if the society is making any attempt to adjust. The obvious analogy, though one which must not be pushed too far, is with habits of eating, walking, writing, etc., which are learned by children and maintained throughout life with no rational reconsideration until some change, physiological or environmental, forces the person to examine whether the development of different habits might be more satisfactory. To discuss a particular culture without reference to the conditions to which it was a response can thus be as senseless as to discuss the sailor's rolling walk without considering conditions at sea, especially if these conditions are no longer present. Accordingly, in evaluating a culture medically or in seeking the cultural determinants of disease, the conditions under which the culture developed are usually relevant, whether these conditions persist or whether they have changed, and although we may occasionally meet an association which persists despite the setting, it is logical to expect that it is the combination of culture and conditions which is pathogenic, rather than either alone.

There are two questions which this paper is expected to tackle. The first is whether there

---

*Reprinted with permission from *The transmission of schizophrenia*, edited by D. Rosenthal and S. S. Kety (1968), Pergamon Press, Limited, and Dr, Murphy.

is sufficient evidence to justify the belief that cultural factors can affect not only the symptomatology of schizophrenia, but its incidence and course. For this, what is required is merely the demonstration of an association between the two variables, plus supporting evidence to suggest that that association is not caused by some third, exraneous factor such as genetic or social selection. If such a demonstration is possible, then even though one cannot say how the two are connected, cultural factors must be kept in mind in discussing the genesis of schizophrenia, whereas if it is not possible then it is better that we put them out of mind since the fewer possibilities we have to juggle with the better. The second question is whether, should an association be found, there is any evidence as to how this might be operating. Here it may be permissible to use less concrete data provided these offer clues to the intervening links in the causal chain.

The first of the two questions sounds relatively easy to answer, since we have a world full of widely different cultures to choose from, and if an association can be established between cultural factors and schizophrenia for any one of these then, theoretically at least, the association becomes potentially present in all the rest. Ideally, however, any such demonstration must in some way manage to exclude such potentially competing explanations as genetic loading of a population, social selection by migration, the stresses of social change and the adverse effects of low or minority status; and this is extremely difficult. It might be thought that the easiest way would be to find remote and exotic people in whom schizophrenia, if not entirely absent, was at least extremely rare. Apart from the problem of excluding a genetic explanation in such a case, however, there is a much greater problem which faces one when one attempts to study schizophrenia in non-westernized peoples, namely the problem of diagnostic criteria. Among such peoples, regardless of continent but with possible exceptions for specific cultures, acute short-lasting psychoses form a major part of all recognized mental disorder, and there is no agreement on where these lie in our current diagnostic classifications. Some psychiatrists include most such cases under schizophrenia on the grounds of their delusional or hallucinatory elements and of the fact that a few of these acute states, indistinguishable from the rest initially, develop into typically chronic schizophrenia later. Other workers, however, call them organic psychoses, incriminating one of the various infections or infestations which nearly every patient in these countries has. Still others regard them as something different from either. The relative number of such conditions is too high for us to treat them as we do borderline schizophrenias in North America, by pretending that they do not make a real difference one way or the other, and their short duration creates serious difficulties for field surveys, which are usually forced to deduce incidence on the basis of prevalence. (This problem will face the Sarawak survey which the Foundations' Fund is supporting.) Study of the longer-term prognosis of these acute states could cast new light on the nature of the functional psychoses, and we are carrying out research into this question at the present time. But the fact remains that until better agreement is reached on the criteria for diagnosing schizophrenia in such peoples an epidemiological approach to that disorder among them is almost impossible.

That sends us back to the examination of relatively lesser differences in rates between population samples whose clinical pictures are more typical. An abundance of potentially useful material exists, but there are virtually no discussions of the comparative merits of the different possible explanations for their findings, so that it has been necessary to do original research for this paper on the more promising sources, research which has unfortunately not usually enabled me to resolve the existing ambiguities. I propose to summarize the evidence on the three peoples regarding whom the case for a cultural influence seems most plausible and then go on to some new data which I am only now working out but which seem to constitute the strongest argument for a cultural influence so far available. I must apologize for the fact that in two of the three illustrations the original work was in part my own, for it is the task of a review paper to give wide coverage to other people's work. It happens, however, that very few researchers have tackled this question systematically, and it is easier for me to assess the influence of extraneous factors in a group which I know than in one which I do not. The three illustrations will all relate to higher-than-average rates of schizophrenia, not to lower-than-average, for the simple reason that the former are fairly self-evident whereas with the latter there is always the suspicion that cases have been missed, and extra work needs to be done to allay that suspicion. There is one well-known instance of a below-average rate of schizophrenia where the extra work had been done and where cultural factors are properly explored, namely the Hutterite survey of Eaton and Weil[5]. Unfortunately, since the original genetic stock of these communities was quite narrow ("In 1950 there were only fifteen patronyms in the entire sect," *op. cit.* p. 32), the possibility of an unusually healthy genetic base cannot be excluded even though the researchers show that the treatment of mentally disturbed people in this culture is tolerant and supportive. Also, I have calculated the 1961 schizophrenia admission rate for the Mennonites and Hutterites combined, from Canada's prairie provinces, and that rate is not significantly below average. Hence although this last finding does not exclude a low rate for the Hutterites alone (Canadian census data do not permit their differentiation from the Mennonites) it makes the attribution of a protective cultural factor doubtful.

The three groups we will be considering are the Tamilians of South India, the southern Irish, and the people of north-west Croatia.

THE TAMIL-SPEAKING PEOPLE OF SOUTH INDIA AND CEYLON

The most incontroversial evidence of an excess liability to schizophrenia in this people comes from data on the student population at the University of Singapore. The upper part of Fig. 15.1 shows the relative incidence of the disorder in the three main ethnic groups attending that institution, as calculated by Z. N. Kadri for 1958–63[8] and by myself for a previous 5-year period. My own rates are based on too few cases to be significant, but they show the same trend as Kadri's data, where the differences are quite significant. Since the students were given free medical attention, since any failure to attend courses had to be explained to the university authorities with medical certificates being passed to Dr. Kadri or myself for checking, and since abnormal behavior or abnormal academic performance on the part of any student usually led to him being referred to the health service, I believe that these differences are not distorted by concealment of non-Indian cases or by other interference with ascertainment. Failure to recognize schizophrenia remains a possible source of error, of course, but this was much more likely with Indian than with Chinese patients owing to the more hysterical quality of the former. In my own first years in Singapore I made this mistake, diagnosing as hysterical neuroses patients who later proved to have schizophenia.[1]

---

[1] My original paper[10] on the Singapore students was written before that realization was made, so that the hysterical quality of Indian psychopathology was stressed there and their liability to schizophrenia overlooked. The original comment on the schizoid character of the Chinese patients remains valid as referring to introversion and seclusiveness, but not if it is thought to imply a liability to schizophrenia.

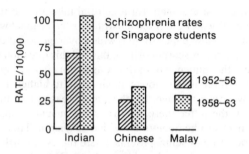

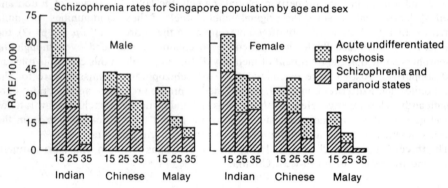

Fig. 15.1(a)   Incidence of schizophrenia in students at the University of Singapore; for two 5-year periods. (Z. N. Kadri[8] and present author.) (b) First admission rates to mental hospital, 1950–1954, for Indian, Chinese, and Malay sections of the population of Singapore; by age and sex; cases diagnosed as schizophrenia, paranoid state and acute undifferentiated psychosis only. (Cases over the age of 44 have been excluded since the "undifferentiated psychosis" group tend after that age to have a more obviously organic basis.)

The excess of Indian over Chinese and Malay rates of schizophrenia among university students is reflected, though to a lesser degree, in the general Singapore population, whether or not one adds to the cases diagnosed as schizophrenia those which we might call the acute undifferentiated psychoses. (In Singapore at that time they were labeled as toxic psychoses, but a specific toxic element was very rarely implicated and discussions with the hospital doctors revealed that they were using this term for any case that showed initial confusion.) However, as the lower part of Fig. 15.1 shows, there is an interesting point about the age distribution of the Indian and other cases, for the Indian rate is especially high only in the youngest age group and in males drops off very sharply thereafter. Furthermore, when rates are calculated both by age and social class, as I have done for total hospital admissions in an earlier paper[11], then for younger men (15–29) the curve is the reverse of the expected, with the highest rates in the highest class and the lowest in class III. This fits with our university findings and might be explained in two very different ways. On the one hand Kadri has shown that virtually all of his Indian cases derived from a particular subgroup of Tamilians, those coming to Singapore not directly from India but from Ceylon, where their ancestors had migrated some centuries previously. These Ceylonese Tamils, as they are called, are found particularly in administrative and professional sections of the middle class and they tend to marry among themselves, so that if there were an inherited liability to schizophrenia in this narrowly based subgroup it could account for some of the peculiarities of schizophrenia distribution. However, that would not explain the differences in the male and female age curves for schizophrenia in the Singapore Indians as a whole or for other peculiarities in the distribution of schizophrenia by occupational group among them. These peculiarities, and the other points remarked on, appear better explained on the basis of the marked and culturally produced difficulties which Tamil youth, from India and from Ceylon alike, have in handling relations with authority. (These difficulties are described in the earlier paper[10]). Moreover, a genetic predisposition to schizophrenia in the small Ceylonese Tamil group, while quite possible, would not explain why in the Indian Army the Tamil-speaking people in the south exhibited a greater predisposition to schizophrenia than the people of other regions and subcultures.

This picture of the mental disorder rates in the Indian Army has to be gathered from a number of sources all of which have some limitations since, as with most wartime military papers, one does not meet accurate data on patients and on the size of the population-at-risk in the same paper. However, from Bhattacharjya[2], Singh[17] and in particular from Hyatt Williams[21], it is clear that the south Indian had more mental disturbance than soldiers from other regions, more difficulties with discipline and authority, and proportionately more schizophrenia in cases coming to psychiatric attention. Hyatt Williams, for instance, found a highly significant difference, as Table 15.1 shows. The difference could still be genetically based, of course, since the southerners are mainly of Dravidian and the northerners of Aryan stock, but the army drew from such a wide population (Madras state alone has 30 million inhabitants) that the odds seem in favor of the sociocultural explanation.

The Indian Army, like Singapore, was westernized in its social structure, and the question may still be asked whether in a more traditional social setting these same Indian groups would have shown the same excess of schizophrenia. There are some indications that in village India, south or north, the risk of schizophrenia is less, although in large cities like Madras it is not. However, the evidence here is too slight to argue from. What can be said is

Table 15.1 Percentage Distribution of Indian Army Patients, by Diagnosis, for Those from South India and for All Others.

Psychiatric Cases Seen on the Arakan (Burma) Front	Indian Army Regional Groups	
	South	All Others
(N)	(86)	(273)
Schizophrenia	19.8%	7.7%
Affective psychoses	14.0%	12.1%
Confusional psychoses	17.4%	12.8%
Hysterical states	38.3%	31.1%
Anxiety states	7.0%	29.3%
Personality disorders	3.5%	7.0%
	100.0%	100.0%

$(\chi^2 = 16.7; n = 1; p = 0.001$ for schizophrenia v. rest.)
Source: From Williams, 1950.

that Indians regardless of region appear to have difficulty in adjusting to Western conditions. For instance, university health services in the United States, Britain, and Australia see more serious disturbance in Indian students than in other Asian or African visitors.[2] But there are too many possible explanations for this to disentangle here. It is sufficient to say that in the conditions described, Tamilians and perhaps other Indians show an excess of schizophrenia with characteristics which cannot easily be accounted for by genetic or other selection, which are not exhibited by other peoples under the same conditions, and which seem easiest explained on the basis of a combination of cultural and social factors.

THE PEOPLE OF NORTH-WESTERN CROATIA

The evidence for an excess of schizophrenia in the people of this region has been accumulated by European psychiatrists since the 1930s and is summarized for the English reader by Crocetti *et al.*[3]. Mainly, this evidence derives from hospital data but statistics from military service tribunals show that the rate of rejection by reason of schizophrenia is twice as high for the relevant population as it is for the rest of the country. Those interested in the detailed checks which Crocetti and his colleagues carried out on their material are referred to the original paper, but it can be broadly summarized by stating that although that material was in many ways incomplete, no evidence could be found to indicate that the difference between the specified population and the rest of Croatia was other than genuine.

A number of possible explanations for the observation have been explored, in each case with negative results. Thus, it was initially believed that the excess might derive from a few isolated and inbred communities, but the researchers have shown that it has a much wider distribution. Then it was thought that since the area had seen much migration, the excess might derive from the immigrants. Analysis of cases, however, showed that they derived much more from the non-migrant than from the migrant group. No one to my knowledge has previously proposed a cultural explanation for the findings, and at first thought this would appear unlikely, since the finding relates not to the total population of Croatia or to a recognized subcultural minority, but to a geographic sector. A limited reading of the history of the region [6], however, led me to realize that the reported boundary between the high and lower rate areas coincides roughly with a geographic and historical division which I believe, on the basis of discussions with Yugoslav colleagues, to have produced sociocultural differences as well.

Briefly, the affected area of Istria and the country round Rijeka (which some of us may recognize better under its former Italian name Fiume) is that part of Yugoslavia which has the strongest ties to the west of Europe and the weakest ties to the rest of the country. A long history of links, first to Venice, then to the Hapsburgs, and then by conquest to Mussolini's Italy, have made the people of this part, so I am told, more "European" and more "civilized" by their own way of thinking than the rest of their countrymen. Moreover, it is this part of Croatia which can be inferred to have been most affected by the historic conflict of loyalties and identities which arose from the Croats being Roman Catholics caught up in national and Pan-Slavic movements which Rome was opposed to.[3] (In Central Croatia, Rome was felt to be further away, and there was until after WW II a greater

---

[2]Various personal communications.

[3]A good description of this problem from an Anglo-Saxon viewpoit is given in Rebecca West's once-famous book *Black Lamb and Grey Falcon* [20].

admixture of Serbian Orthodox influence.) Today this corner of the country is still the one which has the strongest ties to western Europe through tourism, is still the most "civilized" in terms of material riches and property values[17], and still apparently doubtful about its attachment to the centers of national political power, since its officials are the most reluctant to leave their home area for the capital[7]. This long-standing sociocultural ambivalence, if it still persists, could offer a hypothetical link to schizophrenia, as I will attempt to indicate later. Regardless of that hypothesis, however, the fact remains that there are some sociocultural differences between the sector with the high schizophrenia rates and the rest of Croatia, and as long as other explanations for the high rate cannot be found these sociocultural differences have to be accepted as potentially relevant.[4]

THE IRISH CATHOLICS

Evidence suggesting that schizophrenia is unusually frequent in this people can be found on both sides of the Atlantic, and stretches from last century to the present decade, although always the picture is somewhat confused by their much more striking liability to the alcoholic psychoses. The first reference which I have traced in my preparation for this paper is by Spitzka from New York in 1880[18]. There he noted that acute melancholia was particularly frequent in German immigrants, hebephrenia in Jewish ones, and "terminal dementia" in the Irish. By the last term he presumably means chronic schizophrenia, but chronic organic states might also have been included. Each few years more writers present a similar picture, and by 1913 both Pollock for New York[15] and Swift for Massachusetts[19] give sufficiently detailed information to make it almost certain that Irish rates for mental hospital admission were considerably higher than those for other immigrant groups even after alcoholic psychoses had been excluded.

Swift recognized the relevance both of considering the second generation of immigration and of allowing for the age distribution of the different populations but he had no sound means of doing either. Pollock, for the period around 1920[16], and Malzberg for that around 1930[9], did have these means, and in both writers we find the earlier impressions of an Irish liability to schizophrenia confirmed, though the frequency of the disease in the so-called "new" immigration from eastern and southern Europe is beginning to overshadow this. Pollock, for instance, now shows the Irish to have the highest frequency of schizophrenia from among eleven immigrant groups from north-western Europe (roughly, the "old" immigration) but to be overshadowed by many from the "new" groups, the Poles especially[16]. Malzberg, as the figures in Table 15.2 show, found that although the Irish were still the most vulnerable of the cultural groups studied by him from among the second generation of immigration, and still the most vulnerable of female immigrant groups, they were no longer the most vulnerable in the male immigrant population. However, it must be remembered that by the 1920s and 1930s the Irish had a considerable advantage over most other immigrant peoples in New York State, since they were English-speaking and had already gained a solid foothold of political power.

After 1931 the U.S. lost interest in European immigrants and their countries of origin, but

---

[4]Since the above was written I have learned that the excess morbidity in this people applies not only to schizophrenia but to a wide variety of somatic illnesses, and that nutritional factors are now being investigated. While the facts presented above remain correct, therefore, it seems unwise to cite this population as an example of an association between culture and schizophrenia.

Table 15.2 First Admission Rates for Schizophrenia, New York, 1929–31, by Culture of Origin.

Cultural Origin	Immigrants (age-standardized rates)		Native-Born of immigrant parents (Crude Rates) Combined Sexes
	Male	Female	
Irish	29.6	37·4	25·2
English	28.5	23·4	15·9
German	44.8	27.1	21.0
Italian	34.4	26.7	12.2
Scandinavian	40.5	27.8	19.7
Polish	31.7	35.4	not given
Russian	33.9	25.8	not given

Source: Malzberg, 1940.

the story can be taken up elsewhere. First, in Ireland itself it had recently been rediscovered that Ireland had double the number of patients in mental hospitals per 1000 population than England and Wales has [14]. I say rediscovered rather than discovered, for back at the beginning of the century it had been noticed that the rate of insanity in Ireland was 4.7 per 1000 as compared to 3.3 in England, although the latter had the better medical services.[5] In the recent report, however, the matter is taken further, for it is pointed out that Ireland has not only double the English bed occupancy rate, but double the admission rate of England as well, with the proportion diagnosed as schizophrenia among these admissions again being higher than in England [14]. Until new evidence comes in, therefore, we must assume that schizophrenia is genuinely more frequent among the Irish in Éire today than among their English-speaking neighbors, just as it was among the Irish immigrants to the U.S., and as it proves to be among people of Irish Catholic origin in Canada, when compared with those of other English-speaking origin. In the Canadian provinces whose rates I am currently studying they have the highest schizophrenia rate of any origin group from western Europe, and are exceeded only by the Russians and Poles when one looks more widely.[6] These Canadian statistics refer not to the first or to the second generation of immigration only, but to the whole population regardless of how many generations there had been in Canada, and on that basis one would have expected the Irish, with their long settlement, to have been at a definite social advantage over peoples like the Dutch and Scandinavians who arrived later.

The fact that schizophrenia is found with unexpected frequency both in that part of the population that emigrated and in the ancestors of that part that stayed at home suggests strongly that social selection is not an explanation for the foregoing findings, although the social experiences leading up to and deriving from the migration may have some relevance,

---

[5]Noted by Swift in 1913 [19] and discussed from a different angle by O'Doherty [14]. An investigation into the current picture of Éire is being planned and may already have been commenced by Dermott Walsh.

[6]Italians have a higher female rate than the Irish in the provinces studied, but there is reason to believe that this is atypical and that if the Niagara peninsula with its heavy Italian settlement had been included the Italian female rate would have been much lower.

since O'Doherty has shown that it is the Irish counties with the highest schizophrenia rate that produced the highest emigration. The possibility remains that the whole Irish people have a genetic predisposition to the disease, but this is argued against by two factors. One is that the mean age of marriage is late among the southern Irish[1], so that there is less likelihood of the schizophrenic getting married; the other is that while there is this liability among the Roman Catholic southern Irish, there is no evidence of a corresponding tendency in the Protestant northerners. On the last point it must be admitted that the Protestant northerners contain a very much greater admixture of Anglo-Saxon stock than the southerners, but one would have still expected some signs of an inherited racial liability, if such existed. From Northern Ireland I can trace no reference to this and in Canada, though it has not been possible to calculate rates for this subgroup of the total population,[7] the rural survey which will be referred to below did permit the identification of a large Irish Protestant community, and this had the lowest schizophrenia prevalence rate of all the 14 communities studied. Accordingly, while once again an association between culture and schizophrenia cannot positively be established here, it is difficult to think of any characteristic of the Irish which could explain the steady excess of schizophrenia which they have shown and which does not at least partly involve some aspect of their cultural heritage. I do not intend at this point to say what aspect of that heritage I myself suspect may be schizophrenogenic, but there are elements of their family tradition which could be inculpated, and another aspect will be touched on briefly later.[8]

THE ROMAN CATHOLICS IN CANADA

In the foregoing section there had to be an unsatisfactory equating of "peoples" with "cultures," the reason being that official statistics do not usually acknowledge cultural divisions in any other way, and we have needed to use official sources in order to measure large populations and hence eliminate local vagaries. The concept of a "people," however, implies a sharing of a gene pool quite as much as it does a sharing of cultural traditions, and even though I have tried to cite only instances where there are features difficult to explain on a genetic basis, it may be felt that the evidence is inconclusive. There have recently come into my hands, however, data which while not covering any one complete culture, nevertheless involve a cultural element shared by many peoples and not paralleled genetically.

With the Irish and with the Croatians it was noted that the high schizophrenia rates were found in the Catholic sections of a population and were apparently not repeated in the Protestant and Eastern Orthodox sections. In both it was a point of doubtful significance,

---

[7]The above references to the Irish Catholic picture in Canada strictly speaking refer to the picture for the Catholic population of British origin, since this was the only way in which a reliable differentiation could be made. However, the very great majority of Canadians belonging to the Roman Catholic Church and claiming British origin are of Irish descent, so that the groups are approximately equivalent.

[8]During the discussion of this paper Dr. Elliot Mishler raised the question whether the higher Irish rates could be related to the fact that Irish mothers are on average later in commencing child-bearing than mothers in other cultures. The standard texts on schizophrenia all suggest (at least by omission) that there is no association between maternal age and the risk of schizophrenia in the offspring so that this would seem to answer the question. However, although probably not of much relevance to the Irish, there would seem to be grounds for a re-examination of maternal age as a variable, with greater allowance for birth rank. See Moran, P.A.P. *Ann. Hum. Genetics*, **28**, 269 (1965).

since the non-Catholics tended to be of different or more mixed ethnic stock. Among the Singapore Indians I could also have offered rates suggesting that schizophrenia was more frequent in Christians, Catholics in particular, than in the remainder of that population, but there were too many other questions that would have had to be disentangled for this to be worthwhile When Canadian mental hospitalizations for schizophrenia are analyzed by origin and by religion, however, a result is obtained which seems to permit only one explanation, namely that there is some element of Roman Catholic tradition which is more conducive to schizophrenia in Canada than the corresponding aspect of Protestant tradition.

Figure 15.2 presents the relevant comparisons. It will be seen that in every single one of

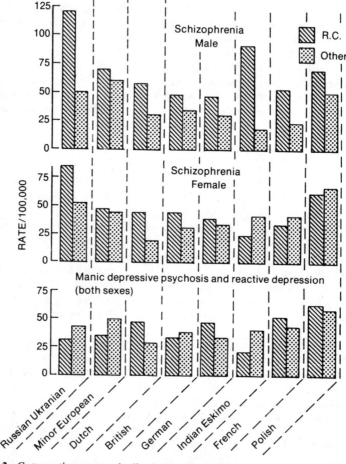

Fig. 15.2 Comparative age-standardized rates of mental hospitalization for scizophrenia and insufficient affective disorders, in Roman Catholic and other sections of the Canadian population, 1961, analyzed by culture of origin. (Data are for 7 provinces only; origin groups with insuffinient Roman Catholics for calculation of representative rates have been excluded; those reporting either Jewish religion of Jewish origin have been excluded also, otherwise all patients and all population not specifically reporting themselves to be Roman Catholic have been included under the category of "other".)

the cultural subgroups of Canadian society in which there is a sufficient proportion of Roman Catholics for their mental hospitalization rates to be worthwhile calculating, the Catholic rate exceeds the non-Catholic with respect to schizophrenia in males. In female schizophrenics the same difference is of doubtful significance, being present in 5 out of the 8 groups only, and in the affective disorders it is absent. Since every patient whose religion is not recorded is assumed to be non-Catholic for this calculation the actual differences in hospitalization rates are probably greater than those shown, and field survey data suggest that if non-hospitalized cases had been included the rates would be wider apart still.[9] The question now is: what does this difference mean and, more pertinently for this paper, can we infer there to be some underlying cultural influence or an influence of a different sort?

The easiest way to approach that question is by asking what alternative hypotheses exist. The idea of a common genetic pool which would be shared by the Catholics from all these different backgrounds but not by the Protestants can be rejected, but there are selective processes which could produce such a result without really implying much relationship to the specific cultural features of the Catholic Church. Thus, mentally disturbed individuals seeking help for their condition sometimes turn to religions other than their own, and certain sects or churches go out of their way to offer such help, thereby increasing the apparent rate of mental disturbance among their members. This is the case with the Jehovah's Witnesses today, and formerly with the Salvation Army, but I have no evidence to suggest that the shift to Catholicism by disturbed individuals in Canada is greater than the shift away from it, so that this does not appear to be the reason for these findings. Another type of shift, namely into the religion of the upper class "establishment," could affect our results in a different way, for this tends to take place in the successful and upwardly mobile, thus increasing the proportion of the healthy in the high-prestige church or sect and reducing that proportion in the churches which the upwardly mobile came from.[10] Such a shift does take place in Canada, with the United Church of Canada being the main recipient, but the shift occurs more strongly away from the smaller Protestant sects than it does from the Roman Catholic Church, and the latter has a higher overall rate for schizophrenia than all but one of the Protestant sects, the exception being the Jehovah's Witnesses mentioned above. Yet a third type of selection is through migration, and if recent immigration to Canada (specifically, to the seven provinces to which Fig. 15.2's data apply) had been predominantly Catholic while earlier migration had been predominantly Protestant within each of the relevant subcultures, then a higher rate of schizophrenia in the Catholics would be expected. There is no evidence to that effect [4], however, and post-war immigration has in any event been mainly to the cities of Toronto and Montreal [4], which had to be excluded from the analysis for Fig. 15.2, owing to incomplete reporting by their hospitals.

These essentially extraneous explanations being rejected, is there any plausible explanation which involves the cultural traditions of the Catholic Church more directly, bearing in mind that the difference applies to males much more than to females? A first point that needs to be remembered here is that cultural attitudes can affect marriage and reproduction and thereby affect the transmission of defective genes. For instance, late marriage, as in the Irish, will tend to reduce the genetic transmission of schizophrenia by restraining some

---

[9]In the "Fourteen Communities Survey" Catholics were found to be less ready to seek psychiatric help than Protestants were, and to have a higher proportion of never-hospitalized mental patients.

[10]This type of shift becomes questionable if one allows for the possibility, suggested by other contributors to this symposium, that there is a genetic association between schizophrenia and creativity.

schizpohrenia-prone from bearing children before the disease has had time to become manifest. Marriage arranged by parents, as in parts of Asia, may have the same effect, since it is usual to investigate the family history of a prospective spouse quite carefully. However, this is not relevant here, since the only recognized influence of this kind among the 8 subcultures, namely that in the Irish, could be expected to operate in the opposite direction, and in any case such an influence would be expected to show its effect equally on men and on women. A second point which needs to be considered, since the common cultural element is religious affiliation, is whether the specifically religious teachings of one church are more schizophrenogenic than that of another; but here again we would need to ask why the effect should show itself more in males than females. Certainly there are religions whose tenets give more support to one sex than to the other, but this does not seem to be the case with Catholicism and Protestantism. However, when we move from the purely religious domain to differences of custom and of broad value orientation, then there are two ways in which Catholicism and Protestantism differ and which might be expected to affect the sexes differently.

One of these differences concerns the celibacy of the priesthood and the fact that in the Catholic Church an important adult male model held before the eyes of a boy is one which excludes marriage and sexuality. Depending on what theory one holds on the genesis of schizophrenia, one can see this as creating problems for the schizophrenia-prone male or as offering him a socially accepted mode of escape from the threats which sexuality and the intimacies of marriage may appear to pose. Hence a hypothesized relation to the incidence of schizophrenia in the two sexes is difficult to propose on that basis. (And moreover, the celibacy of nuns presents girls with similar problems and solutions, though probably to a lesser degree.) The other difference concerns orientations toward independence, work, and social competition. Protestantism stresses independence, private problem-solving and work, while tacitly approving of material acquisitiveness. Catholicism stresses communality, obedience, and greater attention to intangibles. This difference and the subsequent argument that the Protestant ethic is better geared to modern competitive capitalism may appear worked to death, but it still holds some relevance for us here since the Catholic orientation is to some extent in conflict with the wider cultural beliefs of North American society, whereas the Protestant orientation is less so. The Catholic could therefore be said to be faced with greater difficulties in reconciling the expectations impinging on him than the Protestant[15], and the male Catholic can be expected to face more such difficulties than the female, since it is in wider society rather than in the home that the conflict is likely to arise.

Whether or not this last point is relevant to the higher incidence of schizophrenia in Catholic males cannot be established at present; I know of simply no evidence on the matter. The fact remains, however, that Catholic males do have a higher incidence of schizophrenia than Protestant ones, whether we take the hospitalization data for 7 provinces or the field survey data for 14 rural communities, and this difference does not seem to be explainable in any way which would enable us to disregard the cultural teachings of the two groups.

MODES OF OPERATION

These four illustrations offer the strongest evidence presently available for the theory that culture can influence the genesis of schizophrenia. I believe myself that that evidence is sufficient to justify the theory and, furthermore, that it points to culture having an evocative effect rather than merely a distributive one. The illustrations, with the exception of the last, concerned whole peoples and not merely particular strata into which schizophrenia-prone individuals could be expected to drift or to be pushed. However, with the Croatians, the Canadian Catholics and more doubtfully with the Tamils the point was made that their cultural heritages and their present social situations were to some extent in conflict, echoing the earlier remark that we must expect an interaction of sociocultural influences rather than the discovery of constant and independent causal factors. Because cultural traditions are adaptive, any part of such tradition that is strongly evocative of schizophrenia or another mental disorder is likely to become modified, and this is probably one of the reasons why differences in schizophrenia incidence between cultural groups are usually much less than differences between component parts of any one of them.

But now, what evidence is there as to the way in which cultural influences operate with the disease? While there have been some theories on the subject, there are virtually no studies which appear to have investigated the matter, particularly if we confine ourselves to schizophrenia and disregard studies of mental disorder in general. Of course, in one sense all studies into social factors in the genesis of schizophrenia could be cited, since all take place within a particular cultural setting and the social characteristics are never independent of it. This is particularly clear in those studies which have attempted to elucidate the psychodynamics of schizophrenia in the North American Negro. Behind the dramatic foreground action of such studies looms the heavy backdrop of U.S. Anglo-Saxon cultural traditions. Even with such an apparently universal phenomenon as the relation of schizophrenia to social class one can detect a cultural influence. In Singapore quite different associations between schizophrenia and social class appear in the three major peoples, and I suspect that differences which have appeared between British and U.S. findings here may reflect a cultural difference in the way in which class structure is accepted. But with the expectation of some U.S. Negro data, where we would still have some difficulties in deciding which culture we were relating them to—the Negro or the White—the cultural element is not sufficiently explicit for such material to be easily used. Hence, with new apologies for reverting to my own data, I propose to ignore the general literature on social factors and to focus on a single illustration where the relative significance of cultural and other variables was specifically investigated.

The illustration derives from our "Fourteen Communities Survey," which was a field investigation of the key informant type focusing mainly on the active prevalence of psychosis regardless of whether psychiatric care had been received or not. The communities were chosen to represent various cultural traditions and levels of social organization, and attention was especially paid to community-patient relationships. Six of the communities were French-Canadian, three of them chosen to represent the traditional culture and three to represent "border" conditions where that tradition had less hold. The three traditional communities proved to have an extremely high prevalence of schizophrenia in women (13.1 per 1000 adults) and the same phenomenon appeared in each, although they were in different counties and had virtually no recent intermarriage. A review of case material revealed the following features.

The main excess of female cases was found in married women who showed signs of publicly recognizable disorder only after the age of 35. Of the 8 such cases, only one was in a hospital although several were deteriorated to the extent that made such care desirable. All but one had four or more children and in most instances the oldest child had left home or was about to leave. Almost all exhibited delusions of reference and focused these delusions on husband and children. Some had attempted to break with their home and husband by running away (in which case they were hospitalized but soon brought back to look after their children); the others did not make any such "avoidance" gesture but instead accused their husbands or children of misbehavior, attempts at poisoning, etc., and these, since they continued to fulfil their household duties after a fashion, were never hospitalized. In the males of these same communities and in the females of the other communities studied, this picture in this age group was quite rare.

The other excess of female cases was of a more familiar type, occurring in young unmarried women. However, once again the clinical picture was remarkably uniform and quite different from what was shown by the male cases in the same communities. Onset is gradual, with no history of sexual deviancy or of intended marriage but sometimes with a history of the girl trying to establish an independent career in teaching, etc. The career, if embarked on, is abandoned; the girl stays in her parents' home, becomes increasingly withdrawn or increasingly hypochondriacal, and thus slides gradually into a chronic sick-role which may never involve naming the illness and which usually evokes no disapprobation. Some of the women remain in this state, dependent on their parents, keeping apart from community affairs but conforming to its prescribed sick-role behavior, and never being sent to hospital or getting treatment for the psychiatric condition. More usually, however, there is a rebellion against the prescribed role, an exhibition of behavior that is socially disapproved, hospitalization relatively soon after that occurs, and thereafter usually a failure of such attempts as the hospital makes to get the patient back to her family. In the three communities there are eight patients who fit this picture, and what differentiates them from the early-starting male schizophrenics in the same communities is that the males mostly either reintegrate themselves with the community and gradually lose their symptoms or leave it entirely, whereas the females do neither.

Contrasting with these pictures, we found almost no schizophrenia in younger married women, although this was common in the other three French-Canadian communities, and almost none in older single women, although this also was to be found in some other communities.

When the social background to this phenomenon was investigated with the aid of a French-Canadian sociologist, the following was found. The three traditional communities still depict the ideal woman as one who gets married early, has many children, is hardworking, patient, diligent and submissive to her husband. Motherhood is envisaged as a highly rewarding role, and the idea of an independent career for women outside of the religious orders is only now being accepted as a possibility. About a generation ago, however, more schooling became available locally, and since the boys were often taken away to work in the fields while their sisters were left to their classes, the girls became more educated than their brothers and potential husbands. Furthermore, local orders of nuns provided post-school courses in practical nursing, typing, domestic science, etc., and imbued the girls with the idea that this knowledge was there to be made use of, while for the boys local opinion was still maintaining that farming did not require education. For the controlling, organizing type of woman this situation could be and was quite gratifying, for they could marry men less educated than themselves and use their own education to control first their families and then, through their husbands, the male domain of public affairs, while still receiving community approval because they maintained a façade of submission. Such behavior could not be publicly taught or recognized in this male-oriented Catholic society, however, and neither would it satisfy those women who sought a husband to love and respect or those others who were not attracted to marriage at all. A conflict can thus be inferred to have arisen in the minds of many women regarding how to pursue both the ideal of womanhood which the tradition taught and the modern goal of a life which would permit them more use of their new education and more individuality. We find this conflict reflected in the comments of our women informants and in the expressed desire of present-day mothers that their daughters should be able to escape and make a life for themselves. More importantly, however, I believe that we find this conflict reflected in the symptomatology of the female schizophrenics attempting to avoid, to escape from or to destroy the type of marriage which their society sought to tie them to. It is noteworthy that during the early years of marriage and motherhood, when the woman can apply her education to the bringing-up of her young children and can thereby ignore the problems of daily life with an inarticulate and narrow-sighted husband, no schizophrenia makes itself known; only before the decision to marry is made or after the main joys of motherhood are past.

The problem which this generation of women in these villages has been facing might be coloring the symptomatology of the schizophrenics without being at all relevant to the genesis of their disorder. However, in view of the fact that the female rate is double that of the male there and almost double that of the female rate in the "new" French-Canadian villages where a career outside of marriage is much easier to pursue for women, it seems reasonable to believe that the conflict is relevant to the genesis of the disease and not just to its appearances. Moreover, when one looks at the data from the other communities then similar though less striking associations between a conflict of expectations and the onset of schizophrenia appear. That is to say, in the Polish and in the Irish Catholic cases from this survey one can detect a clustering of pathology in sections of the communities that are particularly affected by some cultural inconsistency or conflict of expectations, and a relative absence of schizophrenia in other sections of the population whom the culture either demands very little from or guides very clearly. Details of these other situations can be found in a recent paper[12]; here I wish to indicate what I think they have in common.

The situation in the traditional French-Canadian villages could be described as one of role conflict, but such conflict is too common to be in itself the mediating link we are seeking. Therefore it must be asked what more is present in that situation and in the others. In my opinion one finds the following: a problem of choice which affects the individual deeply; pressure by the community or culture to make some choice; contradictions or confusion in the guidance which the culture provides; chronicity in the sense that the problem persists until a decision is taken. It will be seen, I think, that the type of confrontation which appears to be schizophrenia-evoking in these communities has some similarities to the types of confrontation which are believed to be schizophrenogenic within families and some similarities also to the situations of the peoples cited earlier in this paper. I have suggested elsewhere[13] that it has also similarities to conditions which have been demonstrated in the laboratory to induce pathological thought processes in already schizophrenic subjects. These considerations, however, go beyond the assigned scope of this paper. It is sufficient to say in conclusion that the demonstration of a probable relationship between culture and schizophrenia need not and should not be taken as merely adding one more variable to the already excessive number that apparently must be taken into consideration before schizophrenia can be understood properly. Culture in itself should not be thought of as a factor in the disease; rather it should be thought of as one of a host of variables which can confront the schizophrenia-prone individual with a particular class of experience able to evoke his disease. What is important is to define the characteristics of that class, not to catalogue its innumerable sources.

REFERENCES

1. Arensberg, C. M., & Kimball, S. T. *Family and community in Ireland.* Cambridge, Mass., 1940.
2. Bhattacharjya, B. On the wartime incidence of mental diseases in the Indian army. *Ind. J. Neurol. Psychiat.,* 1949, **1**, 51.

3. Crocetti, G. M. *et al.* Selected aspects of the epidemiology of schizophrenia in Croatia (Yugoslavia). *Milbank Mem. Fund Quarterly*, 1964, **42**, 9–37.
4. Dominion Bureau of Statistics (Canada). *Census of Canada*, 1961 (Section 92–562). Ottawa, 1964.
5. Eaton, J. W., & Weil, R. J. *Culture and mental disorders*. Illinois, 1955.
6. Eterovich, F. H., & Spalatin, C. *Croatia; Land, people, culture*. Toronto, 1964.
7. Fisher, J. C. *Yugoslavia–A multinational state*. San Francisco, 1966.
8. Kadri, Z. N. Schizophrenia in the university students. *Singapore Med. J.*, 1963, **4**, 113–118.
9. Malzberg, B. *Social and biological aspects of mental disease*. Utica, 1940.
10. Murphy, H. B. M. Cultural factors in the mental health of Malayan students. In D. H. Funkenstein (Ed.), *The student and mental health: An international view*. World Federation for Mental Health, 1959. Pp. 164–222.
11. Murphy, H. B. M. The epidemiological approach to transcultural psychiatric research. In de Reuck & Porter (Eds.), *Transcultural Psychiatry, A Ciba Foundation symposium*. London, 1965. Pp. 303–327.
12. Murphy, H. B. M. Canadian rural communities and their schizophrenic patients. Paper presented at a Basic Conference on Human Behavior, McGill University, Montreal, 1967. (a)
13. Murphy, H. B. M. Sociocultural factors in schizophrenia: A compromise theory. In Freyhan & Zubin (Eds.), *Social psychiatry*. American Psychopathological Association, 1967. (b)
14. O'Doherty, E. F. The high proportion of mental hospital beds in the Republic. *Transcult. Psychiat. Res.*, 1965, **2**, 134–136. (Abstract)
15. Pollock, H. M. A statistical study of the foreign-born insane in New York state hospitals. *State Hospitals Bull.* 1913, 10–27 of special number.
16. Pollock, H. M. Frequency of schizophrenia in relation to sex, age, environment, nativity and race. *Schizophrenia* (Assn. Res. Nerv. Ment. Dis., Vol. 5), New York, 1928.
17. Singh, K. Psychiatric practice among Indian troops. *Ind. Med. Gazette*, 1946, **81**, 394.
18. Spitzka, E. C. Race and insanity. *J. Nerv. Ment. Dis.*, 1880, **7**, 342–348.
19. Swift, H. M. Insanity and race. *Am. J. Insanity*, 1913, **70**, 143–154.
20. West, R. *Black lamb and grey falcon*. New York, 1941.
21. Williams, A. H. A psychiatric study of Indian soldiers in the Arakan. *Brit. J. Med. Psychol.*, 1950, **23**, 131.

Suggested Additional Readings

Benedict, P. K., & Jacks, I. Mental illness in primitive societies. *Psychiatry*, 1954, **17**, 377–389.

Chance, N. A. Acculturalization, self-indentification, and personality adjustment. *Americal Anthropologist*, 1965, **67**, 372–393.

Hallowell, A. I. Fear and anxiety as cultural and individual variables in a primitive society. *The Journal of Social Psychology*, 1938, **9**, 25–47.

Hallowell, A. I. Values, acculturation, and mental health. *American Journal of Orthopsychiatry*, 1950, **20**, 732–743.

Kitano, H. H. L. Mental illness in four cultures. *The Journal of Social Psychology*, 1970, **80**, 121–134.

Opler, M. K. (Ed.), *Culture and mental health, cross culture studies.* New York: Macmillan, 1959.

Wittkower, E. D. Perspectives of transcultural psychiatry. *International Journal of Psychiatry*, 1969, **8**, 811–834.

Yap, P. M., & Cantab, B. C. Mental diseases peculiar to certain cultures: A survey of comparative psychiatry, *Journal of Mental Science*, 1951, **97**, 313–327.

Genetic and Biochemical Factors

16

Genetic Research in the Schizophrenic Syndrome*

DAVID ROSENTHAL

In the letter inviting me to write this contribution, I was asked to write about the promise that genetics holds for the understanding, prevention, and treatment of mental illness in general and schizophrenia in particular. That is better than being asked to write about man in relationship to his universe, but not much better. At any rate, I shall try to catch the spirit and intent of the request and address myself to it as best I can.

Before we can talk intelligently about the contributions of genetics to the understanding of schizophrenia, we must first assure ourselves that schizophrenia has some hereditary basis. Without presenting tables and figures or going into great detail about the hundreds of studies concerned with heredity in schizophrenia, let me summarize briefly the main evidence that indicates that schizophrenia does in fact have a genetic basis.

The first body of evidence comes from what we might call consanguinity studies. The nature of the evidence takes two forms. The first is that the incidence of schizophrenia in the immediate families of schizophrenics has repeatedly been found to be much higher than the incidence of the disorder in the general population. This is a consistent finding whether the investigator has a genetic or an environmentalist bias. In fact, investigators who emphasize the *psychological* factors in the etiology of schizophrenia report a much higher incidence of schizophrenic-type pathology in the families that they have studied than do genetic investigators who have not examined the families as intensively.

An additional form of evidence obtained in the consanguinity studies involves a consistent correlation between incidence of schizophrenia in the relatives of schizophrenics and the closeness of the blood relationship to schizophrenic index cases. Thus, the incidence of schizophrenia is higher in the siblings, children, and parents of schizophrenics than in their aunts, uncles, nephews, and nieces. The incidence of the disorder among second-degree relatives is in turn higher than the incidence in the general population, although not very much higher.

This body of evidence can be criticized on two main grounds. The first is methodological. Investigators who have carried out these studies have known the diagnosis of the index case and have primarily had a genetic rather than a psychological orientation to the etiology of schizophrenia. However, the diagnoses have usually been based on hospitalized cases among relatives, and, in the main, the hospital diagnoses corresponded with the diagnosis of schizophrenia made by the investigators. Also, investigators who have a psychological orientation to schizophrenia have reported similar or higher rates of the disorder among first-degree relatives of the probands in their studies. Thus, the general finding of a correlation between incidence of the disorder and degree of consanguinity is probably valid.

The second objection is the more serious one. Here, the argument runs that it is not the genes transmitted from parent to child that are responsible for the mental illness in the

*Reprinted with permission from *The schizophrenic reactions*, edited by R. Cancro (1970), Bruner-Mazel, Inc., and Dr. Rosenthal.

children but rather the type of rearing, the behavioral irrationality, and the chaotic climate of the familial relationships that really induce the behavioral disorder in the child. Investigators favoring this view have had no difficulty in demonstrating the chaos and irrationality that exists in these families. Thus, we have two equally valid bodies of evidence that lead investigators to two different and opposed conclusions. As long as the genetic and psychological variables coexisted in the same family, it was impossible to decide on which one was in fact the culprit factor that induced the psychopathology in the child.

The second body of evidence comes from twin studies which, up until recently, provided the most salient data favoring a genetic basis for the etiology of schizophrenia. In almost all the twin studies done to date, the concordance rate for schizophrenia in monozygotic twins has been appreciably higher than the concordance rate in dizygotic twins. Thus, in ten of eleven studies the rates are in accord with what genetic theory predicts. Although all studies encounter problems of sampling and diagnosis, there is no question but that the *direction* of differences in concordance rates between the two types of twins is valid.

The interpretation of these findings has been a matter of some controversy. One argument holds that psychological factors regarding monozygotic twins are very different from those regarding dizygotic twins. The higher concordance rate for monozygotic pairs might be attributable to the fact that identical twins share a unique and intense identificatory bond. If one member of the pair becomes schizophrenic, the identificatory bond is likely to lead to a similar pattern of psychotic behavior in his co-twin. Thus, the difference in concordance rates between the two types of twins could have a psychological explanation.

However, case reports of monozygotic twins reared apart provide serious difficulties for the identification argument. Sixteen cases of monozygotic pairs reared apart have now been reported in which at least one of the twins was diagnosed as schizophrenic. Among these pairs, ten were concordant and six discordant. The overall concordance rate is comparable to rates obtained for twins reared together. Although there may well have been some sampling bias which led to this concordance rate being inflated, it is clear that an indentificatory bond could hardly have accounted for the many pairs who were concordant. It is difficult to imagine how such a frequency of concordance could have occurred without some common genetic basis.

The third body of evidence comes from studies in which the child generation has not been reared by the parent generation. The child may have been reared in an adoptive home, in foster homes, institutions, or in the homes of relatives. Five such studies have now been reported[9], three of them by my colleagues, including Dr. Seymour Kety, Dr. Paul Wender, and myself. Two of the five studies were carried out in Denmark, one in Iceland, one on the West Coast, and another on the East Coast of the U.S.A. All five studies are consistent in their finding of a higher incidence of schizophrenia or schizophrenic-spectrum disorder among the biological relatives of schizophrenic probands than among relatives who were not biologically related but with whom the subjects studied shared the rearing experience. All five studies differed in the details of their research design, but regardless of whether the schizophrenic index cases were the biological parents of the foster-reared or adopted children, the results point consistently in the same direction. Although one could raise questions about any one of the studies, when the five are considered together they constitute such strong evidence for the genetic hypothesis that it is difficult to see how this hypothesis can now be refuted.

When one considers the combined evidence from the consanguinity studies, the twin studies, and the adoption studies, one must admit that a genetic explanation of all the data is simpler, more parsimonious, and less ad hoc than any environmentalist explanation. This does not mean that environmental factors are not important with respect to the etiology of schizophrenia, but only that they must be considered in conjunction with genetic factors.

Let us assume now that we are all agreed that the case for a hereditary contribution to the etiology of schizophrenia has been proven. How does this knowledge help us to understand the nature of the schizophrenic disturbance? What implications does such knowledge hold for the future planning of research on schizophrenic disorders? Before we can properly appreciate such implications, we ought to know at least three things relevant to the heredity contribution: 1. the mode of inheritance; 2. the genetic or biological unity of schizophrenia; and 3. the specificity of the schizophrenic genotype.

With respect to the mode of inheritance, it is not yet entirely clear whether schizophrenic disorder can be attributed to a single major gene, to a combination of two major genes, or to a number of genes with different effects, all of which may contribute in some degree or dimension to a schizophrenic denouement. Once we accept a genetic hypothesis, whatever the mode of inheritance, we must assume that some sort of metabolic digression has taken place at some time during the development of the affected individual. If the disorder is caused by a single major gene, then investigators who are searching for a specific biochemical abnormality that discriminates schizophrenics from controls may well be on the right track.

However, the genetic research is not as encouraging to such investigators as it once was thought to be. It was not too long ago that genetic investigators were debating with considerable intensity whether the gene that caused schizophrenia was dominant or recessive. The fact that no clear Mendelian distribution of schizophrenia in families could be found did not deter the debate. The theorists spoke in terms of reduced penetrance and modifying genes to account for the deviation from Mendelian distributions. Investigators calculated what the manifestation rate of schizophrenia would have to be for homozygotes and heterozygotes if the gene were recessive or dominant. Some investigators also calculated what the mutation rate for the assumed pathological gene would have to be to maintain the population incidence of the disorder at a constant level.

Single-gene theorists classified the relatives of their probands as either schizophrenic or not schizophrenic and failed to face the possibility that a continuum of schizophrenicity might exist. Of course, there were always some cases who were not clearly schizophrenic but, on the other hand, were not clearly nonschizophrenic either. Investigators would call such cases "doubtful" or "questionable" schizophrenia, and these cases could be included or excluded in the statistical analyses of familial rates, depending on the preference of the investigator or his critics. Different investigators followed different practices in this regard. Cases called schizoid were excluded from such analyses and in fact created difficulty for some investigators since they obviously did not meet the criteria for clear-cut schizophrenia and yet, clinically, looked suspiciously like they belonged with the group of schizophrenics. If they harbored the schizophrenic genotype, why were they not clinically schizophrenic; and if they did not harbor the genotype, why should they have manifested symptoms that appeared to be related to clinical schizophrenia?

If one maintained a theory of recessiveness, one might hold that the schizophrenics had the culprit gene in double dose, whereas the schizoid relatives were heterozygous carriers of the pathological gene. This, in fact, was Kallmann's position[4].

If one supported a dominance theory, then one might maintain that the gene was a partial dominant, that all of the few individuals who were homozygous for the dominant gene were bound to develop clinical schizophrenia, and that most schizophrenics by far would be heterozygous for the dominant gene. Heterozygous carriers, in turn, would manifest a low penetrance so that only a relatively small fraction of them would develop clinical schizophrenia. This, in fact, is the kind of theory that Slater[10] has supported. Although such possible genetic interpretations are desirable, they have tended to alienate nongeneticists and to discourage them from considering any genetic hypothesis in a serious way.

In the 1960s, a polygenic view of schizophrenia attained high popularity among leading investigators in the field. There were many reasons for this. For one thing, such a view was not committed to a yes-or-no conception of schizophrenia. Rather, it viewed schizophrenic disorders as ranging quantitatively along a single continuum. For this reason, the finding in schizophrenic probands' families of cases called questionable or doubtful schizophrenia, or cases called schizoid or paranoid, posed no problem. As a matter of fact, they were to be expected. Those cases who were clinically full-blown schizophrenics merely represented the end point on the continuum. The theory did not have to provide any ad hoc hypotheses such as diminished penetrance or heterozygosity to account for the subschizophrenic cases.

Another factor favoring a switch to polygenic theory was the development in the late fifties and early sixties of new methods and better understanding of quantitative genetics. It became clearer that most traits studied by far in higher order animals had a polygenic basis. Almost all behavioral traits were clearly graded and continuous and therefore polygenically influenced, if genes were relevant at all. Since schizophrenia was a behavioral disorder in the sense that it was defined in terms of specific behaviors, it seemed reasonable to believe that it, too, should have a polygenic basis.

Twin research in the sixties provided additional reasons for thinking that a polygenic view was the correct one. In several studies done during this decade, the modal concordance rate for monozygotic twins was about forty percent. The rates reported were consistently lower than the rates that had been reported in the earlier twin studies, in which the modal rate was about seventy percent. The lower the concordance rate in monozygotic twins, the lower the penetrance that one would have to attribute to a single pathological gene. When the penetrance estimate gets to be lower than fifty percent, then the theory underlying it becomes very shaky indeed.

With respect to heredity-environment consideration, a polygenic view makes it especially important to think about the environmental factors that contribute to the evocation of clinical schizophrenia. As a matter of fact, I have subsumed the polygenic viewpoint under what I call diathesis-stress theory, a term that designates both the hereditary and environmental factors as important agents in the development of schizophrenic disorders.

There is another way of looking at polygenic theory. For example, some strains of mice and rats develop convulsions when subjected to high-pitched tones. In some of the strains, the trait of convulsing is polygenically determined. Although the animals' responses to the high-pitched tones can be graded, the investigators tend to classify their animals in terms of those who develop convulsions and those who do not. Such a trait is called a threshold character. Similarly, schizophrenia might be thought of as a threshold character, a culminating reaction in a polygenically predisposed individual to a high-intensity stress.

A human model for a threshold character may be found in a disorder such as congenital pyloric stenosis. Some geneticists have maintained that this disorder is polygenically based and that the stricture of the pylorus is of a graded character which, when it reaches a certain point, gives rise to the serious clinical symptoms of the disorder. In such a condition, one tends to be concerned primarily with the structural anomaly rather than the developmental metabolic digression that gave rise to it. If the hereditary component in schizophrenia turns out to be a polygenic one, some investigators might feel more confident in finding deviations among schizophrenics in how the central nervous system is put together, or how it is "wired," rather than in finding a specific biochemical abnormality, but, of course, the latter possibility is just as tenable under polygenic theory.

A second way in which genetics may help us to understand schizophrenia has to do with what has traditionally been called the biological or genetic unity of schizophrenia. I use the term only in the sense that it asks this question: What types of clinical syndromes are genetically related to one another and rightly subsumed under the broad category of schizophrenic disorders? More specifically, do the classical subtypes of schizophrenia have a common genetic basis; are process and reactive schizophrenia two separate disorders; or, do patients who fall ill with schizophrenic-like disorders at very early or late ages really belong in a single genetic family of schizophrenias? I shall not review in detail the literature relevant to these problems which can be found elsewhere[8], but shall try to summarize briefly what I think the evidence of past studies leads us to conclude.

With respect to the classical subtypes, we find that paranoid, catatonic, and hebephrenic forms of schizophrenic illness occur repeatedly in the same families. As a matter of fact, one case has been reported in which both parents were paranoid yet they had two children who were hebephrenic[2]. The Genain Quadruplets[7] had a paranoid father and grandmother but all four girls were catatonic-hebephrenic. Such findings suggest that the classical subtypes are genetically related.

However, in studies of monozygotic twins, we find a very strong association within twin pairs with respect to subtype. For example, if one monozygotic twin is catatonic, the probability is very high that his co-twin will be diagnosed catatonic as well. In the case of twins reared together, the possibility clearly exists that the common association and/or rearing induces both twins to develop the same form of illness. From the genetic point of view, the almost constant finding of a common subtype in monozygotic twins suggests genetic specificity with respect to them.

How shall we explain such findings? With respect to the twin studies, it has almost always been the case that the same investigator made the subtype diagnosis for both twins. He may have been influenced in his judgment by the identical appearance of both twins, and his judgment regarding the first twin could have influenced his diagnosis regarding the second twin. Several studies have reported that the reliability of subtype diagnosis is not very high, a fact which indicates that judgments regarding subtype can readily be influenced by extraneous factors. Some of the variation with respect to different subtypes in the same families might possibly be explained on this basis as well.

A polygenic theory of schizophrenia could readily account for the seemingly incompatible findings. One could assume, for example, that individuals characterized as catatonic or hebephrenic had more of the pathological genes than schizophrenics called sample or paranoid. The clinical picture of psychopathology, in fact, tends to be more severe in catatonics and hebephrenics than in cases with simple or paranoid forms of the illness, and the incidence of schizophrenic disorder in their families tends to be higher as well. Individuals in the same family who harbor more or less of the pathological genes might be expected to show different subtype patterns. Monozygotic twins would be expected to have the same clinical picture since they both carry the same number and type of polygenes.

Should cases that have their onset before adolescence be classified as schizophrenic? The evidence suggests that a monozygotic twin with preadolescent schizophrenia is likely to have a co-twin with preadolescent schizophrenia as well. However, about twenty percent of the sick co-twins may develop schizophrenia *after* the onset of adolescence[5]. In addition, a high rate of schizophrenia among the parents of children with prepubertal schizophrenia has been reported as well. As a matter of fact, in one study, eleven percent of prepubertal schizophrenic children had both parents schizophrenic[1]. Thus, these findings suggest that there may be a common genetic anlage for both the pre- and postadolescent forms of schizophrenia. With respect to polygenic theory, the fact that one group of schizophrenics has the onset of the illness so much earlier than the second group suggests that the early onset group may have more of the polygenes. Of course, it is easy to think of environmental explanations of such findings as well.

With respect to early infantile autism, the picture is less clear. One leading investigator[6] found virtually no schizophrenia among the parents of his infant probands whereas a second leading investigator[3] reported an incidence that was quite elevated: twenty-nine percent of the mothers and thirteen percent of the fathers. When the children were divided into cases called organic or nonorganic, as determined by an intensive neurological examination, the rate of schizophrenia in the parents of the nonorganic group was higher than the rate for parents of the organic group. Among the parents of the children called organic, twenty-one percent of the mothers and fifteen percent of the fathers were called schizophrenic. Among the parents of the nonorganic group, forty-four percent of the mothers and eight percent of the fathers were classified as schizophrenic. It is difficult to make genetic sense of a finding in which mothers are five and one-half times more frequent than fathers with respect to schizophrenia, especially in view of the fact that the illness tends to occur in both sexes equally, and only about twice as often in mothers, as compared to fathers, generally.

Without going into the research findings, I shall add that the disorders called schizophreniform psychosis, symptomatic schizophrenia, psychogenic psychosis, a typical, peripheral or reactive schizophrenia, schizo-affective psychosis, borderline schizophrenia, schizoid personality, or paranoid state all seem to be genetically linked to schizophrenia. The studies are many, and the findings not always consistent, but the overall evidence suggests that these disorders do indeed belong in the same genetic family.

Let me add just a few lines on what I call the specificity of the schizophrenic genotype. I use this term to cover the question: Which mental disorders, if any, are genetically distinct from the schizophrenic family of disorders? For historical reasons, I have reference primarily to the disorder called manic-depressive psychosis. With regard to the family studies of both disorders that have been reported to date, the evidence mainly favors the theory that schizophrenia and manic-depressive psychosis are genetically different. By and large, schizophrenia occurs infrequently in the families of manic depressive probands, and very little manic-depressive psychosis occurs among the families of schizophrenics. No clear-cut case has yet been reported of schizophrenia in one twin and manic-depressive psychosis in the monozygotic co-twin.

However, some overlap of the two disorders does occur. Moreover, it is relatively uncommon for schizophrenics to have children with manic-depressive psychosis, whereas manic-depressive parents tend to have schizophrenic children at a rate that is about three to five times higher than the rate of schizophrenia in the general population.

A conclusion that the two disorders are genetically distinct would be based primarily on the pronounced clustering of one illness or the other in different families. The overlap within families that has been reported might have resulted from misdiagnosis in some cases. From a genetic point of view, the spouses of one type of psychotic might sometimes have been carriers of genes implicated in the other disorder. From the environmental side, one might hold that the clinical manifestations are strongly influenced by life experiences of various kinds. Such factors could indeed blur the overall picture, but the evidence for an inherited component in each disorder, especially schizophrenia, is now fairly solid. Any conclusions that we draw with respect to the genetic distinctness of the two disorders, however, must involve some reservation. A review of the literature suggests that further and better research might well enable us to draw clear conclusions with respect to whether schizophrenia and manic-depressive psychosis are indeed two different mental illnesses.

There is some suggestion in the literature, too, that some forms of psychoneurosis and some forms of psychopathy are associated genetically with schizophrenia. Others seem not to be related to schizophrenia at all. For our purposes, however, the question should not be limited to whether or not we can draw definite conclusions about these matters at the present time, but rather whether a clearer understanding of the role of genetics in these disorders will help us to develop a better comprehension of them and perhaps a more sensible nosology as well.

Some implications of genetics for the prevention and treatment of schizophrenic disorders are readily apparent, while others may not be quite as obvious. I shall list and briefly discuss five general implications

1. A genetic basis for a disorder suggests the possibility of identifying a specific metabolic error which causes it. The knowledge that schizophrenic disorders have a genetic basis encourages investigators to carry on not only biochemical research, but also physiological and psycho-physiological research that helps us to obtain a clearer understanding of their functional nature. In addition, such genetic knowledge provides a sound basis for genetic counseling, so that schizophrenics and close relatives of schizophrenics can be advised about the likelihood of having a schizophrenic child. Whether one accepts a genetic or psychological etiology of schizophrenia, it is clear that a high marriage rate for schizophrenics—and possibly for their siblings—will lead to an increased rate of schizophrenia in the next generation. A sound basis for counseling such individuals could prevent an increased incidence from occurring.

2. Now that we have such strong evidence that schizophrenia has a genetic component, we can give thought to identifying who the people are that carry the schizophrenic genotype. For example, my colleagues and I are carrying out a study in which we examine intensively, for two days, individuals who have a high likelihood of being gene carriers. These individuals are adults who had a biological parent that was schizophrenic, but they were not reared by their schizophrenic parent. Instead, they were given up for adoption early in life and reared by adoptive parents.Thus, in their growing-up years, they had no direct personal contact with schizophrenia. We also have a control group of subjects, neither of whose biological parents was known to have had a psychiatric disorder, but these individuals were also reared in adoptive homes.

Through psychological tests and an intensive psychiatric interview, we hope to be able to discriminate the two groups with respect to a number of psychological and behavioral characteristics. If we can make such discriminations, we may be able to describe the basic personality characteristics stemming from the pathological genotype. Positive findings might also provide a sound basis for assuming that a similar identification of gene carriers could be made in individuals who are much younger, perhaps even in infants. Such knowledge, if it can be obtained, is bound to give us a better understanding of what these individuals are like. It could also provide a sound basis for carrying out a rational program of mental hygiene with respect to them.

3. If the effort to identify gene carriers in early life succeeds, we should be in an excellent position to study the effects of different environmental, rearing and experiential factors on the subsequent psychological development of such individuals. For example, my Israeli colleagues and I are carrying out a study in which we examine latency age children who have a schizophrenic parent. Half of these children were born and raised in a *kibbutz* and half in the typical nuclear family situation. We have reason to believe that the child who has a schizophrenic parent but who is reared in a *kibbutz* might fare better than his counterpart in the nuclear family situation. Typically, the child who has a schizophrenic father or mother may be subjected to unusual, bizarre, or confusing behavior on the part of the sick parent, the home may be broken, the sick parent may be absent for long periods of

time because of hospitalization, the child may be forced to live with relatives or friends, in foster homes or in institutions, or in any combination of these.

The child reared in a *kibbutz* has a more stable environment. The sick parent is likely to have less daily contact with him and perhaps, therefore, less influence upon him. During most of the day, the child is under the care of normal caretakers and teachers. He retains a stable set of peers, no matter what happens to the parent. When the parent becomes ill, he or she may be removed to a hospital but the child suffers no serious disruption of any other part of his life. He still has the other parent with him and can visit this parent regularly during the evening as he does ordinarily every day of his life. In his growing-up years, he has normal parent surrogates with whom to identify, as compared to the child in the nuclear family situation whose daily intimate associations may include only a sick parent.

In this study, we have control children as well. One-half of the controls come from the same *kibbutz* as the index case who has a schizophrenic parent. The control child has grown up in exactly the same circumstances as the index child, but the parents of the control child do not have any known psychiatric illness. We also have a control group of children from the towns, who come from the same classrooms as the town index children. These control subjects also have normal parents. The four groups of children are studied intensively over a two-day period. They are brought to examination in pairs and the examiners do not know which one is the index case and which is the control. The children are also observed together in natural situations, often in the same social group.

Not only do we hope to be able to distinguish the children who have a schizophrenic parent from the children who do not with respect to a number of personality characteristics, but the design also permits us to tease out interaction effects between the different types of rearing and the different types of parentage. Thus, we hope to provide clear experimental evidence regarding the nature and direction of some heredity-environment interactions. As a result of this study and, hopefully, other studies carried out in the same vein, we might be able to generate a better understanding of what kinds of environmental factors have what kinds of impact upon the gene-carrying children. Such knowledge should permit us to recommend the kinds of rearing and experiential influences that should be avoided or practiced in order to reduce the possibility of subsequent schizophrenic pathology.

4. Genetic studies of schizophrenia also provide the possibility of a more *positive* outlook regarding such disorders, in that people who are gene-carriers may possess not only a special predisposition toward the development of behaviors we call pathological, but they may also possess special talents and abilities which we should deem to be highly desirable. At least two genetic studies have pointed out that first-degree relatives of schizophrenics were—more often than controls—spontaneous in their behavior, colorful, artistic, and creative. Clinicians have long noted a type of originality in the thinking of some schizophrenics, but in their psychosis the originality was often detrimental to the affected individuals themselves.On the Rorschach, such patients may produce a number of O-minus responses. However, if we are able to identify the gene-carriers early, then we may be in a strategic position to nurture these latent heightened capacities for unusually imaginative and creative thinking. Thus, we could in the future not only help to ward off the development of negative effects, but we could foster as well the positive aspects of the gene-carriers' possible inherent potential.

5. With respect to the implications of genetic studies of schizophrenia for therapy, we can make the following points. First, there is always a possibility that genetic studies in association with biological studies of schizophrenia will lead to new medications that will have a more beneficial effect on clinical symptoms than current drugs have. Certainly, this avenue of research should not be discouraged. Second, if we are able to identify heredity-

environment interactions that influence the development of gene-carriers in a positive or negative way, we might be able to generalize from such findings to techniques of treatment which would be conceptually related to the environmental factors that produced the beneficial effects and avoided the noxious ones. And third, once we recognize the fact that genetic influences are important in schizophrenia, we should try to understand how such influences exert their effect on behavior. With respect to the psychological-behavioral level, it is likely that they increase the probability of certain behaviors occurring while diminishing or precluding the occurrence of other types of behavior. One implication of this hypothesis is that therapists may often have expectations or goals for a patient which he is simply not able to meet. Such impasses may lead to increased feelings of self-derogation in the patient, resentment toward the therapist, and pangs of frustration in the therapist plus feelings of his own ineffectiveness.

Of course, given our current state of knowledge, all the implications of genetics for prevention and treatment that I have listed are highly speculative. However, ongoing research suggests that we may be on the right track and that some of these speculations may be confirmed in the next decade.

REFERENCES

1. Bender, L. Mental illness in childhood and heredity. *Eugenics Quarterly,* 1963; **10,** 1–11.
2. Elsässer, G. *Die Nachkommen geisteskranker Elternpaare.* Stuttgart: Thieme, 1952.
3. Goldfarb, W. The subclassification of psychotic children: Application to a study of longitudinal change. In D. Rosenthal & S. S. Kety (Eds.), *The transmission of schizophrenia.* London: Pergamon, 1968.
4. Kallmann, F. J. The genetic theory of schizophrenia. *American Journal of Psychiatry,* 1946; **103,** 309–322.
5. Kallmann, F. J. & Roth, B. Genetic aspects of preadolescent schizophrenia. *American Journal of Psychiatry,* 1956; **112,** 599–606.
6. Kanner, L. To what extent is early infantile autism determined by constitutional inadequacies? In D. Hooker & C. C. Hare (Eds.), *Genetics and the inheritance of integrated neurological and psychiatric patterns.* Baltimore: Williams & Wilkins, 1954.
7. Rosenthal, D. *The Genain quadruplets.* New York: Basic Books, 1963.
8. Rosenthal, D. *Genetic theory and abnormal behavior.* New York: McGraw-Hill 1970.
9. Rosenthal, D. & Kety, S. S. (Eds.), *The transmission of schizophrenia.* London: Pergamon, 1968.
10. Slater, E. Clinical aspects of genetic mental disorders. In J. N. Cummings & M. Kremer (Eds.), *Biochemical aspects of neurological disorders* (2nd series). Oxford: Blackwell, 1965.

17

Human Chromosome Abnormalities as Related to Physical and Mental Dysfunction*[1]

JOHN H. HELLER

The relationship of human disease syndromes to chromosome aberrations is assuming an increasingly greater role in the detection, diagnosis, treatment and prediction of mental and physical defects in man. By means of karyotype analysis one is enabled to recognize previously unknown syndromes and to differentiate between separate but phenotypically similar entities. Proper diagnosis permits suitable therapeutic measures to be undertaken and enables genetic counselors to assess correct risks in many instances. Recent refinements in sampling embryonic cells by amniocentesis make it feasible to determine, in high risk cases, whether the embryo has a chromosome abnormality or whether it is a male, which has a high risk of sex-linked genetic defect. Termination of pregnancy can be recommended on the basis of this knowledge.

CLASSES OF CHROMOSOME ABNORMALITIES

Chromosome abnormalities have been known in plant and animal species for a very long time. They occur firstly as variations in the number of chromosomes per cell deviating from the normal two sets (maternal and paternal), existing either as complete multiples of sets, a condition called polyploidy (triploidy, tetraploidy, etc.), or as addition or loss of chromosomes within a set, a situation known as aneuploidy (monosomy, trisomy, tetrasomy, etc.). The origin of deviations in chromosome number is known to be through nondisjunction, either during the meiotic divisions in the maturation of the germ cells or during mitotic divisions in the developing individual, or through lagging of chromosomes at anaphase of cell division.

Secondly, chromosome aberrations occur as structural modifications such as duplications, deficiencies, translocations, inversions, isochromosomes, ring chromosomes, etc. These aberrations result from chromosome breakage and reunion in various patterns different from the normal sequence of loci. In most cases especially the "spontaneous" instances, the cause of chromosome breaks is unknown, but many extraneous agents have been demonstrated experimentally to be efficacious in inducing fragmentation. Foremost among these agents is ionizing radiation but many chemical substances (alkylating agents, nitroso-compounds, antibiotics, DNA precursors, etc.) and viruses have been implicated.

*From Heller, J. H., *Journal of Heredity*, 1969, **60**, 239–248. Copyright © 1969 by the American Genetic Association. Reprinted by permission of the American Genetic Association and Dr. Heller.

[1]This paper was prepared in collaboration with Dr. George H. Mickey, the New England Institute, and was presented on August 19, 1969, as the Sixth Wilhelmine E. Key lecture at the annual meetings of the American Institute of Biological Sciences, University of Vermont, Burlington. The key lecture was established by the American Genetic Association through funds bequeathed to the Association by Dr. Wilhelmine E. Key for the support of lectures in human genetics.

GENETIC EFFECTS OF CHROMOSOME ABERRATIONS

The striking genetic alterations accompanying chromosome aberrations were brilliantly analyzed by Blakeslee and coworkers on *Datura,* and by the *Drosophila* workers (Morgan, Bridges, Muller, Sturtevant, Painter, Patterson and many others). The task was greatly facilitated in *Drosophila* by the fortunate circumstance in the larval salivary glands where the giant polytene chromosomes exhibit intimate somatic pairing as well as characteristic banding patterns that permit identification of specific gene loci.

Particularly illuminating were Bridges' analyses of sex chromosomes and sex determination in *Drosophila,* utilizing the phenomenon of nondisjuction of the sex chromosomes and culminating in the genic balance theory of sex determination. In this insect the female normally has two X chromosomes plus the autosomes, and the male has one X and one Y. Two X chromosomes and one Y chromosome results in a female, whereas a chromosome constitution of XO produces a sterile male.

In contrast, the Y chromosome in mammals has a strongly masculinizing influence. The presence of a single Y is sufficient to induce differentiation into a male phenotype in the presence of one to five X chromosomes. The XO constitution differentiates into a female phenotype in both mouse and man.

MAMMALIAN CHROMOSOME STUDIES

The first reported instance of chromosome aberration in mammals was discovered by genetic methods in the waltzing mouse by William H. Gates in 1927[37] and analyzed cytologically by T. S. Painter[68]. Many difficulties in techniques prevented accurate counting and analysis of mammalian chromosomes—large number and relative small size of chromosomes, tendency to clump on fixation, cutting of chromosomes in sectioned material, etc. Even the somatic chromosome number in man was accepted erroneously as 48 until 1956 when Tjio and Levan[88] established the correct count of 46. This count was quickly confirmed by Ford and Hammerton[28], and in 1959 the first positive correlation of a chromosome abnormality and human disease syndrome was made by Lejeune et al.[54] (also Jacobs, et al.[44])— the trisomic number 21 chromosome, and Down's syndrome or mongolism. Shortly thereafter Klinefelter's[46] and Turner's[30] syndromes were identified with XXY and XO sex chromosome constitutions respectively, and in rapid succession reports of many other human chromosome abnormalities appeared, such as trisomy 17, trisomy 18, partial trisomy, ring X chromosome, sex chromosome mosaics, cri-du-chat syndrome, etc.[9, 26].

This sudden explosion of human chromosome studies, in contrast to the long delay of confirmation in human cells of chromosome abnormalities long known in plants and other animals, was made possible by new techniques of preparation. The accumulation of many cells in the metaphase stage of mitosis with colchicine, the use of hypotonic solution to swell the cells and separate chromosomes on the spindle, the discovery that phytohemagglutinin stimulates mammalian peripheral lymphocytes to undergo mitosis, and the method of squashing or spreading on slides of loose cells taken from bone marrow or tissue culture, all contributed to the rapid and accurate analysis of mammalian and human chromosome number and structure.

Karyotype analysis involves the careful comparison of chromosomes in a particular individual to the standard pattern for human cells, including precise measurements of lengths, arm ratios and other morphological features. Special attention is given to comparison of

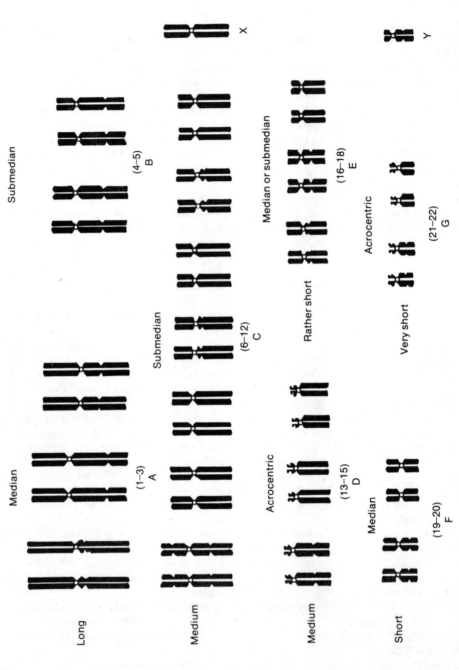

Fig. 17.1 Idiogram of normal male with 22 pairs of autosomes and XY sex chromosome constitution (modified from Patau[69], Sohval[84], Ferguson-Smith *et al.*[27], and Palmer and Funderburk[(68a)]).

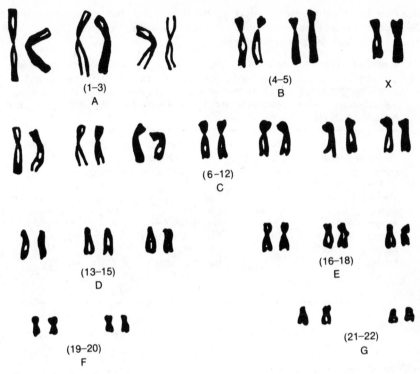

Fig. 17.2 Karyotype of a normal human female with 22 pairs of autosomes and two X chromosomes.

homologous chromosomes where differences may indicate abnormalities. An idiogram is a diagrammatic representation of the entire standard chromosome complement, showing their relative lengths, position of centromeres, arm ratios, satellites, secondary constrictions and other features. Figure 17.1 shows an idiogram of a normal human male with 22 pairs of autosomes and XY sex chromosome constitution. A karyotype is constructed from photographs of chromosomes which are arranged in pairs similar to the idiogram. Figure 17.2 shows a karyotype of a normal human female.

INCIDENCE OF HUMAN CHROMOSOME ANOMALIES

Chromosome anomalies are relatively frequent events. They have been estimated to occur in 0.48 percent of all newborn infants (one in 208)[81]. At least 25 percent of all spontaneous miscarriages result from gross chromosomal errors[13]. The general incidence of chromosome abnormalities in abortuses is more than fifty times the incidence at birth.

Although it is impossible to obtain an accurate total of victims suffering from effects of chromosome aberrations, one can make rough calculations on the basis of their estimated frequencies in the population of the United States assuming that there is no appreciable difference in life expectancy between these individuals and those with normal chromosome complements. Although this assumption probably is unjustifiable, it suffices for this rough calculation. Among the current population of 202 million we arrive at a figure of 1,136,971 total afflicted with chromosome abnormalities. This total probably represents an underestimate since it does not include all types of chromosome aberrations. Table 17.1 indicates totals for a number of specific syndromes.

Table 17.1 Total Frequencies in the United States of Various Types of Chromosomal Abnormalities, Calculated on the Basis of 202 Million Current Population and the Estimated Frequency of Each Abnormality. (It must be noted that the grand total does not include all types of chromosome aberrations, therefore must be lower than the real value.)

Syndrome	Chromosome Number	Estimated Incidence	Calculated Number in U.S.
Down's trisomy 21	47	1 in 700	288,571
Trisomy D	47	1 in 10,000	20,200
Trisomy E	47	1 in 4000	50,500
Trisomy X	47	1 in 10,000 females	101,000
Turner's XO	45	1 in 5000 females	20,200
Klinefelter's XXY	47	1 in 400 males	252,500
Double Y XYY	47	1 in 250 males	404,000
		Total	1,136,971

SYNDROMES RELATED TO AUTOSOME ABNORMALITIES

Down's Syndrome

This defect results from duplication of all or part of autosome 21, either in the trisomic state or as a translocation to another chromosome, usually a 13–15 (D group) or 16–18 (E group) but may be to another G group chromosome. The overall incidence is about 1 in 700 live births[71], but the trisomic type is correlated with age of the mother, having a frequency of about 1 in 2000 in mothers under 30 years of age, and increasing to 1 in 40 in mothers aged 45 or over. The translocation type constitutes about 3.6 percent of cases and is unrelated to the mother's age, but is transmitted in a predictable manner. Among mental retardates mongoloids represent 16.7 percent.

Clinical features include physical peculiarities ranging from slight anomalies to severe malformations in almost every tissue of the body. Typical appearance of a mongoloid shows slanting eyes, saddle nose, often a large ridged tongue that rolls over a protruding lip, a broad, short skull and thick, short hands, feet and trunk. Frequent complications occur: cataract or crossed eyes, congenital heart trouble, hernias, and a marked susceptibility to respiratory infections. They exhibit characteristic dermatoglyphic patterns on palms and soles. Also they have many biochemical deviations from normal, such as decreased blood-calcium levels and diminished excretion of tryptophane metabolites. Early ageing is common.

All mongoloids are mentally retarded; they usually are 3 to 7 years old mentally. Among the relatively intelligent patients, abstract reasoning is exceptionally retarded.

Female mongoloids are fertile and recorded pregnancies have yielded approximately 50 percent mongoloid offspring. Fortunately male mongoloids are sterile. Examination of their testes reveals varying degrees of spermatogenic arrest correlated with the abnormal chromosome features.

Among mongoloids there is a prevalence of leukemia in childhood; the incidence is some twenty times greater than in the general population. Simultaneous occurrence with other syndromes such as Klinefelter's also is found, and many cases of mosaicism have been described.

E Trisomy Syndrome

This is another autosomal anomaly, which involves chromosomes 16, 17 and 18, and is estimated to occur at a frequency of 1 in 4000 live births[20]. Many others die before birth, thus contributing to the large number of miscarriages and stillbirths. These individuals survive only a short time, from one-half day to 1460 days, with an average of 239 days, but females live significantly longer than males.

Trisomy 17 Syndrome

Many serious defects usually are present in afflicted individuals[25]: odd shaped skulls, low-set and malformed ears, triangular mouth with receding chin, webbing of neck, shield-like chest, short stubby fingers, and toes with short nails, webbing of toes, ventricular septal defect and mental retardation, as well as abnormal facies, micrognathia and high arched palate.

Trisomy 18 Syndrome

This anomaly[70, 82] is characterized by multiple congenital defects of which the most prominent clinical features are: mental retardation with moderate hypertonicity, low-set malformed ears, small mandible flexion of fingers with the index finger overlying the third, and severe failure to thrive. It generally results in death in early infancy. Its frequency increases with advanced maternal age. Three times as many females as males have been observed; one would expect that more males with this syndrome will be found among stillbirths and fetal deaths.

D Syndrome

This trisomy[19, 56, 70, 83] involves chromosomes 13, 14 and 15, and has an estimated frequency of about 1 in 10,000 live births. Many others die in utero. Survival time has been reported from 0 to 1000 days, with an average of 131 days.
Clinical features include: microcephaly, eye anomalies (corneal opacities, colobomata, microphthalmia, anophthalmia), cleft lip, cleft palate, brain anomalies (particularly arrhinencephaly) supernumerary digits, renal anomalies (expecially cortical microcysts), and heart anomalies.

Trisomy 22 Syndrome

This syndrome produces mentally retarded, schizoid individuals. Reports of its occurrence are too few to permit an estimate of its frequency in the population.

Cri-du-Chat Syndrome

Lejeune *et al.*[55] first described this anomaly in 1965, which involves a deficiency of the short arm of a B group chromosome, number 5. Translocations appear to be a common cause of the defect, an estimated 13 percent of cases being associated with translocations; described cases have had B/C, B/G, and B/D translocations[23]. The high proportion emphasizes the importance of unbalanced gamete formation in translocation heterozygotes as a cause of this syndrome. Among parents the frequency of male and female carriers is approximately the same, a situation that contrasts with the much greater frequency of female carriers of a D/G translocation among parents of translocation mongolids.

Typical clinical features of cri-du-chat individuals are : low birth weight, severe mental retardation, microcephaly, hypertelorism, retrognathism, downward slanting eyes, epicanthal folds, divergent strabismus, growth retardation, narrow ear canals, pes planus and short metacarpals and metatarsals. About 25 to 30 percent of them have congenital heart disorders. A characteristic cat-like cry in infancy is responsible for the name of the syndrome. The cry is due to a small epiglottis and larynx and an atrophic vestibule. However, this major diagnostic sign disappears after infancy, making identification of older cases difficult.

An estimate of the frequency of this syndrome is given as over 1 percent but less than 10 percent of the severely mentally retarded patients. Many have IQ scores below 10, and most are institutionalized.

Philadelphia Chromosome

Finally, among autosomal aberrations, a deleted chromosome 21 occurs in blood-forming stem cells in red bone marrow. This deletion, which shows up long after birth, appears to be the primary event causing chronic granulocytic leukemia. This aberration was discussed in 1960 by Nowell and Hungerford[67] (also Baikie *et al.*[3]).

SYNDROMES RELATED TO SEX CHROMOSOME ABERRATIONS

The great majority of known chromosomal abnormalities in man involve the sex chromosomes. In one survey (that excluded XYY) it was estimated that abnormalities occurred in 1 out of every 450 births; if the recent estimate of XYY[81] is correct, the frequency actually is much higher. Increased knowledge about sex chromosome aberrations is probably related to the greater concentration of attention on patients with sexual disorders, but is due in part to the ability to detect carriers of an extra X chromosome by the so-called sex chromatin body or Barr body[6]. This structure is a stainable granule at the periphery of a resting nucleus and, according to the Lyon hypothesis[57], is considered to be an inactivated X chromosome. A normal female cell has one Barr body, since it has two X chromosomes, and is said to be sex chromatin positive (or one positive). A normal male cell has no Barr body and is said to be sex chromatin negative.

Klinefelter's Syndrome

The first sex chromosome anomaly described in 1959 by Jacobs and Strong[46] and also by Ford *et al.*[29] was the XXY constitution that is typical of Klinefelter's syndrome. Buccal smears from these patients are sex chromatin positive. They can be tentatively diagnosed by this test along with clinical symptoms. Final confirmation of diagnosis can be achieved by karyotype analysis using either bone marrow aspiration or peripheral blood culture.

Victims of Klinefelter's syndrome are always male but they are generally underde-

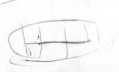

veloped, eunachoid in build, with small external genitalia, very small testes and prostate glands, with underdevelopment of hair on the body, pubic hair and facial hair, frequently with enlarged breasts (gynecomastia), and many have a low IQ.

The classical type with two X chromosomes and one Y chromosome was the first case discovered, but subsequently chromosome compositions of XXXY, XXXXY, XXYY [66] and XXXYY [7, 8, 63, 77] have been reported. In addition, numerous mosaics have been described, including double, triple and quadruple numeric mosaics, as well as combinations of numeric and structural mosaics. These conditions are summarized in Table 17.3. They all resemble the XXY Klinefelter's phenotypically and are considered modified Klinefelter's syndromes. The classical XXY type may have low normal mental development or may be retarded, but other types show increasingly greater mental retardation.

The incidence of Klinefelter's syndrome is estimated to be 1 in 400 male live births, which represents from 1 to 3 percent of mentally deficient patients. This condition also has being correlated with age of the mother: the older the mother, the greater the risk of having such a child. These individuals usually are sterile. Spermatogenesis is generally totally absent. Hyalinization of the semeniferous tubules begins shortly before puberty.

Table 17.2 Reported Sex Chromosomal Constitutions in Klinefelter's Syndrome (modified from Reitalu [77]).

		Sex chromosomal constitution			
Only one karyotype observed per individual		XXY			
		XXYY			
		XXXY			
		XXXYY			
		XXXXY			
Numeric mosaics	Double	XX	XXY		
		XY	XXY		
		XY	XXXY		
		XXY	XXYY		
		XXXY	XXXXY		
		XXXX	XXXXY		
	Triple	XY	XXY	XXYY	
		XX	XXY	XXXY	
		XY	XXY	XXXY	
		XO	XY	XXY	
		XX	XY	XXY	
		XXXY	XXXXY	XXXXYY	
		XXXY	XXXXY	XXXXXY	
	Quadruple	XXY	XY	XX	XO
Numeric and structural mosaics	Double	XXY	XXxY		
	Triple	XY	XXY	XXxY	
		XxY	Xx	XY	

Congenital malformations are rare. Mental retardation is present in approximately 25 percent of affected individuals, and mental illness may be more common than in the general population.

Turner's Syndrome

Female gonadal dysgenesis was described by Turner in 1938 as a syndrome of primary amenorrhea, webbing of the neck, cubitas valgus and short stature, coarctation of aorta, failure of ovarian development and hormonal abnormalities. Patients exhibit sexual infantilism; their breasts are usually underdeveloped, nipples often widely spaced, particularly in those subjects who have a shield or funnel chest deformity. Usually sexual hair is scanty; external genitalia are infantile; labia small or unapparent; clitoris usually normal, although may be enlarged. The uterus is infantile; the tubes long and narrow; the gonads represented by long, narrow, white streaks of connective tissue in normal position of ovary. They are almost always sterile. Hormonal secretions usually are abnormal. Shortness of stature is characteristic and many other skeletal abnormalities occur. Peculiar facies include small mandible, anti-mongolian slant of eyes, depressed corners of mouth, low-set ears, auricles sometimes deformed. Cardiovascular defects are frequent, the most common being coarctation of the aorta. Slight intellectual impairment is found in some patients, particularly those with webbing of the neck.

In 1954 it was discovered that many patients with ovarian agenesis were sex chromatin negative, and in 1959 Ford and colleagues[30] gave the first chromosome analysis showing that Turner's syndrome has the sex chromosome abnormality of only one X chromosome (XO) rather than two X's. It was quickly confirmed by Jacobs and Keay[45] and by Fraccaro et al.[33].

Mosaicism is known to exist—both 45 chromosome cells and 46 chromosome cells occur side by side in tissues of the individual—and can result from nondisjunction in early embryonic development. Isochromosomes sometimes are involved, e.g., creating a situation with 3 long arms of the X chromosome but only 1 short arm.

The incidence of XO Turner's syndrome is estimated as 1 in approximately 5000 women; many die in utero.

Large scale screening of newborn babies by buccal smears can permit detection of chromatin negative females, chromatin positive males, and double, triple, quadruple and quintuple positive cases of either sex[58]. Table 17.3 shows the relationship between sex chromosome complements and sex chromatin pattern.

Triplo-X Syndrome

Females containing three[47], four and five X chromosomes are known[4, 47, 63]. The triplo-X syndrome is thought to have an incidence of about 1 in 800 live female births. This syndrome was first described by Jacobs et al.[47] in 1959. Although it has no distinctive clinical picture, menstrual irregularities may be present, secondary amenorrhea or premature menopause. Most cases have no sexual abnormalities and many are known to have children. The most characteristic feature of 3X females is mental retardation. Quadruple[14] and quintuple-X[50] syndromes are much rarer. These individuals are mentally retarded, usually the more X chromosomes present, the more severe the retardation. Frequently these individuals are fertile.

An extra X chromosome confers twice the usual risk of being admitted to a hospital with some form of mental illness. The loss of an X, on the other hand, has no association with

Table 17.3 The Relationship Between Sex, Sex Chromosome Complement and Sex Chromatin Pattern (Modified from Miller[63]).

Sex Chromatin Pattern	Sexual Phenotype	
	Female	Male
−	XO	XY
−	XY	XYY
	(testicular feminization)	
+	XX	XXY
		XXYY
+ +	XXX	XXXY
		XXXYY
+ + +	XXXX	XXXXY
+ + + +	XXXXX	

mental illness; thus the chance of mental hospital admission is not raised for an XO female. An extra X chromosome also predisposes to mental subnormality. The prevalence of psychosis among patients in hospitals for the subnormal is unusually high in males with two or more X chromosomes.

Numerous other sex chromosome anomalies occur[38], many involving mosaics and structural chromosome aberrations. For example, occasionally an XY embryo will differentiate into a female, a situation referred to as testicular feminization male pseudohermaphrodite (Morris syndrome)[60]. These individuals have only streak gonads and vestigial internal genital organs. They usually have undeveloped breasts and do not menstruate. They are invariably sterile[76].

Still other sexual abnormalities are intersexes and true hermaphrodites, many of which have an XX sex chromosome constitution or are mosaics for sex chromosomes such as XO/XY or XX/XY or more complicated mixtures[31]. Sex chromosome mosaicism is very common. Almost every sex chromosome combination found alone has been found in association with one or more cell lines with a different sex chromosome constitution. These mosaics exhibit quite a variable expression; for example in an XO/XY mosaic the external genitalia can appear female, male or intersexual[85]. *? what a mosaic*

The YY Syndrome

The male with an extra Y chromosome (XYY) has attracted much attention in the public press as well as in scientific circles because of his reputed antisocial, aggressive and criminal tendencies[1, 2, 64]. Although this abnormality belongs in the above category of syndromes related to sex chromosome aberrations, it has been singled out for special discussion because of its social and legal implications.

Evidence supporting the existence of a double Y syndrome has accumulated within the last six years. Studies in Sweden[32] showed an unusually large number of XXYY and XYY men among hard-to-manage patients in mental hospitals. These observations received impressive confirmation in studies of maximum security prisons and hospitals for the criminally insane in Scotland where an astonishingly high frequency (2.9 percent) of XYY males were found[48]. This was over fifty times higher than the then current extimate of 1 in 2000 in the general population. Subsequently many additional studies on the YY syndrome have appeared and a composite picture of the XYY male emerged [5, 15, 19, 21a, 34, 35, 41, 72–75, 78, 80, 92].

The principal features of the extra Y syndrome appear to be exceptional height and a serious personality disorder leading to behavioral disturbances. It seems likely it is the behavior disorder rather than their intellectual incompetence that prevents them from functioning adequately in society[18].

Clinically the XYY males are invariably tall (usually six feet or over) and frequently of below-average intelligence. They are likely to have unusual sexual tastes, often including homosexuality. A history of antisocial behavior, violence and conflict with the police and educational authorities from early years is characteristic[86] of the syndrome.

Although these males usually do not exhibit obvious physical abnormalities [12, 24, 40, 42, 52, 91], several cases of hypogonadisn[11], some with undescended testes, have been reported. Others have epilepsy, malocclusion and arrested development[87], but these symptoms may be fortuitously associated. One case was associated with trisomy 21[61], another with pseudohermaphrodism[35]. The common feature of an acne-scarred face may be related to altered hormone production. The criminally aggressive group were found to have evidence of an increased androgenic steroid production as reflected by high plasma and urinary testosterone levels[12, 43]. If the high level of plasma testosterone is characteristic of XYY individuals, it suggests a mechanism through which this condition may produce behavioral changes, possibly arising at puberty.

Antisocial and aggressive behavior in XYY individuals may appear early in life, however, as evidenced by a case reported by Cowie and Kahn[22]. A prepubertal boy with normal intelligence, at the age of $4\frac{1}{2}$ years, was unmanageable, destructive, mischievous and defiant, overadventurous and without fear. His moods alternated; there were sudden periods of overactivity at irregular intervals when he would pursue his particular antisocial activity with grim intent. Between episodes he appeared happy and constructive. The boy was over the 97th percentile in height for his age, a fact that supports the view that increased height in the XYY syndrome is apparent before puberty.

It has been suggested that the ordinary degree of aggressiveness of a normal XY male is derived from his Y chromosome, and that by adding another Y a double dose of those potencies may facilitate the development of aggressive behavior[65] under certain conditions. A triple dose (XYYY) would be present in the case reported by Townes *et al.*[90].

The first reported case of an XYY constitution[39, 79] was studied because the patient had several abnormal children, although he appeared to be normal himself. Until recently, reports of the XYY constitution have been uncommon, probably because no simple method exists for screening the double-Y condition that is comparable to the buccal smear—sex chromatin body technique for detecting an extra X chromosome. Another possible explanation for the rarity of reports on the XYY karyotype is the absence of a specific phenotype in connection with it. Most syndromes with a chromosome abnormality are ascertained because of some symptom or clinical sign that indicates a need for chromosome analysis. Consequently there have been few studies that place the incidence of this chromosome abnormality in its proper perspective to the population as a whole.

Very recently a study of the karyotypes of 2159 infants born in one year was made by Sergovich *et al.*[81]. These investigators detected 0.48 percent of gross chromosome abnormalities. In this sample the XYY condition appeared in the order of 1 in 250 males, which would make it the most common form of aneuploidy known for man. The previous estimate was about 1 in 2000 males. If this figure of 1/250 is valid for the population as a whole, it means that the great majority of cases go undetected and consequently must be phenotypically normal and behave near enough to the norm to go unrecognized.

Several cases of asymptomatic males have been published, including the first one described (Sandberg *et al.* [79] and Hauschka *et al.* [39]), which proved to be fertile. It appears that the sons of XYY men do not inherit their father's extra Y chromosome [59a].

Another fertile XYY male, reported by Leff and Scott [53], had inferiority feelings, was slightly hypochondriacal and obsessional, and not very aggressive. He gave a general impression of emotional immaturity. He was 6 feet, 6 inches tall, healthy, with normal genitalia and electroencephalogram. His IQ was 118. Wiener and Sutherland [93] discovered by chance an XYY male who was normal; he was 5 feet, $9\frac{1}{2}$ inches tall, with normal genitalia and body hair, normal brain waves, and with an IQ of 97. He exhibited a cheerful disposition and mild temperment, has no apparent behavioral disturbance and never required psychiatric advice. This case supports the idea that an XYY male can lead a normal life.

SOCIAL AND LEGAL IMPLICATIONS OF THE YY SYNDROME

The concept that when a human male receives an extra Y chromosome it may have an important and potentially antisocial effect upon his behavior is supported by impressive evidence [15, 21]. Lejuene states that "There are no born criminals but persons with the XYY defect have considerably higher chances." Price and Whatmore [74] describe these males as psychopaths, "unstable and immature, without feeling or remorse, unable to construct adequate personal relationships, showing a tendency to abscond from institutions and committing apparently motiveless crimes, mostly against property." Casey and coworkers [16] examined the chromosome complements in males 6 feet and over in height and found: 12 XYY among 50 mentally subnormal and 4 XYY among mentally ill patients detained because of antisocial behavior; also 2 XYY among 24 criminals of normal intelligence. They concluded that their results indicate that an extra Y chromosome plays a part in antisocial behavior even in the absence of mental subnormality. The idea that criminals are degenerates because of bad heredity has had wide appeal. There is no doubt that genes do influence to some extent the development of behavior. The influence may be strongly manifested in some cases but not in others. Some individuals appear to be driven to aggressive behavior.

Several spectacular crime cases served to publicize this genetic syndrome, and it has been played up in newspapers, news magazines, radio and television. In 1965 Daniel Hugon, a stablehand, was charged with the murder of a prostitute in a cheap Paris hotel. Following his attempted suicide he was found to have an XYY sex chromosome constitution. Hugon surrendered to the police and his lawyers contended that he was unfit to stand trial because of his genetic abnormality. The prosecution asked for five to ten years; the jury decided to give him seven.

Richard Speck, the convicted murderer of eight nurses in Chicago in 1966, was found to have an XYY sex chromosome constitution. He has all the characteristics of this syndrome found in the Scottish survey: he is 6 feet 2 inches tall, mentally dull, being semiliterate with an IQ of 85, the equivalent of a 13-year-old boy. Speck's face is deeply pitted with acne scars. He has a history of violent acts against women. His aggressive behavior is attested by his record of over 40 arrests. Speck was sentenced to death but the execution has been held up pending an appeal of the conviction.

In Melbourne, Australia, Lawrence Edward Hannell, a 21-year-old laborer on trial for the stabbing of a 77-year-old widow, faced a maximum sentence of death. He was found to have an XYY constitution, mental retardation, an aberrant brain wave pattern, and a neurological disorder. Hannel pleaded not guilty by reason of insanity, and a criminal court jury found him not guilty on the ground that he was insane at the time of the crime.

A second Melbourne criminal with an XYY constitution, Robert Peter Tait, bludgeoned to death an 81-year-old woman in a vicarage where he had gone seeking a handout. He was convicted of murder and sentenced to hang, but his sentence was commuted to life imprisonment.

Another case is that of Raymond Tanner, a convicted sex offender, who pleaded guilty to the beating and rape of a woman in California. He is 6 feet 3 inches tall, mentally disordered, and has an XYY complement. A superior court judge is attempting to decide whether Tanner's plea of guilty to assault with intent to commit rape will stand, or whether he will be allowed to plead innocent by reason of insanity.

Criminal lawyers in the United States have already begun to request genetic studies of their clients. In October of 1968 a lawyer for Sean Farley, a 26-year-old XYY man in New York who was charged with a rape-slaying, maneuvered to raise the issue of his client's genetic defect in court.

Many questions are raised by the double Y syndrome—basic social, legal and ethical questions—which will become more and more insistent as the implications of chromosome abnormalities take root in the public mind. Is an extra Y chromosome causally related to antisocial behavior? Is there a genetic basis for criminal behavior? If a man has an inborn tendency toward criminal behavior, can we fairly hold him legally accountable for his acts? If a criminal's chromosomes are at fault, how can we rehabilitate him?

The evidence to date is inadequate to prove conclusively the validity of the syndrome and convict all of the world's estimated five million XYY males of innate aggressive or criminal tendencies. But if the concept is proved, what then? The first step would seem to be to identify the XYY infants in the general population. This suggests the need for a nationwide program of automatic chromosome analysis of all newborns.

How should society deal with XYY individuals? If they are genetically abnormal, they should not be treated as normal. If the XYY condition dooms a man to a life of crime, he should be restrained but not punished. Mongolism also is a chromosome abnormality, and afflicted individuals are not held responsible for their behavior. Some valuable suggestions on the legal aspects of the double Y syndrome have been published recently by Kennedy McWhirter [59]. Elsewhere, Kessler and Moos [51] claim that definitive concepts relating to the YY syndrome have been accepted prematurely.

If all infants could be karyotyped at birth or soon after, society could be forearmed with information on chromosome abnormalities and perhaps it could institute the proper preventive and other measures at an early age. Although society cannot control the chromosomes (at least at the present time) it can do a great deal to change certain environmental conditions that may encourage XYY individuals to commit criminal acts.

The theory that a genetic abnormality may predispose a man to antisocial behavior, including crimes of violence, is deceptively and attractively simple, but will be difficult to prove. Extensive chromosome screening with prospective follow-up of XYY males will be essential to determine the precise behavioral risk of this group. It is by no means universally accepted yet. Many geneticists urge that we should be cautious in accepting the interpretation that the double Y condition is specifically associated with criminal behavior, and partcularly so with reference to the medicolegal validity of these concepts.

REFERENCES

1. Anonymous. The YY syndrome. *Lancet*, 1966, **1**, 583–584.
2. Anonymous. Criminal behavior—XYY criterion doubtful. *Science News*, 1969, **96**, 2.

3. Baikie, A. G., Court Brown, W. M., Buckton, K. E., Harnden, D. G., Jacobs, P. A., & Tough, I. M. A possible specific chromosome abnormality in human chronic myeloid leukemia. *Nature,* 1960, **188**, 1165–1166.

4. Baikie, A. G., Garson, O. M., Weste, S. M., & Ferguson, J. Numerical abnormalities of the X chromosome. *Lancet,* 1966, **1**, 398–400.

5. Balodimos, M. C., Lisco, H., Irwin, I., Merrill, W., & Dingman, J. F. XYY karyotype in a case of familial hypogonadism, *J. Clin. Endocr.,* 1966, **26**, 443–452.

6. Barr, M. L. Sex chromatin and phenotype in man. *Science,* 1959, **130**, 679.

7. Barr, M. L., & Carr, D. H. Sex chromatin, sex chromosomes and sex anomalies. *Canad. Med. Assn. J.,* 1960, **83**, 979–986.

8. Barr, M. L., Carr, D. H., Soltan, H. C., Wiens, R. G., & Plunkett, E. R. The XXYY variant of Klinefelter's syndrome. *Canad. Med. Assn. J.,* 1964, **90**, 575–580.

9. Belsky, J. L., & Mickey, G. H. Human cytogenetic studies. *Danbury Hospital Bulletin,* 1965, **1**, 19–20.

10. Boczkowski, K., & Casey, M. D. Pattern of DNA replication of the sex chromosomes in three males, two with XYY and one with XXYY karyotype. *Nature,* 1967, **213**, 928–930.

11. Buckton, K. E., Bond, J. A., & McBride, J. A. An XYY sex chromosome complement in a male with hypogonadism. *Human Chromosome Newsletter,* No. 8, December 1962. P. 11.

12. Carakushansky, G., Neu, R. L., & Gardner, L. I. XYY with abnormal genitalia. *Lancet,* 1968, **2**, 1144.

13. Carr, D. H. Chromosome studies in abortuses and stillborn infants. *Lancet,* 1963, **2**, 603–606.

14. Carr, D. H., Barr, M. L., & Plunkett, E. R. An XXXX sex chromosome complex in two mentally defective females. *Canad. Med. Assn. J.,* 1961, **84**, 131–137.

15. Casey, M. D., Blank, C. E., Street, D. R. K., Segall, L. J., McDougall, J. H., McGrath, P. J., & Skinner, J. L. YY chromosomes and antisocial behavior. *Lancet,* 1966, **2**, 859–860.

16. Casey, M. D., Segall, L. J., Street, D. R. K., & Blank, C. E. Sex chromosome abnormalities in two state hospitals for patients requiring special security. *Nature,* 1966, **209**, 641–642.

17. Casey, M. D., Street, D. R. K., Segall, L. J., & Blank, C. E. Patients with sex chromatin abnormality in two state hospitals. *Ann. Human Genet.,* 1968, **32**, 53–63.

18. Close, H. G., Goonetilleke, A. S. R., Jacobs, P. A., & Price, W. H. The incidence of sex chromosomal abnormalities in mentally subnormal males. *Cytogenetics,* 1968, **7**, 277–285.

19. Conan, P. E., & Erkman, B. Frequency and occurrence of chromosomal syndromes. I. D-trisomy. *Amer. J. Human Genet.,* 1966, **18**, 374–386. (a)

20. Conan, P. E., & Erkman, B. Frequency and occurrence of chromosomal syndromes. II. E-trisomy. *Amer. J. Human Genet.,* 1966, **18**, 387–398. (b)

21. Court Brown, W. M. Sex chromosomes and the law. *Lancet,* 1962, **2**, 508–509.

21a. Court Brown, W. M. Males with an XYY sex chromosome complement. *J. Med. Genet.,* 1968, **5**, 341–359.

22. Cowie, J., & Kahn, J. XYY constitution in prepubertal child. *Brit. Med. J.* 1, 1968, **1**, 748–749.

23. de Capoa, A., Warburton, D., Breg, W. R., Miller, D. A., & Miller, O. J. Translocation heterozygosis: A cause of five cases of *cri du chat* syndrome and two cases with a duplication of chromosome number five in three families. *Amer. J. Human Genet.,* 1967, **19**, 586–603.

24. Dent. T., Edwards, J. H., & Delhanty, J. D. A. A partial mongol. *Lancet,* 1963, **2**, 484–487.

25. Edwards, J. H., Harnden, D. G., Cameron, A. H., Crosse, V. M., & Wolff, O. H. A new trisomic syndrome. *Lancet,* 1960, **1**, 787–790.

26. Eggen, R. R. *Chromosome diagnostics in clinical medicine.* Springfield, Ill.: Charles C Thomas, 1965.

27. Ferguson-Smith, M. A., Ferguson-Smith, M. E., Ellis, P. M., & Dickson, M. The sites and relative frequencies of secondary constrictions in human somatic chromosomes. *Cytogenetics,* 1962, **1**, 325–343.

28. Ford, C. E., & Hamerton, J. L. The chromosomes of man. *Nature,* 1956, **178**, 1020–1023.

29. Ford, C. E., Jones, K. W., Miller, O. J., Mittwoch, U., Penrose, L. S., Ridler, M., & Shapiro, A. The chromosomes in a patient showing both mongolism and the Klinefelter syndrome. *Lancet,* 1959, **1**, 709–710.

30. Ford, C. E., Jones, K. W., Polani, P. E., de Almedia, J. C., & Briggs, J. H. A sex-chromosome anomaly in a case of gonadal dysgenesis (Turner's syndrome). *Lancet*, 1959, **1**, 711–713.
31. Ford, C. E., Polani, P. E., Briggs, J. H., & Bishop, P. M. F. A presumptive human XXY/XX mosaic. *Nature*, 1959, **183**, 1030–1032.
32. Forssman, H., & Hambert, G. Incidence of Klinefelter's syndrome among mental patients. *Lancet*, 1963, **1**, 1327.
33. Fraccaro, M., Kaijser, K., & Lindsten, J. Chromosome complement in gonadal dysgenesis (Turner's syndrome). *Lancet*, 1959, **1**, 886.
34. Fraccaro, M., Bott, M. G., Davies, P., & Schutt, W. Mental deficiency and undescended testia in two males with XYY sex chromosomes. *Folia Hereditaria et Pathologica* (Milan), 1962, **11**, 211–220.
35. Franks, R. C., Bunting, K. W., & Engel, E. Male pseudohermaphrodism with XYY sex chromosomes. *J. Clin. Endocr.*, 1967, **27**, 1623–1627.
36. Fraser, J. H., Campbell, J. MacGillivray, R. C., Boyd, E., & Lennox, B. The XXX syndrome—frequency among mental defectives and fertility. *Lancet*, 1960, **2**, 626–627.
37. Gates, W. H. A case of non-disjunction in the mouse. *Genetics*, 1927, **12**, 295–306.
38. Hamerton, J. L. Sex chromatin and human chromosomes. *Inter. Rev. Cytol.*, 1961, **12**, 1–68.
39. Hauschka, T. A., Hasson, J. E., Goldstein, M. N., Koepf, G. F., & Sandberg, A. A. An XYY man with progeny indicating familial tendency to non-disjunction. *Amer. J. Human Genet.*, 1962, **14**, 22–30.
40. Hayward, M. D., & Bower, B. D. Chromosomal trisomy associated with the Sturge-Weber syndrome. *Lancet*, 1960, **2**, 844–846.
41. Hunter, H. Chromatin-positive and XYY boys in approved schools. *Lancet*, 1968, **1**, 816.
42. Hustinx, T. W. J., & van Olphen, A. H. F. An XYY chromosome pattern in a boy with Marfan's syndrome. *Genetics*, 1963, **34**, 262.
43. Ismail, A. A. A., Harkness, R. A., Kirkham, K. E., Loraine, J. A., Whatmore, P. B., & Brittain, R. P. Effect of abnormal sex-chromosome complements on urinary testosterone levels. *Lancet*, 1968, **1**, 220–222.
44. Jacobs, P. A., Baikie, A. G., Court Brown, W. M., & Strong, J. A. The somatic chromosomes in mongolism. *Lancet*, 1959, **1**, 710.
45. Jacobs, P. A., & Keay, A. J. Chromosomes in a child with Bonnevie-Ullrich syndrome. *Lancet*, 1959, **2**, 732.
46. Jacobs, P. A., & Strong, J. A. A case of human inter-sexuality having a possible XXY sex-determining mechanism. *Nature*, 1959, **182**, 302–303.
47. Jacobs, P. A., Baikie, A. G., Court Brown, W. M., MacGregor, T. N., MacLean, N., & Harnden, D. G. Evidence for the existence of the human "super female." *Lancet*, 1959, **2**, 423–425.
48. Jacobs, P. A., Brunton, M., Melville, M. M., Brittain, R. P., & McClemont, W. F. Aggressive behaviour, Mental subnormality and the XYY male. *Nature*, 1965, **208**, 1351–1352.
49. Jacobs, P. A., Price, W. H., Court Brown, W. M., Brittain, R. P., & Whatmore, P. B. Chromosome studies on men in a maximum security hospital. *Ann. Human Genet.*, 1968, **31**, 330–347.
50. Kesaree, N., & Woolley, P. V. A phenotypic female with 49 chromosomes, presumably XXXXX. *J. Prediat.*, 1963, **63**, 1099–1103.
51. Kessler, S., & Moos, R. H. XYY chromosome: Premature conclusions. *Science*, 1969, **165**, 442.
52. Kosenow, W., & Pfeiffer, R. A. YY syndrome with multiple malformations. *Lancet*, 1966, **1**, 1375–1376.
53. Leff, J. P., & Scott, P. D. XYY and intelligence. *Lancet*, 1968, **1**, 645.
54. Lejeune, J., Gautier, N., & Turpin, R. Etude des chromosomes somatiques de neuf enfants monogoliens. *Compt. Rend. Acad. Sci.*, 1959, **248**, 1721–1722.
55. Lejeune, J., Lafourcade, J., Berger, R., & Rethore, M. O. Maladie du cri du chat et sa reciproque. *Ann. Genet.*, 1965, **8**, 11–15.
56. Lubs, H. A., Jr., Koenig, E. V., & Brandt, L. H. Trisomy 13–15: A clinical syndrome. *Lancet*, 1961, **2**, 1001–1002.
57. Lyon, M. F. Gene action in the X-chromosome of the mouse (*Mus musculus* L.). *Nature*, 1961, **190**, 372–373.

58. MacLean, N., Harnden, D. G., Court Brown, W. M., Bond, J., & Mantle, D. J. Sex-chromosome abnormalities in newborn babies. *Lancet*, 1964, **1**, 286–290.
59. McWhirter, K. XYY chromosome and criminal acts. *Science*, 1969, **164**, 1117.
59a. Melnyk, J., Vanasek, F., Thompson, H., & Rucci, A. J. Failure of transmission of supernumerary Y chromosomes in man. American Society of Human Genetics, Annual Meeting, October 1–4, 1969. (Abstract)
60. Mickey, G. H. Chromosome studies in testicular feminization syndrome in human male pseudohermaphrodites. *Mammalian Chromosome Newsletter*, No. 9, 1963. P. 60.
61. Midgeon, B. R. G trisomy in an XYY male. *Human Chromosome Newsletter*, No. 17, 1965.
62. Milcu, M., Nigoescu, I., Maximilian, C., Garoiu, M., Augustin, M., & Iliescu, I. Baiat cu hipospadias si cariotip XYY. *Studio si Cercetari de Endocrinologie* (Bucharest), 1964, **15**, 347–349.
63. Miller, O. J. The sex chromosome anomalies. *Amer. J. Obstet. Gynec.*, 1964, **90**, 1078–1139.
64. Minckler, L. S. Chromosomes of criminals. *Science*, 1969, **163**, 1145.
65. Montagu, A. Chromosomes and crime. *Psychology Today*, 1968, **2**, 43–49.
66. Muldal, S., & Ockey, C. H. The "double male": A new chromosome constitution in Klinefelter's syndrome. *Lancet*, 1960, **2**, 492–493.
67. Nowell, P. C. & Hungerford, D. A. A minute chromosome in human granulocytic leukemia. *Science*, 1960, **132**, 1497.
68. Painter, T. S. The chromosome constitution of Gates "non-disjunction" (v-o) mice. *Genetics*, 1927, **12**, 379–392.
68a. Palmer, C. G., & Funderburk, S. Secondary constrictions in human chromosomes. *Cytogenetics*, 1965, **4**, 261–276.
69. Patau, K. The identification of individual chromosomes, especially in man. *Amer. J. Human Genet.*, 1960, **12**, 250–276.
70. Patau, K., Smith, D. W., Therman, E., Inhorn, S. L., & Wagner, H. P. Multiple congenital anomalies caused by an extra chromosome. *Lancet*, 1960, **1**, 790–793.
71. Penrose, L. S. *The biology of mental defect.* New York: Grune & Stratton, 1949.
72. Pergament, E., Sato, H., Berlow, S., & Mintzer, R. YY syndrome in an American Negro. *Lancet*, 1968, **2**, 281.
73. Pfeiffer, R. A. Der Phanotyp der Chromosomenaberration XYY. *Wochenschrift*, 1966, **91**, 1355–1256.
74. Price, W. H., & Whatmore, P. B. Behaviour disorders and the pattern of crime among XYY males identified at a maximum security hospital. *Brit. Med. J.*, 1967, **1**, 533.
75. Price, W. H., Strong, J. A., Whatmore, P. B., & McClemont, W. F. Criminal patients with XYY sex-chromosome complement, *Lancet*, 1966, **1**, 565–566.
76. Puck, T. T., Robinson, A., & Tjio, J. H. A familial primary amenorrhea due to testicular feminization. A human gene affecting sex differentiation. *Proc. Exper. Biol. Med.*, 1960, **103**, 192–196.
77. Reitalu, J. Chromosome studies in connection with sex chromosomal deviations in man. *Hereditas*, 1968, **59**, 1–48.
78. Ricci, N., & Malacarne, P. An XYY human male. *Lancet*, 1964, **1**, 721.
79. Sandberg, A. A., Koepf, G. F., Ishihara, T., & Hauschka, T. S. An XYY human male. *Lancet*, 1961, **2**, 488–489.
80. Sandberg, A. A., Ishihara, T., Crosswhite, L. H., & Koepf, G. F. XYY genotype. *New Eng. J. Med.*, 1963, **268**, 585–589.
81. Sergovich, F., Valentine, G. H., Chem, A. T. L., Kinch, R. A. H., & Smout, M. S. Chromosome aberrations in 2159 consecutive newborn babies. *New Eng. J. Med.*, 1969, **280**, 851–855.
82. Smith, D. W., Patau, K., & Therman, E. The 18 trisomy syndrome and the D₁ trisomy syndrome. *Amer. J. Dis. Child.*, 1961, **102**, 587.
83. Smith, D. W., Patau, K., Therman, E., Inhorn, S. L., & Demars, R. I. The D₁ trisomy syndrome. *J. Pediat.*, 1963, **62**, 326–341.
84. Sohval, A. R. Sex chromatin, chromosomes and male infertility. *Fertility and Sterility*, 1963, **14**, 180–207. (a)
85. Sohval, A. R. Chromosomes and sex chromatin in normal and anomalous sexual development. *Physiol. Rev.*, 1963, **43**, 306–356. (b)

86. Telfer, M. A., Baker, D., Clark, G. R., & Richardson, C. E. Incidence of gross chromosomal errors among tall criminal American males. *Science*, 1968, **159**, 1249–1250.
87. Thorburn, M. J., Chutkan, W., Richards, R., & Bell, R. XYY sex chromosomes in a Jamaican with orthopaedic abnormalities. *J. Med. Genet.*, 1968, **5**, 215–219.
88. Tjio, J. H., & Levan, A. The chromosome number of man. *Hereditas*, 1956, **42**, 1–6.
89. Tjio, J. H., Puck, T. T., & Robinson, A. The somatic chromosomal constitution of some human subjects with genetics defects. *Proc. Natl. Acad. Sci.*, 1959, **45**, 1008–1016.
90. Townes, P. L., Ziegler, N. A., & Lenhard, L. W. A patient with 48 chromosomes (XYYY). *Lancet*, 1965, **1**, 1041–1043.
91. Vignetti, P., Capotorti, L., & Ferrante, E. XYY chromosomal constitution with genital abnormality. *Lancet*, 1964, **2**, 588–589.
92. Welch, J. P., Borgaonkar, D. S., & Herr, H. M. Psychopathy, mental deficiency, aggressiveness and the XYY syndrome. *Nature*, 1967, **214**, 500–501.
93. Wiener, S., & Sutherland, G. A normal XYY man. *Lancet*, 1968, **2**, 1352.

18

The Biochemistry of Mental Disorders*

WHO SCIENTIFIC GROUP

Biochemical research on mental illnesses has shown that many of them may be caused by purely chemical deficiencies and thus perhaps more readily treated. The . . . report[1] of a WHO Scientific Group[2] reviews the present situation in neurochemistry and makes proposals for promoting this important new branch of study.

Many mental disorders may be caused by purely chemical deficiencies in the brain or body or by an imbalance of enzyme systems, a knowledge of which could lead directly to successful remedies. Indeed, this has already been achieved for hepatolenticular degeneration (Wilson's disease). Biochemists are accordingly trying to apply to mental illnesses the approach that has proved so successful with rickets, diabetes, and pernicious anaemia, in all of which the discovery of specific biochemical deficiencies quickly led to rational therapy.

With the refinement of both clinical and laboratory methods during the past two decades, there has been a great expansion of biochemical research in psychiatry, and many interesting data have come to light.

MENTAL RETARDATION

A significant proportion of cases of mental retardation are associated with inherited metabolic disease, and in many of them an enzyme deficiency has been demonstrated. The basic defect is often not in the brain at all but in some other organ, usually the liver. The biochemical abnormalities in many inborn errors of metabolism are well understood, but little is known about the way in which the function of the brain is disturbed.

In investigating the pathogenesis of a mental defect it is informative to compare mentally retarded patients with others suffering from the same disease who are not mentally retarded.

The analysis of biopsy and autopsy material from the brain by various techniques is now a well-established method of investigating degenerative disorders of the nervous system. It

---

*From the *WHO Chronicle*, 1970 (January), **24**, 6–10. Copyright © 1970 by the World Health Organization. Reprinted by permission of the World Health Organization.

[1]WHO Scientific Group on the Biochemistry of Mental Disorders (1969) *Report*, Geneva (*Wld Hlth Org. techn. Rep. Ser.*, No. 427).

[2]Members: Dr. J. Durell, USA (*Rapporteur*); Dr. L. R. Gjessing, Norway (*Chairman*); Dr. J. Jacob, France; Dr. R. Rajalakshmi, India; Dr. M. Schou, Denmark; Dr. T. L. Sourkes, Canada (*Vice-Chairman*); Dr. J. Stern, United Kingdom; Dr. H. Utena, Japan; Dr. M. Vartanjan, USSR. Representative of the World Psychiatric Association: Dr. W. Linford Rees. Secretariat: Dr. S. S. Kety (*Temporary Adviser*); Dr. B. A. Lebedev, WHO (*Secretary*); Dr. D. Richter (*Temporary Adviser*).

is sometimes possible to arrive at a diagnosis by examining the nerve cells of rectal biopsy material or of the appendix.

Inborn errors affecting the metabolism of essential amino acids can be treated by including in the diet a protein substitute that provides just enough of the appropriate amino acid to permit growth. Most experts agree that the majority of children with classical phenylketonuria benefit from this treatment if it is started early.

During the pregnancy of an untreated phenylketonuric mother, the fetus is exposed to a high concentration of phenylalanine, and the child is liable to be severely retarded. The developing brain seems to be particularly vulnerable to a high level of phenylalanine.

The treatment of inborn errors has not been confined to phenylketonuria. Significant successes have also been achieved with maple syrup urine disease, homocystinuria, galactosaemia, and tyrosinosis, and the incidence of mental deficiency resulting from other biochemical causes, such as hyperbilirubinaemia, hypoglycaemia, and lead poisoning, has been reduced. Work on several other diseases indicates that they are caused by the hereditary absence of specific enzymes, some of which have been tentatively identified.

The early treatment of neurometabolic diseases, where such treatment is available, may save a child's life or prevent permanent damage to its brain. For this reason the mass screening of newborn infants is carried out in a number of countries. Specialized laboratories must be ready to help in establishing the diagnosis and in controlling treatment, since the wrong diet can be dangerous. The problems of mass screening are largely economic and administrative, and every country must decide what proportion of its health resources can be spared for this purpose.

In many retarded patients the insult to the brain occurs before birth—particularly during the first three months of gestation—or in the perinatal period. When the brain is examined years later, the original pathological process may be masked by scarring and degenerative changes. A systematic study of the developing human brain is urgently needed, particularly since much of the required information cannot be obtained from animal experiments. Fetuses from spontaneous and induced abortions and stillborn infants should provide suitable material for study.

NUTRITIONAL FACTORS

The brain has a high metabolic rate in comparision with other organs; it has a high rate of protein turnover and synthesizes many substances locally. It is thus particularly susceptible to the effects of malnutrition. Deficiencies in calories, protein, vitamins, and minerals are all associated with clinical symptoms suggesting central nervous system (CNS) disorders. Intellectual retardation in children and suboptimal function in adults resulting from undernutrition probably account for a larger number of these disorders than all other causes put together.

The apathy and mental confusion of the starving or chronically undernourished person and his inability to concentrate on a task are well known from the experience of prisoners of war and from studies of human volunteers subjected to undernutrition. There is a reduction in the basal metabolic rate and voluntary activity. Although the undernourished person may do heavy muscular labor of a repetitive kind, he cannot be bothered to undertake the simplest inessential task. Animal studies suggest that the effect of calorie undernutrition is less serious than that of protein deficiency, but apathy and decreased activity caused by undernutrition of any type may result in an artificial restriction of psychological stimulation during crucial stages of development.

Protein deficiency in animals can produce abnormal electroencephalographic (EEG) patterns, and changes have been reported in the nerve cells and neuroglial cells of the spinal cord including chromatolysis, foaming of the cytoplasm, an increased number of oligodendroglial cells, degeneration of Nissl structures, neuronal loss, and fibrous gliosis. Protein-deficient animals show tremors, drowsiness, poor motor coordination, impaired psychological performance, and delayed maturation. The effects are greater if the mothers have also been subjected to deficiency. Many of the changes are partly or fully reversible.

A child suffering from kwashiorkor exhibits severe apathy and irritability. He shows an abnormal EEG pattern, and in untreated cases the electrical activity of the brain stops before that of the heart. There are important differences between marasmus and kwashiorkor. In marasmus, the serum protein and enzymes are less affected and the serum amino acid levels are higher. Vitamin A absorption is normal in the child with marasmus, and disorders of the eyes due to a deficiency of vitamin A are consequently less frequent than in kwashiorkor. These differences can be expected to result in differences in psychological development. However, apathy is found in both conditions.

The effects of nutritional deficiency and the extent to which they are reversible are believed to depend on the age of onset. Some workers believe that malnutrition before the age of six months produces irreversible changes. This might occur in some deficiencies but not in others. Malnutrition and poor psychological environment often exist together, and nutritional amelioration without improvement of the psychological environment may have no effect on psychological status. Well-nourished children brought up in a restricted environment such as an orphanage also show evidence of retarded development.

Vitamin deficiencies are responsible, in part at least, for illnesses such as beriberi, pellagra, and pernicious anaemia, all of which are associated with dysfunction of the central nervous system.

The role of vitamin A deficiency in the functioning of the photoreceptor cells of the eye is well known, and poor sensitivity to light can have serious effects on CNS functions by restricting the psychological stimulation necessary for normal CNS development. The effect of vitamin A deficiency on the development of the skeleton, including the vertebrae and skull, can also cause CNS abnormalities. This vitamin is necessary for the formation and closure of the neural tube and also appears to exert an indirect effect on the central nervous system through its interaction with the thyroid hormone.

A severe deficiency of vitamin D combined with a deficiency of calcium sufficient to lower serum calcium levels results in tetany and death.

Subjects suffering from thiamine deficiency show anxiety, depression, irritability, and increased sensitivity to noise and pain. Loss of tendon reflexes, paralysis, and death follow in severe cases. Supplementation with thiamine improves a number of psychological functions in children.

A deficiency of iodine during the prenatal period is a cause of cretinism, the basic features of which are irreversible changes in mental development, abnormalities of hearing and speech, neuromuscular disorders, impairment of physical development, and hypothyroidism. Cretinism has now largely disappeared wherever iodized salt is used.

The amount of biochemical work that has been carried out on the brain, although it may appear impressive at first sight, is actually insufficient to give even a superficial knowledge of the effects of nutritional deficiencies on structural and biochemical changes in the brain and their association with specific clinical symptoms, to say nothing of the mechanisms involved. Only a few studies of brain biochemistry in relation to malnutrition have been carried out, and these have been largely confined to brain lipids. It would be desirable to study the electrophysiological, histological, biochemical, and behavioral effects of nutritional deficiencies in animals and to correlate them as far as possible with observations in human subjects.

AFFECTIVE DISORDERS

Various biochemical studies have indicated the presence in the brain of amines located in specific clusters of neurons, the distribution of which has been partially mapped out, and there appears to be a relationship between affective states and the synthesis, storage, metabolism, and release of such amines. Furthermore, it has been noted that monoamines in peripheral synapses as well as in the brain are significantly affected by most of the procedures used in altering mood, including electroconvulsive treatment and chemotherapy. The drugs that cause these effects include the two main groups of antidepressants—tricyclic compounds of the imipramine type and monoamine oxidase inhibitors. This finding, which suggests that the drugs affect mood by acting on cerebral monoamines, may provide a clue to the biochemical basis of affective disorders. Research is now progressing on the composition of cerebrospinal fluid from manic and depressed patients. A comparison of the amines and amine metabolites in the brains of persons who commit suicide with those in the brains of people who die suddenly from other causes indicates a lowering of serotonin and 5-hydroxyindolacetic acid in the former.

It has been noted repeatedly in patients suffering from manic-depressive psychoses that phase changes in the affective state are accompanied by changes in water balance, but it is not known whether the changes in water balance and distribution also involve the brain.

There is strong evidence that the distribution of sodium and possibly potassium in the body tissues may differ significantly in manic patients, depressed patients, and normal subjects. The interpretation of these findings, which have been made with isotope dilution methods, is complicated by the binding of sodium in bone and by the non-homogeneity of the extracellular fluid. The findings themselves, however, are unchallenged and have been supported by recent observations of changes in the sodium content of the saliva of depressed patients.

The administration of lithium salts is of particular promise for the treatment of affective disorders. Lithium counteracts mania in a highly specific way, without producing lethargy or sedation. Its continued administration in doses that do not interfere with normal mental processes may prevent relapses in cases of recurrent manic-depressive psychosis. It has been reported that not only manias but depressions are prevented, and this may be true both for patients with depressions only (unipolar type) and for those with manias and depressions (bipolar type).

Lithium differs radically from other psychotropic drugs, and current research has revealed lithium effects on cerebral monoamines, adrenocortical function, and total body water and also on the intermediate metabolism of carbohydrates, amino acids, and phospholipids. It is conceivable that lithium ions in the brain serve to stabilize functions that depend on particular molecular structures involving protein, water, and electrolytes.

PERIODIC PSYCHOSES

Several psychiatric syndromes can take a periodic course—for example, mania, melancholia, and paranoia—and the periodicity is often quite independent of external events, highly regular, and constant over years. The length of the period differs from person to person and may be days, weeks, or years.

The study of periodic psychoses rather than chronic psychoses has the advantage that the patient serves as his own control and observations can be made on what occurs during the interval and the transition from the interval to the psychosis. Experimental interventions can be planned to test hypotheses on the biochemical mechanisms.

In periodic catatonia, which has been extensively studied, there are pronounced changes in many physiological functions. Similar changes are observed in the fasting blood sugar, serum fatty acids, electrolytes, acid-base equilibrium, diuresis, urinary pigments, steroids, and thiocyanate. Changes in the nitrogen balance seem to be characteristic for periodic catatonia, and it was this finding that provided a rational basis for giving thyroid hormone to patients. When this was done, retention of nitrogen did not recur, and in many patients the periods of mental disturbance disappeared, together with the biochemical and neurophysiological changes.

Longitudinal studies need to be carried out on patients with periodic psychoses and serial determinations made of enzyme activities and metabolites in body fluids both with and without the administration of drugs or radioactive compounds. It is also important to study the periodic changes in behavior and sleep, especially the sleeping EEG pattern in the different phases. Further insight into the pathogenesis of periodic psychoses may lead to greater understanding of the acute and chronic functional psychoses.

SCHIZOPHRENIA

There is considerable evidence that genetic factors are important in schizophrenia, and consequently there is good reason to suspect the existence of a biological abnormality, although none has yet been identified. Abnormalities have been sought in the concentration of catecholamines or indolamine or their derivatives, and a "transmethylation hypothesis" has been proposed to account for the disease. According to this hypothesis, an abnormal endogenous methylated amine acts as a psychotogen, producing the symptoms of schizophrenia. This view is supported by the finding that the administration of methionine coupled with a monoamine oxidase inhibitor leads to an exacerbation of symptoms in some schizophrenics.

METHODS OF CLINICAL INVESTIGATION

It is sometimes assumed that any biochemical disorder associated with psychiatric illness is most likely to be found in the brain. This is not necessarily true, since it is possible to postulate primary disorders in other organs that would influence the physiology of the brain, as is the case in phenylketonuria. Again abnormalities that occur in various bodily tissues may have more profound effects on the brain than on other organs—hence the relevance of studies of body fluids such as blood, urine, and cerebrospinal fluid and of tissues other than brain tissue.

It is commonly believed that cerebrospinal fluid is a better indicator of cerebral metabolism than are other body fluids, but it is interesting to note that there have been several reports of the presence in urine of a compound that is believed primarily to reflect brain metabolism, namely 3-methoxy-4-hydroxyphenylglycol. Low urinary levels of this substance have been reported in depressed patients, and if this is confirmed it might provide important evidence relating depression to altered CNS norepinephrine metabolism.

Mental illnesses being partly hereditary, it is likely that biochemical abnormalities will be found, but such abnormalities may be detectable only under certain conditions—for example, if an adaptive enzyme is involved. Since hormones are intimately involved in enzyme control mechanisms, it is not difficult to imagine biochemical abnormalities that are apparent only in stressful situations—perhaps only when the patient is acutely ill.

Many investigations of biochemical factors are cross-sectional in design—that is to say the factors are measured in a group of patients and compared with normal values or with those obtained from a control sample. One of the problems of this method is the difficulty of defining a homogeneous population, and biochemical abnormalities may go undetected unless they are particularly marked.

If the biochemical abnormality is not constant but varies with the intensity of the symptoms, a longitudinal study is indicated. Changes in biochemical factors are correlated with changes in the clinical state, and the values obtained in a symptom-free period serve as controls for those obtained during symptomatic periods.

Research in neurochemistry advances understanding of the structural components of the nervous system in relation to their function at the macroscopic, cellular, and subcellular levels. Consequently it supplies essential information about the substratum of mental activities. Progress in the conquest of mental illness will continue to depend on the accumulation of such fundamental knowledge and on its application to particular clinical problems.

19

Biochemical Hypotheses and Studies*

SEYMOUR S. KETY

Biochemistry, which has had notable success in elucidating etiologic factors in many areas of medicine, has also been brought to bear on the problem of schizophrenia. Although these efforts have not to date been successful in demonstrating a biochemical "lesion," a number of arguments can be made to support the viewpoint that chemical factors operate significantly and specifically in schizophrenia.

Perhaps the strongest of these arguments is the good evidence for the operation of genetic factors in the transmission of schizophrenia[92], consisting of a higher concordance rate for the disorder in the monozygotic twins of afflicted individuals[43, 57, 59, 67, 99] and in the biologic families of schizophrenics where early adoption or removal from their natural parents has served to disentangle the operation of genetic and environmental factors in its transmission[50, 64, 93].

Another argument which has been used is the ability of a number of exogenous chemical substances (iodides, mescaline, LSD, amphetamine, iproniazid, psilocybin) or some endogenous biochemical disturbances (porphyria, thyroid disorders) to produce psychoses resembling schizophrenia in some or many of its features.

Biochemical hypotheses and findings related to schizophrenia have been the subject of several exhaustive and critical reviews of which only a few are cited for further reference[22, 61, 63, 109]. In spite of the large number of abnormal chemical findings which have been reported in schizophrenia, few have been independently confirmed and on none is there general agreement with regard to its significance. This may be attributed to the operation of an inordinate number of variables, difficult to control, which are associated with the clinical studies of schizophrenia.

Despite the phenomenologic similarities which permitted the concept of schizophrenia to emerge, there is little evidence that all of its forms have a common etiology or pathogenesis. Errors involved in the study of relatively small samples from heterogeneous populations may help to explain the frequency with which findings of one group fail to be confirmed by another.

Most biochemical research in schizophrenia has been carried out in patients with a long history of hospitalization in institutions where overcrowding is difficult to avoid and hygienic standards cannot always be maintained. It is easy to imagine the spread of chronic infections such as infectious hepatitis among such patients, and one wonders how often this may account for findings attributable to disturbed hepatic function or elevated plasma titres of antibody globulins. Even in the absence of previous or current infection, the development of a characteristic pattern of intestinal flora in a group of patients living together for long periods of time may occasionally contribute to the findings of what appear to be deviant metabolic pathways.

---

*From *The Schizophrenic Syndrome*, edited by Bellak, L., and Loeb, L. Reprinted by permission of Grune & Stratton, Inc., Publisher, and Dr. Kety.

The variety and quality of the diet of the institutionalized schizophrenic is rarely comparable to that of the nonhospitalized normal control. In the case of the acute schizophrenic, the weeks of continual turmoil which precede recognition of the disorder are hardly conducive to a normal dietary intake. It is not surprising that a dietary vitamin deficiency has been found to account for at least one biochemical abnormality which had been attributed to schizophrenia[77] Horwitt[55] found signs of liver dysfunction during long periods of borderline protein ingestion.

Emotional stress is known to cause profound changes in man, in adrenocortical and thyroid function, in excretion of water, electrolytes, creatinine, epinephrine and norepinephrine, to mention only a few recently reported findings. On the other hand, physical inactivity would be expected to produce changes in a number of body functions. Schizophrenic illness is often characterized by indolence and lack of exercise or by marked emotional disturbance in the basal state and frequently exaggerated anxiety in response to routine and research procedures. The disturbances in behavior and activity which mark the schizophrenic process would also be expected to cause deviations from the normal in many biochemical and metabolic measures: in urinary volume and concentration, in energy and nitrogen metabolism, in the state and activity of numerous organ systems and metabolic pathways. The biochemical changes which are secondary to the psychologic and behavioral state of the patient are often of interest in themselves; it is important, however, not to attribute to them etiologic roles.

Another incidental feature of the schizophrenic patient which differentiates him from the normal control and from many other types of patient is the long list of therapies to which he may have been exposed. The ataractic drugs which are often used over extended periods of time are particularly prone to produce metabolites which appear in the urine and interfere with a number of chemical determinations long after the drug has been withdrawn.

With this combination of many variables and the subjective judgments necessary for diagnosis and the evaluation of clinical course, it is not unexpected that subjective bias would from time to time affect the results of research in schizophrenia and make even more necessary in that field than in many others the employment of rigorous research design.

ENERGY METABOLISM

A decrease in basal metabolism was found in schizophrenia by earlier workers, although more recent work has not confirmed this[89], and hypotheses attributing the disease to disturbances in the fundamental mechanisms of energy supply or conversion in the brain have been formulated but on the basis of rather inadequate evidence. Kelsey and co-workers[60] found a decreased B.M.R. [basal metabolism rate] in their series of schizophrenics to be associated with an increased uptake of ^{131}I by the thyroid, correctable by the addition of iodine to the diet, and attributed to a lack of that element in the institutional diet. Periodic catatonia and some other schizophreniform psychoses seem to be associated with disturbances in thyroxine or thyrotropic hormone regulation[21, 40], but little evidence exists to suggest that such disturbances are characteristic of schizophrenia generally.

The oxygen consumption and blood flow of the brain as a whole have been found to lie within the normal range in a variety of forms of schizophrenia[65], and although localized changes in these functions have sometimes been postulated, there is no evidence to support this supposition. The clear consciousness usually present in schizophrenia does not suggest the manifestation of cerebral anoxia.

Richter[89] has pointed out the uncontrolled factors in earlier work which implicated a defect in carbohydrate metabolism as a characteristic of the schizophrenic process. The finding in schizophrenia of an abnormal glucose tolerance in conjunction with other evidence of hepatic dysfunction, or evidence of a retarded metabolism of lactate by the schizophrenic [2], does not completely exclude incidental hepatic disease, nutritional deficiencies or the psychophysiologic influences on carbohydrate metabolism as possible sources of error. Horwitt and associates [56] were able to demonstrate and correct similar abnormalities by altering the dietary intake of the B group of vitamins.

A deficiency of glucose-6-phosphate dehydrogenase, known to occur in 10–20 percent of American Negroes, has been found to show an incidence significantly different from normal in Negro catatonic and paranoid schizophrenics [19], an observation which has recieved partial confirmation by an independent group [29]. Findings that schizophrenia is associated with cellular changes in oxidative phosphorylation or in the uptake [44] or metabolism of glucose [35] require further confirmation [17].

It is difficult to believe that a generalized defect in energy metabolism, a process fundamental to every cell in the body, could be responsible for the highly specialized features of schizophrenia. For this reason, perhaps, interest has developed in other aspects of metabolism, the substrates or products of which appear to have some special role in the brain.

PROTEIN

Although Gjessing [10] found definite alterations in bodily nitrogen balance correlated with and sometimes preceding the changes in mental state of periodic catatonics, there has been no evidence to indicate a major change in protein metabolism for schizophrenia generally. On the other hand, some interest has been focused recently on more specific protein constituents or the metabolism of particular amino acids or their amines.

Interest in the possible presence of an abnormal protein constituent of blood of schizophrenics was stimulated by a report, in 1958, that a serum fraction obtained from schizophrenic patients was capable of causing some of the symptoms of that disorder when injected into nonschizophrenic volunteers [49]. This material, which was given the name "taraxein," appeared to have some relationship to ceruloplasmin, the copper-containing globulin of normal plasma which the same group had found to be elevated in schizophrenia [71] and, upon its intravenous injection, to produce rapid clinical improvement [18]. Very recently, Martens [76], in a thorough examination of the relationships between ceruloplasmin and schizophrenia, has reported an equivalent elevation of serum copper in that disorder and in delirium tremens. In a controlled, double blind series he was unable to confirm the earlier report of clinical improvement following intravenous injections of ceruloplasmin. One attempt to replicate the production of psychotic symptoms in volunteers by means of taraxein was not successful [91], and to date the original findings have not been confirmed in a significant and well controlled series.

A number of groups, however, have reported evidence compatible with the thesis that an abnormal protein is present to a greater extent in the blood of some schizophrenics than in normals and that this substance is capable of producing certain behavioral, metabolic, or cellular changes in lower animals. Haddad and Rabe [45], replicating and extending an earlier report by Malis [73], found some evidence for an antigenic abnormality in the pooled serum of chronically ill schizophrenic patients. More recent studies by this group using different immunologic methods have yielded negative results which they do not regard as conclusive. Faurbye, Lundberg, and Jensen [23] were unable to confirm Malis' results.

Using another approach, Vartanyan[108] has found evidence for an immunologic abnormality in schizophrenia. Heath and co-workers[47] have advanced an auto-immune concept as the biologic basis of schizophrenia. The studies with fluorescent antibodies, electrophysiologic, immunologic and behavioral observations, on which the concept is based, await independent confirmation. Precipitin reactions have yielded positive[79] and negative[58, 84, 90] results with respect to the occurrence of specific proteins in the serum of schizophrenics.

Fessel and co-workers[26, 28] have reported increases in 4S and 19S macroglobulins in a considerable proportion of schizophrenic patients and the ability to differentiate schizophrenic from manic-depressive patients on this basis. Mental stress in nonpsychotic individuals was found to elevate the same macroglobulins[27]. Certain of these findings have been confirmed by two independent groups[66, 97]. Gammack and Hector[37], while failing to confirm Fessel's findings, observed a highly significant increase in the α-globulin fraction and the haptoglobin component in the serum of schizophrenics. They also questioned the specificity of such findings which occur frequently in many types of chronic disease. Others have not confirmed this increase in haptoglobins[72]. It seems fair to conclude that to the present time no abnormal protein characteristic of schizophrenia has been characterized by physico-chemical technics.

Some special properties of the plasma of schizophrenics have been reported by workers using various biologic assays. Bishop[11] has reported evidence for the effect of plasma from schizophrenic patients upon learning and retention of learning in the rat. Other investigators[8, 112] found a slowing of rope climbing activity in rats injected with whole serum or certain fractions from schizophrenic patients as compared with normal fractions. The specificity of this response for schizophrenia has not been demonstrated and later findings were not confirmatory[96]. German[38] reported an effect of serum of schizophrenics on cortical evoked responses in rats which in later, more rigorously controlled studies he and his associates were unable to confirm[39]. In well controlled studies of the effects of plasma from psychotic patients on behavior, Ferguson and Fisher[25] have reported observations using a precision timing task in cebus monkeys in which a highly significant delay in responsiveness was produced by the injection of plasma from some newly admitted catatonic patients. It is of interest that in their studies plasma from normal individuals under preoperative stress produced a similar but not as marked slowing of response.

Frohman and his associates[34] have reported increases in the ratio of lactate-to-pyruvate in the medium after chicken erythrocytes are incubated with plasma or plasma fractions of some schizophrenic patients as compared to normal controls. Mangoni and associates[74] have been unable to confirm this. In a subsequent paper, Frohman and associates[36] were able to demonstrate this difference in the lactate : pyruvate ratio only when the subjects had engaged in moderate exercise before the blood samples were drawn; no appreciable difference was found when the subjects were at complete rest, in normal activity, or exercising vigorously. This, plus the fact that exercise affected the lactate: pyruvate ratio in the incubation mixture more than did the presence or absence of schizophrenia, suggests the need for better definition of what may be a large number of variables involved in this reaction.

Recently, Ryan, Brown, and Durell[94] have succeeded in clarifying some of the fundamental processes involved in the ability of human plasma to affect the lactate production of chicken erythrocytes, which appears to be the determining variable of the lactate : pyruvate ratio. In their test system, lactate production by aerobic glycolysis did not occur in completely intact erythrocytes but was contingent upon and correlated with hemolysis.

This, in turn, was caused by a complement-requiring antibody present in variable titre in all human plasma tested. The plasma of schizophrenics could not be reliably distinguished from that of nonschizophrenic patients from the same hospital[95]. Turner and Chipps[107] found a higher heterophile hemolysin titre in the blood of schizophrenics than of nonschizophrenics. Chronic alcoholics, however, also showed a higher titre of the hemolysin. Although Frohman and his associates have consistently found this phenomenon with higher frequency among schizophrenics, a possibility which remains to be ruled out is that the titre of this antibody is more closely related to a history of chronic hospitalization and greater exposure to a variety of antigens than to the presence of schizophrenia. An interesting further possibility is the significantly greater antibody responsiveness of schizophrenic patients than normal or depressed individuals to a standard antigen challenge [33a].

The evidence with regard to the biologic or behavioral effects of the plasma of schizophrenics is far from conclusive at the present time. Most of the effects reported have failed of confirmation and none have been shown to be properties of plasma which are characteristic of schizophrenia.

Further work is necessary to determine to what extent the abnormalities in plasma found by physico-chemical analysis, when they are confirmed, are characteristic of schizophrenia or a reflection of the stress, exposure to chronic endemic infections, dietary or other adventitious factors which accompany the disorder and are associated with chronic institutionalization[61].

AMINO ACIDS AND AMINES

Although an earlier report indicated abnormalities in amino acid excretion in schizophrenia[114], this has not been further confirmed. Much interest, on the other hand, has been attached to the possibility that abnormal metabolism of one or another amine could be of etiologic importance in schizophrenia[51]. The great sensitivity and relative nonspecificity of chromatographic methods and the ease with which findings may be affected by exogenous factors such as diet or drugs increase the likelihood of false positives in this area, and great caution must be exercised in identifying the particular metabolite which appears to be involved or interpreting the significance which should be attached to it[42, 75].

The significance of an unidentified Ehrlich positive substance ("the mauve spot") attributed to a new form of schizophrenia by Hoffer and Osmond[52] has been brought into question by O'Reilly and his associates[80, 81] who found it with high frequency in the urines of patients with affective psychosis, alcoholism, psychoneurosis, personality disorders, and cancer.

TRANSMETHYLATION

In 1952, Osmond and Smythies[82] pointed out some similarities between mescaline psychosis and schizophrenia and between that drug and epinephrine. They included a biochemical note by Harley-Mason which stated, in part:

It is extremely probable that the final stage in the biogenesis of adrenaline is a transmethylation of noradrenaline, the methyl group arising from methionine or choline. It is just possible that a pathological disordering of its transmethylation mechanism might lead to methylation of one or both of its phenolic hydroxyl groups instead of its amino group. . . . Methylation of phenolic hydroxyl groups in the animal body is of rare occurrence but a significant case has been reported recently. . . . It is particularly interesting to note that out of a series of phenylethylamine derivations tested by Noteboom, 3,4-dimethoxyphenylethylamine was the most potent in producing catatonia in animals.

Since that time the transmethylation of norepinephrine to epinephrine has been established[12], while Axelrod, Senoh, and Witkop[5] have demonstrated the O-methylation of both catecholamines as an important step in their normal metabolism.

The suggestion that pathologic transmethylation may occur in schizophrenia was further strengthened by the recognition that a number of psychotomimetic agents, in addition to mescaline, were methylated congeners of normal body metabolites. On this basis, Hoffer and associates[53] used niacin and niacinamide, methyl accepters, in an effort to inhibit competitively the possible abnormal process. They reported beneficial results which have not been independently confirmed. In 1961, Pollin, Cardon, and Kety[86] tested this hypothesis by administering large doses of L-methionine to chronic schizophrenic patients in conjunction with a monoamine oxidase inhibitor to permit the accumulation of any monoamines formed. This substance is an essential precursor of S-adenosylmethionine, the active substance which was shown by Cantoni[18] to transfer its methyl group to accepter compounds in the process of transmethylation. In some of the patients during the administration of the L-methionine there was a brief intensification of psychosis which involved an exacerbation of some of the schizophrenic symptoms. No other amino acids tested (glycine, tyrosine, phenylalanine, tryptophan, histidine, glutamine) were associated with this phenomenon. The intensification of psychosis in schizophrenics with methionine has since, in essence, been confirmed by four other groups[1, 15, 46, 83] and, in addition, Brune and Himwich[16] found that betaine, another methyl donor, was equally effective in accentuating psychotic symptoms in schizophrenics. Baldessarini and Kopin[6] found that feeding L-methionine to rats produced a significant increase in S-adenosylmethionine concentration in the liver and brain. Axelrod[4] demonstrated the presence in normal mammalian tissue of enzyme capable of methylating normal metabolites, i.e., tryptamine and serotonin to their dimethyl derivatives for which psychotomimetic properties have been reported.

DIMETHOXYPHENYLETHYLAMINE

In 1962, Friedhoff and Van Winkle[32] examined the urine of patients with early schizophrenia and reported the occurrence of 3,4-dimethoxyphenylethylamine (DMPEA), to which Harley-Mason had alluded as a possible abnormally methylated metabolite. This compound is a dimethylated derivative of dopamine and closely related to mescaline, which represents a trimethylated congener of this biogenic amine.

Since 1962 a number of groups have attempted to confirm the excretion of DMPEA in schizophrenia and further to define the variables which affect it. Friedhoff and Van Winkle[32] had found it in the urine of 15 of 19 schizophrenics and in none of 14 normal urines. Kuehl and associates[68] confirmed its presence in 7 of 22 schizophrenics and none of 10 normals. Takesada and associates[105] found it in 70 of 78 (90 percent) schizophrenics but also in 35 of 67, or 52 percent, of normals. Faurbye and Pind[24], who modified the method to increase its sensitivity and to avoid interference by phenothiazine metabolites, were unable to detect DMPEA in the urine of 15 schizophrenics and 10 normals. Perry, Hansen, and Macintyre[85] were unable to find the compound in 10 schizophrenics on a diet free of fruits and vegetables. After finding DMPEA in the urine of 4 out of 6 schizophrenics and 2 of 3 controls, Studnitz and Nyman[104] demonstrated its disappearance when the same individuals were placed on a pure carbohydrate regimen.

In an extensive series in which biochemical determinations and psychiatric diagnoses were made independently, Bourdillon and his associates[14] reported the presence of a "pink spot" having some of the characteristics of DMPEA in the urines of 46 of 84 (55 percent) schizophrenics, while it was absent in all of 17 nonschizophrenic patients and 149 normal controls. A second experiment with less striking results showed a low incidence (3 percent) of the spot in the urine of paranoid patients and a 29 percent incidence in nonparanoid schizopherenics. Drug administration which was not controlled could have been different in type of drug or dosage for different diagnostic categories. Drugs or their metabolites are known to interfere with DMPEA determinations, and at least one group[24] has observed a phenothiazine metabolite with Rf value and color reactions similar to DMPEA which persisted in the urine for as long as 25 days after withdrawal of the drug. Williams[110] has examined the technic used by Bourdillon and found it relatively insensitive to DMPEA. Further studies by his group[111] and by others using more specific technics[7, 13] have indicated that Bourdillon's "pink spot" was not, in fact, DMPEA and that DMPEA is not excreted in abnormal amounts by schizophrenics. Friedhoff[33], on the other hand, on the basis of its behavior in six solvent systems, a number of color reactions, thin layer and gas chromatography and melting point determinations, has concluded that the material he has found in the urine of schizophrenics is identical to DMPEA. Although this substance, when administered to schizophrenics is rapidly converted to 3,4-dimethoxyphenyl-acetic acid[31], Kuehl and associates[69] could not detect a significant difference in the excretion of that acid between normal subjects and schizophrenics.

These findings—the intensification of psychosis in schizophrenics by methionine or betaine, the increase in S-adenosylmethionine in the brain and liver of rats by methionine feeding, the existence of at least one enzyme capable of transmethylating normal metabolites to psychoto-mimetic compounds, the evidence obtained by some workers for the excretion of DMPEA in a substantial number of schizophrenics— are compatible with the hypothesis that the process of biologic transmethylation is somehow disturbed in schizophrenia with the production or persistence of excessive amounts of methylated derivatives of normal metabolites capable of inducing some of the symptoms of schizophrenia. That hypothesis, however, is far from having been validated. Although methionine and betaine are the only ones of a large number of amino acids which have been shown capable of briefly exacerbating psychosis in some schizophrenics, it has not been established that the clinical changes resulted from any specific methylated derivatives, and the possibility that this was a nonspecific toxic psychosis or a peculiarly schizophrenic response to nonspecific toxic changes has not been ruled out. Haydu *et al.*[46], who confirm the ability of methionine to exacerbate schizophrenic symptomatology, found an ameliorating effect from hydroxychloroquine and suggest that the clinical effects of these agents result from their activation or suppression of thiol groups. A special sensitivity of schizophrenics to methionine has not been established although a similar regimen of methionine without iproniazid in a small number of normal volunteers produced no hint of a psychotic reaction[62]. The accumulated evidence for the excretion of dimethoxyphenylethylamine in association with some forms of schizophrenia is as yet inconclusive. Several groups have been unable to confirm it and the possibility that it is an artifact of drug therapy has not been completely ruled out. There is evidence that some dietary factors are necessary for its appearance although the same is true for phenylketonuria and does not argue against its significance or relevance to schizophrenia. On parenteral administration to man, DMPEA has not been shown to produce perceptible mental effects[31], but this does not preclude an effect from higher concentrations locally within the brain. The transmethylation hypothesis appears to require and merit further examination and development.

INDOLEAMINES

Although Woolley[113] was impressed with indirect evidence for the possibility of a disorder in serotonin metabolism in schizophrenia, significant differences between schizophrenic and normal populations with respect to this amine or its metabolites have not been established[61]. Earlier findings of indolic compounds (indole acetamide and 6-hydroxyskatole) with abnormal frequency in the urine of schizophrenics[78, 101] have more recently been found to a similar extent in the urine of other types of mental patient and are probably to be attributed to exogenous or nondisease-related factors[20, 100, 115].

Tryptamine excretion may have some significance in schizophrenia since an increase has been found to occur in such patients before a period of exacerbation[9]. An increase in urinary tryptophan metabolites has also been observed following the administration of methionine[10, 102, 103] and it has been suggested that the conversion of tryptamine to its hallucinogenic methylated derivative may occur. Aside from one positive report[30] the search for dimethyltryptamine or dimethylserotonin in the urine of schizophrenics has yielded negative results[98, 102, 106].

EPINEPHRINE

The hypothesis that adrenochrome or other abnormal metabolites of circulating epinephrine were formed in schizophrenia and accounted for many of the symptoms[54] has received careful scrutiny made possible by the recently acquired knowledge of the normal metabolism of this hormone[3]. No evidence was found for the abnormal metabolism of labeled epinephrine infused into schizophrenic patients[88], and in one study which accounted almost entirely for the excreted label in terms of unchanged epinephrine and four metabolites (3-methoxy-4-hydroxymandelic acid, metanephrine, 3,4-dihydroxymandelic acid, and 3-methoxy-4-hydroxyphenyglycol), no qualitative or quantitative differences were found in this pattern between chronic schizophrenics and normal volunteers[70]. The infusion of epinephrine into schizophrenics was not found to intensify the psychosis[87] which would have been expected if the psychosis were associated with abnormal metabolites of circulating epinephrine.

Although it would be difficult to demonstrate that a definitive increase in our knowledge of biochemical mechanisms in the schizophrenic psychoses has occurred in the past decade, substantial progress has nonetheless been made. There is an increasing awareness of the complexity of the problem and of the sophistication of research design necessary to cope with it. Most important, there has been a burgeoning of fundamental knowledge in biochemistry and neurochemistry and their interaction with behavior on which depend meaningful hypotheses relating to schizophrenia and from which may eventually come an understanding of whatever biochemical mechanisms operate significantly in its etiology, pathogenesis, or therapy.

Before the etiology of any syndrome has been established, it is idle to regard it as a single disease, and, in the case of schizophrenia, the striking resemblance which certain temporal lobe epilepsies or chronic intoxications (bromidism, iodism, amphetamine psychosis, porphyria) bear to it makes tenable the possibility that the syndrome may emerge from different etiologic pathways. Recognition of such a possibility aids in the interpretation of genetic and biologic findings and would facilitate the characterization of more specific subgroups.

Those interested in exploring the biologic aspects of schizophrenic disorders cannot with impunity ignore the psychologic, social, and other environmental factors which operate significantly at various stages of their development. Leaving aside etiologic considerations, it is clear that exogenous factors may precipitate, intensify, or ameliorate the symptoms and confound the biologic picture. To what extent the classical psychologic features of chronic schizophrenia are created by prolonged isolation and hospitalization will become apparent with the increasing adoption of community-oriented treatment. Examples are readily found in which uncontrolled nutritional, infectious, or pharmacologic variables may have accounted for specific biochemical abnormalities in populations of chronic schizophrenics. These secondary variables are so manifold that it is hard to imagine a design which could anticipate and control them all, and successive studies concentrating on particularly relevant controls will probably continue to be called for. There is, in addition, much to be said for broadening the scope of the typical sample from chronic hospitalized schizophrenia to the early, more acute, remitting, episodic, or periodic forms [21, 41] in which it may not only be possible to obviate some of the difficulties imposed by chronic hospitalization and drug administration but, by study of the same patient in psychotic and nonpsychotic states, to avoid the effects of interindividual variance.

An unavoidable difficulty at the present time is the fact that the crucial processes of diagnosis and evaluation of change are based almost entirely on subjective estimates. It is not insensitivity which diminishes the reliability of such measures as much as their vulnerability to bias; failure to recognize and guard against this source of error probably accounts for much of the inconsistency in the study of schizophrenia not only from biologic but also from sociologic and psychologic points of view.

The single-gene-single-enzyme concept of the biologic disorder in schizophrenia was encouraged by the very high concordance rate found in monozygotic twins in earlier studies. More recent twin studies in which selective bias in sampling has been more effectively controlled have yielded a concordance rate of 40 percent or less. Studies with adopted schizophrenics [64, 93] where environmental factors can be more successfully controlled have still reinforced the importance of genetic factors but have emphasized the genetic transmission of a vulnerability to schizophrenia or to a variety of personality or character disorders. This suggests that personality or intelligence may be more appropriate models for schizophrenia than phenylketonuria. A polygenic inadequacy interacting with particular life situations seems more compatible with all of the evidence [92]. The biologic component of the schizophreniform illnesses may lie in the mechanisms which underlie arousal, inhibition, perception, cognition, affect, or the complex relationships among them, all of which appear to be involved at one time or another. Although a single chemical substance such as mescaline or lysergic acid diethylamide may produce disturbances in all of these areas, it would be well to keep in mind the possibility that more complex neurochemical, neurophysiologic and psychologic interactions may form the biologic substrate of schizophrenia.

REFERENCES

1. Alexander, F., Curtis, G. C., Sprince, H., & Crosley, A. P. L-methionine and L-tryptophan feedings in nonpsychotic and schizophrenic patients with and without tranylcypromine. *J. Nerv. Ment. Dis.*, 1963, **137**, 135–142.

2. Altschule, M. D., Henneman, D. H., Holliday, P., & Goncz, R. -M. Carbohydrate metabolism in brain disease. VI. Lactate metabolism after infusion of sodium d-lactate in manic-depressive and schizophrenic psychoses. *AMA. Arch. Intern. Med.*, 1956, **98**, 35–38.
3. Axelrod, J. Metabolism of epinephrine and other sympathomimetic amines. *Physiol. Rev.*, 1959, **39**, 751–776.
4. Axelrod, J. Enzymatic formation of psychotomimetic metabolites from normally occurring compounds. *Science*, 1961, **134**, 343.
5. Axelrod, J., Senoh, S., & Witkop, B. O-methylation of catecholamines *in vivo. J. Biol. Chem.*, 1958, **233**, 697–701.
6. Baldessarini, R. J., & Kopin, I. J. Assay of tissue levels of S-adenosylmethionine. *Anal. Biochem.*, 1963, **6**, 289–292.
7. Bell, C. E., & Somerville, A. R. Identity of the "pink spot." *Nature*, 1966, **211**, 1405–1406.
8. Bergen, J. F., Pennell, R. B., Saravis, C. A., & Hoagland, H. Further experiments with plasma protiens from schizophrenics. In R. G. Heath (Ed.), *Serological fractions in schizophrenia.* New York: Harper & Row, 1963. pp. 67–76.
9. Berlet, H. H., Bull, C., Himwich, H. E., Spaide, J., Tourlentes, T. T., & Valverde, J. M. Endogenous metabolic factor in schizophrenic behavior. *Science*, 1964, **144**, 311–313.
10. Berlet, H. H., Matsumoto, K., Pscheidt, G. R., Spaide, J., Bull, C., & Himwich, H. E. Biochemical correlates of behavior in schizophrenic patients. *Arch. Gen. Psychist.* 1965, **13**, 521–531.
11. Bishop, M. P. Effects of plasma from schizophrenia subjects upon learning and retention in the rat. In R. G. Heath (Ed.), *Serological fractions in schizophrenia.* New York: Harper & Row, 1963. pp. 77–91.
12. Blaschko, H. The devlopment of current concepts of catecholamine formation. *Pharmacol. Rev.*, 1959, **11**, 307–316.
13. Boulton, A. A., & Felton, C. A. The "pink spot" and schizophrenia. *Nature*, 1966, **211**, 1404–1405.
14. Bourdillon, R. E., Clarke, C. A., Ridges, A. P., Sheppard, P. M., Harper, P., & Leslie, S. A. "Pink spot" in the urine of schizophrenics. *Nature*, 1965, **208**, 453–455.
15. Brune, G. G., & Himwich, H. E. Effects of methioine loading on the behavior of schizophrenic patients. *J. Nerv. Ment. Dis.*, 1962, **134**, 447–450.
16. Brune, G. G., & Himwich, H. E. Biogenic amines and behavior in schizophrenic patients. In *Recent advances in biological psychiatry.* Vol. V. New York: Plenum Press, 1963. pp. 144–160.
17. Buhler, D. R., & Ihler, G. S. Effect of plasma from normal and schizophrenic subjects on the oxidation of labeled glucose by chicken erythrocytes. *J. Lab. Clin. Med.*, 1963, **62**, 306–318.
18. Cantoni, G. L. S-Adenosylmethinine: A new intermediate formed enzymatically from L-methionine and adenosine-triphosphate. *J. Biol. Chem.*, 1953, **204**, 403–416.
19. Dern, R. J., Glynn, M. F., & Brewer, G. J. Studies on the influence of hereditary G-6-PD deficiency in the expression of schizophrenic patterns. *Clin. Res.*, 1962, **10**, 80.
20. Dohan, F. C., Ewing, J., Graff, H., & Sprince, H. Schizophrenia: 6-hydroxyskatole and environment. *Arch. Gen. Psychiat.*, 1964, **10**, 420–422.
21. Durell, J., Lidow, L. S., Kellam, S. F., & Shader, R. I. Interrelationships between regulation of thyroid gland function and psychosis. *Res. Publ. Ass. Res. Nerv. Ment., Dis.*, 1966, **43**, 387–399.
22. Durell, J., & Schildkraut, J. J. Biochemical studies of the schizophrenic and affective disorders. In S. Arieti (Ed.), *American handbook of psychiatry.* Vol. III. New York: Basic Books, 1966. Pp. 423–457.
23. Faurbye, A., Lundberg, L., & Jensen, K. A. Studies on the antigen demonstrated by Malis in serum from schizophrenic patients. *Acta Path. Microbiol. Scand.*, 1964, **61**, 633–651.
24. Faurbye, A., & Pind, K. Investigation on the occurrence of the dopamine metabolite 3,4-dimethoxyphenylethylamine in the urine of schizophrenics. *Acta Psychiat. Scand.*, 1964, **40**, 240–243.
25. Ferguson, D. C., & Fisher, A. E. Behavior disruption in cebus monkeys as a function of injected substances. *Science.* 1963, **139**, 1281–1282.
26. Fessel, W. J. Macroglobulin elevations in functional mental illness. *Nature.* 1962, **193**, 1005. (a)
27. Fessel, W. J. Mental stress, blood proteins and the hypothalamus: Experimental results showing effect of mental stress upon 4S and 19S proteins. *Arch. Gen. Psychiat.*, 1962, **7**, 427–435. (b)

28. Fessel, W. J. & Grunbaum, B. W. Electrophoretic and analytical ultracentrifuge studies in sera of psychotic patients: Elevation of gamma globulins and macroglobulins, and splitting of alpha₂ globulins. *Ann. Intern. Med.*, 1961, **54**, 1134–1145.

29. Fieve, R. R., Brauninger, G., Fleiss, J., & Cohen, G. Glucose-6-phosphate dehydrogenase deficiency and schizophrenic behavior. *J. Psychiat. Res.*, 1965, **3**, 255–262.

30. Fischer, E., Fernández Lagravere, T. A., Vázquez. A. J., & Di Stefano, A. O. A bufotenin-like substance in the urine of schizophrenics. *J. Nerv. Ment. Dis.*, 1961, **133**, 441–444.

31. Friedhoff, A. J., & Hollister, L. E. Comparison of the metabolism of 3,4-dimethoxyphenylethylamine and mescaline in humans. *Biochem. Pharmacol.*, 1966, **15**, 269–273.

32. Friedhoff, A. J., & Van Winkle, E. The characteristics of an amine found in the urine of schizophrenic patients. *J. Nerv. Ment. Dis.*, 1962, **135**, 550–555.

33. Friedhoff, A. J., & Van Winkle, E. New developments in the investigation of the relationship of 3,4-dimethoxyphenylethylamine to schizophrenia. In H. E. Himwich, S. S. Kety, & J. R. Smythies (Eds.), *Amines and schizophrenia.* Oxford: Pergamon Press, 1967. Pp. 19–21.

33a. Friedman, S. B., Cohen, J., & Iker, H. Antibody response to cholera vaccine. Differences between depressed, schizophrenic, and normal subjects. *Arch. Gen. Psychiat.*, 1967, **16**, 312–315.

34. Frohman, C. E., Czajkowski, N. P., Luby, E. D., Gottlieb, J. S., & Senf, R. Further evidence of a plasma factor in schizophrenia. *Arch. Gen. Psychiat.*, 1960, **2**, 263–267.

35. Frohman, C. E., Latham, L. K., Beckett, P. G. S., & Gottlieb, J. S. Evidence of plasma factor in schizophenia. *Arch. Gen. Psychiat.*, 1960, **2**, 255–262.

36. Frohman, C. E., Latham, L. K., Warner, K. A., Brosius, C. O., Beckett, P. G. S., & Gottlieb, J. S. Motor activity in schizophrenia: Effect on plasma factor. *Arch. Gen. Psychiat.*, 1963, **9**, 83–88.

37. Gammack, D. B., & Hector, R. I. A study of serum proteins in acute schizophrenia. *Clin. Sci.*, 1965, **28**, 469–475.

38. German, G. A. Effects of serum from schizophrenics on evoked cortical potentials in the rat. *Brit. J. Psychiat.*, 1963, **109**, 616–623.

39. German, G. A., Antebi, R. N., Dear, E. M. A., & McCance, C. A further study of the effects of serum from schizophrenics on evoked cortical potentials in the rat. *Brit. J. Psychiat.*, 1965, **111**, 345–347.

40. Gjessing, R. Disturbances of somatic functions in catatonia with a periodic course, and their compensation. *J. Ment. Sci:*, 1938, **84**, 608–621.

41. Gjessing, L. R. Studies of periodic catatonia. II The urinary excretion of phenolic amines and acids with and without loads of different drugs. *J. Psychiat., Res.*, 1964, **2**, 149–162.

42. Goldenberg, H., Fishman, V., Whittier, J., & Brinitzer, W. Urinary aromatic excretion patterns in schizophrenia *Arch. Gen. Psychiat.*, 1960, **2**, 221–230.

43. Gottesman, I. I., & Shields, J. Schizophrenia in twins: Sixteen years' consecutive admissions to a psychiatric clinic. *Dis. Nerv. Syst.*, 1966, **27** (Suppl.), 11–19.

44. Haavaldsen, R., Lingjaerde, O., & Walaas, O. Disturbances of carbohydrate metabolism in schizophrenics: Effect of serum fractions from schizophrenics on glucose uptake of rat diaphragm *in vitro. Confin. Neurol.*, 1958, **18**, 270.

45. Haddad, R. K., & Rabe, A. An antigenic abnormality in the serum of chronically ill schizophrenic patients. In R. G. Heath (Ed.), *Serological fractions in schizophrenia.* New York: Harper & Row, 1963. Pp. 151–157.

46. Haydu, G. G., Dhrymiotis, A., Korenyi, C., & Goldschmidt, L. Effects of methionine and hydroxychloroquine in schizophrenia. *Amer. J. Psychiat.*, 1965, **122**, 560–564.

47. Heath, R. G. & Krupp, I. M. The biologic basis of schizophrenia: An autoimmune concept. In O. Walaas (Ed.), *Molecular basis of some aspects of mental activity.* Vol. II. London: Academic Press, 1967. Pp. 313–344.

48. Heath, R. G., Leach, B. E., Byers, L. W., Martens, S., & Feigley, C. A. Pharmacological and biological psychotherapy. *Amer. J. Psychiat.*, 1958, **114**, 683–689.

49. Heath, R. G., Martens, S., Leach, B. E., Cohen, M., & Feigley, C. A. Behavioral changes in nonpsychotic volunteers following the adminstration of taraxein, the substance obtained from serum of schizophrenic patients. *Amer. J. Psychiat.*, 1958, **114**, 917–920.

50. Heston, L. L. Psychiatric disorders in foster home reared children of schizophrenic mothers. *Brit. J. Psychiat.*, 1966, **112**, 819–825.

51. Himwich, H. E., Kety, S. S., & Smythies, J. R. (Eds.), *Amines and schizophrenia.* Oxford: Pergamon Press, 1967.
52. Hoffer, A., & Osmond, H. Malvaria: A new psychiatric disease. *Acta Psychiat. Scand.*, 1963, **39**, 335–366.
53. Hoffer, A., Osmond, H., Callbeck, M. J., & Kahan, I. Treatment of schizophrenia with nicotinic acid and nicotinamide. *J. Clin. Exp. Psychopathol.*, 1957, **18**, 131–158.
54. Hoffer, A., Osmond, H., & Smythies, J. Schizophrenia: A new approach. II. Result of a year's research. *J. Ment. Sci.*, 1954, **100**, 29–45.
55. Horwitt, M. K. Report of Elgin Project No. 3 with emphasis on liver dysfunction. In Nutrition Symposium Series No. 7. New York: National Vitamin Foundation, 1953, pp. 67–83.
56. Horwitt, M. K., Liebert, E., Kreisler, O., & Wittman, P. Investigations of human requirements for B-complex vitamins. In National Research Council Bulletin No. 116. Washington, D.C.: National Academy of Sciences, 1948.
57. Inouye, E. Similarity and dissimilarity of schizophrenia in twins. *Proceedings of the Third World Congress of Psychiatry.* Montreal, 1961, **1**, 524–530.
58. Jensen, K., Clausen, J., & Osterman, E. Serum and cerebrospinal fluid proteins in schizophrenia. *Acta Psychiat. Scand.*, 1964, **40**, 280–286.
59. Kallmann, F. J. The genetic theory of schizophrenia. An analysis of 691 schizophrenic twin index families. *Amer. J. Psychiat.*, 1946, **103**, 309–322.
60. Kelsey, F. O., Gullock, A. H., & Kelsey, F. E. Thyroid activity in hospitalized psychiatric patients. *AMA Arch. Neurol. Psychiat.*, 1957, **77**, 543–548.
61. Kety, S. S. Biochemical theories of schizophrenia. *Science*, 1959, **129**, 1528–1532, 1590–1596.
62. Kety, S. S. Possible relation of central amines to behavior in schizophrenic patients. *Fed. Proc.*, 1961, **20**, 894–896.
63. Kety, S. S. Current biochemical approaches to schizophrenia. *New Eng. J. Med.*, 1967, **276**, 325–311.
64. Kety, S. S., Rosenthal, D., Wender, P. H., & Schulsinger, F. The types and prevalence of mental illness in biological and adoptive families of adopted schizophrenics. *J. Psychiat. Res.*, 1968, **6** (Suppl.), 345–362.
65. Kety, S. S., Woodford, R. B., Harmel, M. H., Freyhan, F. A., Appel, K. E., & Schmidt, C. F. Cerebral blood flow and metabolism in schizophrenia. The effects of barbiturate semi-narcosis, insulin coma and electroshock. *Amer. J. Psychiat.*, 1948, **104**, 765–770.
66. Kopeloff, L. M., & Fischel, E. Serum levels of bactericidin and globulin in schizophrenia. *Arch. Gen. Psychiat.*, 1963 **9**, 524–528.
67. Kringlen, E. Schizophrenia in twins: An epidemiological–clinical study. *Psychiatry*, 1966, **29**, 172–184.
68. Kuehl, F. A., Jr., Hichens, M., Ormond, R. E., Meisinger, M. A. P., Gale, P. H., Cirillo, V. J., & Brink, N. G. Para-O-methylation of dopamine in schizophrenic and normal individuals. *Nature*, 1964, **203**, 154–155.
69. Kuehl, F. A., Jr., Ormond, R. E., & Vandenheuvel, W. J. A. Occurrence of 3,4-dimethoxyphenylacetic acid in urines of normal and schizophrenic individuals. *Nature*, 1966, **211**, 606–608.
70. LaBrosse, E. H., Mann, J. D., & Kety, S. S. The physiological and psychological effects of intravenously administered epinephrine and its metabolism in normal and schizophrenic men. III. Metabolism of 7-H^3-epinephrine as determined in studies on blood and urine. *J. Psychiat. Res.*, 1961, **1**, 68–75.
71. Leach, B. E., Cohen, M., Heath, R. G., & Martens, S. Studies of the role of ceruloplasmin and albumin in adrenaline metabolism. *AMA Arch. Neurol. Psychiat.*, 1956, **76**, 635–642.
72. Lovegrove, T. D., & Nicholls, D. M. Haptoglobin subtypes in a schizophrenic and control population. *J. Nerv. Ment. Dis.*, 1965, **141**, 195–196.
73. Malis, C. Y. *K etiologii schizofrenii.* Moscow: Medgiz, 1959.
74. Mangoni, A., Balazs, R., & Coppen, A. J. The effect of plasma from schizophrenic patients on the chicken erythocyte system. *Brit. J. Psychiat.*, 1963, **109**, 231–234.
75. Mann, J. D., & LaBrosse, E. H. Urinary excretion of phenolic acids by normal and schizophrenic male patients. *Arch. Gen. Psychiat.*, 1959, **1**, 547–551.

76. Martens, S. Effects of exogenous human ceruloplasmin in the schizophrenia syndrome. Stockholm: Tryckei Balder AB, 1966.

77. McDonald, R. K., Weise, V. K., Evans, F. T., & Patrick, R. W. Studies on plasma ascorbic acid and ceruloplasmin levels in schizophrenia. In J. Folch-Pi (Ed.), *Chemical Pathology of the nervous system*. Oxford: Pergamon Press, 1961. Pp. 404–412.

78. Nakao, A., & Ball, M. The appearance of a skatole derivative in the urine of schizophrenics. *J. Nerv. Ment. Dis.*, 1960, **130**, 417–419.

79. Noval, J. J., & Mao, T. S. S. Abnormal immunological reaction of schizophrenic serum. *Fed. Proc.*, 1966, **25**, 560.

80. O'Reilly, P. O., Ernest, M., & Hughes, G. The incidence of malvaria. *Brit. J. Psychiat.*, 1965, **111**, 741–744.

81. O'Reilly, P. O., Hughes, G., & Russell, S., & Ernest, M. The mauve factor: An evaluation. *Dis. Nerv. Syst.*, 1965, **26**, 562–568.

82. Osmond, H., & Smythies, J. Schizophrenia: A new approach. *J. Ment. Sci.*, 1952, **98**, 309–315.

83. Park, L., Baldessarini, R. J., & Kety, S. S. Methionine effects on chronic schizophrenics. *Arch. Gen. Psychiat.*, 1965, **12**, 346–351.

84. Pennell, R. B., Pawlus, C., Saravis, C. A., & Scrimshaw, G. Further characterization of a human plasma component which influences animal behavior. *Trans. NY Acad. Sci.*, 1965, **28**, 47–58.

85. Perry, T. L., Hansen, S., & Macintyre, L. Failure to detect 3,4-dimethoxyphenylethylamine in the urine of schizophrenics. *Nature*, 1964, **202**, 519–520.

86. Pollin, W., Cardon, P. V., & Kety, S. S. Effects of amino acid feedings in schizophrenic patients treated with iproniazid. *Science*, 1961, **133**, 104–105.

87. Pollin, W., & Goldin, S. The physiological and psychological effects of intravenously administered epinephrine and its metabolism in normal and schizophrenic men. II. Psychiatric observations. *J. Psychiat. Res.*, 1961, **1**, 50–67.

88. Resnick, O., & Elmadjian, F. Excretion and metabolism of dl-epinephrine-7-C^{14}-d-bitartrate infused into schizophrenic patients. *Amer. J. Physiol.*, 1956, **187**, 626.

89. Richter, D. Biochemical aspects of schizophrenia. In D. Richter (Ed.), *Schizophrenia: Somatic aspects*. London: Pergamon Press, 1957. Pp. 53–75.

90. Rieder, H. P., Ritzel, G., Spiegelberg, H., & Gnirss, F. Serologische Versuche zum Nachweis von "Taraxein." *Experientia*, 1960, **16**, 561–562.

91. Robins, E., Smith, K., & Lowe, I. P. Discussion of clinical studies with taraxein. In H. A. Abramson (Ed.), *Neuropharmacology: Transactions of the Fourth Conference*. New York: Josiah Macy Jr. Foundation, 1957. Pp. 123–135.

92. Rosenthal, D., & Kety, S. S. (Eds.), The transmission of schizophrenia, *J. Psychiat. Res.*, 1968, **6**, (Suppl.).

93. Rosenthal, D., Wender, P. H., Kety, S. S., Schulsinger, F., Welner, J., & Østergaard, L. Schizophrenics' offspring reared in adoptive homes. *J. Psychiat. Res.*, 1968, 6 (Suppl.), 377–392.

94. Ryan, J. W., Brown, J. D., & Durell, J. Antibodies affecting metabolism of chicken erythrocytes: Examination of schizophrenic and other subjects. *Science*, 1966, **151**, 1408–1410.

95. Ryan, J. W., Steinberg, H. R., Green, R., Brown, J. D., & Durell, J. Controlled study of effects of plasma of schizophrenic and non-schizophrenic psychiatric patients on chicken erythrocytes. *J. Psychiat. Res.*, 1968, **6**, 33–44.

96. Sanders, B. E., Small, S. M., Ayers, W. J., Oh, Y. H., & Axelrod, S. Additional studies on plasma proteins obtained from schizophrenics and controls. *Trans. NY Acad. Sci.*, 1965, **28**, 22–39.

97. Sapira, J. D. Immunoelectrophoresis of the serum of psychotic patients. *Arch. Gen. Psychiat.*, 1964, **10**, 196–198.

98. Siegel, M. A sensitive method for the detection of N,N-dimethylserotonin (bufotenin) in urine; failure to demonstrate its presence in the urine of schizophrenic and normal subjects. *J. Psychiat. Res.*, 1965, **3**, 205–211.

99. Slater, E. *Psychotic and neurotic illnesses in twins*. London: Stationery Office, 1953.

100. Sohler, A., Noval, J. J., & Renz, R. H. 6-Hydroxyskatole sulfate excretion in schizophrenia. *J. Nerv. Ment. Dis.*, 1963, **137**, 591–596.

101. Sprince, H., Houser, E., Jameson, D., & Dohan, F. C. Differential extraction of indoles from the urine of schizophrenic and normal subjects. *Arch. Gen. Psychiat.*, 1960, **2**, 268–270.

102. Sprince, H., Parker, C. M., Jameson, D., & Alexander, F. Urinary indoles in schizophrenic and psychoneurotic patients after administration of tranylcypromine (parnate) and methionine or trypophan. *J. Nerv. Ment. Dis.*, 1963, **137**, 246–251.
103. Sprince, H., Parker, C. M. Jameson, D., & Josephs, J. A. Effect of methionine on nicotinic acid and indoleacetic acid pathways of tryptophan metabolism *in vivo*. *Proc. Exp. Biol. Med.*, 1965, **119**, 942–946.
104. Studnitz, W. V., & Nyman, G. E. Excretion of 3,4-dimethoxyphenylethylamine in schizophrenia. *Acta Psychiat. Scand.*, 1965, **41**, 117–121.
105. Takesada, M., Kakimoto, Y., Sano, I., & Kaneko, Z. 3,4-Dimethoxyphenylethylamine and other amines in the urine of schizophrenic patients. *Nature*, 1963, **199**, 203–204.
106. Takesada, M., Miyamoto, E., Kakimoto, Y., Sano, I., & Kaneko, Z. Phenolic and indole amines in the urine of schizophrenics. *Nature*, 1965, **207**, 1199–1200.
107. Turner, W. J., & Chipps, H. I. A heterophil hemolysin in human blood. I. Distribution in schizophrenics and nonschizophrenics. *Arch. Gen. Psychiat.*, 1966, **15**, 373–377.
108. Vartanyan, M. E. Immunological investigation of schizophrenia. *Zh. Nevropat. Psikhiat. Korsakov*, 1963, **63**, 3–12.
109. Weil-Malherbe, H. The biochemistry of the functional psychoses. In *Advances in enzymology.* Vol. XXIX. New York: Interscience, 1967. Pp. 479–553.
110. Williams, C. H. The pink spot. *Lancet*, 1966, 1, 599–600.
111. Williams, C. H., Gibson, J. G., & McCormick, W. O. 3,4-Dimethoxyphenylethylamine in schizophrenia. *Nature*, 1966, **211**, 1195.
112. Winter, C. A., Flataker, L., Boger W. P., Smith, E. V. C., & Sanders, B. E. The effects of blood serum and of serum fractions from schizophrenic donors upon the performance of trained rats. In J. Folch-Pi (Ed.), *Chemical pathology of the nervous system.* Oxford: Pergamon Press, 1961. Pp. 641–646.
113. Woolley, D. W. *The biochemical bases of psychoses.* New York: Wiley, 1962.
114. Young, H. K., Berry, H. K., Beerstecher, E., & Berry, J. S. Metabolic patterns of schizophrenic and control groups. (Biochemical Institute Studies IV, University of Texas Publ. No. 5109). Austin: University of Texas, 1951. Pp. 189–197.
115. Yuwiler, A., & Good, M. H. Chromatographic study of "Reigelhaupt" chromogens in urine. *J. Psychiat. Res.*, 1962, 1, 215–227.

Suggested Additional Readings

Bleuler, M. A 23-year longitudinal study of 208 schizophrenics and impressions in regard to the nature of schizophrenia. In D. Rosenthal & S. S. Kety (Eds.), *Transmission of schizophrenia*. Oxford: Pergamon Press, 1968.

Eiduson, B. T., Eiduson, S. & Geller, E. Biochemistry, genetics and the nature-nurture problem. *American Journal of Psychiatry*, 1962, **119**, 342–350.

Forssman, H. The mental implications of sex chromosome aberrations. *British Journal of Psychiatry*, 1970, **117**, 353–363.

Jackson, D. D. A critique of the literature on the genetics of schizophrenia. In D. D. Jackson (Ed.), *The etiology of schizophrenia*. New York: Basic Books, 1960.

Jacobs, P. A., Price, W. H., Court Brown, W. M., Brittain, R. P., & Whatmore, P. B. Chromosome studies on men in a maximum security hospital. *Annals of Human Genetics*, 1968, **31**, 339–347.

Kallmann, F. J. The genetics of human behavior. *American Journal of Psychiatry*, 1956, **113**, 496–501.

Kety, S. S. Biochemical theories of schizophrenia. Part II. *Science*, 1959, **129**, 1590–1596.

Kringlen, E. Schizophrenia in twins: An epidemiological-clinical study. *Psychiatry*, 1966, **29**, 172–184.

Meehl, P. E. Schizotaxia, schiotypy, schizophrenia. *American Psychologist*, 1962, **17**, 827–838.

Montagu, A. Chromosomes and crime. *Readings in clinical psychology today*. Del Mar, Calif.: CRM Books, 1970. Pp. 153–159.

Owen, D. R. The 47, XYY male: A review. *Psychological Bulletin*, 1972, **78**, 209–233.

Woolley, D. W. *The biochemical bases of psychoses*. New York: Wiley, 1962.

Wyatt, R. J., Termini, B. A, & Davis, J. Biochemical and sleep studies of schizophrenia: A review of the literature—1960–1970. *Schizophrenia Bulletin*, 1971, No. 4, 10–66.

UNIT III

Drug Usage and Alcoholism

INTRODUCTION

There is little doubt that we are a drug using society.

During the past two decades, mental health professionals have become increasingly concerned about our use and abuse of drugs. Most recently, this concern has been directed toward the use of those drugs which have been labeled as "dangerous," "hallucinogenic," "narcotic," etc., as well as the use of alcohol. The problem of alcohol consumption is not new, but the increased public awareness of the extent to which people in our society have drinking problems is new. This awareness has resulted in the recognition of alcohol abuse as a public health problem in need of research to determine its causes, biological and psychological effects, and treatment.

The public has also recognized that drug use is a serious health problem and that continued research is needed to assess its effects, causes, and treatment. This unit presents a series of articles which discuss the use of drugs and alcohol, the major emphasis being on drug use.

Article 20 by Helen H. Nowlis provides an overview of drug use in our society. She states that drugs have their effects only after they have interacted with the biological, psychological, social, and other aspects of an organism. Thus, it is important *not* to consider the effects of drugs in a vacuum but with respect to the organism's internal and external environment. Drugs, including those that are medically or nonmedically approved, provide risks for the user. Whether drugs are declared "dangerous" or "illegal" seems to be determined by whether society considers their use to be appropriate or inappropriate. In addition to discussing briefly the non-narcotic drugs used in our society (e.g., alcohol, marijuana, ups, downs, LSD-like drugs, and solvents), Nowlis presents some issues regarding their use and raises some questions concerning the criteria that should be used to judge their acceptability.

Article 21 is about the use of marijuana. Much has been written in the popular press about the rapid spread of marijuana use in this country. Estimates of its use among various groups of college students have ranged from one-third to one-half, these figures including any student who has reportedly tried it at least once.

Overall estimates of the number of people in the United States who have ever used it range from fifteen to twenty-four million. What seem to be lacking in many of the popular writings, however, are the findings of controlled laboratory research on the physiological and behavioral consequences of using marijuana. Once these facts are known, we should be better able to judge the desirability of incorporating the use of this drug into our social system.

In an attempt to obtain these facts, the federal government has contracted with a number of scientists to study the effects of marijuana on the physiology and behavior of humans and animals. The results of the initial research were made public by the Secretary of the Department of Health, Education and Welfare in a series of reports to Congress (National Institute of Mental Health, 1971, 1972). A summarization of the most recent report is presented in Article 21.

The use of d-lysergic acid diethylamide (LSD) in our society is the cause of much concern to the public as well as among health professionals. As with marijuana, the use of this drug is illegal in the United States. LSD, though not used as frequently as marijuana, has received a great deal of attention because of its hallucinogenic properties and the claims about its effects on chromosomes. Experiments approved by the federal government have been conducted on this drug for a number of years because of its possible use in the treatment of mental illness and alcoholism and in helping scientists understand the possible biochemical factors related to the development of schizophrenia.

A fair amount of research has been conducted on the psychological, biological, and genetic effects of LSD in animals and humans. One of the major concerns of these studies relates to the possibility that LSD produces chromosomal damage in the gamete cells of users as well as congenital malformations in the children of parents who took the drug prior to conception or of mothers who took it during pregnancy. In Article 22, José Egozcue and Samuel Irwin discuss the effects of LSD on chromosomes. After reviewing much of the research on this subject, these investigators, though not denying the reports of a high incidence of birth defects, spontaneous abortions, stillbirths, etc. associated with LSD users, conclude that we do not have sufficient knowledge of the effects of this drug to make any final judgment about its causal connection to chromosomal damage in gamete cells, to any type of birth defect, or to spontaneous abortions or miscarriages.

The most frequently used narcotic drug, heroin, is discussed in Article 23, by Harvey W. Feldman. This drug, as well as other opium-derived drugs, is made from the juice of the poppy fruit. Estimates of the number of narcotic addicts in the United States range from about 68,000 to 200,000, with approximately 95 percent of these people using heroin. Feldman states that traditionally experimentation with, and the use of, various drugs have been attributed to the user's particular personality characteristics. According to Feldman, these explanations have neglected other important causal factors. He feels that the willingness of people to initially try heroin should also be explained in terms of the sociology of the slum environment. He sees the action-seeking ideology of many slum residents as providing young people with role models and information regarding how to survive in "street life." These youths are expected to be tough, strong, and daring. Those who do not accept the ideology are labeled as outcasts or deviant and stand a good chance of being ignored by others in the neighborhood. Within this framework, Feldman describes how slum youth are introduced to heroin use, how they develop a physical dependence on it and begin to adopt the behavior patterns of the drug-using subculture. In summary, he views the social context of these youth as being a major contributor to the development of their heroin addiction.

Article 24 by Kenneth L. Jones, Louis W. Shainberg, and Curtis O. Byer is concerned with alcoholism. Research has shown that approximately 70 percent of American adults drink occasionally, and about 5 percent of American adults are alcoholics. Jones *et al.* describe succinctly the various phases leading to what they label complete alcohol addiction and discuss the symptoms of alcoholism. They maintain that the alcoholic can be treated successfully during any phase of his problem, but he must be motivated to change his behavior patterns.

REFERENCES

National Institute of Mental Health. *Marijuana and health.* Washington, D.C.: U.S. Government Printing Office, 1971.

National Institute of Mental Health. *Marijuana and health.* Washington, D.C.: U.S. Government Printing Office, 1972.

function of drugs
interact w/organism
amounts, patterns, frequently + setting
of drugs
meaning + function of use to
ind.

20

Perspectives on Drug Use*

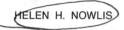

HELEN H. NOWLIS

Drug use sounds like a fairly unitary phenomenon which ought to be, and unfortunately often is, rather simply described. It is in fact an extremely complex set of phenomena. This complexity is a function of drugs themselves and how they interact with the organism, the amounts and patterns and frequency and settings of use of different drugs, and of the meaning and function of drug use to the individual and to society. Lack of recognition of these complexities is one of the main reasons for current confusion and controversy and for ineffective individual and social action.

Society at large has fallen into an either-or trap and has failed to make the discriminations so necessary for understanding and for intelligent action. Most people believe that drugs are either good or bad, safe or dangerous, that individuals are drug users or non-users. Any meaningful discussion of drug use must be based on careful discriminations among drugs and types of drug use, among people who use and how and why they use.

There are some inescapable facts about drugs and drug action and about people and the things they do. They are not the "facts" most people seek. For a variety of historical and psychological reasons most people find it difficult to think of drug effects in terms of probabilities and uncertainities, of dose-response curves, of multiple effects (some desirable and some undesirable), of reactions which vary from individual to individual and from time to time in the same individual. None of these are consistent with the widely held view of drugs as magic potions having within them great power over man and beast for good or for evil. Drugs have no effects until they interact with an organism—biologically, psychologically, and socially defined. Organisms, especially when they are human, are large or small, old or young, healthy or sick, happy or depressed, cautious or adventuresome, anxious or secure. Human organisms have language. They live in cultures and subcultures. All of these variations and many more influence the drug-person interaction. Drugs do not have the ability to level these variations. In fact, they often enhance them.

Whether the goal is to describe why, how, and with what effect man uses chemicals, to control certain types of drug use, or to predict or influence drug use in the future, we must try to discriminate clearly between what chemicals do and what people do. Both are important but they must not be confused.

A Drug Is a Drug

The title of this special issue [of the *Journal of Social Issues*] carefully avoids the word "drug." One can speculate that this was in order to include among man's chemical comforts

---

*From Nowlis, H. H., *Journal of Social Issues*, 1971, 27, 7–22. Copyright © 1971 by the Society for the Psychological Study of Social Issues. Reprinted by permission of the Society for the Psychological Study of Social Issues and Dr. Nowlis.

a number of chemicals which many resist labeling as drugs and which are called beverages or cigarettes. Or perhaps it was to single out those chemicals which, among other things, alter man's mood, feeling, or perception. In either case it avoids a word that currently arouses so much feeling and emotion that it has a drug-like effect in many. It may, however, be the better part of wisdom to try to rehabilitate the term, difficult as that will be. As long as chemical comforts include substances which are called drugs, whether they be medicines and "good" or socially disapproved substances and "bad," along with substances called beverages and cigarettes, there is a great temptation to believe that they are indeed different and act according to different principles.

From a strictly scientific point of view, *drug* is defined as any substance which by its chemical nature affects the structure or function of the living organism. This definition is objective. It is not based on value judgments about proper and improper, legal and illegal reasons for use. It includes medicines, both prescription and over-the-counter, socially disapproved substances which are increasingly and indiscriminately labeled "narcotics," beverage alcohol, caffeine, cigarettes, and even foods. It also includes many agricultural and industrial chemicals and pollutants. It provides a basis from which to consider any special class of substance no matter how it is classified or for what purpose it is used and assumes that all chemicals act according to the same basic principles.

Biochemical Changes and Behavioral Changes

All drugs are chemicals or contain chemicals which interact with the complex biochemical system that is the living organism. Changes in that biochemical system are related to changes in the perceptions, feelings, and behavior of the organism in ways we as yet see only in a mirror darkly.

Changes in perceptions, feelings, and behavior are a function of complex interactions among the nature of the substance, the amount present in the body at any time, the route and speed of administration of the substance, the physiological characteristics and current physiological state of the individual, the psychological characteristics and current psychological state of the individual, the physical and social setting of the individual when he takes the substance, the reasons why he takes the substance, and what he expects the changes will be.

For every substance there is a dose response curve. This is simply a way of describing the modal response of a given population to increasing amounts of that substance. It is a statistical abstraction with all that that implies. There are three critical points on such a curve. The first is the "effective" dose (ED50), which depends on what effect one is seeking or is ready to observe or measure. ED50 is the dosage level required to produce the desired effect in 50 percent of a given population; by definition this also means that 50 percent did not show the particular effect at ED50. It does not mean that there were not other effects at dosages smaller than ED50. The second critical point is the "toxic" dose (TD50), which—again—depends on what effects one defines as toxic. The third is the lethal dose (LD50). Although defining the response in this instance presents no problems the actual dose is, as in the other two instances, a statistical abstraction. LD50 is that dosage by which, not at which, 50 percent of a given group of animals die. To complicate matters further even this determination may change by a wide margin if the animals are tested under stress, i.e., crowded into a small cage rather than housed normally. Even in medicine the safety of a drug is a function of the distance on the dose response curve between the effective dose and the toxic dose, and this will vary from individual to individual.

All drugs have multiple effects, most of which are termed "side effects." Some of these side effects are harmful, some simply annoying; many of them occur in some people at dosage levels below those effective for the desired effect. Some are ignored or tolerated because the desired effect is valued; some are not tolerated because the sought-for effect is not considered of sufficient value. A widely used minor tranquilizer, at dosage levels considered effective in relieving psychic tension and resultant somatic symptoms, may in some individuals also produce such side effects as drowsiness, confusion, double vision, nausea, fatigue, depression, jaundice, skin rash, ataxia, slurred speech, tremor, dizziness, and such paradoxical reactions as acute hyperexcited states, anxiety, insomnia, hallucinations, rage. Reducing the dosage level may reduce or eliminate many of these side effects, but at the same time the desired effect may be eliminated.

The principal reason why drugs do not have predictable and reliable effects is because the other term in the drug-organism interaction is so complex and so variable. Except in high dosages, the effect of many drugs is more a function of non-drug factors than of the drug itself. So important are these factors that in many instances a placebo, or sugar pill, can produce "drug effects."

Individuals vary in weight, age, sex, sickness and health, in the way in which they react to their perception of physiological and psychological changes in themselves and their physical and social environment, and in the meaning and significance of these perceptions to their personal and social adjustment. These are all influential factors in determining the response to any drug. Few have any difficulty recognizing and accepting this with regard to alcohol. Having ingested the same amount of alcohol, some individuals will be gay and talkative, some relaxed and drowsy, some loud and boisterous, some aggressive, some abusive, some destructive. The difference is not the drug or the amount of the drug but the individual and the situation. But we call alcohol a beverage.

All of these principles apply to all drugs but they are especially influential when drugs act primarily on the central nervous system and modify mood, feeling, and perception. How they act and where they act within this system is in most cases still a matter of hypothesis. How biochemical changes in the central nervous system are related to changes in behavior is still in the realm of conjecture. From the point of view of man's voluntary use of chemicals, the key factor is that they produce changes, at least some of which are valued.

The effects of psychoactive drugs, like those of all drugs, are dose related. At low or moderate doses they are, even more than other drugs, a result of non-drug factors such as the psychological characteristics of the individual, the reasons why he uses the drug, what he expects the effects will be, the physical and social setting in which he uses it, how he perceives its use or non-use as instrumental in contributing to or interfering with his important goals, how his friends, his subculture, and his society define and respond to his drug use. These psychological and social factors not only influence the reaction to a specific drug but they are key factors in determining use or non-use, choice of substance, and pattern and circumstances of use.

Drugs Used for Medical Reasons

The major drugs currently used, both legally and illegally, are chemical comforters. The largest single class of prescriptions is for mood changing drugs—for pain relievers, tranquilizers, anti-depressants, anti-anxiety drugs, stimulants, and sedatives. Alcohol and caffeine are almost universally used, and cigarette consumption remains high despite vigorous efforts to halt it. A high proportion of over-the-counter drugs fall in the same category as their names attest.

All of these substances are increasingly used on a daily basis for varying periods of time, regularly enough and for long enough to be described validly as resulting in psychological dependence and, with prolonged use of increasing amounts of some, physiological dependence.

In the majority of instances these drugs are used by adults. Except for alcohol, caffeine, and nicotine, which are not considered drugs, they are deemed to be appropriate treatment for legitimate complaints and to contribute to the effective functioning of the individual in society—as long as they have the approval of the medical profession.

In the case of alcohol and caffeine, both have been institutionalized socially rather than through medicine even though both drugs are or have been used medically. Both are used by most people as contributing to personal and social functioning. Excessive use of either may interfere, in a given individual, with his personal and social functioning.

It is important to reiterate that all of these drugs act according to the principles discussed above. Their effects are a function of dose. For each there is an effective dose, a toxic dose, and, for most, a lethal dose. All of them have multiple effects. Their side effects are often critical, including such common effects as drowsiness, distractibility, irritability, temporary lapse of memory, and, more rarely, hallucinations, intoxication, hyperexcitability, and similar phenomena. The effects of all of them at moderate dose levels are highly dependent on non-drug factors. At high dose levels, and for some individuals at much lower levels, all may be dangerous. Some have been demonstrated to produce a statistically significant increase in chromosome breakage in white blood cells. Some, when taken during certain critical periods of pregnancy, produce a statistically significant increase in fetal deformities.

Drugs Used for Non-Medical Reasons

Many of these same drugs and a host of others are used by the young and the not-so-young without benefit of prescription and for non-medical reasons. The reasons for use are still primarily to change mood or feeling but often not changes which society considers appropriate. Under such circumstances the drugs are declared illegal and dangerous and their use criminal. Once this happens, their use is viewed from a totally different perspective. There is preoccupation with toxic reactions, with the effects of high dosages, and with psychological dependence. There is a great interest in and concern for who uses them, how often, and why. Many are persuaded that these drugs, or even the same drugs they use for approved reasons, are a completely different kind which act according to different principles.

All of these drugs have dose-response curves—effective, toxic, and lethal. The effects of all are influenced by the non-drug factors discussed above; all have multiple effects; all have side effects, some of which may be harmful and some of which can be ignored; at high dose levels and for some individuals at much lower dose levels, all may be dangerous. Some probably increase the probability of chromosome breakage in white blood cells; it is likely that some increase the probability of fetal deformities during critical periods of pregnancy.

All Drugs Involve Risk

All of this would suggest that there should be relatively more concern than is currently held for drugs used for medically approved reasons, and relatively less concern than the current level of panic for drugs used for non-medically approved reasons. *But there should be great concern for both.* All drugs involve risks, some more than others. The real questions are: how much risk for what benefit? and who should decide and on what basis? These are "people problems," not drug problems.

Risk-Benefit Decisions Are Value Judgements

The discomforts of man are myriad. Throughout history he has sought relief from cold, hunger, deprivation, anxiety, pain, and boredom, primarily through whatever substances were available to him in his environment. In most instances these were plants which contained a variety of chemical substances which were identified only long after their use was established. Their effects were originally discovered by trial and error, and their virtues and dangers, whether real or imagined, became part of the lore of a group. Their continued use and spread was a function of the prevalence of the particular need that they were believed to fulfill and its relationship to the needs and values of the group or the society in which they were used.

Since as drugs they had effects other than those which were sought and their effects varied with amount, frequency of use, the characteristics of the user, the set and the setting in which they were used, different individuals and groups of individuals made different value judgments as to the appropriateness of the benefits and the seriousness of the risks.

Through much the same basic processes, modern man has used a wide variety of chemical substances and the use of each substance or class of substances has been institutionalized. Societies have decided what needs are legitimate, what effects are valuable, what risks are tolerable. These decisions are usually made on the basis of the general attitudes, values, and beliefs which characterize the society or powerful groups within it. They are based on value judgments about specific drugs, about drug effects, about the reasons for using drugs, and about the people who use or do not use them. These judgments lie in the eye of the beholder, not in the drug.

It is a basic psychological principle that man does not ordinarily continue to do something that does not fulfill some need, real or imagined. To persist, behavior must be reinforced. To the extent that it does fulfill a need he will continue to do it, often at risk, unless it interferes with some more important need. If drug use does not fulfill some need it will be abandoned. The need may be closely related to real or imagined effects of the drug or may be social rather than chemical. Society's (or a subculture's) definition of and response to use of a given substance, rather than any pharmacological or psychological effects of that substance, may give it meaning which determines the decision either to try, to stop, or to continue use. Use of specific substances may determine group membership or status within a group or among groups. It may function as either sign or symptom of rebellion, alienation, independence, sophistication. Persistence in or abandonment of a variety of behaviors is an important, though indirect, statement about individual and social values.

DRUGS CURRENTLY USED

Presently man seeks comfort with a wide variety of chemicals. Merely to describe the incidence or prevalence of the use or non-use of specific substances is not very useful even if it could be done reliably and validly. It may, in fact, lead to false conclusions. In order to describe use, it is essential to define use and to make distinctions among drugs and among patterns of use of specific drugs. Using LSD daily is a very different phenomenon than using marijuana daily. Smoking three joints in one evening once a week has a different meaning than one joint three times a week.

Until recently, and even now except for some conducted scientifically, surveys have tended to distinguish only between any use and non-use, and between legal or illegal drugs or drug use. Legal is defined as for medically approved reasons and with medical supervision, however indirect. Illegal is defined as for non-medically approved reasons or having no medically accepted uses. The criteria of use vs. non-use and legal vs. illegal substances make for very strange bedfellows and serve primarily as an imperfect measure of the prevalence of one particular category of deviant behavior.

Useful and meaningful assessments which can provide a basis for understanding and influencing drug use or abuse must, at a minimum, distinguish among drugs, or at least functionally meaningful groups of drugs, and among patterns of use of specific drugs or meaningful groups of drugs. Additionally it is helpful if the various uses of any specific drug are considered in the context of all similar drugs and use by any particular group in context of use by all groups.

Alcohol

Any survey of drugs which does not begin with alcohol can lead only to a distorted picture of drug use. Alcohol is the most commonly used comforter. It is usually the first non-medical drug to be used. Acute and chronic effects of various patterns of use are well documented. The British Medical Council on Alcoholism (*New York Times*, 1970) has estimated that there are 300,000 teenage alcoholics (without defining "alcoholic"). The Council is reported to consider that youthful alcoholism is a medical and social problem that surpasses narcotic addiction and that the potential teenage drinking problem should give far more cause for alarm than does drug addiction.

But alcohol is a drug! It is the fact that a psychoactive drug is being used in amounts and with a frequency which can result in all of the things implied in the designation as alcoholic which is significant, not simply that it is alcohol.

Virtually every survey of adolescent drug use which has included alcohol use and has inquired into outcomes indicates that some use of alcohol is almost universal, and that adolescents report more bad outcomes from both single and repeated use of alcohol than of any other drug.

Marijuana

The next most frequently and widely used non-medical drug is marijuana. Estimates as to the number of Americans who have utilized marijuana at least once range from 12 to 20 million. All surveys indicate tremendous variations from region to region, community to community. The National Institute of Mental Health has estimated (February, 1970), on the basis of all of the information available to it, that between 20 to 40 percent of all high school and college students have tried marijuana. Of this number, 65 percent had used marijuana less than ten times, 25 percent occasionally when it was available, and 10 percent as often as once a week. The most that this indicates is that between 7 and 14 percent of students find marijuana *use* (not to be necessarily equated with the effects of marijuana as a drug) rewarding enough to use it occasionally, and 2 to 4 percent gain satisfaction sufficient to use it as often as once a week—at considerable legal risk. The more challenging figure, given current societal beliefs and reactions, is the 50 to 60 percent who never try or who try and do not continue to use it.

Since marijuana is a drug, or more accurately a plant which contains a number of drugs, it is not surprising that, as is true of all drugs, excessive amounts may produce toxic reactions. Side effects may be annoying to some, harmful to others, and lead to panic reactions in the unwary.

Ups

"Ups" are primarily those drugs which are classified as stimulants. Caffeine, now institutionalized through the American breakfast, coffee break, and coffee shop, has at times in its history been illegal and painted as a villain. In amounts usually ingested, it is for most people a mild stimulant. For some, even small amounts cause sleeplessness, jitteriness, irritability, or an upset stomach. It is sold over-the-counter in concentrated form and is used in combination drugs to counteract the drowsiness which is often a side effect of a number of commonly used medications.

Various forms of amphetamines (e.g., Benzedrine, Dexedrine, Methedrine) are used both legally and illegally. They are classified as stimulants because of their action on the central nervous system. They also produce constriction of peripheral blood vessels, increase blood pressure and heart rate, relax smooth muscles of the stomach, intestines, and bladder, and suppress appetite. Which is effect and which is side effect depends on why they are taken. Because of their appetite suppressing effect they are widely used in weight reduction programs. Though perhaps helpful in temporarily suppressing appetite, they also produce feelings of energy and alertness, reduction in distractibility, relief of depression, and talkativeness in many individuals. Many who start using amphetamines for appetite reduction continue using them for these stimulant effects.

Prolonged use of amphetamines in excessively high dosages may result, in some individuals, in development of psychotic symptoms with predominance of paranoid or persecutory ideas. When injected in high doses frequently over a period of several days ("speeding") the result is long periods of activity and wakefulness during which little food is eaten. At the end of such an episode there is a "crash." This may be accompanied in some individuals by severe depression. When the response to that depression is more speed, as is often the case, a difficult and dangerous cycle may begin.

Although legally classified as a narcotic, cocaine is a stimulant. Derived from the coca leaf, it has long been used to mask hunger and fatigue and to produce feelings of energy and power. Use of cocaine has recently increased in some areas.

Downs

"Downs" are usually equated with sedatives such as the barbiturates. If classified on the basis of how those who use them feel, rather than on the basis of chemical structure or medical use, they include alcohol, barbiturates, minor tranquilizers, and the opiates. Medical and pharmacological arguments as to whether a substance is a sedative, a hypnotic, a hypnotic sedative, a depressant, or a narcotic (defined as producing sleep and stupor and relieving pain) are of little interest to the growing number of amateur pharmacologists. To them they are all Downs. The important fact is that they bring you down when you are up too high. Like alcohol, in sufficient amounts they all produce intoxication in some individuals.

It is significant that at least part of the increase in use of heroin is a result of its use to "come down" from a speed trip. It is possible that the "street pharmacology" may result in classifications of drugs which will prove more useful in terms of understanding and influencing non-medical drug use.

Contrary to popular belief, alcohol is a "downer" and, it should be noted, illegal for those under a certain age (18 or 21, depending on state laws).

LSD-like Drugs

An increasing group of substances, almost all of which were originally of plant origin, have at least one thing in common. Their major effect is to change perceptions and to dissolve, at least temporarily, habitual ways of looking at the world and at one's self. There are more scientific ways of describing them, but, again reverting to the pragmatic street pharmacology, they are good for "tripping," for exploring, for getting outside of one's self, for getting new insights, for "getting off the natural." For years prisoners have sought any means to "get off the natural," including raiding the kitchen for nutmeg.

To call these substances psychotomimetics, psychodysleptics, hallucinogens, or psychedelics is to invite argument. In some individuals under some circumstances, they result in reactions which resemble psychoses. In many individuals at some dosage levels, there are most certainly deviations from "normal" in perception and functioning which are exactly what is sought. They, like many other drugs, may produce hallucinations or pseudohallucinations in some individuals at some dosage level, but this does not help in understanding their use or their appeal. Many insist that their effects are mind-manifesting (psychedelic). To use any one of these terms involves a value judgment based, in most instances, on overgeneralization without regard for dose and for individual differences in response.

Included in this group of substances are LSD, mescaline, psilocybin, THC[9] (Δ^9-Trans-tetrahydracannabinol derived from cannabis), to mention only a few. Street pharmacologists have discovered or produced others which are primarily combinations of these with a variety of other drugs—STP, LBJ, FDA, PCP, HOG, PEACE, the list is endless. They appear, cause a flurry in establishment circles while they are analyzed, result in some sick young people, and generally go away, or, what is most alarming, go down the age scale.

Solvents

Among younger adolescents in some areas, airplane glue and a number of solvents are inhaled, primarily for their intoxicating effect. Getting drunk or feeling dizzy has always appealed to some youngsters. Alcohol has been and still is the drug of choice. Perhaps because they are easier for a youngster to obtain, perhaps because they are defined as more daring, solvents of all kinds are used for this purpose.

It is becoming increasingly academic to engage in scientific discussions of the properties and actions of any of these substances. They are available only on the black market and the only assurance that they are what they are thought to be and contain any approximation of the dose reported is what someone told someone who says so. Except for amphetamines, barbiturates, and other drugs produced legally but diverted into the illegal market there is virtually no quality control. Although mescaline would seem to be replacing LSD as a drug of choice, there is very little if any pure mescaline on the market.

BEYOND DRUGS TO PEOPLE

In order to understand current non-medical drug use it is necessary to go far beyond the cataloguing of substances (pharmacologically defined where possible), the listing of effects, and the counting of users and non-users of each. The focus must shift from drugs to people, go beyond pharmacological effects to the meaning and function of drug use. The response of society and of various social groups is crucial in determining that meaning.

Just as there is a dose response curve for drugs, there is a use response curve for drug use. This curve is also a statistical abstraction hiding tremendous individual variability, and it too has at least three critical points: initial use, continued use, and compulsive use.

Initial use has less to do with a drug and its pharmacological action than with the significance of drug use and expectations of effect. It involves an individual and his beliefs about a drug and its effects, and it involves society and how it defines that drug and its users. Reasons for experimenting include curiosity, a desire for some physical, psychological, or social change, social pressure, and communicating to friends, family, or society something about one's identity. Of significance are social definitions of drug use as adult, daring, deviant, "cool." Choice of substance is a function of availability, of beliefs about the effects, and of the status of use of the substance as socially defined.

The majority of experimenters do not become users. Curiosity is satisfied; status is gained; it did not do what it was supposed to do; it was unpleasant or frightening; it is not worth the risk.

Whether an individual continues to use a substance is determined by the degree to which it serves some personal or socially meaningful function, the degree to which its use brings about some physical, psychological, or social change, real or imagined, which is perceived as more pleasant than unpleasant, more desirable or functional than undesirable or dysfunctional. Desirable and functional need not correspond to stated social norms.

The reasons for continuing may or may not be related to reasons for trying. In the process of use, new functions of use may develop. These may lead to continued use, to intensified use, or to abandoning use. What started from curiosity may be continued because it was fun, because it provided acceptance into a group, or because it made one feel better.

The majority of users remain at the moderate level, using moderately and on "appropriate" occasions, as in the case of alcohol. They are able to enjoy whatever benefits they find and avoid the hazards of excessive amounts and frequency of use. For them their drug use does not become a central factor in their lives.

When use goes beyond moderate in amount and frequency and appropriate in occasion, two factors become crucial. The first is the centrality of the function served by the drug use and the second involves characteristics of the particular substance used. Drug use which serves an important function for a given individual usually requires repeated use since its effects are necessarily temporary and in most instances do nothing more than produce a temporary change. Relief of persisting pain, anxiety, or depression, escape from unpleasant realities, avoidance of painful experiences, support of a social role or identity, or any of the central personal and social functions drug use can appear to serve, require continued drug use.   ? physiological dependence.

Some drugs, notably opiates, alcohol, barbiturates, amphetamines, and nicotine, produce tolerance. With repeated frequent use, increasing amounts are required to produce the same effect. Not only do these drugs produce tolerance but, if used in sufficient amounts with sufficient frequency over a long enough period of time, they produce physiological dependence. The drug must be used to feel normal and to avoid being physically ill. The amount, frequency, and length of use necessary to produce physiological dependence varies with the drug and with the individual.

Physical and psychological dependence on a drug which at best provides temporary relief of symptoms or escape from reality, especially if that drug is illegal and expensive, is

after moderate
centrality + characteristics

good for neither the individual nor society. But relatively few who use it become dependent in this sense.

THE REAL DRUG PROBLEM

Historically, the use of drugs outside of medicine has served to explain all manner of social deviance. In the process it has become a symbol and a means of communicating deviance. As such it can also serve as a badge and a rallying point for groups that wish to proclaim their deviance. A number of different groups have adopted drug use both as a rationale for particular subcultures and as a response to the problems encountered in being deviant.

LSD was not what Timothy Leary and the League for Spiritual Discovery were all about. The League was a direct attack on majority values which were considered to be hypocritical. Marijuana was not what the hippies were all about. The original hippie movement was a rebellion against and a retreat from a dominant society which, in their eyes, was not living according to the values it proclaimed.

Man has always sought chemical comforts. Which chemical for which discomfort has varied from time to time and from place to place. Until recently, on balance, man has mostly used the chemical comforts with reasonable intelligence, in moderate amounts, and on appropriate occasions, in order to make life more pleasant, to feel better, to relieve temporary malaise, to facilitate social activity, and to solidify groups. He probably always will. But something new has been added. Technology has produced a bewildering array of new and complex drugs specifically fashioned to do particular things. When these drugs are used to prevent or to cure states agreed upon as disease we hail them. When they produce side effects which for some become main effects, i.e., sought in their own right, we become uneasy. When they are used to change mood or modify behavior, to get high, to improve memory, to reduce aggression, to make the unruly manageable, serious questions are raised.

According to what criteria are effects to be judged acceptable or unacceptable? Is it desirable to improve memory or intelligence, to reduce aggression? Who shall decide, the individual or society? Who within society? Who shall decide which drugs shall be developed for which purposes? These questions are already with us and are at the heart of the current "drug problem."

In order to approach an intelligent consideration of these issues there must be an understanding of what drugs are and how they act, what drugs do and what people do, the complex personal factors which influence the outcomes of drug use, the role of society's definition of and response to any particular drug use by any particular group in determining the nature and extent of the outcomes of that use. As the nature of the biochemical organism is better understood, and it will be, and as the relationship of biochemical changes to changes in behavior is pursued, and it is being pursued, the nature and range of possible behavior modification will be expanded and the challenges increased.

SUMMARY

Some of man's chemical comforts are called drugs, some are not; some are illegal and some are legal. Regardless of label or of legal status, all are drugs and all act according to the same basic principles. The effects of all are a function of complex interactions between an amount and pattern of use of the substance and the individual, physiologically, psychologically, and socially defined. The meaning and function, real or imagined, that effect and use of a drug serve for a given individual or group of individuals determine to a major degree the substance used, the pattern and frequency of use, and the outcomes of use. Meaning and function may be determined by either personal or social factors.

Drugs currently in use, both legally and illegally, are primarily Ups, Downs, or any of a variety of substances which change perceptions of the self or of the social or physical environment. Choice of substance is a function of the individual's reasons for use and his beliefs about the effectiveness of a given substance in relation to those reasons. Amount and pattern of use are more important than the mere fact of use. Distinctions must be made at least among experimenters, regular users, and compulsive users. The definition of each will vary from substance to substance.

All drugs involve risks at some dosage level, in some people, under some circumstances. The real question is: How much risk should be tolerated for what benefit and who should decide? This is a question of values, not of drugs.

REFERENCES

The New York Times, July 31, 1970.
NIMH Report, February 1970.

21

Marihuana and Health:
Summary of Findings*

NATIONAL INSTITUTE OF MENTAL HEALTH

During the year since submission to the Congress of the first annual report on Marihuana and Health our knowledge of this complex issue has been significantly advanced in almost all aspects. We have a far better picture of the extent of present usage in the United States, of the basic nature of the material. Much of the essential basic research on short-term effects in animal and man has been done. Well controlled studies of more extensive human use in a laboratory setting are underway and two overseas studies of long-term, chronic users are nearing completion. Nevertheless, even as the extent of the problem has grown so has our awareness of its complexity and of the difficulties of studying it.

In this summary of the second annual report we will attempt to describe the present state of our knowledge, to summarize the progress made in the past year and to again translate the disparate and necessarily technical data into as reasonable an answer as possible to the question: What are the health implications of marihuana use for the American people?

Despite the advances of the past year, any simple answer to this disarmingly simple question is not likely to be possible now or in the near future. It is increasingly apparent that any satisfactory answer will have to take into account the many contexts of use, the purposes of use, the age, sex, physical, and psychological characteristics of the user, the material, its dosage and frequency of use, the route of use, etc. Even in assessing the immediate effects of marihuana on mental or physical performance it has become increasingly apparent that effects can vary greatly depending on the complexity of the task, the expectations of the user, the cultural context of use, user motivation, and the stage and level of intoxication of the user.

EXTENT, PATTERNS, AND SOCIAL CONTEXT OF USE IN THE UNITED STATES

Much additional data has been gathered with respect to the extent of American marihuana use since last reporting. Nationwide studies of high school and college level youth have reported preliminary findings and there is now data on use in the general population and among employed groups. As use in the United States has increased, increasing sophistication is being shown in assessing such use. Researchers are going considerably beyond the oversimplified question, "Have you ever used marihuana?" to inquire into the frequency of use, the level of use and the circumstances surrounding use. We are more confident that data is reported with reasonable consistency although more needs to be done to correlate reported use with actual use.

---

*From *Marihuana and Health.* Second Annual Report to Congress, Washington, D.C.: U.S. Government Printing Office, 1972.

There is every indication that use has increased and is very widespread. In teenage and young adult groups use is very extensive; in some groups as high as 90 percent have used marihuana at some time. Even among young people, however, use is by no means evenly distributed in all areas of the country. For example, one national survey reveals that among persons 18–29 years there is three times the percentage (over a third of the total age group) who "have used" in the West as compared with the other regions of the country sampled.

Among a still younger age group, the 12–17 year olds, a nationwide study has indicated that nearly one in four in the West has used the drug, a slightly lower percentage in the northeast and more than one in ten "have used" in other parts of the country. It is noteworthy in all studies that where the percentage of those who "have ever used" is large, so too is the percentage who make regular use of marihuana.

Based on converging evidence from several recent surveys, we estimate the total number in the United States who have ever used marihuana to be 15 to 20 million. A very recently released National Commission on Marihuana and Drug Abuse survey has estimated that the total number at present may well exceed 24 million. Exact figures, of course, depend heavily on the date of the survey, the methodology employed and the underlying statistical assumptions which are made. Estimates may thus be expected to vary considerably from survey to survey depending on all these aspects. While many people experiment and do not continue, over half are estimated to use the drug one or more times per month. About one in four of those who use that often do so three times a week or more. Since users fall heavily into the teenage, young adult group, we are talking principally about youth. It should be emphasized that even among youth, however, there is considerable variation from school to school. High school rates of having ever used range from as low as five percent to as high as 90 percent.

Last year it was noted that one northern California county that might be a bellwether of marihuana use more generally had experienced a leveling off of drug use among high school students during the preceding year. The most recent annual survey of student use in this county now indicates sizable increases, especially in marihuana use, at all grade levels. About half "had used" at some time in the year. On the senior high level at the time of the survey (late spring, 1971) a third to a half of those who reported having used marihuana in the preceding school year had used it fifty or more times during the year. Even among junior high students in this high-use county, a third to a half of the users had done so ten or more times (13–29 percent had used at some point in the year).

Studies indicate that among college students 31 percent had reported having used marihuana by 1970. During 1971 this figure increased to 44 percent of the total college group. Even among four medical schools surveyed from one on six to seven out of ten students had tried marihuana with as many as nearly half in one school currently using.

Several studies suggest, not unexpectedly, that the more psychologically disturbed or socially unstable are more likely to make regular, heavy use of marihuana. School dropouts are more likely to be using marihuana as are those from disturbed families.

While the amount of data on minority group use is small, at least one study of Mexican-American youth in California suggests that among that group use was no higher than among high school youth in California generally.

Much remains to be learned about the relationship of drug use to vocational adjustment and job performance. One study conducted in New York State showed wide variation in the percentage of those in various occupations who had made use of marihuana one or more times per month. The range was from one in seven sales workers who had used it to no reported use among the farmers sampled. Among regular users who actually used marihuana on the job, nearly half of those who had used and were employed in sales had smoked at work. About a fifth of those users in professional and managerial occupations had done so, but only 3 percent of those users employed in service and protective work had ever made use of marihuana in the work situation. There is no evidence in this study bearing on the issue of work effectiveness or industrial safety as related to drug use.

While heavier marihuana use is clearly associated with the use of other drugs as well—those who use it regularly are far more likely than nonusers to have experimented with other illicit drugs—there is no evidence that the drug itself "causes" such use. More frequent users are likely to find drug use appealing or to spend time with others who do so or in settings where other drugs are readily available. Marihuana use does not appear to have a casual role in the commission of crimes. . . .

PRECLINICAL RESEARCH IN ANIMALS

Animal research, generally supported by limited clinical observation in humans, has clearly established that the margin of safety with cannabis and its synthetic psychoactive ingredient THC (delta-9-tetrahydrocannabinol) is very high. This work on the toxicology of the substances has laid the groundwork for the systematic study of more extended periods of carefully controlled administration in humans.

Work in animals has also shown that cannabis and its original constituents are rapidly transformed in the body into metabolites which are persistently present for several days. The implications of this persistence are unclear although it is possible that these metabolites may affect the later use of further amounts of cannabis or interact with other drugs taken in presently unknown ways. It may also be that it is the metabolites rather than the original drug constituents which are responsible for the drug's effects. Improved knowledge of the chemistry of these bio-transformation products may provide the key to a relatively simple test of the fact and level of marihuana intoxication. Persistence of these products may also permit detection of previous intoxication days after the initial event.

Studies of the distribution of the drug, radioactively labelled, have shown that its metabolites tend to concentrate in areas of the brain related to those functions affected by the drug. Despite this gross correspondence of drug concentration to brain function, much still remains to be learned about the specific mode of action of marihuana.

TOLERANCE

The issue of tolerance to cannabis has been an object of considerable discussion. By tolerance is meant a need which develops over a time, as a result of repeated use, for increasing quantities of a drug to produce a similar effect. Users have frequently reported that those who are experienced require smaller amounts of cannabis to achieve the same effect than do novices. This so-called "reverse tolerance" is an effect unlike that of most other drugs. Whether this reverse tolerance is based on metabolic and distribution changes after repeated use or is the result of a learning process has not yet been determined.

Reports from countries where use is traditional suggest a level of use that would be highly unpleasant for the inexperienced user. This suggests that tolerance, at least for the effects which are perceived subjectively as unpleasant, does develop. Whatever the subjective impressions of drug effects, it seems clear that experienced marihuana users can also tolerate larger doses in the sense that disruption of their performance on various intellectual, perceptual and psychomotor tasks is less than for the inexperienced.

In animals, for the most part, the evidence is clear that tolerance to certain effects of cannabis develops. It has been found in most species tested and is large. It is noteworthy, however, that in animals as well as humans tolerance may develop for some aspects of the drug's effects but not for others. Whatever the ultimate resolution of the tolerance question, it appears unlikely that in man a degree of tolerance comparable to that for opiates will be found.

EFFECTS IN MAN

Research of the past year has underscored the necessity of taking into account multiple aspects of the individual and the drug taking situation in evaluating marihuana's effects. These include such varied aspects as the characteristics of the material itself, the dose and route of administration, the individual's metabolic rate, his prior experience with the drug, his set (personal expectations) and the setting in which the drug is used.

While there is little doubt that the major psychoactive ingredient in marihuana is delta-9-THC, there is still considerable uncertainty regarding the biologic activity of the many other marihuana constituents. Of the two usual ways in which marihuana is consumed by man, smoking is by far the more common in the United States. As compared to eating the material, smoking results in considerably more rapid absorption, with the onset of effects typically occurring within a few minutes. The quantity required for a given effect is significantly smaller when smoked and since the onset is rapid, the user can more readily control the drug's effects than if the drug is eaten. By contrast, when consumed orally it may require from a half to over two hours to feel the drug's effects which tend to peak later and to persist longer. In experimental studies with humans, it has become increasingly apparent that in the use of the synthetic THC the choice of the substance in which to administer the material orally makes a substantial difference in how rapidly and completely the THC itself is absorbed.

Experienced users appear to metabolize the drug more rapidly than do less experienced although the exact significance of this is unclear. It may partially explain the greater sensitivity or "reverse tolerance" that users have reported. Much remains to be done to clarify some of the implications of cannabis metabolism in man.

By now the acute effects of marihuana have been generally well elucidated. Subjective effects are highly variable partly depending on the user's expectations and the setting in which he consumes the drug. Experienced users report such subjective effects as: an awareness of subtlety of meaning in sight and sound and an increasing vividness of such experiences. Frequently users report enhanced sensations of touch, taste and smell. Alteration of time perspective with an apparent slowing down of the time sense is almost universally reported. A sense of enhanced social awareness is often reported with low dosages, but at higher levels this is apparently diminished and there may be social withdrawal. Although emotional reactions reported by regular users are usually pleasant, one in five experienced users in one study reported having at times experienced temporarily overwhelming negative feelings.

Several studies have underscored the critical role of attitude and expectation in determining effects at least at low to moderate dosage levels. Such expectations can result in the individual having subjective reactions to an inactive material that are similar or identical to the active drug.

The two most consistent physiological effects of marihuana continue to be an increase in pulse rate and a characteristic reddening of the eyes. The latter occurs even with oral dosages, indicating that it is not primarily the result of smoke irritation. Although marihuana users, frequently report substantially increased hunger at the time of use, there is no evidence that marihuana lowers blood sugar. It may be that the effects on appetite are an indirect result of an enhancement of the subjective sense of taste leading in some to increased food consumption.

Neurological correlates of marihuana use seem minimal although it is possible that marihuana-induced drowsiness may obscure small drug-related effects on the electroencephalograph. There is some EEG evidence that tends to objectively confirm the report of users that they have an enhanced ability to ignore outside stimuli while high.

Effects on Intellectual and Psychomotor Performance

More recent findings continue to confirm earlier reported observations that acute marihuana intoxication causes a deterioration in intellectual and psychomotor performance which is heavily dose-related as well as dependent on the complexity of the task. The more complex and demanding the task, the greater is the deterioration in performance. When alcohol and marihuana are consumed together the decrement in performance is greater than when either is used alone. To some degree at least, experienced users seem better able to compensate for part of the effect of marihuana than do inexperienced users.

Marihuana clearly has an acute effect on short term memory, a fact which has now been confirmed by many investigators. One explanation for this impairment is that the drug reduces the ability to concentrate while intoxicated, preventing the implicit rehearsal that may be essential to remembering newly acquired information.

Driver Performance

Driver Performance has been of considerable research interest and such research is continuing. There is, however, increased reason for believing a motorist's performance is significantly impaired by marihuana intoxication.

Although initial research suggested relatively slight impairment of performance on a driver simulator, more recent work suggests that this may not be the case. An increase in time required for braking has been reported as has a marked increase in glare recovery time which persists for several hours following intoxication. Research on driving tasks more closely resembling actual driving conditions is going on. Such studies seek to more accurately specify the degree of impairment likely under varying conditions. It should be noted that the performance of a highly motivated test subject under laboratory conditions may be considerably less impaired than that of a driver functioning under more typical driving conditions. Under usual driving circumstances multiple distractions are common and the driver may be less motivated. The possibility of a spontaneous recurrence of an earlier drug experience (a so-called "flashback"), related to the use of marihuana and other hallucinogens and which interfered with driving, has been raised by some case reports. Evidence for the frequency of such phenomena in this or other contexts is generally lacking.

Acute Physical Toxicity

Death from an overdose of cannabis is apparently extremely rare and difficult to confirm. This is consistent with animal data which indicates the margin of safety with cannabis or its synthetic equivalents is quite high. Nausea, dizziness and a heavy drugged feeling have been reported usually as a result of an inadvertent overdose. There have, however, been a number of cases of acute collapse following an attempt to inject marihuana intravenously or some preparation made from it. It is not clear whether these were the result of an acute overdose of cannabis constituents *per se* or a combination of other factors related to the injection process. In view of the hazards, such intravenous use seems especially dangerous. While there has been one case report of epileptic seizures temporally related to marihuana use, there have been other past reports of the efficacy of cannabis as an anti-seizure medication in children. In general, it appears that acute toxic physical reactions to marihuana are relatively rare.

Chronic Physical Effects

Frequent, relatively heavy use of cannabis is still rather uncommon in the United States. Thus, observations on the implications of such use are derived from cultures very different from our own. The marked differences in diet, living standards including level of medical care and in patterns of use make it difficult to apply overseas observations to our own domestic situation. Nevertheless, such observations may provide valuable clues to the possible implications of American use and, when combined with the results of other research, may be quite valuable.

While respiratory complaints have long been reported as a result of cannabis use, it is not always certain to what degree this is the result of the drug or the tobacco with which it is frequently mixed. In an American military sample of heavy hashish smokers, complaints of bronchitis, asthma, and nose and throat inflammation were common and reported to improve upon discontinuing the drug. While there have been reports of impaired liver function as well, upon closer examination these seemed to be more closely related to alcohol use than to cannabis use.

Blood circulatory difficulties in the legs have been reported in a North African sample of users, as have arterial changes among some young multiple drug users in the United States, but the role of cannabis in these is still unclear.

There has also been a report of slurred speech, staggering gait, hand tremors and difficulties in depth perception in a few adolescent patients, but the exact significance is difficult to evaluate since these patients were also using other drugs.

One of the most serious reports is a recent one based on some very recent British work which, using radiographic techniques, found evidence of cerebral atrophy in ten young cannabis smokers. However, some researchers have questioned where such techniques can be used to demonstrate cerebral atrophy. Unfortunately, the subjects were multiple drug users, with 8 out of 10 admitting to the use of amphetamines a drug which some reports have implicated in organic brain changes. The comparison group was not altogether appropriate and thus the role of cannabis remains uncertain. Because of the seriousness of the finding, however, this work will be followed up by careful animal research as well as further clinical studies to explore this serious possibility. The authors themselves caution against overinterpretation of their work and emphasize the need for additional research.

Preliminary findings of a study of 31 male chronic hashish users in Greece and of a similarly sized Jamaican sample of intensively studied cannabis users are noteworthy for the relative absence of pathology in these chronic using groups. It should, however, be emphasized that the samples are small and the data are preliminary. Given the small size of the samples, rarer or less obvious consequences of use may be missed. Larger scale epidemiological studies of chronic users are planned to overcome the limitations of smaller pilot efforts.

Genetics and Birth Defects

Among the most serious consequences that might ensue from the use of any drug are persistent changes in the genetic heritage of users or the production of birth anomalies as a result of drug use by parents. The amount of evidence bearing on this question is modest. What work has been done has found little evidence of chromosomal abnormalities in marihuana users as compared to matching nonuser controls. With respect to birth defects that might be the result of maternal cannabis use during pregnancy, there have been several case reports but it is impossible to be certain whether there is a differential rate of such defects between users and nonusers. It is known that in animals THC can cross the placental barrier and enter fetal circulation. Once again it must be emphasized that the potential seriousness of the effect makes the use of marihuana (or other drugs) of unknown potential for producing birth defects unwise. This is especially true for women during their reproductive years.

Cannabis and Psychiatric Illness

Any discussion of the relationship of cannabis use to psychiatric illness must take into account the formidable difficulties of establishing the role of any drug as a causal factor in mental illness. It is typically extremely difficult to separate the role of the drug from the many other factors that may play a role in the etiology of a specific disorder. In addition, in those countries in which chronic cannabis use is common, epidemiological surveys are virtually nonexistent and adequate diagnostic evaluation is more often the exception than the rule. As a result, the diagnosis of cannabis psychosis may be used as a catchall description for all those with a known history of cannabis use who are also emotionally disturbed. Finally, we are aware that non-drug factors such as the pre-existing psychological state of the user and the circumstances surrounding use can be of fundamental importance in determining the user's response to the drug.

Cannabis psychosis has been used as a diagnosis for many years in countries in which cannabis use is traditional. During the nineteenth century, it was popularly believed in India that marihuana produced mental illness. The Indian Hemp Commission, upon learning that such a diagnosis was frequently based on the impressions of laymen, did a careful analysis of its own and concluded that drug use was a factor in no more than between seven and thirteen percent of admissions to Indian mental hospitals. In other countries estimates of the percentage of admissions that are cannabis related range from 2 to 3 percent in South Africa to as high as 17 percent in Morocco. In most reports, it is simply impossible to distinguish between illness resulting primarily from toxic effects of cannabis and an aggravation of a previously existing serious mental disturbance.

Diagnosis is typically most heavily based on a history of drug use although attempts have been made to take into consideration the duration of the illness and its failure to develop into a long lasting schizophrenic picture. Symptoms which have been emphasized in the Eastern literature have included: acute or subacute onset of confusion, visual and auditory hallucinations and paranoid ideation sometimes accompanied by agitation and aggression.

In the 1930s, toxic psychoses were reported among some marihuana users who were described as recovering in a few days. During the experimental phase of the investigation conducted by the La Guardia Commission, psychotic episodes were reported by one in nine of the 77 subjects studied. Beginning in the late 1960s there has been a spate of reports of adverse psychological consequences of use on the United States. Unfortunately, few of these provide any indication of how frequently such reactions occur in a large population of users. A wide range of symptoms have been reported, most more nearly resembling a panic state than full-blown mental illness. There is, however, little question that given a sufficiently high dose, hallucinations and delusions can occur. While such adverse psychological reactions are more common with the inexperienced and when inadvertently high doses are ingested, they occasionally occur even with low doses. Reports typically are of individuals who have sought treatment for their difficulties and it is usually difficult to be sure how much of the pathology displayed is the result of previously existing personality problems rather than "caused" by marihuana use. There is some evidence that when a sample of frequent marihuana users is matched with their non-using friends, the amount of psychiatric symptomatology found in both groups is greater than in youth generally. This suggests that heavy marihuana users may be drawn from a population with an above average amount of pre-existing psychopathology. Thus, use, especially in association with other drugs, may more typically aggravate already existing psychiatric problems rather than in itself causing such illness.

There have been a number of reports on adverse psychiatric reactions to marihuana use in Vietnam among American troops. Onset was usually acute and, again, the reports suggest that pre-existing pathology is an important non-drug factor. Almost certainly many of those most attracted to drug use are individuals who have personality problems. In some cases, the drug is sought with a conscious hope that it will be psychotherapeutic.

While marihuana use has been widely described in the Eastern literature and to some extent more recently in the West as resulting in a loss of motivation, the question of its role in the process is still unresolved. Many of those most attracted to its use are "amotivated" by conventional standards. The time and effort required to obtain drug supplies and use them may also further erode the expression of more conventional motivation. There is also the definite possibility that the drug and the personality of the user interact in such a way to further intensify the loss of conventional motivation.

THERAPEUTIC USES OF CANNABIS

While use of cannibis is not a medically accepted mode of treatment for any illness in the United States today, the drug has had an ancient tradition of medical use. Even today in much of the world where Western medical practice has made only modest inroads, cannabis retains an important role in self-medication and in folk or native medicine. The range of diseases and other medical conditions for which it has been and continues to be used is very long. For much of the nineteenth century and well into the twentieth, cannabis was a recognized part of the physician's armamentarium against illness although its lack of water solubility and its variable potency were problems. Gradually, it was supplanted in Western medicine by drugs that were more consistent in their effects or more conveniently used. Since most of the early reports of use were clinical case reports rather than drug tests conducted under carefully controlled conditions, the relevance of this older literature to potential modern use is questionable.

During the early 1940s the development of "Synhexyl," a drug clinically related to marihuana, generated some interest in medical uses. Some attempts were made to use it in the treatment of depression, the treatment of alcoholism and in preventing epileptic seizures. Results of these limited studies were reported to be generally favorable. Some later research demonstrated that cannabis preparations had an antibacterial action in the treatment of dermatological conditions as well as in the treatment of otitis and sinusitis.

More recently, with the increase in illicit use and the development of a synthetic form of

THC, there has been a revival of interest in potential therapeutic uses. In addition to the experimental uses reported in last year's report, there has been a continued interest in the drug's possible therapeutic value in the treatment of depression and in the possible development of an antihypertensive agent. Most recently, it has been found that marihuana reduces intraocular pressure. This observation holds forth the promise that cannabis or some chemically related synthetic may prove useful in the treatment of glaucoma. With the greatly expanded research effort into marihuana and related synthetic materials, there is a strong possibility that cannabis derivatives, very possibly in chemically modified form, will once again achieve medical acceptance in the treatment of a variety of conditions.

FUTURE RESEARCH DIRECTIONS

As our knowledge of the properties of marihuana and related materials has expanded so has our awareness of the many questions that require answers in assessing the health implications of their use. The overall question of what dosages, frequency and duration of use are clearly likely to be injurious to health in various groups remains unresolved.

Because the material in its natural state is quite variable, more needs to be learned about it since the implications of use for different types of marihuana may not be the same. The mode of actions of the drug and its many components needs to be elucidated. Little, for example, is presently known about the effects of marihuana on the biochemistry of the brain.

The whole question of interaction between marihuana use and that of other drugs is an important one. Some of the reports of adverse effects may be the consequence of multiple drug use in which one or more other psychoactive drugs in combination with cannabis are more injurious in combination than alone.

The recent report of brain atrophy possibly related to marihuana use needs to be carefully followed up in animals and further clinical studies. Adequate assessment of the psychiatric risks of use require that we do better epidemiological studies to determine the incidence of the adverse consequences that have been reported to date. It would be especially valuable to know the extent to which such adverse consequences occur in those without evident pre-existing psychopathology.

The limitations of relatively small scale, intensive studies of chronic users require that we do more extensive studies of larger populations in order to determine what, if any, are implications of use that may otherwise go undetected. We know, for example, that some of the most serious effects of other drugs (e.g. tobacco and birth control pills) in widespread use would not have been determined but for larger scale study of their use.

Present longitudinal studies of American users should be expanded to determine the longer term implications of use that may not be evident over a shorter time span. Although there is some reason to suspect that many young people, for example, modify their patterns and level of use of marihuana over time, we know little about the factors that influence changes or what changes typically occur.

While we know something about the social conditions of use much more should be learned about the social reinforcements of use—i.e. what are the factors in the user's relationship to others that tend to foster beginning use and to perpetuate various patterns of use.

More needs to be learned about the implications of use for such areas as the operation of motor vehicles, traffic accidents and industrial safety and performance. The economic implications of use should also be explored.

Studies of cultures other than our own may be useful in improving our social means of control not only of marihuana but of other drugs as well.

The extent of need for and the most effective means of treatment for the heavy user of cannabis needs to be explored, since it is evident that with a general increase in the numbers who have ever used has also come a significant expansion in the number who use extensively.

Finally, preliminary indications of possible therapeutic implications for the use of cannabis or its derivatives require careful exploration.

22

LSD-25 Effects on Chromosomes:
A Review*

JOSÉ EGOZCUE and SAMUEL IRWIN

Following the first observation in 1967 of chromosomal damage induced by LSD-25, the scientific community divided itself over the validity and the medical implications of that observation. The many issues surrounding the genetic effects of LSD, including the consequences of the drug's use during pregnancy, have yet to be resolved. What follows is a brief review of the major and more recent developments in the field that attempts to bring the issues and data into a more critical focus.

In 1967, Cohen and his colleagues[7] reported that LSD-25 caused chromosomal damage to human leukocytes *in vitro.* Shortly afterwards, Irwin and Egozcue[20] described chromosomal damage in the leukocytes of LSD users. Several earlier reports had shown hereditary syndromes exhibiting such increased chromosomal aberrations to be correlated with an increased incidence of cancer and leukemia[4–5, 14–16, 26–27, 30, 32]. This suggested that the use of LSD might similarly result in an increased incidence of neoplasia and leukemia among its users. The presence of chromosomal aberrations in LSD users was later confirmed by several investigators[1, 8, 10, 19]; negative results have been reported by others[24, 29].

The possibility that LSD might produce congenital malformations was raised not only by the presence of chromosomal breaks in users of the drug, but by the presence of chromosomal aberrations in some children exposed to the drug *in utero* [8, 10] and by reports of malformations induced by LSD in experimental animals[2, 3, 13]. Since then, the results in experimental animals have been questioned by Warkany and Takacs[31] and by Fabro and Sieber[12]. Reports of malformations in humans[17, 33] based on LSD consumption by the mothers of two malformed children have also been questioned, but such reports cannot be ignored.

CHROMOSOMAL BREAKAGE IN SOMATIC TISSUES

In spite of some negative reports[24, 29] the weight of evidence suggests that LSD can and does produce chromosomal aberrations in *circulating blood cells* [1, 7–10, 18–20, 23, 25, 33]. Since the first studies were conducted in individuals who ingested illicit LSD[8, 10, 20], it seemed possible that impurities in the LSD might be responsible for the chromosomal breaks[10]. However, studies *in vitro* and *in vivo* with pure LSD, using human[7] and

---

*From Egozcue, J. and Irwin, S., *Journal of Psychedelic Drugs*, 1970, **3**, 10–12. Copyright © 1970 by the Student Association for the Study of Hallucinogens. Reprinted by permission of the Student Association for the Study of Hallucinogens, and Dr. Egozcue.

Macaca mulatta [11] blood cells, showed that pure LSD could produce chromosomal breaks in circulating leukocytes.

Studies in mice [11, 22] indicated that bone marrow was not affected, although Cohen and Mukherjee [6] reported positive results. That bone marrow is probably not affected in humans is supported by the findings of Hungerford and his colleagues [19] who found that the increase in chromosomal breaks in patients treated with LSD disappeared in a few months. On the other hand, studies in children exposed to the drug *in utero* [8, 10] showed that chromosomal aberrations could be found in circulating blood cells as late as $2\frac{1}{2}$ years after exposure to the drug. The preference of LSD for producing damage in circulating blood cells is supported by the fact that rhesus macaques (*Macaca mulatta*) treated with LSD did not show an increase in chromosomal breaks in other tissues while chromosome damage in their circulating leukocytes increased [11]. LSD-induced breaks in skin fibroblasts were reported by Abbo and his co-workers [1].

CHROMOSOMAL BREAKAGE IN GERM TISSUES

Studies of LSD's effect on germinal cells have been conducted only in experimental animals, and the results are far from conclusive. While two studies found an increase in chromosomal anomalies in male mice treated with 25 micrograms per kilogram [6] and 1 milligram per kilogram [28] of LSD, Jagiello and Polani [22] could not find such anomalies in male and female mice treated with doses of the drug as high as 1 milligram per kilogram. Our own study [11] in male mice treated with up to 60 micrograms per kilogram of LSD was also negative, as were our studies with monkeys (*Macaca mulatta*) given weekly doses of 40 micrograms per kilogram orally for 4 weeks. The only human study of LSD and germ cells, published by Hulten and his colleagues [18] also reported negative findings.

CONGENITAL MALFORMATIONS

The capacity of LSD to produce congenital malformations has not been well established. While Alexander and co-workers [2], Auerbach and Rugowski [3] and Geber [13] were able to produce stunted growth and a number of malformations in mice, rats and hamsters, negative results were reported in rats by Warkany and Takacs [31], and in rabbits by Fabro and Sieber [12]. The two cases of malformations described in humans [17, 33] failed to establish a clear relationship between use of the drug and the production of malformations. Jacobson [21] reported brain and skull defects rarely observed otherwise in 4 of 14 therapeutically aborted fetuses of LSD-using mothers, and alluded to a higher incidence of spontaneous abortions. However, no one to date has conclusively proven that any birth defect is directly attributable to parental use of LSD.

CONCLUSIONS

Although a large number of studies have been devoted to the possible production of chromosomal aberrations by LSD, clear-cut answers have not been forthcoming. The existing evidence strongly suggests that LSD can and does produce chromosomal aberrations in circulating leukocytes of users, of some patients treated with the pure drug and of children exposed to the drug *in utero*. Without corresponding aberrations in the bone marrow, however, chromosomal changes in circulating leukocytes are unlikely to have any serious medical consequences. Regarding meiotic chromosomes, the varied results obtained may be due to differences in sensitivity of the strains of mice used in the experiments. Our own experiments in monkeys were negative, but one cannot extrapolate safely from animals to man. The only published meiotic study in humans was negative. Yet, even if a chemical causes no gross chromosome abnormalities, it may still produce gene or point mutations in the chromosomes of somatic or germinal cells. The production of these phenomena by LSD remains to be demonstrated. An unusually high incidence of spontaneous abortions, miscarriages or stillbirths among pregnant LSD-users could be evidence of such mutations. It may also be related to the uterine-specific actions of lysergic acid and its derivatives. For the time being, it seems wiser to maintain a wait-and-see attitude.

REFERENCES

1. Abbo, G., Norris, A., & Zellweger, H. Lysergic acid diethylamide (LSD-25) and chromosome breaks. *Humangenetik*, 1968, **6**, 253–258.
2. Alexander, G. J., Miles, B. E., Gold, G. M., & Alexander, R. B. LSD injection early in pregnancy produces abnormalities in offspring of rats. *Science*, 1967, **157**, 459–460. (L7. D34)
3. Auerbach, R., & Rugowski, J. A. Lysergic acid diethylamide: Effect on embryos. *Science*, 1967, **157**, 1325–1326. (L7. D18)
4. Bloom, G. E., Warner, S., Gerald, P. S., & Diamond, L. K. Chromosome abnormalities in constitutional aplastic anemia. *New. Eng. J. Med.*, 1966, **274**, 8–14.
5. Buckton, K. E., Jacobs, P. A., Court Brown, W. M., & Doll, R. Study of chromosome damage persisting after X-ray therapy for ankylosing spondylitis. *Lancet*, 1962, **2**, 676–682.
6. Cohen, M. M., & Mukerjee, A. B. Meiotic chromosome damage induced by LSD-25. *Nature*, 1968, **219**, 1072–1074. (L7. D48)
7. Cohen, M. M., Marinello, M. J., & Back, N. Chromosomal damage in human leukocytes induced by lysergic acid diethylamide. *Science*, 1967, **157**, 1417–1419. (L7. D15)
8. Cohen, M. M., Hirschhorn, K., & Frosch, W. A. In vivo and in vitro chromosomal damage induced by LSD-25. *New Eng. J. Med.*, 1967, **277**, 1043–1049. (L7. D26)
9. Egozcue, J., & Fowlis, M. J. Transporte placentario de la d-dietilamida del acido lisergico (LSD-25). *Acta Obst. Ginec. Hisp. Lus.*, 1969, **2**, 135–146.
10. Egozcue, J., Irwin, S., & Maruffo, C. A. Chromosomal damage in LSD users. *J.A.M.A.*, 1968, **204**, 214–218. (L7. D37)
11. Egozcue, J., & Irwin, S. Effect of LSD-25 on mitotic and meiotic chromosomes of mice and monkeys. *Humangenetik*, 1969, **8**, 86–93. (L7. Q128)
12. Fabro, S. & Sieber, S. M. Is lysergide a teratogen? *Lancet*, 1968, **1**, 639.
13. Geber, W. F. Congenital malformations induced by mescaline, lysergic acid diethylamide and bromolysergic acid in the hamster. *Science*, 1967, **158**, 265–267. (H3. D3)
14. German, J., Archibald, R., & Bloom, D. Chromosomal breakage in a rare and probably genetically determined syndrome of man. *Science*, 1965, **148**, 506–507.
15. German, J., & Grippa, L. P. Chromosomal breakage in diplid cell lines from Bloom's syndrome and Fanconi's anemia. *Ann. Genet.*, 1966, **9**, 143–154.
16. Hecht, F., Koler, F. D., Rigas, D. A., Dahnke, G. S., Case, M. P., Tisdale, V., & Miller, R. W. Leukemia and lymphocytes in ataxia-telangiectasia. *Lancet*, 1966, **2**, 1193.
17. Hecht, F., Beals, R. K., Lees, M. H., Jolly, H., & Roberts, P. Lysergic acid diethylamide and cannabis as possible teratogens in man. *Lancet*, 1968, **2**, 1087. (H3. Q19)
18. Hulten, M., Lindsten, J., Lidberg, L., & Ekelund, H. Studies on mitotic and meiotic chromosomes in subjects exposed to LSD. *Ann. Genet.*, 1968, **11**, 201–210.
19. Hungerford, D. A., Taylor, K. M., Shagass, C., LaBadie, G., Balaban, G. B., & Paton, G. R. Cytogenic effects of LSD-25 therapy in man. *J.A.M.A.*, 1968, **206**, 2287–2291. (L7. Q15)

20. Irwin, S., & Egozcue, J. Chromosomal abnormalities in leukocytes from LSD-25 users. *Science*, 1967, **157**, 313–314. (L7. Q37)

21. Jacobson, C. B. Chemical mutagens—An expanding roster of suspects. *Chem. Eng. News*, 1969, **47**, 54–68.

22. Jagiello, G., & Polani, P. E. Mouse germ cells and LSD-25. *Cytogenetics*, 1969, **8**, 136–147.

23. Kato, T., & Jarvik, L. F. LSD-25 and genetic damage. *Dis. Nerv. Syst.*, 1969, **30**, 42–46. (L7. D67)

24. Loughman, W. D., Sargent, T. W., & Israelstam, D. M. Leukocytes of humans exposed to lysergic acid diethylamide: Lack of chromosomal damage. *Science*, 1967, **158**, 508–510. (L7. Q85)

25. Nielsen, J., Friedrich, U., Jacobsen, E., & Tsuboi, T. Lysergide and chromosome abnormalities. *Brit. Med. J.*, 1968, **2**, 801–803. (L7. D69)

26. Sawitsky, A., Bloom, D., & German, J. Chromosomal breakage and acute leukemia in congenital telangiectatic erythema and stunted growth. *Ann. Intern. Med.*, 1966, **65**, 487–495.

27. Schroeder, T. M., Anschutz, F., & Knopp, A. Spontane chromosomenaberrationen bei Familiarer Panmyelopathie. *Humangenetik*, 1964, **1**, 194–196.

28. Skakkebaek, N. E., Philip, J., & Rafaelsen, O. J. LSD in mice: Abnormalities in meiotic chromosomes. *Science*, 1968, **160**, 1246–1248. (L7. Q66)

29. Sparkes, R. S., Melnyk, J., Bozzetti, L. P. Chromosomal effect in vivo of exposure of lysergic acid diethylamide. *Science*, 1968, **160**, 1343–1345. (L7. Q34)

30. Swift, M. R., & Hirschhorn, K. Fanconi's anemia: Inherited susceptibility to chromosome breakage in various tissues. *Ann. Intern. Med.*, 1966, **65**, 496–503.

31. Warkany, J., & Takacs, E. Lysergic acid diethylamide (LSD): No teratogenicity in rats. *Science*, 1968, **159**, 731–732. (L7. Q32)

32. Wolman, S. R., Hirschhorn, K., & Todaro, G. J. Early chromosomal changes in SV-40-infected human fibroblast culture. *Cytogenetics*, 1964, **3**, 45–61.

33. Zellweger, H., McDonald, J. S., & Abbo, G. Is lysergic acid diethylamide a teratogen? *Lancet*, 1967, **2**, 1066–1068. (L7. D32)

23

Ideological Supports to Becoming and Remaining a Heroin Addict*

HARVEY W. FELDMAN

Causal explanations of the spread of drug use in slum neighborhoods have depended heavily on either psychological or psychiatric theories of behavior. In near unanimity, investigators of all institutional and professional persuasions have described the drug user as maladjusted, hostile, immature, dependent, manipulative, narcissistic—or any number of other reprehensible traits that place the blame for drug experimentation on the personality weaknesses of the individual user (Larrimore & Brill, 1960; Kuh, 1961; Diskind, 1962; Chein et al., 1964, pp. 193–226; Yablonsky, 1965; Meiselas, 1966). Up to the present, only a few researchers have examined the drug user in his home community (Finestone, 1957; Ray, 1964; Fiddle, 1965; Preble, 1966; Blumer et al., 1967). The failure to explore how features in the slum neighborhood may contribute to the spread of drug use developed from two major research difficulties: (1) the investigators, for the most part, were attached to large institutions specializing in the treatment of addicts; or (2) they were educated to seek causal explanations in the pathology of individuals, a kind of trained incapacity (cf. Burke, 1954, pp. 49–57) that disallowed creative use of social information about life styles in the slums. For the investigators attached to large institutions, direct observations of the slums were physically beyond their vision. For the professionals dependent on a medical model of disease theory (i.e., the belief that emotional disturbance causes disruption of normal personality growth comparable to a germ causing illness in the physical organism) the limits of perception were narrowed to individual weaknesses. This was true even for those investigators who located themselves in a slum environment (Kron & Brown, 1965). The major consequence of these difficulties was the failure to explain how drug use could spread in near epidemic proportions. To observe that emotional pathology is widespread among slum dwellers, or that the general population has a predisposition to addiction, does little to explain how a large minority of slum residents become drug addicts while others, often members of the same family, do not. Nor does listing a series of pathological symptoms explain why some persons who possess them choose deviant careers in drug addiction rather than pursue other deviant routes such as child molesters, Skid Row bums, or homosexuals, when these same reprehensible traits are employed to describe them.

Part of the causal explanation of a slum youth's movement into illicit drug use should involve an understanding of his immediate social context, the slum environment, which provides major clues to what constitutes acceptable and unacceptable behavior. In the local neighborhood, he learns how prestige may be gained or lost. In essence, he develops a way of viewing his world, an ideology that helps him make social choices so that life is meaningful within his network of relationships.

---

*From Feldman, H. W., *Journal of Health and Social Behavior*, 1968, **9**, 131–139. Copyright © 1968 by the American Sociological Association, Reprinted by permission of the American Sociological Association, and Dr. Feldman.

When an individual accepts the opportunity to use drugs, he must fit the act into some set of existing beliefs so that his first step toward highly censured behavior can be justified to himself and to important others in his life. In the beginning, he must be able to define drug use as consistent with his understanding of how status and prestige are earned within his social network. Once, however, he experiences the physical impact of a drug, other causal explanations may be necessary to understand how he goes about continuing or quitting further drug experimentation (Becker, 1963b pp. 19–39).

When I speak of ideology I do not have in mind the full-blown intellectual set of justifying propositions that behavioral scientists usually attach to social movements like Marxian Communism, the Black Muslims, or others from the genre of true believers. My notion is closer to the layman's and means simply, "the doctrines, opinions, or ways of thinking of an individual or class, etc.," as defined in *Webster's New World Dictionary*, College Edition, 1964.

I would like to emphasize the tentative nature of my conclusions. They have been developed primarily from my six years of working as a neighborhood social worker with a settlement house in the Lower East Side of New York City from 1958 to 1962. More recent data were gathered at the drug addiction ward in an eastern state mental hospital. Other data include recently published firsthand accounts of either slum life or heroin addiction (Hughes, 1961; Larner & Tefferteller, 1964; Malcolm X, 1964; Brown, 1965). The primary aim of this paper is to provide a preliminary way of analyzing the use of heroin among lower socio-economic males by focusing attention on features of slum life that are crucial to understanding the causes of initial experimentation.

CONDITIONS IN THE PRE-DRUG PHASE THAT SUPPORT EXPERIMENTATION WITH NARCOTICS

When drug use moves into a slum neighborhood, it does not seem to be a slowly mounting phenomenon. One second it is a small and new spark; in the next, new users emerge almost daily. Chein (1964) referred to drug use in deprived areas as "epidemic," probably because he borrowed the concept of epidemiology from public health. Claude Brown (1965) called it "the plague" because he saw one or more drug users including his own younger brother, in almost every family he knew in Harlem.

Sociologically, two important questions must be raised regarding a causal explanation for the instant recruitment pattern of new drug users: (1) Who are these eager recruits and how do they go about flooding into experimentation with heroin? (2) Once the first wave of addicts passes and the physical and social consequences become pathetically visible, how do new recruits become involved when role models of failure stand slumped in just about every doorway? An assessment of the action-seeking ideology of a large minority of slum residents may provide important clues.

Gans (1962, pp. 24–32) described the life style of action-seeking Italians as "dominated by the adventurous episode" and claimed the goal of action was "an opportunity for thrills, and a chance to face and overcome a challenge." Miller (1958, pp. 8–12) noted among Negroes a concern for excitement and a high regard for toughness. Reissman (1962, pp. 26–30) in his participant observation of Puerto Ricans in New York City described their preference for physical strength and excitement that counteracted the hum-drum of daily life. These descriptive qualities may be summed up in a lower socio-ecomonic ideology that prepares and guides the youth in slum neighborhoods to compete and survive in "street life." It is "on the street" that qualities of excitement, feats of strength, and the day-to-day thrills get played out to whatever important audience happens to watch.)

In the folklore of the streets, where reputations of the young may prescribe the degree of deference or disrespect for the total family, there are pressures on adolescent boys to live up to the ideals of toughness, strength, daring, and the willingness to challenge the bleak fate of being poor. Some youths achieve high status reputations built on these qualities. Some do not. Persons who do not subscribe to the ideology, who turn their backs on the beliefs of their neighbors, are sometimes called middle-class oriented or upward mobile by sociologists. In the language of the streets, they are called: "chicken" [archaic], "punk," "square," or "faggot," They and members of their families may be ignored, ridiculed, or exploited. Those youths who energetically thrust themselves into the slum neighborhood ideology seek to establish their reputations according to an ideal type: the *stand-up cat.* Puerto Ricans call him a "maucho." Negroes may refer to him as "a bad-ass nigger." And Italians call him a "guy with a pair of balls." But across the boards, he is a stand-up cat.

The stand-up cat requires fortuitous situations in which he can prove his daring, strength, predilection for excitement, and ultimate toughness. If the situations do not arise—and they seem to occur with frequent regularity—the stand-up cat may arrange them. The situations are primarily dangerous where severe bodily damage may result. More important, the situations provide tests for the stand-up cat recruit, tests in which he demonstrates well or badly his commitment to what he believes is the code of the streets. If arrested in a shared delinquent act, he does not "rat out" his friends and remains tight-lipped in the face of clever or brutal police tactics. In fight or theft episodes, the stand-up cat controls his fears, most often with bravado and a quiet ruthlessness. In the extreme, he gives the impression and sometimes genuinely believes that he is prepared to die. Preferably, the odds of triumph are not in his favor. Victories in such situations permit him to join the list of heroes in the myths and folk tales told by witnesses and those persons not in attendance who enjoy embellished truth.

Just how a young person finds himself in situations where his stand-up cat aspirations can be tested seems to be socially induced so that side-stepping these periodic and recurring moments of truth is almost inescapable unless the youth willingly readjusts his level of aspiration. He then risks being called "punk" or "faggot," both painful assaults on his manhood.

By the time the action-seeking youth reaches adolescence, he has practiced the mannerisms, adopted the clothing style, and selected an argot congruent with toughness and strength. If he is Puerto Rican or Negro, he has perfected a style of walking described as "walking with a bad bop." The slant of the shoulders and a rhythmic swagger emanate confidence. White youth—Italian or Irish or Polish—may shape their hair styles in what prison officials sometimes call a Tony Curtis cut. In times of situationally induced conflict, where the proof is in the action, all of them have mastered the offensive "bad look" that was brought to public attention when Sonny Liston outstared Floyd Patterson at the weigh-in for the heavyweight championship.

When drugs are introduced into a neighborhood, the first users seem to be older adolescents whose stand-up cat reputations have been indisputably earned. Usually one or two of them serve as distributors of drugs to friends, the middlemen between an illicit supply and the emerging market. They serve two important functions, at least temporarily: a) as proven stand-up cats, they can be trusted as distributors by adult lower-level underworld suppliers; b) as sponsors, they can create a market through their selection of younger recruits who desire approval and recognition from the older stand-up cats. For a period of time, the middlemen appear to be enormous financial successes as they reap the profits from their first gusher. One user-seller whom I knew at this stage of his career earned $500 a week and enough heroin to supply his personal use. For a while, his obvious increase in wealth made him the envy of every stand-up cat who dreamed of a "big score."

Younger recruits, eager for association with the successful, get selected not through any screening committee necessarily, but on the basis of their availability to the older user-seller and their general reputation as aspiring stand-up cats. As promising candidates who can widen the market for the older distributor, a young stand-up cat can gain sponsorship and enter a business arrangement where the profits, if not as lucrative as his sponsor's, compare favorably to mugging, "rolling queers," or being unemployed. He himself may or may not use drugs; but if he does, the sales talk on its benefits has greater credibility. As leaders among their own age peers, they can cajole, entice through withholding, or employ any number of other psychological inducements that make drug use sound and look attractive to action-seeking friends who want in on reckless fads. The side-bet on winning a reputation as a stand-up cat seems to explain the literal rush toward beginning drug use when heroin is first introduced into a slum neighborhood (Becker, 1960a). This aspect of anticipatory excitement usually gets masked in *ex post facto* reports by self-confirmed addicts, probably because in the later stages of a drug-using career a profound weariness sets in. Recalling the early eagerness may seem just plain foolish to addicts; and since addicts are usually in some condition of confinement or are obviously in some complicated legal or personal entanglement, they may wish to disguise or deny their impatient rush to experiment with heroin because it sounds foolish and illogical to the listener and detracts from the cool image addicts eventually fashion for themselves.

In the fall of 1958, I witnessed what Claude Brown has called "the plague" get ushered into a neighborhood on the Lower East Side of New York City. It began with a group of young-adult Italian boys. Soon, some of the older adolescents, all core members of a fighting gang, began to show signs of skin-popping heroin. Their drowsy appearance, puffed eyes and noses, and persistent vomiting in the settlement house hallways made it evident that their change in behavior was physically induced and dramatic. The younger boys, somewhat fearful of seizing their first opportunity and possibly excluded because of their youth, modified the real drug experience by sniffing cleaning fluid. They, too, soon experimented with heroin. Because I was an adult, and, more pertinently, a social worker from a middle-class world, the boys colluded to keep their behavior a secret from me. But I was working on the streets at the time, and they could not contain their excitement with this new form of adventurous episode. Their yearning to experiment with drugs would have made a scientist hot on the trail of a new discovery seem like a dispassionate observer. Brown (1965, pp. 263–264) has described the quality of determination among young Negroes who pursued the image of the stand-up cat when the drug experience became a fad among older role models. His description differed from what I saw in only ethnicity:

> When I came home, Kid and Butch and Danny weren't smoking reefers anymore. I'd have a smoke, but they were doing other things. And the first thing that Danny told me was that they were using something they called "horse." ... It seemed that they were saying this was something I wasn't old enough for. But I wanted to do the same things they were doing. ... All the older cats were using horse. The younger cats were still smoking reefers, drinking wine, and stuff like that. But I didn't want to be young. I wanted to be old. And the first time Danny spoke to me about it, I knew I was going to get some horse somehow, somewhere—soon.
>
> Horse was a new thing, not only in our neighborhood but in Brooklyn, the Bronx, and every place I went, uptown and downtown. It was like horse had just taken over. Everybody was talking about it. All the hip people were using it and snorting it and getting this new high. To know what was going on and to be in on things, you had to do that. And the only way I could come out of

Wiltwyck and be up to date, the only way to take up where I had left off and be the same hip guy I was before I went to Wiltwyck, was to get in on the hippest thing, and the hippest thing was horse.

Within six months or less after the first wave of drug users, non-users, both young and old, begin to develop negative responses. By then, they had seen their friends withdraw into a silent, itchy nod. They had usually been the victims of a series of small loans which addicts almost never repay. If the non-users were young and without a stand-up cat reputation of their own, they may have been forced to give money to addicts whose former reputations provided their own intimidation. They had seen addicts arrested and jailed. They began to know that heroin had addicting qualities and that the pains of withdrawal were ugly. And if they had not witnessed it firsthand, they knew at least one young addict who had died of an overdose, and probably three or four others who barely survived.

Still, in the face of evidence, new and eager recruits experiment. For the first wave of users, some measure of ignorance may provide an excuse for not understanding the addicting power of opiate-type drugs. Several times I had heard confirmed addicts, as they looked back on their introduction to heroin, say something like: "If I had known I was going to get strung out [heavily addicted], maybe, I'm not sure, but maybe I would have stayed away from drugs." The same excuse, however, seems less valid for users who know about the physical consequences of heroin addiction and have highly visible examples in their home neighborhoods. Again, the stand-up cat notion may be helpful in understanding this development.

Interest in drug use arises partly from a prospective stand-up cat's disillusionment with his former heroes, who in the past seemed invincible. Now, after a period of drug use, they have declined in the young stand-up cat's own status system. Instead of the hero's going out and taking money like he used to, he may implore or ask in such a way that the younger boy begins to feel his mastery over someone whom he had previously respected and feared. The youth may even chance his strength against the addict by showing open disrespect or by actually fighting him with the result that the drug user gets stripped of his toughness in much the same manner that heavyweight champions provide stepping stones for rising young boxers. Because addicts get to be known for their unwillingness to fight, victories over them seem partially hollow. For the youth to become truly a stand-up cat, he must fight more worthy opponents, championship material, whoever they may be. And since he has seen previous stand-up cats buckle to the strength of heroin, the lure it holds as a route to prestige and status among action-seeking peers is enhanced. His challenge is to triumph in a situation where previous heroes have failed. Using heroin, controlling its addictive effects, and eventually stopping becomes the test of toughness, of danger, and of chancing what for others has been the inevitability of fate. A common report from workers in the field who have attempted to intercede with adolescent heroin users has been the youthful certainty that they can control their use of heroin and avoid addiction. Foremost in the adolescent's belief is a firm conviction that he is too strong, too tough, too much of a stand-up cat ever to be defeated by a chemical.

Operating in his favor are other role models, older time-tested stand-up cats who cut short their drug-using careers, who had, in fact, used drugs for a longer or shorter duration and stopped. They had, as well, known or heard of other users—like Ray Charles, Billie Holliday, and Lenny Bruce—who managed to control their drug consumption or had become famous in the popular arts despite a known history of drug use. These examples provide the young recruit with proof that one or two shots of heroin, or even continued use over a period of time, does not necessarily lead to the "living death" popularly preached. While the odds may be heavily against avoiding addiction and its negative social consequences, heavy odds make the possibility of triumph for the stand-up cat even more inviting.

THE INITIAL FAVORABLE SHOT AND SHORTLY AFTER

Assessing the effects of the initial favorable shot of heroin becomes a complicated matter for any social scientist. Heroin has chemical properties whose effects on the physical organism are not clearly understood by laboratory technicians or physiologists. Most important, perhaps, is the tension-relieving quality, the immediate impact of relaxation on the stand-up cat whose ideology has kept him constantly prepared for one kind of battle or another. Further, the drug delivers with a potency a warm, lazy elation, a feeling of ecstatic comfort one user described by saying: "I didn't know I could feel that good." This impact may be felt on the first snort, the first intramuscular injection, or later, after several experiments. It may be followed by nausea and vomiting, but the flash of exultation is crucial to continuance. At this juncture a favorable physical response to the effects of heroin is an important contingency in the career of the heroin addict. To the best of my knowledge, there is no adequate explanation—psychological, physical or social—to predict who will respond favorably and who will merely get nauseous. One boy whom I knew described his quitting by explaining that he failed to experience the pleasurable physical effects his friends described and merely got sick; since the financial cost was high for self-induced nausea, he stopped taking heroin. Since the persons who quit heroin use early in their career seldom come to official attention or get labeled as drug addicts, they are less available to social investigators. Presently, explanations for their failure to advance along the more or less typical career line remain a social and psychological mystery. The few ex-experimenters I knew, however, never lost their stand-up cat reputations. In fact, their reputations were enhanced, enough so that some of them were permitted to assume the stance of the "square." But my cases for now are too few for generalization.

For the experimenters who respond favorably to the effects of heroin, a new world opens. Their favorable response falls into that twilight area where external social forces merge with the intra-personal whirl of emotions. Heroin, with a magical *flash*, provides an emotional well-being, a peace and calm the stand-up cat may never have known in the past. In a sense, the alerted readiness to display toughness, the poised tenseness of being prepared to fight anyone at anytime, the ubiquitous fear about dying from a knife wound or a gunshot are washed away. In its place, the user feels a warm immunity from danger, even if the danger is close at hand. Under such heavy sedation, who, he may ask, could feel the pain anyway? Even the most articulate users lose their flow of words when attempting to describe the first time heroin took its comforting effects. One user described his initial favorable reaction: "Like I was in heaven; I just fell in love with it." Although the career lines of the female addict undoubtedly differ from the male's, they share in common the same enthusiastic description of the initial flash. "Janet Clark," the anonymous respondent of *The Fantastic Lodge*, describing her initial flash, departed from her usual concrete clarity into a language of abstract sensations (Hughes, 1961, pp. 99):

> But this second time I made it. I got my first flash and I never felt anything like that before. I dug it, completely. And if I thought the world had been all right when I snorted, it was insane and solid and smooth and crazy when I made it in my arm.

The *flash*—the odd combination of a cocoon-comfort and an inexplicable physical ascendency to a "high"—provides the major incentive for the new experimenter to move to the next phase of his career. Without it, use of drugs would be merely a profitless activity where the social rewards were heavily overshadowed by the dangers. Pursuit of "the high" becomes paramount. Some older drug addicts believe that the initial flash can never be duplicated. In fact, some of them believe that their total careers have been dedicated to the re-creation of those first, glorious feelings.

In this new phase, the drug user begins to learn the ropes of becoming a successful drug consumer (Geer *et al.*, 1968). Because he spends a substantial amount of time and energy learning how to insure the possibility of continued drug use, he starts neglecting his non-drug-using friends. The process of disengagement with non-users and movement toward involvement in a drug-consuming subculture may be abrupt, or it may extend over a period of time. The user may maintain substantial contact with non-using friends, or he may attempt to separate himself completely. The variables involved are undoubtedly numerous although a critical one may well be the way the former reference group defined and responded to drug-using behavior (Chein *et al.*,. 1964, pp. 181–185). Built into that definition would be a continued or declining commitment to the stand-up cat ideology. My tentative hypothesis on the process of disengagement would be phrased something like this: Where adherence of the former reference group to the stand-up cat ideology is strong, the quicker the beginning drug user (while he is learning the ropes) will disengage himself from his non-using friends. Conversely, he will thrust himself into a new ideology consistent with the pleasurable effects of heroin.

During the disengagement the drug user begins to revise his attitudes about the stand-up cat ideology. To a greater or lesser extent, a kind of reaction formation sets in. Movement away from the stand-up cat ideology can be measured in qualities of temperature. Where the stand-up cat was admired for his bursts of hot hate, the new image ideal is admired for his coolness (Finestone, 1957). Instead of brutality and physical strength, the new drug user prefers to be seen as slick and clever. Fighting becomes an unprofitable choice of behavior unless it involves access to drugs. The drug effect moves to the top of his priority list. With the discovery that an injection of heroin can trigger off an inner world of excitement and calm, being a stand-up cat begins to seem as foolish as Don Quixote's attempt to revive knighthood. He starts to lose his belief that walking away from a fight will make him a "punk" or a "faggot." He doesn't even believe that discretion is the better part of valor. He simply believes, finally, that fighting is silly, very uncool, especially when his "high" can be achieved—so he thinks at this stage of his career—with far less risk to life and limb.

As the drug user learns the ropes, he starts to reshuffle his itinerary. The amount of time he spends with non-drug-using friends lessens as the time he spends with other drug users increases. Slowly, his selection of new friends is based almost exclusively on their involvement with drugs. Friendship patterns extend cross-culturally and include ethnic groups toward whom the user in his pre-drug days may have felt strong antipathy. It was not unusual, for example, to see some former members of an Italian gang in close association with former members of a Puerto Rican or Negro gang, all of whom, prior to drug use, were sworn enemies. Drug use provided a new experiential bond. As members of a drug subculture they may laugh together about their wild and foolish escapades when they hunted one another with guns.

As an apprentice, the beginning drug user has much to learn. This paper will not detail the learning-the-ropes phase; but the beginning drug user is not unlike other apprentices entering an occupation. He begins to note that the social system in which he must survive is far more complicated than he first imagined. In addition to learning how to gain maximal pleasure from drugs, he learns how to secure them, how to prepare them, and how to provide himself with the financial resources that insure a continuing supply. If he does not master these basic skills, he is dependent on more knowledgeable drug users. Like the college student who must learn to think for himself, the drug user must move toward more independent operations. To gain acceptance in his academic community, he, too, begins to distinguish between the prosaic and the profound. He may choose a specialty, and he guards against the exploitation of his teachers. He realizes that the social forces of the larger society have assembled a counteracting system to prevent him from enjoying his heroin. And eventually he learns how to manage the system and be managed by it.

SUMMARY

The specific aim of this paper has been the attempt to provide causal explanations for the movement of a large minority of slum youth into drug experimentation by shifting the emphasis away from notions of psychological predisposition or social structural weaknesses of slum neighborhoods toward procedural issues of how drug users, both before and after drug experimentation, interact with important members of their social network and move toward an addicted identity. In this way, drug experimentation can be seen as growing out of an ideological seed-bed where rewards of high status and prestige are conferred upon action-seeking youth who strive to become stand-up cats by becoming involved in behavior that is exciting, daring, tough, and dangerous. Rather than viewing drug experimentation as the result of acting-out internal problems or the consequence of failure in legitimate or illegitimate social structures, drug users play an active, conscious role in their introduction into drug use by striving toward the high status of a stand-up cat. Achieving the status, to a large degree, depends on the response of age peers and older role models. The enthusiasm to achieve the status of stand-up cat may explain the speed with which heroin use can spread through a slum neighborhood so that observers refer to it as "an epidemic" or "plague."

Moving along the career line toward confirmed use depends upon the user's having a positive physical response to heroin and learning how to enjoy the effects of "the high." Once the user finds pleasure in drug use and prefers his dreamy state to the action world of non-using friends, he disengages himself from the usual routines of the stand-up cat and begins to learn the ropes of a drug-consuming subculture in which he renounces his stand-up cat ideology and learns to believe in a new ideology that is consistent with the pleasurable effects of heroin. The speed with which the new drug user disengages himself from his former reference group depends upon the way the members adhere to the ideology of the stand-up cat.

My observations support neither the usual psychiatric view that drug use emerges from attempts to resolve internal emotional problems nor the Cloward-Ohlin (1960) thesis that heroin use is a retreatist adaptation to a youth's double failure in legitimate and illegitimate opportunity structures of the slums. The user turns to drugs, not as a result of anomie, but rather to capitalize on a new mode of enhancing his status and prestige with a social system where the highest prizes go to persons who demonstrate attributes of toughness, daring, and adventure. Within the life style of the stand-up cat, movement into heroin use is one route to becoming a " somebody" in the eyes of the important people who comprise the slum social network.

REFERENCES

Becker, H. S. Notes on the concept of commitment. *American Journal of Sociology*, 1960, **66**, 32–40. (a) Becker, H. S. *Outsiders: Studies in the sociology of deviance.* New York: Free Press, 1963. (b)

Blumer, H., *et al. The world of youthful drug use.* Berkeley: University of California, 1967.

Brown, C. *Manchild in the promised land.* New York: Macmillan, 1965.

Burke, K. *Permanence and change:* Pp. 37–49. *An anatomy of purpose.* Los Altos, California: Hermes Publications, 1954.

Chein, I., *et al. The road to H: Narcotics, delinquency and social policy.* New York: Basic Books, 1964.

Cloward, R. A., & Ohlin, L. E. *Delinquency and opportunity: A theory of delinquent gangs.* New York: Free Press, 1960.

Diskind, M. H. The New York experiment: A summary of New York State Parole Division special narcotic project program. *The Proceedings of the White House Conference on Narcotic and Drug Abuse.* Washington, D.C.: United States Government Printing Office, 1962. Pp. 77–80.

Fiddle, S. The addict culture and movement into and out of hospitals. Quoted in E. M. Schur, *Crimes without victims,* Englewood Cliffs, N.J.: Prentice-Hall, 1965. Pp. 141–145.

Finestone, H. Cats, kicks, and color. *Social Problems* 1957, **5**, 3–13.

Gans, H. J. *The urban villagers: Group and class in the life of Italian-Americans.* New York: Free Press, 1962.

Geer, B. *et al.* Learning the ropes: Situational learning in four occupational training programs. In I. Deutscher & E. Thompson (Eds.), *Among the poor: Studies of the urban poor.* New York: Basic Books, 1968.

Hughes, H. M. *The fantastic lodge.* Derby, Conn.: Monarch Books, 1961.

Kron, Y. J., & Brown, E. M. *Mainline to nowhere: The making of a heroin addict.* Cleveland, Ohio: World, 1965.

Kuh, R. H. A prosecutor's thoughts concerning addiction. *The Journal of Criminal Law, Criminology, and Police Science,* 1961, **53**, 321–327.

Larrimore, G. W., & Brill, H. The British narcotics system: Report of a study. *New York State Journal of Medicine,* 1960, **60** 107–115.

Larner, J., & Tefferteller, R. *The addict in the streets.* New York: Grove Press, 1964.

Malcolm X (with the assistance of Alex Haley) *The autobiography of Malcolm X.* New York: Grove Press, 1964.

Meiselas, H. Narcotic addiction program of the New York State Department of Mental Hygiene. In *Rehabilitating the Narcotic Addict.* Washington, D. C.: United States Government Printing Office, 1966. Pp. 141–148.

Miller, W. B. The lower-class culture as a generating milieu of gang delinquency. *The Journal of Social Issues.* 1958, **3**; 5–19.

Preble, E. Social and cultural factors related to narcotic use among Puerto Ricans in New York City. *The International Journal of the Addictions,* 1966, **1**, 30–41.

Ray, M. B. The cycle of abstinence and relapse among heroin addicts. *Social Problems* 1961, 132–140.

Reissman, F. *The culturally deprived child.* New York: Harper and Brothers, 1962.

Yablonsky, L. *The tunnel back: Synanon.* New York: Macmillan, 1965.

24

Alcoholism*

KENNETH L. JONES, LEWIS W. SHAINBERG and CURTIS O. BYER

NATURE AND EXTENT OF ALCOHOLISM

Even among recognized authorities, there are various concepts as to what constitutes an alcoholic. Some authorities use a highly restrictive definition of alcoholism; others define it in a very general way. An example of a relatively restrictive definition is that of M. E. Chafetz and H. W. Demone, who view alcoholism as

...a chronic behavioral disorder manifested by undue preoccupation with alcohol to the detriment of physical and mental health, by a loss of control when drinking has begun, although it may not be carried to the point of intoxication and by a self-destructive attitude in dealing with relationships and life situations.[1]

An example of a more general definition of alcoholism is that of O. Diethelm, who considers an alcoholic to be an individual who

...uses alcohol to such an extent that it interferes with a successful life (including physical, personality, and social aspects) and is either not able to recognize this effect or is not able to control his alcohol consumption, although he knows its disastrous results.[2]

It can be seen that both definitions emphasize not how much a person drinks, but the effects of his drinking. There are some persons who cannot be classified as alcoholics who actually drink more than others who can be so classified.

There is no established system for reporting the incidence of alcoholism in the United States. Thus, any figures given for the prevalence of alcoholism are estimates. Since much alcoholism escapes medical or legal detection and since there are various definitions of "alcoholism," it is to be expected that a wide range occurs among published estimates as to the extent of alcoholism in the United States. The consensus of the estimates, however, seems to be that about 5 percent of the adults in the United States are alcoholics. It is also estimated that about 70 percent of the adults in the United States are at least occasional users of alcoholic beverages. So among those adults who do use alcoholic beverages, about one in fourteen is an alcoholic....

*Pp. 138–145, from *Drugs and alcohol,* 2nd ed. by Kenneth L. Jones, Lewis W. Shainberg, Curtis O. Byer. Copyright © 1969, 1973 by Kenneth L. Jones, Lewis W. Shainberg, and Curtis O. Byer. Reprinted by permission of Harper & Row, Publishers, Inc. (Photograph has been omitted.)

[1]M. E. Chafetz and H. W. Demone, Jr. *Alcoholism and Society,* New York, Oxford, 1962.
[2]O. Diethelm. *Etiology of Chronic Alcoholism,* Springfield, Ill.: Thomas, 1955.

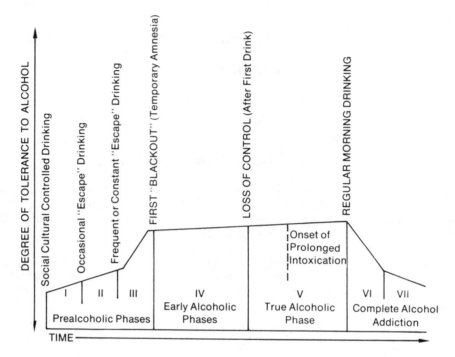

Fig. 24.1

PHASES OF ALCOHOLISM

Since at least one in every fourteen drinkers eventually becomes an alcoholic, it is important that anyone who uses alcoholic beverages be able to recognize the signs and symptoms of impending and early alcoholism. Hopefully, if a person noticed these symptoms in himself and knew what they meant, he might have the good judgment to cease drinking before he reached a more advanced stage of alcoholism.

A classic research project in which the late Dr. E. M. Jellinek interviewed over 2000 alcoholics revealed that most alcoholics pass through definite progressive stages with characteristic symptoms. This progression is graphically represented in Fig. 24.1. On this graph, time proceeds from left to right. There can be no fixed scale of months or years, since some alcoholics make the entire progression in a matter of months while others may take many years to reach the same point. Dr. Jellinek pointed out that the development of alcoholism in women is frequently more rapid than in men, with the stages less clear-cut. The vertical line on the graph indicates the relative degree of alcohol tolerance, in other words, the amount of alcohol required to reach a given degree of intoxication.

Prealcoholic Phases

During the course of social drinking, most people learn the feeling of escape from everyday cares that alcohol can provide (Phase I on Fig. 24.1). When an individual occasionally drinks for the specific purpose of escape from tensions he has progressed to the second prealcoholic phase. About 20 percent of all drinkers fall into this category. In the person destined for alcoholism, this escape drinking gradually becomes more and more frequent (Phase III).

As drinking becomes more frequent, a person develops an increased tolerance for alcohol, that is, he must drink more in order to achieve the same effect. At first tolerance increases gradually; then it often takes a sudden jump. (A high level of tolerance is maintained until in late alcoholism there is a marked loss of tolerance)(Phases VI and VII).

Alcoholic Blackouts

Soon after his increase in tolerance, the frequent drinker may experience his first *alcoholic blackout* (Phase IV). A blackout is a period of temporary amnesia occuring when a person is drinking. In contrast to passing out, which results in unconsciousness, a person in an alcoholic blackout is still conscious of what he is doing at the time and may be doing all the things he might normally do. But after he comes out of his blackout, he has no memory of anything that took place during the blackout. Anyone who drinks too much will pass out, but only the alcoholic or near-alcoholic blacks out. The mechanism of the blackout is not yet definitely known. It may have a physiological origin or it may be a psychological ego-defense mechanism.

Loss of Control

Another major milestone in the development of alcoholism is loss of control (Phase V). This means the loss of the ability to drink in a moderate, controlled manner. It does not mean that the individual feels compelled to start drinking, but when he does start, he cannot stop after a predetermined, moderate amount of alcohol. He may continue to drink until he becomes quite intoxicated or gets sick. The period of drinking may last for a few hours or become a binge, lasting for days or weeks. The individual can choose when he starts his drinking, but not when he stops it. By any definition of alcoholism, this individual is now an alcoholic.

Other Signs of Alcoholism

Many other symptoms are characteristic of the alcoholic. These symptoms are arranged in sequence from the characteristics of early alcoholism to those of late alcoholism. In a given individual, these symptoms may not occur in this exact order, but are usually in about this sequence.

1. *Secret Drinking.* The alcoholic often "sneaks" his drinks, so that others will not know how much he is drinking.

2. *Preoccupation with Alcohol.* The personal aspects of social functions become secondary to the opportunity for drinking. For example, when an alcoholic is invited to a party, he is more interested in the fact that drinks will be available than in who will be there.

3. *Gulping the first few drinks.* The alcoholic drinks for the quickest possible effect.

4. *Guilt Feelings About Drinking.* As the alcoholic begins to realize that his drinking habits are not normal, he develops vague conscious or subconscious feelings of guilt, which may lead to several outward symptoms.

(a) *Avoids Talking About Alcohol.* The person who eagerly talks about his drinking is seldom a problem drinker. The alcoholic, in contrast, does not like to discuss drinking because he is afraid he will be criticized for his excessive drinking.

(b) *Rationalizes His Drinking Behavior.* The alcoholic always has a "reason" for drinking, which is actually an excuse, a rationalization. It never occurs to the normal
drinker to offer a reason for his drinking. For the alcoholic, good news and bad news
are both valid reasons for drinking. He drinks to celebrate his accomplishments or to
drown his sorrows. These rationalizations are needed primarily for the protection of
his own ego and only secondarily as alibis to his family and associates.

(c) *Exhibits Grandiose Behavior.* The alcoholic often goes through overly extravagant
and generous periods, during which he throws money around in a showy way. He
may buy drinks for perfect strangers and leave unusually large tips. The purpose of
such display is not so much to impress others as it is to reassure himself that he is
really not such a bad guy after all. This is part of the system of rationalization
which strongly influences the life of the alcoholic and serves to protect his ego.

(d) *Has Periods of Remorse.* Often the guilt feelings of the alcoholic lead to periods of
persistent remorse, which may have the unfortunate effect of leading him on to still
more drinking.

5. *Periods of Total Abstinence.* As a result of social pressures or his own concern, the
alcoholic may go "on the wagon." For several weeks or months he does not take a drink.
Then he usually resumes drinking with renewed vigor because he is satisfied that he can
still live without alcohol. Hence the oft-repeated reassurance, "I can take it or leave it,"
becomes the theme song of the alcoholic.

6. *Changing Drinking Patterns.* The alcoholic feels that there must be some way in
which he can drink without loss of control. In attempting to drink in a normal, controlled
manner, he frequently varies his drinking pattern, trying different types of liquor, different
mixers, or different times or places. Of course, none of these changes helps.

7. *Behavior Becomes Alcohol Centered.* This symptom is characterized by a marked
loss of interest in anything other than alcohol. Personal appearance is neglected, as is the
maintenance of living quarters and possessions. There is a deterioration in interpersonal relationships. Instead of worrying about how his drinking is affecting his activities, the
alcoholic avoids activities which might interfere with his drinking. The alcoholic becomes
increasingly egocentric.

8. *Effects on the Family.* The family members of the alcoholic often change their habits.
They may withdraw into the home for fear of embarrassment or, in contrast, may become
very active in outside interests as a means of escape from the home environment. Financial
problems are usually a way of life for the family of the alcoholic.

9. *Unreasonable Resentments.* The alcoholic often builds up tremendous feelings of
resentment and self-pity. He spends much time brooding over minor or imaginary injus-
tices he has suffered.

10. *Hiding Bottles.* The many jokes and cartoons about alcoholics hiding (and losing)
their bottles have a factual basis. The alcoholic often takes elaborate precautions to avoid
running out of liquor.

11. *Neglect of Proper Nutrition.* The chronic alcoholic typically has little interest in
food, deriving most of his Calories from alcoholic beverages which are very poor sources
of vitamins, minerals, and proteins. He may suffer from serious malnutrition, which may
actually cause more physical damage than the toxic effect of alcohol.

12. *Decrease in Sexual Drive.* As a result of his deteriorating physical and emotional
condition, the alcoholic may suffer a decrease in sexual drive. This decrease often leads to
alcoholic jealousy, in which the spouse of the alcoholic is accused of having extramarital
affairs. The marriage which has managed to survive to this point is often shattered by such
jealousy.

13. *Regular Morning Drinking.* Alcohol can be an addictive substance. After years of heavy drinking, a level of addiction may be reached which requires the constant presence of alcohol in the body to prevent withdrawal symptoms. This level of dependence indicates chronic alcohol addiction (Phase VI on Fig. 24.1).The alcoholic must now start his day with a drink…. If the fully addicted alcoholic is deprived of alcohol, his first withdrawal symptom is usually a shaking of the hands, arms, and body. His mood may be one of apprehension or fear and he may suffer hallucinations. The alcoholic at this stage should not be forced to sober up without medical assistance, as there is a chance he will go into convulsions and perhaps even die.

14. *Intoxication During Working Hours.* Another result of the addiction aspect of alcoholism occurs when the alcoholic finds himself intoxicated in the morning on a working day and either misses work or sneaks drinks while on the job. This is the "beginning of the end" of his job.

15. *Loss of Tolerance.* After a long term of heavy drinking, the alcoholic loses the tolerance to alcohol he previously had acquired. This loss is possibly connected to a decrease in the ability of the liver to oxidize alcohol. Following this loss of tolerance, he becomes intoxicated on less liquor than before and sobers up much more slowly. He is able to remain intoxicated at all times with only a moderate total consumption of alcohol.

16. *Mental Impairment.* Many alcoholics eventually suffer a severe disintegration of personality. If drinking continues after this symptom appears, there may be permanent brain damage. It is believed that this brain damage is due to the combined effect of severe dietary deficiency plus the direct effect of alcohol.

A type of psychosis which commonly appears in late alcoholics is *delirium tremens,* the "DT's." This is a temporary condition, lasting only from two to ten days, but there may be repeated attacks. An attack may be triggered by injury, illness, or withdrawal from alcohol. The symptoms may include confusion, vivid visual hallucinations, fear, apprehension, restlessness, and sleeplessness. There may even be convulsions similar to epileptic seizures. The attack ends with a period of deep sleep….

Fortunately, it is not necessary for an alcoholic to go through the entire course of the disease of alcoholism. An alcoholic can be successfully treated at any stage if he is willing to admit that he has a drinking problem and if he really wants to do something about it….

Suggested Additional Readings

Aaronson, B., & Osmond, H. *Psychedelics.* New York: Anchor Books, 1970.

Alcohol and alcoholism. Washington, D.C.: United States Government Printing Office, 1968.

Black, P. (Ed.) *Drugs and the brain.* Baltimore: John Hopkins University Press, 1969.

Chafetz, M. F. *Liquor, servant of man.* Boston: Little, Brown, 1965.

Chafetz, M. L., & Hill, M. J. The alcoholic in society. In A. Grunebaum (Ed.), *The practice of community mental health.* Boston: Little, Brown, 1970.

Chein, I., Gerard, D. L., Lee, R. S., & Rosenfeld, E. *The road to H.* New York: Basic Books, 1964.

Crancer, A., Jr., Kille, N. M., Delay, J. C., Wallace, J. E., & Haykin, M. D. Comparison of the effects of marijuana and alcohol in simulated driving performance. Science, 1969, **164**, 851–854.

Farber, L. H. Ours is the addicted society. *The New York Times Magazine,* December 11, 1966.

Jellinek, E. M. Phases of alcohol addiction. *Quarterly Journal of Studies on Alcohol,* 1952, **13**, 673–684.

Jellinek, E. M. *The disease concept of alcoholism.* Highland Park, N.J.: Hillhouse Press, 1960.

Keniston, K. Heads and seekers: Drugs on campus, countercultures and American society. *The American Scholar,* 1968–1969 (*Winter*), **38**, 99–112.

McGlothlin, W., Cohen, S., & McGlothlin, M. Long lasting effects of LSD on normals. *Archives of General Psychiatry,* 1967, **17**, 521–532.

Nowlis, H. H. *Drugs on the college campus.* New York: Anchor Books, 1969.

Richards, L. G., & Carroll, E. E. Illicit drug use and addiction in the United States. *Public Health Reports,* 1970, **85**, 1035–1941.

Roueche, B. *Alcohol.* New York: Grove Press, 1960.

Smart, R. G., & Jones, D. Illicit LSD users: Their personality characteristics and psychopathology. *Journal of Abnormal Psychology,* 1970, **75**, 286–292.

Snyder, S. H. *Uses of marijuana.* New York: Oxford University Press, 1971.

Task Force on Narcotics and Drug Abuse, the President's Commission on Law Enforcement and the Administration of Justice. *Task force report: Narcotics and drug abuse.* Wahington, D.C.: United States Government Printing Office, 1967.

Weil, A. T., Zinberg, N. E., & Nelson, J. M. Clinical and psychological effects of marihuana in man. *Science,* 1968, **162**, 1234–1242.

Weil, A. T. & Zinberg, N. E. Acute effects of marijuana on speech. *Nature,* 1969, **212**, 434–437.

Weil, A. T. Adverse reactions to marijuana. *New England Journal of Medicine,* 1970, **282**, 997–1000.

Wikler, A. *Opiate addiction.* Springfield, Ill.: Charles C. Thomas, 1953.

UNIT IV

Perspectives in the Treatment of Abnormal Behavior

INTRODUCTION

As previously pointed out, there have been many changes in the study of abnormal psychology over the past 20 years. One of the areas in which these changes are most noticeable is in the treatment of maladaptive behavior. Prior to 1950, the most prominent way in which patients were treated was through the use of techniques derived from psychoanalytically oriented theories or, in the case of many patients who were in psychiatric hospitals, through the use of custodial care and attention.

In the early 1950s, two significant developments in the mental health field radically changed the treatment of patients. The first was the introduction of tranquilizing drugs, sedatives, and antidepressants, the effects of which were striking. Antidepressant drugs, for example, were found to make chronically depressed patients more lively, while tranquilizers made combative and hyperactive patients more relaxed and caused the hallucinatory activity and illogical speech of many patients to decrease. The use of these and other drugs demonstrated that the symptomatic behaviors of patients could be modified by pharmacological means.

The second major factor was the growing disenchantment on the part of many mental health professionals with the traditional, psychoanalytically derived, therapy procedures. This disenchantment led to the development of alternative therapeutic models and techniques, and to a greater use of group treatment methods.

Various individual and group therapeutic approaches being used in the treatment of maladaptive behavior are presented in this unit. The three major therapeutic approaches—chemotherapy, individual therapy, and group therapy—are each considered in a separate section, and a fourth section is devoted to treatment procedures with special populations.

Chemotherapy

In the first section, the use of drugs in the treatment of maladaptive behavior is discussed in an excellent article by Elton B. McNeil. He describes the types of drugs currently used and some of the problems associated with the introduction

295

and utilization of these drugs. McNeil also discusses the use of drugs in the treatment of children with emotional difficulties as well as the various problems and uncertainties which arise in prescribing such drugs.

Individual Therapy Approaches

The articles in the second section represent various individually oriented therapeutic models currently used in the treatment of maladaptive behavior. Article 26 by Lewis R. Wolberg describes *psychoanalysis.* This therapy procedure is based on the *medical model* (discussed in Unit I), and assumes that treatment should be directed toward discovering the underlying cause of a patient's maladaptive behavior. Therapy is not concerned with treating a patient's symptoms, but helping him develop insight into why he behaves the way he does.

The patient is helped to gain this insight by talking to the therapist about his basic feelings toward others, his likes, dislikes, fears, etc. All of this takes place in a setting that is confidential and with a therapist who is skilled, trustful, and nonjudgmental. It is not uncommon for this therapy to last for many years, with the patient seeing the therapist from one to five times a week.

Wolberg notes that psychoanalytic therapy is based on Freud's theory of the libido and his theory of psychosexual development. The therapist encourages the patient to free associate about his problems, and utilizes such therapeutic tools as transference, interpretation, and dream analysis. Each of these techniques helps the patient bring various repressed feelings to consciousness, so that he can develop insight into his present difficulties, resolve them, and mature psychologically.

In contrast to the procedures based on the medical model, the therapy techniques described in Article 27 by Teodoro Ayllon and Jack Michael, and in Article 28 by Joseph Wolpe are based on the *behavioral model.* This model is not based on the assumption that there is an underlying cause for a patient's maladaptive behavior. Advocates of this approach maintain that a patient's maladaptive behavior is a sample of the way he behaves in similar environmental situations, and that this behavior is determined by certain events in these situations. Therapy is thus directed toward modifying specific maladaptive behaviors and the environmental events that precipitate and maintain them, not toward trying to help the patient gain insight into why he behaves the way he does.

Also, according to the behavioral model, therapy should treat maladaptive behaviors separately. If, for example, a patient has a fear of close interpersonal relationships, continually bites his fingernails, and is afraid to talk back to people who criticize him unjustly, the clinician who follows this model would treat each of these maladaptive behaviors separately. He would not make the assumption that they are all surface manifestations of a single underlying cause and proceed to treat this underlying cause.

One of the criticisms of the behavioral model relates to a theorized condition called "symptom substitution." This is an hypothesized condition derived from the medical model and refers to the belief that if the therapist treats a patient's symptoms directly without also treating their underlying cause(s), the patient will develop other maladaptive behaviors to replace those which were successfully treated. Thus, according to this belief, only after the underlying cause has been successfully treated will the patient stop developing symptoms.

Advocates of the behavioral model do not accept this belief, since they maintain that there is no underlying cause for maladaptive behavior. These clinicians (e.g., Ullmann & Krasner, 1965) do not deny that new maladaptive behaviors can develop after therapy has stopped, nor do they deny that a patient's previous symptoms can return after the completion of therapy; however, they do not explain the occurrence of these behaviors in terms of symptom substitution. Instead, they discuss them in relation to people (or objects) in the patient's environment who, for example, have rewarded him for behaving in an unacceptable manner. Alternatively, they discuss the occurrence of other (new) maladaptive behaviors in terms of their having been in the person's repertoire, but having increased in frequency when his prominent maladaptive behavior was successfully eliminated.

The behavioral model evolved largely from the area of experimental psychology called learning theory and conditioning. Models of this type fall into one of two major treatment categories. The first category makes use of procedures which have been derived from B. F. Skinner's (e.g., Skinner, 1938, 1953) operant conditioning approach. The second category is based on the learning theory positions of such theorists as Ivan Pavlov (e.g., Pavlov, 1927) and Clark Hull (e.g., Hull, 1943). The various therapy procedures included in these categories are commonly referred to as *behavior therapy.*

Article 27 discusses the use of techniques based on operant conditioning as a means of treating patients in a psychiatric hospital. By Teodoro Ayllon and Jack Michael, it represents one of the pioneering studies that used behavior therapy techniques to modify the maladaptive behaviors of adult psychiatric patients.

Article 28 by Joseph Wolpe then describes additional behavior therapy methods, including the procedure he developed called *systematic desensitization.* In this procedure the therapist systematically pairs certain imagined scenes that are anxiety-provoking for the patient with deep muscle relaxation, so that the patient learns to inhibit the anxiety response that these imagined scenes evoked previously.

A treatment method derived from *both* learning theory and psychoanalytic theory is discussed in Article 29, by Thomas G. Stampfl and Donald J. Levis. In this procedure, called *implosive therapy,* the patient's internal emotional responses (e.g., anxiety) to particular situations are dealt with by requesting him to imagine scenes that are directly related to his phobia and then have him imagine scenes which are based on the therapist's psychoanalytic interpretations of his maladaptive behavior.

Article 30 describes a therapy procedure consistent with the third major therapy model—the *humanistic model.* This approach, like the medical model, is based on the assumption that there is an underlying cause to a person's maladaptive behavior, but the theorized origin of the maladaptive behavior is different. Instead of assuming that maladaptive behavior is caused by unconscious motives that are primarily sexual in origin, the therapist following this model assumes that such maladaptation occurs as a result of the incongruencies between an individual's self-concept and his experiences. Also, unlike the psychoanalytic position, the therapist following this model treats the patient in the here and now rather than concentrating on past events (e.g., the patient's childhood).

In this final selection, Carl Rogers discusses his therapeutic approach, *client-centered therapy*. This form of therapy relies on the patient's capacity to help himself. The therapist does not try to direct the patient, but tries to understand him by adopting the way in which he perceives the world. This is accomplished through the therapist's being nonjudgmental and showing positive regard for the patient, as well as his being genuine and demonstrating an emphatic understanding of the patient's problems. Rogers also describes the process of therapy and the changes in the patient's personality which result from this therapy procedure. For example, the patient is more congruent with his experiences and less defensive; his perceptions are more realistic and objective; he is more accepting of others; and he has a higher degree of self-regard and is more confident and self-directed.

Group Therapy Approaches

The third section is addressed to group therapy procedures. The treatment of patients on an individual basis takes a significant amount of a therapist's time. As a result, a large number of people who are in need of therapy do not receive it. Moreover, as many therapists point out, some adjustment problems can be dealt with best in a group situation rather than on an individual basis. These and other factors stimulated the growth of group treatment techniques.

The types of group procedures used are as varied as those developed for individual therapy. Four techniques are described in this section. Article 31 by Louis Wender tells of the use of *group psychotherapy* within a psychoanalytically oriented framework with hospitalized patients. In this approach, group inter-action is emphasized and the therapy procedure is briefer than individual psychoanalysis. As in individual psychoanalytically oriented therapy, one finds catharsis, transference, and various defense mechanisms at work in those patients undergoing this kind of treatment. Wender also discusses the dynamics present in this form of therapy.

Another group approach is presented in Article 32 by John M. Atthowe, Jr. and Leonard Krasner. They discuss the preliminary results of a research project which applied a behavioral model to the treatment of hospitalized psychiatric patients. The program was initiated in an attempt to modify the maladaptive behavior of patients viewed as chronic cases, and to generate self-care activities in these patients. To accomplish this, a *token-economy system* was created on the ward where the patients lived. They were rewarded with tokens (e.g., colored file cards) whenever they behaved in an adaptive manner and were charged tokens for various items, events, and activities (e.g., cigarettes, candy, watching televison, going to a movie, etc.) that were desirable to them. The authors discuss the preliminary results of this research project as well as the implications of their findings.

Article 33 by Carl Rogers describes a recently developed group treatment technique known as the *encounter group*. Rogers focuses on the process and interactions which take place in the group and discusses their effects on the members of the group. He states that even though there is a potential for negative results, the encounter group appears to help rehumanize interpersonal relationships in a majority of cases.

An innovative group treatment approach is discussed in Article 34 by Nicholas Hobbs. He outlines a program for the treatment of emotionally disturbed children. This program, which was labeled Re-ED (for the reeducation of emotionally disturbed children), developed from the position that psychiatric hospitals, detention homes, etc., have not been helpful in the treatment of disturbed children. The general assumption of this project, according to Hobbs, is that the child is considered an inseparable part of a small social system, made up of his family, his neighborhood and community, his school, and himself, and that the goal is to get each part of this system working reasonably well in order to modify the child's maladaptive behaviors. To start the system working, Hobbs and his associates worked with each of its components and, in addition, placed the child in a small group in a residential treatment center with teacher-counselors. The center was designed so that the child could continue his education, succeed in what he did, develop trust in others, learn to control his maladaptive behaviors and mature socially. The implications of this program are also discussed.

Therapy Approaches with Special Populations

The final section is concerned with the development and use of treatment techniques with individuals and groups who have not always been considered an integral part of abnormal psychology, but in recent years have become of interest to clinicians. These include such groups as alcoholics, drug addicts, geriatric patients and senior citizens, the physically disabled, and the mentally retarded.

Treatment of one of our society's most frequent behavior problems is discussed in Article 35, published by the National Institute of Mental Health. It reviews the types of therapy approaches available for the treatment of alcoholics, along with the probable costs and possible results of such treatment. Three main aspects of treatment are dealt with: symptom withdrawal in a hospital setting (also called detoxification), drug therapy (making use of drugs that help the person to relax in situations that usually cause him to drink and the use of drugs that make him nauseous if he drinks), and psychotherapy (to help him resolve some of his psychological problems and learn to accept himself). According to this article, however, the success of any treatment program depends to a large extent on the motivation of the patient and the expertise of the therapist.

Article 36 by Joseph A. Skelly and Alexander Bassin describes a therapy program for drug addicts that has become a model for many current drug treatment programs. Prior to the development of Daytop Lodge in New York and Synanon in California, the treatment of drug addicts was not very successful. Daytop Lodge is a therapeutic community, the purpose of which is to alter the addict's value system through a process of resocialization. Conformity to the values of the community is emphasized, and deviance is met with public renunciation. The formal therapy used is based on encounter group practices.

Article 37 by Ogden R. Lindsley discusses ways in which clinicians can help the elderly, a group our society has tended to neglect over the years. Lindsley suggests that we consider the development and use of prosthetic environments for the aged. The development of these environments would be based on operant conditioning techniques. This suggestion follows directly from his theory of aging, a condition he describes as the accumulation of behavioral deficits, with such deficits becoming noticeable when adequate prosthetic devices are no longer available.

Article 38 by Lee Myerson, Nancy Kerr, and Jack L. Michael is addressed to the treatment of another special group, namely, mentally retarded and physically disabled children. Meyerson *et al.* present an alternative approach to the traditional way that professionals in rehabilitation centers have worked with these children. Specifically, they discuss a treatment program based on the behavioral model in which operant conditioning techniques are used. To illustrate the application of this treatment program, the authors present some case studies and an interesting discussion of the merits and criticisms of this approach.

REFERENCES

Hull, C. *Principles of behavior.* New York: Appleton-Century-Crofts, 1943.
Pavlov, I. P. *Conditioned reflexes.* Translated by G. V. Anrep. London: Oxford University press, 1927. 1938.
Skinner, B. F. *The behavior of organisms.* New York: Appleton-Century-Crofts, 1968.
Skinner, B. F. *Science and human behavior.* New York: Macmillan, 1953
Ullmann, L. & Krasner, L. *Case studies in behavior modification.* New York: Holt, Rinehart & Winston, 1965.

Chemotherapy

25

Chemotherapy

ELTON B. McNEIL

The discovery of psychoactive chemicals offered a way out for therapists caught in the bear-trap of unresponsive cases that were excessively demanding of time and effort with little to justify this expenditure. If you were of an age to witness the magical transformation of hospital wards as the psychochemical era was ushered in, you might better comprehend the importance of the event. Patients once uncontrollable and intractable became docile, almost rational, and manageable, if not curable, The first application of the stimulants, depressants, and tranquilizers in mental hospitals was shockingly random and indiscriminate considering that so little was known of their effect on various patterns of disorder. Treatment today is much more sophisticated; the unwanted and unexpected side effects are fewer, interaction effect of various drugs is better understood, and the results achieved in the drugged state are better controlled.

[handwritten margin note: ON WARDS DULLED PATIENTS]

Drugs gave the harried ward physician time to pause and make a new evaluation of the complex problem of caring for an increasing number of severely disturbed human beings pumped into the mental hospitals by an expanding population. Drugs were as old as man foraging among the shrubs, plants, and roots of antiquity seeking relief from painful difficulties, and modern physicians have re-examined the old-wives' tales of leaf, root, and fermented juice cures of the ancients in the search for new compounds for remedy of emotional disorder,

The history of drug use in therapy is one of a sudden and explosive proliferation of a multitude of psychoactive agents, most of which were over-promoted by the drug companies. As Peterson (1966) indicated, "In common with virtually all new medical treatments, the considerable real worth of these drugs in the treatment of mental disorders was at first exaggerated through the use of inadequately designed research. Only 10 of the roughly 1,000 studies concerned with chlorpromazine therapy that were published between 1952 and 1956, for example, could be described as controlled" (p. 19). Research with drugs has hardly been a model of scientific excellence.

Placebos and their effects make the task of evaluation of drug therapy particularly difficult. Almost the entire catalogue of possible symptoms a human being can experience seems to be capable of relief by the harmless "sugar pill" doctors have employed for hundreds of years to achieve peace of mind for their patients) The magic of the placebo is amazing. Placebos even produce "side effects" of a kind that would be reasonable if the patient had been administered an actual medicine. In a study of thousands of patients, over 60 percent reported relief from headaches after getting placebos, and similar percentages of relief have been reported for neuroses, colds, coughs, gastro-intestinal disorders, and a variety of other illnesses.

When drugs are evaluated scientifically, attention must be paid to this psychic compo-

---

nent of scientific findings. All too often the enthusiasm of the researcher bent on proving his point interferes with an objective appraisal of the effects of the drug. Another peril is the conduct of research "in house" by drug companies with a vested interest in the compound. The general practitioner, harried by a multitude of responsibilities, may take at face value the questionable scientific findings presented in glowing terms in the drug company's brochure.

Peterson (1966) observes that despite these problems of evaluation there are several advantages to the use of drugs in therapy. Both clinically and scientifically, drugs have the advantage of control of the intensity and duration of treatment, and they cost less in time, effort, and money. Drugs can be an adjunct to other forms of therapy and produce effects (unlike psychosurgery where the act once done cannot be reconsidered) which can often be reversed.

THE TRANQUILIZERS

It is conceptually convenient to cast complex drugs into simple categories in which a single effect is ascribed to a single drug, but this seldom matches the fact of drug use. The first antidepressants, for example, increased the motor activity of patients but, at the same time, left them with depressive thoughts. Drugs, it was suggested, make the patient more "reactive" to stimuli but do little to change the content of his thoughts and perceptions.

There is no drug that acts on behavior alone; all drugs alter body chemistry and change the internal physical balance. The action of the drug differs from the drug's effect. Thus, tranquilizers (ataractics) are designed to have an effect on the patient's level of anxiety, but they may also have a sedative side effect. The patient may not, subjectively, be able to tell if he is tranquil or merely sleepy. The effect of either action may be a desired one, however.

The sedatives (barbiturates) produce an effect that resembles the tranquility of other drugs. They were first used medically in 1903 as a means of chemical restraint to replace the unpopular physical restraints (strait-jackets, etc.) long in use in asylums (Sharoff, 1967). The use of barbiturates was soon extended to include the treatment of schizophrenias of all

TRANQUILIZERS

The Phenothiazines		Rauwolfia Alkaloids
Sparine		Serpasil
Vesperin		Harmonyl
Mellaril		Moderil
Compazine		Raudixin
Dartac		
Stelazine		
Permitil		
Thorazine		
	Minor Tranquilizers	
Librium	Softran	Listica
Valium	Soavitil	Levetran
Serax	Trancopal	Quiactin
Miltown, Equanil	Levanil	Ultran
Solacen	Striatran	Sycotrol

kinds by continuous sedation for long periods of time. Today, sedatives (Nembutal, Amytal, Phenobarbital, etc.) are used to take the sting out of the psychic pains of rage, anxiety, guilt, and other unpleasant emotions. Restlessness and instability decrease when the depressant effect of these drugs occurs, but there is seldom a freeing of the patient from his psychotic symptoms. Sedatives are used primarily to deal with crisis situations in which unusual emotional stress is being experienced or is anticipated.

Tranquilizers are usually subdivided into major and minor, or strong and weak, categories. It is estimated that tranquilizers constitute about 10 per cent of the nearly 65 million prescriptions dispensed each year by pharmacists and that, for the general practitioner of medicine, tranquilizing agents make up the third most common drug prescribed. The bulk of this mass of "tranquility pills" being taken to calm our society is made up of minor tranquilizers. Surprisingly, there is no reliable evidence that these minor tranquilizers are any better than the harmless sugar coated placebos.

The tranquilizers are about a decade and a half old, dating from about 1953, and they are probably improperly named (Denber, 1967). It is true they appear to make agitated patients more "tranquil" but it is the progressive disappearance of symptoms in acute and chronic psychoses that makes the "tranquilizers" so valuable. Thus, the drugs are anti-anxiety and anti-psychotic in action. A detailed account of which drug is proper for which particular set of psychotic symptoms is not possible. Each drug does not have nearly so specific an action and, as we have seen, diagnosis and symptom description is far from an exact science.

Denber (1967) suggests that the following are among the many conditions appropriate for tranquilizer therapy: acute schizophrenia; manic, involutional, and senile psychoses; agitated depression; acute alcoholic and epileptic psychoses; psychoses due to mental deficiency or organic brain disorder. This prescription of tranquilizers applies equally to those displaying borderline psychotic symptoms. In short, tranquilizers are used with almost all kinds of disorder. Denber's list of symptoms so treatable (regardless of diagnosis) include tension, anxiety, hyperactivity, agitation, impulsiveness, aggressiveness, and auditory or visual hallucinations.

It is apparent that a great deal of art and trial and error characterize the use of psychoactive chemicals. As Fink and Itil (1967) observed, "The ways in which the organic therapies of schizophrenia are associated with alterations in behavior are unclear . . . [and] duration of illness, length of hospitalization, type of onset, previous treatment, age, social class, and educational level influence the selection of treatment" (pp. 661–62). Some tranquilizers are known to have antidepressant effects as well, and this further scrambles the hoped for treatment utopia of one patient-one pill.

The tranquilizers once in most frequent use with psychotic patients were reserpine and chlorpromazine. Reserpine comes from the snakeroot plant (rauwolfia) and has been used in India for thousands of years. This drug was used initially to treat high blood pressure (hypertension) and to calm anxious and agitated patients. Its effectiveness was questioned by researchers (Segal & Shapiro, 1959), since placebos properly administered seemed to produce much the same benefit for patients.

Chlorpromazine was described as the drug that produces "indifference." It was used to limit anxiety and agitation in patients. Recently, it has been administered in combination with other drugs and has produced better results than a simple placebo (Fink, Klein, & Kramer, 1963). A number of controlled, long-term studies report an adequate level of effectiveness of chlorpromazine (Caffey, Diamond, Frank, Grasberger, Herman, Klett, & Rothstein, 1964; Casey, Bennett, Lindley, Hollister, Gordon, & Springer, 1960).

The rauwolfia derivatives have fallen into some disfavor in recent years, and the use of phenothiazines has increased accordingly. This has occured primarily because the phenothiazines have produced fewer side effects and more immediate results in the patient.

As we noted earlier, a simple schema of one drug-one patient is unworkable. Thus, no simple chart of psychosis and appropriate drug dosage level can be presented. In general, however, the major tranquilizers are administered to those with acute or chronic psychoses, agitated depressions, and organic brain disorders of many kinds. The rauwolfia compounds are used for both acute and chronic schizophrenia and for agitated states apparent in the manic psychoses or senile conditions. The minor tranquilizers are most often administered to neurotic rather than psychotic patients, but they have been used adjunctively with major tranquilizers.

Scientific assessment of the effect of tranquilizers on psychotics has most often failed to indicate that one drug is markedly better than the next for a specific disorder. All seem, in varying degrees, to produce the necessary sedative, tranquilizing, and anti-psychotic effects.

THE ANTIDEPRESSANTS

In the late 1950s the antidepressant drugs were discovered as an enlightened accident in the search for new and better tranquilizers. These new drugs acted as antidepressants, stimulants, or euphoria-producers in distressed patients but had no significant effect when administered to "normals." Since depression ranks close to schizophrenia as a serious mental health problem, these discoveries marked an important therapeutic stride forward.

Depression can exist as a separate symptom of psychological difficulty, of course, but it is often an important component of syndromes such as psychosis, organic brain disease, and the like. Some remedy for this condition was available before the discovery of the antidepressants in the form of amphetamine substitutes (Ritalin, Meratran). These mood-elevators, however, often had fairly severe side-reactions (jumpiness, insomnia, loss of appetite, jitters, etc.); the euphoria lasted only a few hours and was followed by an even deeper depression. Increased tolerance was usual and the escalation of dosage needed to produce an effect was excessive. Substitutes for the amphetamines proved to be little better than the originals.

The common antidepressants in use today are:

Marsilid	Niamid
Nardil	Parnate
Marplan	Tofranil
Elavil	Norpramin
Auentyl	Ritalin
Deaner	Dexedrine
Benzedrine	

The antidepressants are particularly useful in depressions marked by anxiety. These drugs trigger a chemical state of alertness in the brain that is reflected in the patient's behavior and rouses him from his inattention to the outside world. Yet, we must be aware that nearly 30 percent of depressed patients report improvement in response to the administration of simple placebos (Cole & Davis, 1967), and this fact makes it difficult to appraise the true effect of antidepressant drugs.

The most promising effects of antidepressants are to be found in the affective disorders.

Paranoid patients and classic schizophrenics of all kinds respond less well and sometimes suffer adverse effects (Hordern, Burt, & Holt, 1965; Marks & Pare, 1965). Electroconvulsive treatment for acute depressions seems still to hold a therapeutic edge over drug application since, if possible suicide is an important consideration, electroconvulsion seems to lift the depression with greater speed and certainty. Energizers, such as imipramine, phenelzine, and ipronizaid, have been compared favorably with placebo administration and electric shock (Wechsler, Grosser, & Greenblatt, 1965).

Any attempt to evaluate the many studies of antidepressants fails to be convincing at this moment, however, since one type of antidepressant may be completely ineffective with a particular patient while another very similar drug will produce dramatic effects in him. Antidepressants have been combined experimentally with tranquilizers (one for the anxiety and one for the depression), but no trustworthy and controlled studies of the outcome have yet appeared. In something of the same fashion, electroshock therapy and antidepressants have been used in combination. A burst of enthusiastic studies followed the combined application of these remedies, but conflicting and contradictory results with these combinations suggest that the hope that drugs could replace electroshock therapy or at least decrease the number of treatments necessary has yet to be realized.

The discovery of psychoactive drugs has made an astounding difference in our capacity to treat seriously disordered mental patients. Drug therapy still has the quality of an experimental art about it, and it will be some time before we sort out the ever-increasing mass of newly synthesized compounds in terms of which drug, or combination of drugs, best fits which diagnostic categories. The integration of drugs and psychotherapy has yet to be completely explored and remains a vital next step in our understanding of the treatment of severe mental disorder (Lesse, 1966).

DRUGS AND CHILD THERAPY

Drugs have become an integral part of the treatment of disturbed children despite the fact that the child, as a growing organism, presents quite special problems in evaluating the effect of the drug (Fish, 1967; Fisher, 1959). When children display excessive activity and excitement or are chronically anxious, impulsive, or irritable (over-reactive), drugs are increasingly prescribed. The theoretical basis for this hasty application of drug therapy rests on the assumption that the child needs to be returned to a "normal" state as quickly as possible in order not to warp the course of his development.

The goal of drug therapy is to reduce or modify symptoms in order to facilitate the execution of a comprehensive plan of therapy that may include psychotherapy and/or manipulation or alteration of the child's environment. Therapists agree chemicals alone cannot undo attitudes and patterns of learned behavior that are a part of the child's disturbance.

The phenothiazine compounds (tranquilizers) are recommended for children with schizophrenia or organic brain disease. If the schizophrenic child patient fails to respond, the rauwolfia alkaloids are suggested despite the fact they have a less reliable action (Fish, 1967). For older children (adolescents) stimulants, antidepressants, and tranquilizers are used very much in the same fashion as for adults. This delicate therapeutic task of drugging children should not be viewed lightly by the therapist. In the words of Barbara Fish (1967):

> Drugs would destroy therapy if the doctor used them as a quick expedient to avoid responsibility for the child's complex problems in living or if he saw drugs as the ultimate weapon of authority to enforce compliance on a problem child or if he felt drugs were a measure of desperation to be used

only after all other measures had failed. Children differ from adults only in that they are frequently more acutely aware of the doctor's unconscious intent and are less tolerant of his rationalizations [p. 1471].

An interesting sidelight to this observation is that again and again results obtained by drugs are inexplicably opposite from those intended by the chemical therapy. Some violently hyperactive children can receive a mixture of powerful sedatives and tranquilizers only to display even more frantic and frenetic behavior. Then, for reasons that remain unknown, they are calmed and "slowed down" when their medication is shifted to an energizing drug such as benzedrine. There is an appalling shortage of adequate information about drug action in both adults and children, but it seems somehow less ethical to drug uncomprehending children in our present state of scientific ignorance.

REFERENCES

Caffey, E. M., Jr., Diamond, L. S., Frank, T. V., Grasberger, J. C., Herman, L., Klett, C. J., & Rothstein, C. Discontinuation or reduction of chemotherapy in chronic schizophrenics. *J. chronic Diseases*, 1964, **17**, 347–1358.

Casey, J. F., Bennett, I. F., Lindley, C. J., Hollister, L. E., Gordon, M. H., & Springer, N. N. Drug therapy in schizophrenia. *A.M.A. Arch. gen. Psychiatr.*, 1960, **2** 210–220.

Cole, J. O., & Davis, J. M. Antidepressant drugs. In A. M. Freedman & H. I. Kaplan (Eds.), *Psychiatry.* Baltimore: Williams & Wilkins, 1967. Pp. 676–688.

Denber, H. C. B. Tranquillizers in psychiatry. In A. M. Freedman & H. I. Kaplan (Eds.), *Psychiatry.* Baltimore: Williams & Wilkins, 1967. Pp. 1251–1263.

Fink, M. & Itil, T. M. Schizophrenia. VI. Organic therapy. In A. M. Freedman & H. I. Kaplan (Eds.), *Psychiatry.* Baltimore: Williams & Wilkins, 1967. Pp. 661–664.

Fink, M., Klein, D. F., & Kramer, J. C. Clinical efficacy of chlorpromazine-procyclidene combination, imipramine and placebo in depressive disorders. *Psychopharmacologia*, 1963, **7**, 27–38.

Fish, B. Organic therapies. In A. M. Freedman & H. I. Kaplan (Eds.), *Psychiatry.* Baltimore: Williams & Wilkins, 1967. Pp. 1468–1472.

Fisher, S. *Child research in psychopharmacology.* Springfield, Ill. : Charles C Thomas, 1959.

Hordern, A., Burt, C. G., & Holt, N. F. *Depressive states.* Springfield, Ill. : Charles C Thomas, 1965.

Lesse, S. Psychotherapy plus drugs in severe depressions: Technique. *Compreh. Psychiatr.*, 1966, **1**, 224–231.

Marks, J. & Pare, C. M. B. *The scientific basis of drug therapy in psychiatry.* New York: Pergamon Press, 1965.

Peterson, E. *Psychopharmacology.* Dubuque, Iowa: William C. Brown, 1966.

Segal, M. M. & Shapiro, K. L. A clinical comparison study of the effects of reserpine and placebo on anxiety. *A.M.A. Arch. Neurol. Psychiatr.*, 1959, **81**, 392–398.

Sharoff, R. L. Sedatives. In A. M. Freedman & H. I. Kaplan (Eds.), *Psychiatry.* Baltimore: Williams & Wilkins, 1967. Pp. 1275–1277.

Wechsler, H., Grosser, G. H & Greenblatt, M. Research evaluating antidepressant medications on hospitalized mental patients: A survey of published reports during a five-year period. *J. Nerv. Ment. Dis.*, 1965, **141**, 231–239.

Suggested Additional Readings

Blair, D. *Modern drugs for the treatment of mental illness.* London: Staples Press, 1963.

Caldwell, W. V. *LSD psychotherapy.* New York: Grove Press, 1968.

Dally, P. *Chemotherapy of psychiatric disorders.* New York: Plenum Press, 1967.

Davis, J. M. Efficacy of tranquilizing and anti-depressant drugs. *Archives of General Psychiatry,* 1965, **13**, 552–572.

Dews, P. B. Psychopharmacology. In A. J. Bachrach (Ed.), *Experimental foundations of clinical psychology.* New York: Basic Books, 1962

Eiduson, S., Geller, E., Yuwiler, A., & Eiduson, B. T. *Biochemistry and behavior.* New York: Van Nostrand, 1964.

Freedman, A. M. & Kaplan, H. I. (Eds.) *Psychiatry.* Baltimore: Williams & Wilkins., 1967.

Marks, J. & Pare, C. M. B. *The scientific basis of drug therapy in psychiatry.* New York: Pergamon Press, 1965.

Peterson, E. *Psychopharmacology.* Dubuque, Iowa: William C. Brown, 1966.

Rickels, K. *Non-specific factors in drug therapy.* Springfield, Ill. : Charles C Thomas, 1968.

Shepherd, M., Lader, M., & Rodnight, R. *Clinical psychopharmacology.* London: English Universities Press, 1968.

Wittenborn, J. R. & May, P. R. A. *Prediction of response to pharmacotherapy.* Springfield, Ill.: Charles C. Thomas, 1966.

Individual Therapy Approaches

26

Freudian Psychoanalysis*

LEWIS R. WOLBERG

... Freudian psychoanalytic therapy is based on the libido theory...., It rests on the hypothesis that neurotic illness is nurtured by the repression of vital aspects of the self and its experiences; particularly oral, anal and sexual (including Oedipal) experiences in relation to important parental agencies. This repression is sponsored by fear of the loss of love or of punishment from the parents, which has been internalized in the super-ego. Repressed feelings, attitudes and fears, and the early experiences associated with them, continue to strive for conscious recognition, but are kept from awareness by dread of repetition of parental loss of love or punishment now invested in the super-ego. The removal from the mainstream of consciousness makes it impossible for the individual to come to grips with basic conflicts. These remain in their pristine state, uncorrected by reality and by later experiences. The energy required to maintain repression, as well as to sustain other defenses against anxiety, robs the individual of energy that could be utilized to nurture psychosexual development.

Therapy, of necessity, consists of restoring to consciousness that which was removed by repression, and which has been draining off energies needed to foster personality growth. In therapy, the relationship with the therapist helps strengthen the ego to a point where it can eventually cope with anxiety, mobilized by the return of the repressed to awareness. It is essential that the patient recognize the derivatives of the repressed, since these represent in an attenuated form, the warded-off material. To minimize the distortion of these derivatives, the obtrusion of current situations and other reality influences must be kept at a minimum. This is fostered by certain technical procedures, such as "free association," the assumption of the couch position, passivity of the therapist, encouragement of transference, the use of dreams, and the focusing of the interview away from reality considerations.

The basis of Freudian psychoanalysis lies in what is perhaps Freud's most vital discovery, that of transference. As has previously been indicated, Freud found that the patient, if not interfered with, inevitably projected into the therapeutic situation, feelings and attitudes that were parcels of his past. Sometimes transference manifestations became so intense that the patient actually reproduced and reenacted with the therapist important conflictual situations and traumatic experiences (transference neurosis) which had been subject to infantile amnesia. By recovering and recognizing these repressed experiences and conflictual situations that had never been resolved, and by living them through with a new, less neurotic and non-punitive parental agency, the super-ego was believed to undergo modification. The individual became tolerant of his id, and more capable of altering ego defenses that had crippled his adaptation. There occurred, finally, a mastery of his early conflicts and a liberation of fixated libido which could then enter into the development of a mature personality.

---

*From Wolberg, L. R., *Techniques of psychotherapy*, Copyright © 1954 by Grune & Stratton, Inc. Reprinted by permission of Grune & Stratton, Inc., publishers, and Dr. Wolberg.

Since the Oedipus complex is considered by Freud to be the nucleus of every neurosis, its analysis and resolution in transference constitutes a primary focus. Where the Oedipus complex is not revealed, where its pathologic manifestations are not thoroughly analyzed and worked through, and where forgotten memories of early childhood experiences are not restored, treatment is considered incomplete.

Because Freudian psychoanalysis *is* transference analysis, all means of facilitating transference are employed. These include the assumption by the therapist of an extremely passive role, the verbalization by the patient of a special kind of communication—"free association"—the analysis of dream material, the maintenance of an intense contact with the patient on the basis of no less than five visits weekly, and the employment of the recumbent couch position.

Passivity on the part of the therapist is judiciously maintained even through long periods of silence. The therapist also refrains from reacting emotionally, or responding positively or negatively to any verbalized or non-verbalized attitude or feeling expressed by the patient. Strict anonymity is observed, no personal information being supplied to the patient irrespective of how importunate he may become. A non-judgmental, non-punitive, non-condoning attitude by the therapist is adhered to, dogmatic utterances of any kind being forbidden.

The only "rule" the patient is asked to obey is the "basic rule" or "fundamental rule" of verbalizing whatever comes to his mind, however fleeting, repulsive or seemingly inconsequential it may seem (free association). This undirected kind of thinking is a most important means of tapping the unconscious, and of reviving unconscious conflicts and the memories that are related to their origin. Most importantly, free association, like passivity, enhances the evolution of transference. So long as the patient continues to associate freely, the therapist keeps silent, even though entire sessions may pass without a comment. The therapist fights off all temptations toward "small talk" or impulses to expound on theory. Only when resistances to free association develop, does he interfere, and only until the patient proceeds with his verbalizations.

Dream analysis is utilized constantly as another means of penetrating the unconscious. By activating repressed material and working on defenses as they are revealed in dream structure, the therapist aids the development of transference.

The frequency of visits in Freudian psychoanalysis is important. To encourage transference, no fewer than five visits weekly are required. In some cases four visits may suffice. Fewer visits than this encourage "acting-out" and other resistances to transference.

The use of the recumbent couch position enables the patient to concentrate on the task of free association with as few encumbrances of reality as possible. It helps the therapist, also, to focus on the unconscious content underlying the patient's verbalizations without having to adjust himself to the demands such as would exist in a face-to-face position. Concentrating on his inner life, rather than on external reality, helps to bring on the phenomenon of transference.

During the early stages of analysis, the main task is to observe—from his free associations and dreams—unconscious conflicts, and the types of defenses employed by the patient, which form a kind of blueprint of the unconscious problems of the patient. This blueprint is utilized later at the stage of transference. Since repression is threatened by the operation of exploring the unconscious, anxiety is apt to appear, stimulating defensive mechanisms. These function as resistances to productivity, and even to verbalization. Free association may consequently cease, and the patient may exhibit other manifestations that oppose cooperation with the treatment endeavor. Such resistances are dealt with by interpretation. Through interpretation the patient is brought to an awareness of how and why he is resisting, and the conflicts that make resistance necessary.

Sooner or later the patient will "transfer" past attitudes and feelings into the present relationship with the analyst. Observance of the "basic rule," the attack on his resistances through interpretation, and the consideration of unconscious material in dreams and free associations, remove habitual protective devices and façades that permit the patient to maintain a conventional relationship. Toward the therapist he is most apt to express strivings rooted in past experiences, perhaps even reproducing his past in the present. Thus, a revival of pathogenic past conflicts develops. Unlike supportive and reeducative therapy, in which transference may be utilized as a therapeutic vehicle, the transference is interpreted to the patient in order to expose its nature. This is the chief means of resolving resistance, of bringing the individual to an awareness of the warded off content, and of realizing the historical origin of his conflicts.

The development of transference may occur insidiously and manifest itself indirectly, or it may suddenly break out in stark form. It often shows itself in changes in the content of free associations, from inner feelings and past relationships with parents, to more innocuous topics, like current events and situations. This shift is evidence of resistance to deeper material activated by the erupting transference feelings. Sometimes free association may cease entirely, with long stubborn silences prevailing which are engendered by an inability to talk about feelings in relation to the therapist. The purpose of superficial talk or silence is to keep from awareness repressed emotions and forgotten memories associated with early childhood, particularly the Oedipus complex. Until these can be brought out into the open, the emotions relating to them discharged, and the associated memories revived, the conflictual base of neurosis will remain. The transference neurosis offers an opportunity for this revival, since, in the relationship with the therapist, the patient will "act-out" his loves, fears and hates, which were characteristic of his own experiences during the Oedipal period.

Transference, however, acts as a source of powerful resistances that impede therapeutic progress. Once the patient is in the grip of such resistances, he is usually determined to cling to them at the expense of any other motivation, including that of getting well. On the positive side, transference is important diagnostically, since it reveals a most accurate picture of the patient's inner conflicts. Additionally, it induces a coming to grips with and a working-through in a much more favorable setting of those unresolved conflicts that have blocked maturation. The resolution of transference is felt by Freudian psychoanalysts to be the most powerful vehicle known today for producing structural alterations in the personality.

Active interpretations of the transference are essential to its resolution. These include the interpretation of its manifestations, its origin, and its original and present purposes. The working-through of transference is accompanied by a recollection of forgotten infantile and childhood experiences—a recounting of distortions in relationships with parents or parental surrogates. Interpretations will usually be denied at first as part of the resistance manifestation. Acknowledgment of the unreal nature of transference is usually opposed by the patient, because this either constitutes too great a threat for him, or because he does not want to relinquish transference gratifications which are deemed essential to life itself. So long as he continues to accept transference as factual, the analysis will remain interminable, unless forcefully terminated by either participant. With persistence on the part of the therapist, interpretations usually take hold, and the patient is rewarded with greater insight, an increased sense of mastery, liberation from neurotic symptoms, and a genuine growth in maturity.

The therapist must also constantly guard against manifestations of counter-transference, which may be both disguised and varied, and which are mobilized by unresolved problems and pressing needs within the therapist himself. Common forms of counter-transference

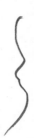

are subtle sadistic attacks on the patient, impulses to be pompous and omnipotent, or desires to reject the patient or to detach oneself from the relationship. Because of counter-transference, a personal analysis is considered essential for the analyst in order that he can deal with his own unconscious tendencies and resistances precipitated by his contact with his patients.

As the ego of the patient is strengthened by an alliance with the therapist, it becomes more and more capable of tolerating less and less distorted derivatives of unconscious conflict. The continued interpretation by the therapist of the patient's unconscious feelings and attitudes, as well as the defensive devices that he employs against them, enables the patient to work-through his problems by seeing how they condition every aspect of his life. In the medium of the therapeutic relationship, the individual is helped to come to grips with early fears and misconceptions, resolving these by living them through in the transference. The patient is finally able to resolve libidinal fixations, and to liberate energy that should originally have gone into the formation of a mature sexual organization[1–22].

REFERENCES

1. Balint, M. The final goal of psychoanalytic treatment. *Internat. J. Psycho-Analysis*, 1936, **17**.
2. Berg, C. *Psychotherapy-Practice and theory.* New York: Norton, 1948. Pp. 349–357.
3. Bibring-Lehner, G. A contribution to the subject of transference resistance. *Internat. J. Psycho-Analysis*, 1936, **17**, 181–189.
4. Fenichel, O. *Problems of psychoanalytic technique.* Albany, N.Y.: The Psychoanalytic Quarterly, Inc., 1941.
5. Freud, S. *A general introduction to psychoanalysis.* New York: Boni & Liveright, 1920.
6. Freud, S. Papers on technique. In *Collected papers.* Vol. 2. London: Hogarth Press, 1924.
7. Freud, S. *New introductory lectures on psychoanalysis.* New York: Norton, 1933.
8. Freud, S. Analysis terminable and interminable. *Internat. J. Psycho-Analysis*, 1937, **18**, 373–405.
9. Glover, E. Lectures on technique in psychoanalysis. *Internat. J. Psycho-Analysis*, 1924, **8**, 1–4.
10. Glover, E., Fenichel, O., Strachey, J., Bergler, E., Nunberg, H., & Bibring, E. On the theory of therapeutic results of psychoanalysis. (Symposium) *Internat. J. Psycho-Analysis*, 1937, **18**, 125–189.
11. Jones, E. The relation of technique to theory. *Internat. J. Psycho-Analysis*, 1924, 8, 1–4.
12. Kubie, L. *Practical and theoretical aspects of psychoanalysis.* New York: International Universities Press, 1950.
13. La Forgue, R. Exceptions to the fundamental rule of psychoanalysis. *Internat. J. Psycho-Analysis*, 1937, **18**.
14. Lorand, S. *Technique of psychoanalytic therapy.* New York: International Universities Press, 1946.
15. Nunberg, H. Practice and theory of psychoanalysis. *Nerv. & Ment. Dis. Monog.*, 1948, No. 74.
16. Schmidegerg, M. The mode of operation of psychoanalytic therapy. *Internat. J. Psycho-Analysis*, 1938, **19**.
17. Searl, M. N. Some queries on principles of technique. *Internat. J. Psycho-Analysis*, 1936, 17.
18. Sharpe, E. F. The technique of psychoanalysis. *Internat. J. Psycho-Analysis*, 1931, **12**.
19. Sterba, R. The dynamics of the dissolution of the transference resistance. *Psychiatric. Quart.*, 1940, **9**.
20. Stern, A. On the counter-transference in psychoanalysis. *Psychoanalyt. Rev.*, 1924, **9**, 166–174.
21. Strachey, J. The nature of the therapeutic action of psychoanalysis. *Internat. J. Psycho-Analysis*, 1934, **15**, 127.
22. Zilboorg, G. The fundamental conflict with psychoanalysis. *Internat. J. Psycho-Analysis*, 1939, **20**, 480–492.

27

The Psychiatric Nurse as a Behavioral Engineer*†

TEODORO AYLLON and JACK MICHAEL

The behavior which leads to a person's admission to a mental hospital often involves danger to himself or others, withdrawal from normal social functions, or a dramatic change from his usual mode of behaving. The professional staff of the psychiatric hospital directs its major efforts toward the discovery of the flaw in the patient's mental apparatus which presumably underlies his disturbing and dangerous behavior. Following the medical paradigm, it is presumed that once the basic dysfunction has been properly identified the appropriate treatment will be undertaken and the various manifestations of the dysfunction will disappear.

While diagnosis is being made and during subsequent treatment, the patient is under the daily care of the psychiatric nurses[1] in the ward. There, he often exhibits annoying and disrupting behavior which is usually regarded as a further manifestation of his basic diffi- culty. This behavior is sometimes identical with that which led to his admission; but at other times it seems to originate and develop within the hospital setting. Although it is still regarded as a reflection of his basic problem, this disruptive behavior may become so persistent that it engages the full energies of the nurses, and postpones, sometimes perma- nently, any effort on their part to deal with the so-called basic problem.

Disrupting behaviors usually consist in the patient's failure to engage in activities which are considered normal and necessary; or his persistent engagement in activities that are harmful to himself or other patients, or disrupting in other ways. For example, failures to eat, dress, bathe, interact socially with other patients, and walk without being led are invariably disruptive. Hoarding various objects, hitting, pinching, spitting on other patients, constant attention-seeking actions with respect to the nurses, upsetting chairs in the day- room, scraping paint from the walls, breaking windows, stuffing paper in the mouth and ears, walking on haunches or while in a squatting position are disruptive when they occur frequently and persistently.

At present, no systematic approach to such problems is available to the nurses. A psychodynamic interpretation is often given by psychiatrists and psychologists; and, for

---

*From Ayllon, T., and Michael, J., *Journal of the Experimental Analysis of Behavior*, 1959, **2**, 323–334. Copyright © 1959 by the Society for the Experimental Analysis of Behavior. Reprinted by permission of the Society for the Experimental Analysis of Behavior, Inc., and Dr. Ayllon.

†This paper contains a portion of the data from a doctoral dissertation submitted to the Department of Psychology, University of Houston, in partial fulfillment of the requirements for the Ph.D. degree in August, 1959. Grateful acknowledgment is due to the members of the doctoral committee for their help and encouragement, and also to Drs. H. Osmond and I. Clancey, Superintendent and Clinical Director of the Saskatchewan Hospital, for making research at this institution possible.

Additional information and related research can be found in *The Token Economy: A Motivational System for Therapy and Rehabilitation* by T. Ayllon and N. H. Azrin published by Appleton-Century- Crofts, 1968.

[1]As used in this paper, "psychiatric nurse" is a generic term including all those who actually work on the ward (aides, psychiatric nurses, and registered nurses).

that matter, the nurses sometimes construct "depth" interpretations themselves. These interpretations seldom suggest any specific remedial actions to the nurses, who then have no other recourse than to act on the basis of common sense, or to take advantage of the physical therapy in vogue. From the point of view of modern behavior theory, such strong behaviors, or behavioral deficits, may be considered the result of events occurring in the patient's immediate or historical environment rather than the manifestations of his mental disorder. The present research represents an attempt to discover and manipulate some of these environmental variables for the purpose of modifying the problem behavior.

RESEARCH SETTING

The research was carried out at the Saskatchewan Hospital, Weyburn, Saskatchewan, Canada. It is a psychiatric hospital with approximately 1500 patients. Its most relevant features in terms of the present experiment are:

1. The nurses are trained as psychiatric nurses in a 3-year program.

2. They are responsible for the patients in their wards and enjoy a high degree of autonomy with respect to the treatment of a patient. The psychiatrists in the hospital function as advisers to the nursing staff. This means that psychiatrists do not give orders, but simply offer advice upon request from the psychiatric nurses.

3. The nurses administer incoming and outgoing mail for the patients, visitor traffic, ground passes, paroles, and even discharge, although the last is often carried out after consultation with a psychiatrist. The nurses also conduct group therapy under the supervision of the psychiatric staff.

The official position of the senior author, hereafter referred to as *E*, was that of a clinical psychologist, who designed and supervised operant-conditioning "therapy" as applied by the nurses. Once his advice had been accepted, the nurses were responsible for carrying out the procedures specified by *E*. It was the privilege of the nurses to discontinue any treatment when they believed it was no longer necessary, when they were unable to implement it because of lack of staff, or when other ward difficulties made the treatment impossible. Whenever termination became necessary, *E* was given appropriate notice.

SUBJECTS

The subjects used in this investigation were all patients in the hospital. Of the total 19 patients, 14 had been classified as schizophrenic and 5 as mentally defective. Except for one female patient who was resident for only 7 months, all patients had been hospitalized for several years. Each subject presented a persistent behavior problem for which he had been referred to *E* by the nursing staff. None of the *S*s was presently receiving psychotherapy, electroconvulsive therapy, or any kind of individual treatment.

The behaviors which were studied do not represent the most serious problems encountered in a typical psychiatric hospital. They were selected mainly because their persistence allowed them to survive several attempts at altering them.

PROCEDURE

Prior to a systematic observational study of the patient's behavior the nurses were asked about the kind and frequency of naturally occurring reinforcement obtained by the patient, the duration and frequency of the problem behavior, and the possibility of controlling the reinforcement. Next, a period of systematic observation of each patient was undertaken prior to treatment. This was done to obtain objective information on the frequency of the behavior that was a problem to the nurses, and to determine what other behaviors were emitted by the patient.

Depending on the type of behavior, two methods were used for recording it. If the behavior involved interaction with a nurse, it was recorded every time it occurred. Entering the nurses' office, and eating regular meals are examples of such behavior.

Behavior which did not naturally involve contact with the nurse was recorded by a timesampling technique. The nurse who was in charge of the program was supplied with a mimeographed record form. She sought out the patient at regular intervals; and without interaction with him, she recorded the behavior taking place at that time. She did not actually describe the behavior occurring, but rather classified it in terms of a pre-established trichotomy: (a) the undesirable behavior; (b) incompatible behavior which could ultimately displace the undesirable behavior; and (c) incompatible behavior which was not considered shapeable, such as sleeping, eating, and dressing. (Although these latter acts are certainly susceptible to the influence of reinforcement, they were regarded as neutral behaviors in the present research.) The period of observation varied from 1 to 3 minutes. After making an observation, the nurse resumed her regular ward activities until the next interval was reached, whereupon she again sought out the patient. Except for one patient, who was observed every 15 minutes, such observations were made every 30 minutes.

The relevant aspect of the data obtained by the time-check recording is the proportion of the total number of observations (excluding observations of neutral behavior) during which the patient was engaging in the behavior being altered. This will be called the relative frequency of the behavior. As an example, on the first day of the program of extinction for psychotic talk in the case of Helen (see below), 17 nonneutral behaviors were recorded. Of these, nine were classed as psychotic talk and eight as sensible talk; the relative frequency of psychotic talk was 0.53.

Although it would have been desirable, a long pretreatment period of observation was precluded by the newness of this approach and the necessity of obtaining the voluntary cooperation of the nurses.

After the pretreatment study had been completed, E instructed the ward nurses in the specific program that was to be carried out. In all cases the instruction was given at ward meetings and usually involved the cooperation of only two shifts, the 7 a.m. to 3 p.m., and 3 p.m. to 11 p.m., since the patients were usually asleep during the 11 p.m. to 7 a.m. shift.

The pretreatment studies indicated that what maintained undesirable behavior in most of the patients was the attention or social approval of the nurses toward that behavior. Therefore, the emphasis in instructing the nursing staff was on the operation of giving or withholding social reinforcement contingent upon a desired class of behavior. What follows illustrates the tenor of E's somewhat informal instructions to the nurses. "Reinforcement is something you do for or with a patient, for example, offering candy or a cigarette. Any way you convey attention to the patient is reinforcing. Patients may be reinforced if you answer their questions, talk to them, or let them know by your reaction that you are aware of their presence. The common-sense expression 'pay no attention' is perhaps closest to what must be done to discourage the patient's behavior. When we say 'do not reinforce a behavior,' we are actually saying 'ignore the behavior and act deaf and blind whenever it occurs.'"

When reinforcement was given on a fixed-interval basis, the nurse was instructed to observe the patient for about 1 to 3 minutes at regular intervals, just as in the pretreatment observation period. If desirable behavior was occurring at the time of observation, she would reinforce it; if not, she would go on about her duties and check again after the next interval had passed. Strictly speaking, this is fixed interval with a limited-hold contingency (Ferster & Skinner, 1957). During a program of extinction the nurse checked as above; however, instead of reinforcing the patient when he exhibited the behavior being altered, she simply recorded it and continued her other work. Except for specific directions for two patients, the nurses were not given instructions on the operation of aversive control.

The programs requiring time-sample observations started after breakfast (around 9 a.m.) and ended at bedtime (around 9 p.m.), and were usually carried out by only one of the 6 to 12 nurses on each shift. Because of the daily shift changes, the monthly ward rotations, and a systematic effort to give everyone experience at this new duty, no patient's program was followed by any one nurse for any considerable length of time. Nineteen, as a minimum, different nurses were involved in carrying out each patient's program. Over 100 different nurses participated in the entire research project.

Most social ward activities took place in the dayroom, which was a large living room containing a television set, card tables, magazines, and games. It was here that reinforcement was given for social behaviors toward patients, and for nonsocial behaviors which were strengthened to compete with undesirable behaviors. The fact that the research was carried out in five wards distributed far from each other in a four-floor building made it impossible for *E* to observe all the nurses involved in the research at any one time. Because of the constant change in nursing personnel, most of *E*'s time was spent in instructing new people in the routines of the programs. In addition, since *E* did not train the nurses extensively, he observed them, often without their knowledge, and supervised them in record keeping, administering reinforcement, extinction, etc. That the nurses performed effectively when *E* was absent can be at least partially determined by the ultimate results.

RESULTS

The results will be summarized in terms of the type of behavior problem and the operations used in altering the behavior. In general, the time required to change a specific behavior ranged from 6 to 11 weeks. The operations were in force for 24 hours a day, 7 days a week.

Strong Behavior Treated by Extinction, or Extinction Combined with Reinforcement for Incompatible Behavior

In the five cases treated with this program, the reinforcer was the attention of the nurses; and the withholding of this reinforcer resulted in the expected decline in frequency. The changes occurring in three of the behavior problems, scrubbing the floor, spending too much time in the bathroom, and one of the two cases of entering the nurses' offices, were not complicated by uncontrollable variables. Lucille's case is presented in detail as representative of these three. The interpretation of the changes occurring in the other two behavior problems, entering the nurses' offices, and psychotic verbal behavior, is not so clear-cut. Helen's case illustrates this point. For details concerning the cases not discussed in this paper, see Ayllon (1959).

Lucille   Lucille's frequent visits to the nurses' office interrupted and interfered with their work. She had been doing this for 2 years. During this time, she had been told that she was not expected to spend her time in the nurses' office. Frequently, she was taken by the hand or pushed back bodily into the ward. Because the patient was classified as mentally defective, the nurses had resigned themselves to tolerating her behavior. As one of the

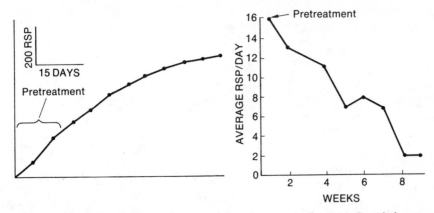

Fig. 27.1   Extinction of the response "entering the nurses' office." (a) Cumulative record, (b) conventional record.

nurses put it, "It's difficult to tell her anything because she can't understand—she's too dumb."

The following instructions were given to the nurses: "During this program the patient must not be given reinforcement (attention) for entering the nurses' office. Tally every time she enters the office."

The pretreatment study indicated that she entered the office on an average of 16 times a day. As Fig. 27.1b shows, the average frequency was down to two entries per day by the seventh week of extinction, and the program was terminated. Figure 27.1a shows the same data plotted cumulatively.

Helen   This patient's psychotic talk had persisted for at least 3 years. It had become so annoying during the last 4 months prior to treatment that other patients had on several occasions beaten her in an effort to keep her quiet. She was described by one of the psychiatrists as a "delusional" patient who "feels she must push her troubles onto somebody else, and by doing this she feels she is free." Her conversation centered around her illegitimate child and the men she claimed were constantly pursuing her. It was the nurses' impression that the patient had "nothing else to talk about."

A 5-day pretreatment observation of the patient was made at 30-minute intervals to compare the relative frequencies of psychotic and sensible content in her talk. Some of the nurses reported that, previously, when the patient started her psychotic talk, they listened to her in an effort to get at the "roots of her problem." A few nurses stated that they did not listen to what she was saying but simply nodded and remarked, "Yes, I understand," or some such comment, the purpose of which was to steer the patient's conversation onto some other topic. These reports suggested that the psychotic talk was being maintained by the nurses' reaction to it. While it is recognized that a distinction between psychotic and normal talk is somewhat arbitrary, this case was included in the research because of its value as a problem involving primarily verbal behavior.

The following instructions were given to the nurses: "During this program the patient must not be given reinforcement (attention) for her psychotic talk (about her illegitimate child and the men chasing her). Check the patient every 30 minutes, and (a) tally for psychotic talk; and (b) reinforce (and tally) sensible talk. If another patient fights with her, avoid making an issue of it. Simply stop the other patient from hurting her, but do so with a matter-of-fact attitude."

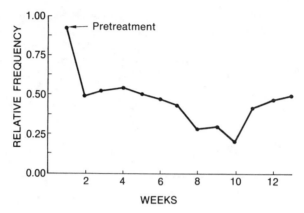

Fig. 27.2   Extinction of psychotic talk.

The 5-day observation period resulted in a relative frequency of psychotic talk of 0.91. During treatment (Fig. 27.2), the relative frequency dropped to less than 0.25; but, later on, it rose to a value exceeded only by the pretreatment level. The sudden increase in the patient's psychotic talk in the ninth week probably occurred because the patient had been talking to a social worker, who, unknown to the nurses, had been reinforcing her psychotic talk. The reinforcement obtained from the social worker appeared to generalize to her interaction with other patients and nurses. The patient herself told one of the nurses, "Well you're not listening to me. I'll have to go and see Miss———[the social worker] again, 'cause she told me that if she would listen to my past she could help me."

In addition to the reinforcement attributable to the social worker, two other instances of bootleg reinforcement came to light. One instance occurred when a hospital employee came to visit the ward, and, another, when volunteer ladies came to entertain the patients. These occasions were impossible to control, and indicate some of the difficulties of long-term control over verbal behavior.

It is of interest to note that since the reinforcement program began, the patient has not been attacked by the other patients and is only rarely abused verbally. These improvements were commented upon by the nurses, who were nevertheless somewhat disappointed. On the basis of the improvement shown in verbal behavior, the nurses had expected a dramatic over-all change which did not occur.

Strong Behavior Treated by Strengthening Incompatible Behavior

This case represented an attempt to control violent behavior by strengthening an incompatible class of responses, and to recondition normal social approaches while the violence was under control. The first phase was quite successful; but errors in strategy plagued the last half of the program, and it was terminated by the nurses because the patient became more violent.

The immediate reason for referral was that the patient, Dotty, had become increasingly violent over the last 5 years, and recently attacked several patients and hospital personnel without any apparent reason. Since admission and up to the present, she had received many electroconvulsive-therapy treatments aimed at reducing this violence, with little or no success. In 1947, a physician recommended her as a good case for psychosurgery. In

December of the same year, she attempted to strangle her mother who was visiting her at the time. In July 1948, the patient had a leucotomy. The situation had recently become so serious that at the least suspicious move on her part the nurses would put her in the seclusion room. She spent from 3 to 12 hours in that room.

A 5-day pretreatment study, at 15-minute intervals, indicated that one of the nonviolent behaviors exhibited fairly often was "being on the floor" in the dayroom. The response included lying, squatting, kneeling, and sitting on the floor. Strengthening this class of responses would control the violence and, at the same time, permit the emotional behavior of other patients and nurses toward her to extinguish. To strengthen the patient's own social behavior, her approaches to the nurses were to be reinforced. The response "approach to nurse" was defined as spontaneous requests, questions or comments made by the patient to the nurse. Ultimately, the plan was to discontinue reinforcing being on the floor once the patient-nurse social interaction appeared somewhat normal. Presumably, this would have further increased the probability of approach to the nurses.

For the duration of the program, continuous social reinforcement was to be available for her approach to the nurses. Social reinforcement was to be available for the first 4 weeks only, on a fixed interval of 15 minutes, contingent on the response being on the floor. For the last 4 weeks, social reinforcement was to be withheld for being on the floor.

The following instructions were given to the nurses first 4 weeks of the program: "Reinforce (and tally) her approaches to you every time they occur. Check the patient every 15 minutes, and reinforce (and tally) the behavior being on the floor."

From the fifth week on the instructions were modified as follows: "Continue reinforcing (and tallying) her approaches to you every time they occur. Check the patient every 15 minutes, and tally but do not reinforce the behavior being on the floor."

During the period of reinforcement, as shown in Fig. 27.3, the relative frequency of the response being on the floor increased from the pretreatment level of less than 0.10 to a

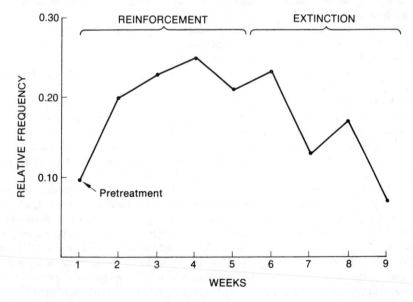

Fig. 27.3 Reinforcement and subsequent extinction of the response "being on the floor."

value of 0.21. During the succeeding 4 weeks of extinction, the frequency of being on the floor returned to the pretreatment level.

It was clear that being on the floor was incompatible with the fighting behavior and that the latter could be controlled by reinforcing the former. During the period of reinforcement for being on the floor, she attacked a patient once; but during the period of extinction, she made eight attacks on others. Her approaches to nurses increased over-all during the 4 weeks of reinforcement, but they decreased during the last 4 weeks, even though they were still being reinforced. This decrease paralleled the decrease in being on the floor. While being on the floor was undergoing extinction, attacks on the patients and nurses increased in frequency, and the nurses decided to return to the practice of restraining the patient. The program was terminated at this point.

The patient's failure to make the transition from being on the floor to approaching the nurses suggests that the latter response was poorly chosen. It was relatively incompatible with being on the floor. This meant that a previously reinforced response would have to be extinguished before the transition was possible, and this, too, was poor strategy with a violent patient.

Weak Behavior Strengthened by Escape and Avoidance Conditioning

Two female patients generally refused to eat unless aided by the nurses. One, Janet, had to be forcefully taken to the dining room, where she would permit the nurses to spoonfeed her. The other patient, Mary, was spoonfed in a room adjacent to the dining room. Both patients had little social contact with others and were reported to be relatively indifferent to attention by the nurses. Both were also reported to care only for the neat and clean appearance of their clothing. Mary had been at the hospital for 7 months, and Janet had been there for 28 years. These two patients were in different wards and apparently did not know each other.

The program involved a combination of escape and avoidance conditioning, with food spilling as the aversive stimulus. All spoonfeeding was to be accompanied by some food spilling which the patient could escape by feeding herself after the first spilling, or avoid by feeding herself the entire meal. Social reinforcement was to be given contingent on feeding herself.

It was hoped that once self-feeding began to occur with some regularity, it would come under the control of environmental variables which maintain this behavior in most people, such as convenience, social stimulation at meal time, etc. In both cases, the program ultimately resulted in complete self-feeding, which now has been maintained for over 10 months. Janet's behavior change was complicated by a history of religious fasting, and her change took a little longer. Mary's case will be given here in detail.

The following instructions were given to the nurses: "Continue spoonfeeding the patient; but from now on, do it in such a careless way that the patient will have a few drops of food fall on her dress. Be sure not to overdo the food dropping, since what we want to convey to the patient is that it is difficult to spoonfeed a grown-up person, and not that we are mean to her. What we expect is that the patient will find it difficult to depend on your skill to feed her. You will still be feeding her, but you will simply be less efficient in doing a good job of it. As the patient likes having her clothes clean, she will have to choose between feeding herself and keeping her clothes clean, or being fed by others and risking getting her clothes soiled. Whenever she eats on her own, be sure to stay with her for a while (3 minutes is enough), talking to her, or simply being seated with her. We do this to reinforce her eating on her own. In the experience of the patient, people become nicer when she eats on her own."

During the 8-day pretreatment study, the patient ate 5 meals on her own, was spoonfed 12, and refused to eat 7. Her weight at this time was 99 pounds. Her typical reaction to the schedule was as follows: The nurse would start spoonfeeding her; but after one or two "good" spoonfuls, the nurse would carelessly drop some food on her dress. This was continued until either the patient requested the spoon, or the nurse continued spoonfeeding her the entire meal.The behaviors the patient adopted included (a) reaching for the spoon after a few drops had fallen on her dress; (b) eating completely on her own; (c) closing her mouth so that spoonfeeding was terminated; or (d) being spoonfed the entire meal. Upon starting the schedule, the most frequent of all these alternatives was the first; but after a while, the patient ate on her own immediately. The relevant data are shown in Fig. 27.4. On the 12th day, the patient ate all three meals on her own for the first time. Four meals were refused out of the last 24: one meal was missed because she stated she didn't like "liver" and the other three because she said she was not hungry. Her weight when she left the hospital was 120 pounds, a gain of 21 pounds over her pretreatment weight.

Mary's relapse in the fifth week, after she had been eating well for 2 weeks, was quite unexpected. No reasonable explanation is suggested by a study of her daily records; but, after she had been spoonfed several meals in a row, the rumor developed that someone had informed the patient that the food spilling was not accidental. In any event, the failure to feed herself lasted only about 5 days.

Since the patient's hospital admission had been based on her refusal to eat, accompanied by statements that the food was poisoned, the success of the program led to her discharge. It is to be noted that although nothing was done to deal directly with her claims that the food was poisoned, these statements dropped out of her repertoire as she began to eat on her own.

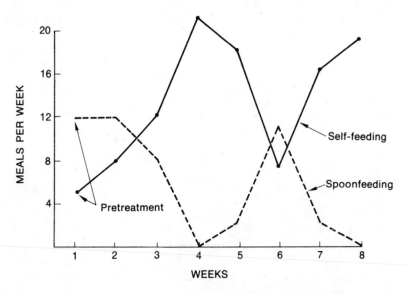

Fig. 27.4 Escape and avoidance conditioning of self-feeding.

Strong Behavior Weakened Through a Combination of Extinction for Social Attention and Stimulus Satiation

For 5 years, several mentally defective patients in the same ward, Harry, Joe, Tom, and Mac, had collected papers, rubbish, and magazines and carried these around with them inside their clothing next to their body. The most serious offender was Harry, whose hoarding resulted in skin rashes. He carried so much trash and so persistently that for the last 5 years the nurses routinely "dejunked" him several times during the day and before he went to bed.

An analysis of the situation indicated that the patient's hoarding behavior was probably maintained by the attention he derived because of it and by the actual scarcity of printed matter. There were few papers or magazines in the ward. Some were brought in occasionally; but since they were often torn up and quickly disappeared, the nurses did not bring them in very often.

It was expected that flooding the ward with magazines would decrease the hoarding behavior after the paradigm of satiation. Similarly, the availability of many magazines was expected to result in their being the major object of hoarding. The latter would facilitate an easier measurement of this behavior.

In addition, social reinforcement was to be withheld for hoarding magazines and rubbish. The results for all patients were essentially similar: a gradual decrease in hoarding. After 9 weeks of satiation and extinction, the program was terminated, since hoarding was no longer a problem. This improvement has been maintained for the last 6 months.

The following instructions were given to the nurses: "During this program the patients Harry, Mac, Joe, and Tom must not be given reinforcement (attention) for hoarding. There will be a full supply of magazines in the dayroom. Every night, after all patients have gone to bed, replenish the magazine supply in the dayroom. Every night while the patients are in bed, check their clothes to record the amount of hoarding. Do not, however, take their hoarding from them."

The original plan was to count the number of magazines in the patients' clothing after they had gone to bed. This is, in fact, the dependent variable shown in Fig. 27.5 for Joe,

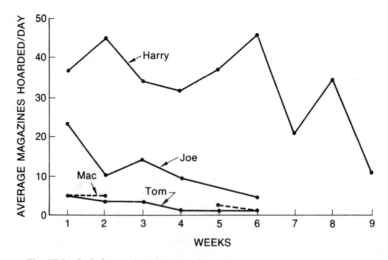

Fig. 27.5 Satiation and extinction of two forms of magazine hoarding.

Tom, and Mac. The recording for Harry had to be changed, however; after 4 days of the program, he no longer carried the rubbish or magazines in his clothing. Instead, he kept a stack of magazines on his lap while he was sitting in the dayroom. The number of magazines in his stack was counted when he left the dayroom for supper, and this is the dependent variable shown for Harry in Fig. 27.5. (Mac was out of the ward for 3 weeks because of illness.)

Prior to the program, one of the nurses questioned the possibility and even advisability of changing Harry's behavior. Her argument was that "behavior has its roots in the personality of the individual. The fact that he hoards so much indicates that Harry has a strong need for security. I don't see how we are going to change this need, and I also wonder if it is a good thing to do that." This was a point of view commonly encountered, especially regarding relatively nonverbal patients.

It would seem in this case that Harry transferred his security needs from hoarding rubbish and magazines to sitting in the dayroom and looking at magazines, especially during T.V. commercials. The transfer occurred with no apparent signs of discomfort on his part.

Other Cases

Combinations of extinction, reinforcement, and avoidance programs were set up for three patients; in two of these the problem behavior was eliminated in only a few weeks. The program of the third patient was followed for 20 days and then terminated since he had shown no changes by that time. An interpretation of the outcome of each of these programs is rendered questionable by the number of controlling variables involved and the nature of the changes.

The pretreatment study of four additional patients showed that the problem behavior of three of them did not occur often enough to justify carrying through a program; and in the fourth case, no easily controllable variables were available and, again, no program was undertaken.

DISCUSSION

On the basis of this work, further research along the same lines is now under way.[2] The present results are presented in this preliminary form in the hopes that they will provide encouragement to those who are in a position to conduct similar research. Therefore, it will be useful to mention a few other aspects of this work.

A major problem concerns the use of nurses as experimental assistants as well as substitutes for the recording and programming apparatus of the laboratory. There is no question as to the greater reliability of the ordinary laboratory component. In large part, however, the nurses' failures in carrying out E's instructions were unsystematic with respect to the results obtained, and although undesirable, they do not by any means render this kind of work uninterpretable. Systematic errors in observation can be reduced to some extent by dealing with response classes that are relatively easily identified. But, of course, this problem will become more serious as efforts are made to alter more subtle aspects of behavior. Perhaps the only solution is to be dissatisfied with one's techniques and principles until the behavioral changes are so obvious as to render statistical analysis superfluous.

―――――――

[2]This new project is supported by a grant from the Commonwealth Fund, and is being conducted under the auspices of the Saskatchewan Hospital, Weyburn, Saskatchewan, Canada.

Another question concerns the acceptability of this approach to the hospital staff. The nurses and psychiatrists who were familiar with the "reinforcement programs," as they were called, were given questionnaires and interviews to determine their attitudes toward this work. The results indicate a mildly favorable reception in general, with some enthusiastic support from both nurses and psychiatrists.

Regarding time actually spent in carrying out the programs, it might seem unreasonable to expect the already overworked nurse to devote 2 or 3 minutes every half-hour to observation and recording. However, this is only about 40 minutes of an 8-hour shift; and, besides, much of her work stems from patients' behavior problems, the elimination of which would make the 40 minutes an excellent investment of time.

Two sources of possible misunderstanding between *E* and nurses should be pointed out. First, when nurses were asked about the sort of problems they had in the ward, if no dramatic behaviors, such as attempts at suicide, or violent acts, had been recently reported, they often denied having any problems. Problems also went unrecognized because they were considered unsolvable. For example, since most nurses attributed the behavior of a patient to his diagnosis or age, little or no effort was made to discover and manipulate possibly relevant environmental variables.

Second, even after a behavior had been modified, it was not uncommon to hear nurses remark, "We've changed her behavior. So what? She's still psychotic." It seemed that once a persistent problem behavior was eliminated, its previous importance was forgotten and other undesirable aspects of the patient's repertoire were assumed to be the most important ones. In general, their specific expectations were unclear or unverbalized, and they tended to be somewhat dissatisfied with any change less than total "cure."

Finally, an objection often raised against this approach is that the behavior changes may be only temporary. However, permanent elimination of ward behavior problems requires a permanent elimination of the environmental variables that shape them up and maintain them. The clinical belief that a favorable behavioral change, if properly accomplished, will be permanent probably rests on a faulty evaluation of the role of environmental variables in controlling behavior. Certainly, it is not based on any actual accomplishments in the field of mental health.

REFERENCES

Ayllon, T. The application of reinforcement theory toward behavior problems. Unpublished doctoral dissertation, University of Houston, 1959.

Ferster, C. B., & Skinner, B. F. *Schedules of reinforcement.* New York: Appleton-Century-Crofts, 1957.

28

Basic Principles and Practices of Behavior Therapy of Neuroses*[1]

JOSEPH WOLPE

Behavior therapy or conditioning therapy was formally introduced to American psychiatry 14 years ago [21]. The term *behavior therapy* was first used by Skinner and Lindsley [16] and subsequently popularized by Eysenck [3, 4, 5]. It denotes the use of experimentally established principles of learning for the purpose of changing unadaptive behavior. Behavior therapy is thus an applied science, in every way parallel to other modern technologies and in particular to the technologies constituting medical therapeutics. Therapeutic possibilities emerge when we know the lawful relations of organismic processes. In the psychotherapeutic field the lawful relations that are most often relevant are those established by experimental psychology.

Persistent maladaptive (unadaptive) *anxiety* responses are the nucleus of most cases that are labeled "neurotic," and therefore much of the effort of behavior therapists has been directed toward overcoming them. "Anxiety" is defined as a particular organism's characteristic pattern of autonomic responses to noxious stimulation [22]. Anxiety is conditionable; conditioned anxiety responses are in fact far more common than unconditioned ones. Anxiety responses are called maladaptive when they have been conditioned to stimulus situations that do not pose any objective threat. It is implicit in this formulation that neurotic responses are not ways of avoiding stress; they *are* stress responses.

Behavior therapy of human neuroses had its origin in observations of animal neuroses [20, 22]. An animal placed in a confined environment and subjected to either strong ambivalent stimulation or noxious stimulation acquires a persistent habit of responding with marked anxiety to the environment concerned, and with weaker anxiety to other environments according to their similarity to the original one.

The most effective way of procuring unlearning is to feed the animal repeatedly while it is in an environment which evokes *weak* anxiety. The effect of this is to diminish progressively—ultimately to zero—the strength of the anxiety response to the particular stimulus. Increasingly "strong" stimulus situations are successively dealt with in the same way, so that finally the animal shows no anxiety to any of the situations to which anxiety has been conditioned. The basis of this gradual elimination of the anxiety response habit is considered to be an example [22], at a more complex level, of the phenomenon of *reciprocal inhibition* described by Sherrington [15]. Each time the animal eats, the anxiety response is to some extent inhibited, and each occasion of inhibition diminishes the anxiety habit. Apparently the evocation of a response that inhibits anxiety weakens the bond between the anxiety-evoking stimulus and the anxiety response.

*Reprinted from *The American Journal of Psychiatry*, volume 125, pages 1242–1247, 1969. Copyright © 1969, the American Psychiatric Association.
[1] Read at the 124th annual meeting of the American Psychiatric Association, Boston, Mass., May 13–17, 1968.

Human neuroses resemble those of the animal in all basic respects [26]. Even though not all human neuroses present themselves as anxiety states, anxiety underlies most of them. For example, the patient with a stutter is not as a rule aware of the stimuli that produce the anxiety that is usually a necessary condition for stuttering. Indeed, he may not realize that he has any special anxiety in the situations in which he stutters, even though he can contrast them with other situations in which his speech is normal. Investigation generally shows that there is an emotional undercurrent, the intensity of which determines the degree of stutter.

The same is true of a host of other conditions in which the main presenting complaint is not anxiety—obsessions and compulsions, psychosomatic states, character neuroses, impotence, frigidity, homosexuality, and many others. The key to recovery is generally the deconditioning of anxiety. This is why a detailed behavioral analysis is an essential prerequisite to effective behavior therapy. The behavior therapist makes a practice of obtaining a detailed life history and a full account of the present life situation and administers various questionnaires designed to reveal stimulus situations conditioned to neurotic anxiety responses [27].

METHODS OF BEHAVIOR THERAPY

Many of the methods of behavior therapy derive from the therapeutic experiments with animals described above. They exemplify reciprocal inhibition (counterconditioning). Other methods derive from positive reinforcement, experimental extinction, and various other experimental paradigms [27].

Counterconditioning by the Emotions of Life Situations

Where neurotic responses are conditioned to situations involving direct interpersonal relations, the essence of reciprocal inhibition therapy has been to inhibit anxiety by the instigation of patterns of motor behavior that express anger (or whatever other feelings may be relevant). The repeated exercise of these patterns in the proper context weakens the anxiety response habit.

For example, a patient may need to be taught how to stand up for his rights when somebody gets in front of him in a line. The teaching will be either by direct instruction and exhortation or by actual rehearsal of the desired new behavior in the consulting room. A recent patient had become so intent on acceding to his wife's requirements that his own needs were completely subordinated. He repeatedly went into states of depression that he attempted to relieve by heavy drinking. He was shown how to assert himself appropriately—for example, by refusing to allow whatever he might be doing, such as reading the newspaper, to be interrupted by his wife's demands for conversation. By dint of a program along these lines he achieved reasonable control of this interpersonal situation and stopped having depressions.

Sexual responses are used to overcome anxiety responses to sexual situations that are the basis of impotence or premature ejaculation. The essence of treatment is to control sexual approaches so that anxiety is never permitted to be strong. Inhibition of anxiety can then be obtained by the parasympathetic dominated sexual arousal and the anxiety response habit can consequently be weakened.

Tactics vary from case to case but always involve the cooperation of the spouse. The therapist must determine at what point in the patient's sexual approach there are the first indications of anxiety. He then instructs the patient to take love-making no farther than this point, having obtained the acquiescence of the spouse. In the course of a few amorous sessions, anxiety usually ceases to be felt at the permitted point, and then the patient is permitted to go on to the next stage. Usually several preliminary stages need to be passed before coitus is attempted; and it, too, requires a succession of graded steps.

Systematic Desensitization Based on Relaxation

Neurotic anxiety responses conditioned to stimuli other than those arising from direct interpersonal relations (e.g., phobic responses) do not lend themselves to behavioral treatment in the life situation of the patient. In such cases, reciprocal inhibition of anxiety must be obtained by methods that do not involve motor activity on the part of the patient toward the fearful object. In the earliest deliberate example of therapy on this basis, the anxiety of phobic children was inhibited by eating[8], very much as in the case of the experimental neuroses described above.

Deep muscle relaxation[7] has had the widest use in this way, mainly in a method known as *systematic desensitization* [21, 22, 27]. In brief, desensitization consists of repeatedly presenting to the imagination of the deeply relaxed patient the feeblest item in a list of anxiety-evoking stimuli until no more anxiety is evoked either as reported by the patient or as psychophysiologically recorded. The next higher item in the list is then presented—again until the anxiety response to it is extinct. The procedure is continued until eventually even the strongest of the anxiety-evoking stimuli fails to evoke any stir of anxiety in the patient. It is almost always found in those subjects in whom imagined scenes have initially evoked anxiety that a situation that no longer evokes it in imagination also ceases to evoke it when encountered in reality.

Variants of Systematic Desensitization

Other inhibitors of anxiety may also be employed therapeutically in a systematic way. In some patients the therapeutic situation itself evokes anxiety-inhibiting emotions. These are very likely the usual basis of whatever therapeutic changes result from therapies other than behavior therapy. They must also account for part of the success of behavior therapy[22]. But they can in addition be deliberately used in behavior therapy—usually in what is called desensitization in vivo, in which real stimuli take the place of imaginary ones, and the anxiety may be inhibited by these emotions.

For example, a patient who has a fear of humiliation at making mistakes is made to perform minor errors and then progressively more serious ones in the presence of the therapist—in each instance until all feelings of anxiety disappear. To the extent that this succeeds it is probably due to the anxiety being inhibited by competing interpersonal emotions. Tests of this assumption are now being planned.

Use has also been made of the observation that anxiety can be inhibited by cutaneous stimulation by nonaversive electric shocks. The therapist arranges for these to break in on the anxiety evoked by images from hierarchies by getting the patient to signal when the image is clear, and then delivering two or three shocks in quick succession. This apparently weakens anxiety on the basis of *external inhibition* [13].

Another method of procuring inhibition of anxiety depends on presenting a neutral stimulus just before the cessation of a strong continuous current to the forearm. The effect of this is to condition cessation (inhibition) of anxiety to the neutral stimulus[21, 22, 27]. The conditioned stimulus can then be systematically used to inhibit neurotic anxieties in the life situation.

Avoidance Conditioning

Avoidance (aversive) conditioning is an application of the reciprocal inhibition principle to overcoming responses other than anxiety. A noxious stimulus—usually a strongly unpleasant electric shock—is administered to the patient in an appropriate time relation to the stimulus to which avoidance conditioning is desired. It has been effectively used to overcome obsessional thinking, compulsive acts, fetishes, and homosexuality. It is, however, not always successful for reasons that are often quite clear.

Homosexuality, for example, is often based on neurotic interpersonal anxiety, which should be treated by deconditioning the anxiety[17]. But when aversion is used for homosexuality, the most promising technique consists of administering a very unpleasant shock as long as a homosexual figure is projected onto a screen and terminating the shock at the appearance of an attractive female[8]. Further details and other applications have been discussed in my book, *The Practice of Behavior Therapy* [27].

Experimental Extinction

Experimental extinction is the breaking of a habit through repeated performance of the relevant response without reinforcement (reward). The therapeutic use of extinction was formally introduced by Dunlap[2] under the name "negative practice."

The method did not then achieve much popularity, but recently there has been renewed interest in it, mainly in the context of the treatment of tics. The patient is instructed to perform deliberately the undesired movement very many times, and in the course of some weeks it may be found that spontaneous evocations of the tic have decreased, perhaps markedly[14, 18, 28]. Kondas[10] has reported that many resistent tics can be cured if the negative practice is accompanied by a strong aversive stimulus that is terminated each time the practice stops. (cf. anxiety-relief conditioning described above).

Positive Reinforcement

The deconditioning of unadaptive autonomic response habits is the central approach to behavior therapy of neuroses, but it is often also necessary to condition new motor habits. This often occurs as a result of the same measures that break down the anxiety habit. For example, in assertive training (see above), simultaneously with the counterconditioning of anxiety, motor (operant) habits of assertion are conditioned. They are reinforced by the rewarding consequences of the assertive act, such as gaining control of a situation.

But operant conditioning can also be effected on its own. Anorexia nervosa has been successfully treated by arranging for eating to be followed by social rewards such as the use of a radio or company and withholding the rewards when the patient does not eat[1]. The same principles have been effective in a variety of cases. For example, Williams[19] has described how tantrum behavior is completely under the control of the adult attention it elicits.

RESULTS OF BEHAVIOR THERAPY

The distinctive feature of behavior therapy is that the therapist selects his targets and plans his strategy in respect to each of them. He can sometimes—for example, in desensitization of classical phobias—even calculate the quantitative relations between number of therapeutic operations and amount of change[24].

Statistical Data

R. P. Knight's[9] five criteria—symptomatic improvement, increased productiveness, improved adjustment and pleasure in sex, improved interpersonal relationships, and ability to handle ordinary psychological conflicts and reasonable reality stresses—have been generally adopted by behavior therapists. By these criteria, the results of behavior therapy of neurosis have been quite notably good. For example, in several series of neurotic patients totaling 618 cases, about 87 percent either apparently recovered or were much improved[27]. In the last published series of my own[22], the median number of sessions for 88 cases was 23. (Follow-up studies in this as in other series have shown neither the spontaneous relapses nor the symptom substitutions that psychoanalytically oriented colleagues have prognosticated.)

Compare these results with the 60 percent "cured" or "greatly improved" among the *completely analyzed* patients in the study of the Central Fact-Finding Committee of the American Psychoanalytic Association. While the psychoanalyzed patients were treated an average of four times a week for three to four years, i.e., about 700 sessions, and the average course of behavior therapy covered about 30 sessions[22], it is fair to point out that the comparison is not a controlled one.

A controlled comparative study is currently under way in the department of psychiatry at Temple University. Meanwhile, laboratory controlled studies have been distinctly favorable to behavior therapy. Paul[12] found that "dynamically" trained therapists did significantly better with systematic desensitization than with their own insight-giving techniques in treating fears of public speaking. Moore[11] reported a controlled study of cases of asthma in a London clinic. One schedule she employed was relaxation training; the second was support and suggestion under relaxation; and the third was systematic desensitization. In terms of both immediate and delayed effects, desensitization was clearly superior to the other two methods. In terms of maximum peak flow of respired air the difference was significant at 0.001.

One popular fallacy about behavior therapy is that it is useful in its place—for simple cases but not for complex ones. In 1964 I made a reexamination[25] of some previously published results dividing 86 cases into simple and complex. A neurosis was regarded as complex if it had one or more of the following features: (a) a wide range of stimuli, conditioned to neurotic responses (not just one), (b) reactions to which the conditioned stimuli are obscure and determined with difficulty, (c) reactions that include unadaptiveness in important areas of general behavior (character neuroses), (d) obsessional neuroses, and (e) reactions that include pervasive anxiety.)

Of the 86 cases reviewed, 65 were complex in one or more of the senses defined. Fifty-eight of these (89 percent) were judged either apparently cured or much improved. This percentage was exactly the same as that obtained for the whole group. However, the median number of sessions for the complex group was 29 and the mean 54.8 in contrast to a median for the noncomplex remainder of 11.5 and a mean of 14.9. Thus, while complex cases responded to behavior therapy as often as simple ones did, therapy took longer.

HOW FUNDAMENTAL ARE THE EFFECTS OF BEHAVIOR THERAPY?

It is sometimes contended that behavior therapy is superficial and possibly even dangerous because it does not attempt to deal with the "basic dynamic conflict" that is alleged to underlie neuroses. In particular, it is prognosticated that recovery will be followed by relapse or symptom substitution sooner or later. A survey[23] of the results of follow-up studies on neuroses successfully treated by a variety of methods not concerned with the dynamic conflict revealed only a 1.6 percent incidence of relapse or symptom substitution. Skilled behavior therapists hardly ever encounter relapse or symptom substitution.

The weight of the evidence is thus that neuroses are indeed nothing but habits—the results of conditioning—often very complex conditioning. The implication is that a therapy based on principles of conditioning is fundamental therapy.

REFERENCES

1. Bachrach, A. J., Erwin, W. J., & Mohr, J. P. The control of eating behavior in an anorexia by operant conditioning techniques. In L. Ullman & L. Krasner (Eds.), *Case studies in behavior modification* New York,: Holt, Rinehart & Winston, 1965.
2. Dunlap, K. *Habits, their making and unmaking.* New York: Liveright, 1932.
3. Eysenck, H. J. Learning theory and behaviour therapy. *J. Ment. Sci.*, 1959, **105**, 61–75.
4. Eysenck, H. J. *Behavior therapy and the neuroses.* New York: Pergamon Press, 1960.
5. Eysenck, H. J. *Experiments in behavior therapy.* Oxford: Pergamon Press, 1965.
6. Feldman, M. P., & MacColloch, M. J. The application of anticipatory avoidance learning to the treatment of homosexuality. I. Theory, technique, and preliminary results. *Behav. Res. Ther.*, 1965, 2 165–183.
7. Jacobson, E. *Progressive relaxation.* Chicago: University of Chicago Press, 1938.
8. Jones, M. D. A laboratory study of fear. The case of Peter. *J. Genet. Psychol.*, 1924, **31**, 308–315
9. Knight, R. P. Evaluation of the results of psychoanalytic therapy. *Amer. J. Psychiat.*, 1941, **98**, 434–446.
10. Kondas, O. The possibilities of applying experimentally created procedures when eliminating tics. *Studia Psychol.*, 1965, **7**, 221–229.
11. Moore, N. Behaviour therapy in bronchial asthma: A controlled study. *J. Psychosom, Res.*, 1965, **9**, 257–276.
12. Paul, G. L. *Insight vs. desensitization in psychotherapy: An experiment in anxiety reduction.* Stanford, Calif.: Stanford University Press, 1966.
13. Pavlov, I. P. *Conditioned reflexes.* Translated by G. V. Anrep. New York: Liveright, 1927.
14. Rafi, A. A. Learning theory and the treatment of tics. *J. Psychosom. Res.*, 1962, **6**, 71–76.
15. Sherrington, C. S. *Integration action of the nervous system.* New Haven; Conn.: Yale University Press, 1906.
16. Skinner, B. F., & Lindsley, O. *Studies in behavior therapy, Status reports II and III.* (Naval Research Contact N5 ori-7662) 1954.
17. Stephenson, I., & Wolpe, J. Recovery from sexual deviations through overcoming nonsexual neurotic responses. *Amer. J. Psychiat.*, 1960, **116**, 737–742.
18. Walton, D. Experimental Psychology and the treatment of a tiquer. *J. Child Psychol. Psychiat.*, 1961, **2**, 148–155.
19. Williams, C. D. The elimination of tantrum behavior by extinction procedures. *J.Abnorm. Soc. Psychol.*, 1959, **59**, 269.
20. Wolpe, J. Experimental neuroses as learned behavior. *Brit. J. Psychol.*, 1952, **43**, 243–268.
21. Wolpe, J. Reciprocal inhibition as the main basis of psytherapeutic effects. *Arch. Neurol. Psychiat.*, 1954, **72**, 205–226.
22. Wolpe, J. *Psychotherapy by reciprocal inhibition.* Stanford, Calif.: Stanford University Press, 1958.
23. Wolpe, J. The prognosis in unpsychoanalyzed recovery from neurosis. *Amer. J. Psychiat.*, 1961, **118**, 35–39.
24. Wolpe, J. Quantitative relationships in the systematic desensitization of phobias. *Amer. J. Psychiat.*, 1963, **119**, 1062–1068.

25. Wolpe, J. Behavior therapy in complex neurotic states. *Brit. J. Psychiat.*, 1964, **110**, 28–34.
26. Wolpe, J. Parallels between animal and human neuroses. In P. Hoch & J. Zubin (Eds.), *Comparative psychopathology*. New York: Grune & Stratton, 1967.
27. Wolpe, J. *The practice of behavior therapy*. New York: Pergamon Press, 1968.
28. Yates, A. J. The application of learning theory to the treatment of tics. *J. Abnorm. Soc. Psychol.*, 1958, **56**, 175–182.

Phobic Patients: Treatment with the Learning Theory Approach of Implosive Therapy*

THOMAS G. STAMPFL and DONALD J. LEVIS

Unlike other behavioral therapies which adhere to a learning orientation, Implosive Therapy (IT) incorporates into its model some of the general concepts of psychodynamic personality theory (Stampfl, 1967; Levis, 1967; Stampfl & Levis, 1967a, 1967b, 1968). The learning position upon which Implosive Therapy is based, although differing in some essential details, is similar to the analyses proposed by Dollard and Miller (1950), Mowrer (1939, 1960a, 1960b), and Shoben (1949).

The theoretical model adopted distinguishes between two different response categories which are considered learned by the patient. Briefly, the first response category involves the conditioning of fear to specific stimuli or stimulus compounds; the second category deals with attempts of the organism to reduce or control that fear. The first category involving the negative affective response is assumed to be elicited by stimuli previously considered "neutral," which have acquired their fear-producing potential as a result of having closely preceded the onset of a painful state, such as external injury or organic deprivation. In principle, the model presupposes that humans acquire anxieties much like the laboratory animal who can be conditioned to respond with fear or anxiety to a light, buzzer, or tone which has been paired with the primary noxious stimulus of electric shock. This analysis heavily relies upon the concepts of stimulus generalization, higher order conditioning, response mediated generalization, and/or the principle of redintegration to account for the etiology of a fear reaction elicited by a particular stimulus situation.

Symptoms and defense mechanisms comprise the second response category. They are interpreted as conditioned avoidance responses designed to remove or reduce the presence of the anxiety-provoking stimuli. The reinforcement for such behavior is reduction of anxiety. Symptoms which are operating effectively are relatively successful in minimizing or eliminating affectively charged stimulus patterns. However, when a relative failure of avoidance occurs, the anxiety stimuli continue to be activated.

According to the model, in order to effectively remove the symptom it is necessary to extinguish the conditioned emotional response which activates and provides the reinforcement for strengthening the avoidance behavior. Therefore, it is essential to have some understanding of what stimulus patterns are being avoided. In the case of phobic objects or situations (e.g., high buildings, thunderstorms, water, airplanes, animals), a systematic analysis of the symptom-contingent cues surrounding the phobic situation can aid considerably in determining the stimulus properties (visual, tactual, auditory) directly correlated with the avoidance response. However, it is assumed that the symptom-contingent cues comprise only one of a number of the stimulus patterns that are avoided.

---

*From Stampfl, T. G. and Levis, D. J., Voices, 1967, 23–27. Copyright © 1967 by the American Academy of Psychotherapists. Reprinted by permission of the American Academy of Psychotherapists and Dr. Stampfl.

The phobic object is believed to be avoided not only because of previous conditioning to this complex but also because the phobic stimulus pattern functions as a signal for the onset of additional "dangerous" associations. In learning terminology, the phobic event activates or redintegrates cues (thoughts, memories, images) which have been more completely avoided (repressed). These additional stimulus patterns are considered to be sequentially ordered in terms of their aversiveness and in terms of their accessibility to the level of verbal report. The more intense the aversive loading of these cues, the greater the tendency to avoid.

Clinically speaking, the supposition seems tenable that additional fear-eliciting stimuli exist beyond the immediate stimulation provided by the phobic object itself. Phobic patients frequently report experiencing an intense subjective reaction which contains strong emotional components of impending disaster. An example of what is meant is illustrated in Leonard's (1927, pp. 304–307) report of his phobic reaction to a locomotive. The incident described is that of hearing the whistle of a locomotive located a half-mile across the lake.

> Then on the tracks from behind Eagle Heights and the woods across the lake comes the freight-train, blowing its whistle. . . . The cabin of that locomotive feels right over my head, as if about to engulf me. I am obsessed with a feeling as of a big circle, hogshead, cistern-hole or what not, in air just in front of me. The train feels as if it were about to rush over me. . . so intensely in contradiction to what the eye sees is the testimony of the feeling of that cabin over my head, of that strange huge circle hovering at me.

The train whistle was not the only cue to which Leonard responded. The whistle apparently activated a number of additional internal conditioned cues (e.g., the reported feeling that the cabin is over his head; the strange huge circle hovering) which at the time had no external representation. Considerable anxiety was reported experienced at the introduction of these cues. "My God, won't that train go away! I smash a wooden box to pieces, board by board, against my knee to occupy myself against panic."

Leonard's attempt to avoid the elicitation of these stimuli may have prevented additional conditioned cues from becoming exposed. The nature of additional stimulus patterns which may be functioning below his level of verbal report can be hypothesized. These patterns most likely would involve thoughts or images about severe bodily injury and mutilation. A psychodynamic position might even suggest cues associated with fear of castration, masochistic wishes, or perhaps an unconscious desire for punishment stimulated by forbidden wishes associated with sex or aggression.

If the above assumption is correct that additional cues exist which have not as yet been exposed, the anxiety attached to these cues are prevented from extinguishing (Solomon & Wynne's principle of anxiety conservation, 1954). In most phobic cases the amount of exposure to cues also is markedly reduced because of rapid avoidance. To extinguish these cues, it is only necessary, according to the present model, to present them in the absence of primary reinforcement (painful physical injury or physical states of deprivation). Support for a nonreinforcement procedure of extinction comes from such studies as Black (1958), Denny, Koons, and Mason (1959), Hunt, Jernberg, and Brady (1952), Knapp (1965), and Weinberger (1965). Additional evidence by Lowenfeld, Rubenfeld, and Guthrie (1956), and Wall and Guthrie (1959) suggests that enhanced perceptual clarity of the feared stimuli also facilitates the extinction process.

The strategy of the Implosive therapist is to reexpose to the patient conditioned stimuli he is presumed to be avoiding. To achieve this goal, the therapist suggests to the patient scenes which incorporate the symptom-contingent cues and the hypothesized anxiety-arousing stimuli. The patient is asked to experience the cues in imagery and the anxiety associated with these cues. (It is assumed that events reproduced in imagery provide a more adequate method of representing the properties of the feared stimuli than mere verbal statements.) The images, thoughts, and/or verbal statements introduced by the therapist are considered extinguishable since they do not impart any physical injury to the organism. Each repetition of the cues leads to a decrement of the elicited anxiety through extinction by nonreinforcement.

The therapist may make use of clinical interviews and/or diagnostic material in order to identify the more dynamic cues the patient is avoiding. That is, the "meaning" of the phobic object or situation may include cues which are related to bodily injury, aggression, sex, dependency, or other conflicts not readily identifiable by the patient. Since many of these cues are assumed to have been highly correlated with actual physical pain (primary reinforcement), the Implosive therapist routinely attempts to introduce in imagery conditioned cues associated with primary bodily injury and with states of deprivation. Although the cues of this nature suggested by the therapist may differ from the actual conditioning events, considerable generalization of extinction across this class of cues is expected.

A summary of the treatment procedure is given in the following seven steps.

1. The therapist attempts to identify the stimuli related to the phobic object. Such an analysis should incorporate symptom-contingent cues as well as additional hypothesized cues believed to be motivating the symptomatology.

2. The patient is given training in visualizing essentially "neutral," nonthreatening scenes in imagery.

3. The patient is asked to imagine scenes which incorporate cues directly related to the phobic situation. For example, in the case of acrophobia, the following sequence of scenes might be presented: (a) A tall building is described which the patient sees himself visualizing from a distance; (b) he walks closer and closer toward the building until he is standing in front of it; (c) he enters into the building and climbs the stairs to the roof of the building, periodically looking down as he climbs; (d) he walks over to the edge of the roof and looks down, seeing the street below. Each step of the way is described by the therapist with great clarity and in considerable detail.

4. With each set of fearful scenes introduced, the patient is urged not to avoid these cues while they are being presented and, indeed, to experience as much anxiety as possible. He is also instructed to attend to the sensory manifestations of the anxiety that he experiences, since the feedback from the anxiety state itself also can function as a cue.

5. Each scene is repeated until some anxiety reduction has occurred.

6. After repeated exposure to the symptom-contingent cues, the therapist progressively introduces additional associative cues activated by the phobic situation, as well as the clinically hypothesized cues thought to be associated with the phobic object. For example, if fear of bodily injury is hypothesized in the acrophobic case, scenes might be presented in which the patient is asked to visualize himself jumping off the tall building. A detailed description of the patient falling, of the ground getting closer and closer, and of his hitting the ground is described. The impact of the fall, the feeling of bones breaking, the pouring out of blood, and other bodily injury cues are included.

7. The therapist trains the patient to work through the scenes by himself so that additional repetitions in the form of a homework assignment can be given outside the therapy session.

Clinical experience with the above method suggests that it is an effective technique for eliminating phobic symptoms. However, considerable caution is needed in the evaluation of any psychotherapeutic technique until a sufficient number of well-controlled experimental studies with adequate follow-ups have been completed. Presently three studies designed to reduce fear of rats and snakes in phobic college students have been completed (Kirchner & Hogan, 1966; Hogan & Kirchner, 1967a, 1967b). The data indicate that the above technique is at least initially effective with this type of population. Studies by Hogan (1966) and Levis and Carrera (1967) with psychotic and neurotic patients, respectively, suggest an even wider range of applicability.

REFERENCES

Black, A. H. The extinction of avoidance responses under curare. *Journal of Comparative and Physiological Psychology*, 1958, **51**, 519–524.

Denny, M. R., Koons, P. B., & Mason, J. E. Extinction of avoidance as a function of the escape situation. *Journal of Comparative and Physiological Psychology*, 1959, **52**, 212–214.

Dollard, J., & Miller, N. E. *Personality and psychotherapy*. New York: McGraw-Hill, 1950.

Hogan, R. A. Implosive therapy in the short term treatment of psychotics. *Psychotherapy: Theory, Research and Practice*, 1966, **3**, 25–31.

Hogan, R. A., & Kirchner, J. H. A preliminary report of the extinction of learned fears via short term implosive therapy. *Journal of Abnormal Psychology*, 1967, **72**, 106–109. (a)

Hogan, R. A., & Kirchner, J. H. A comparison of implosive, eclectic verbal, and biblio therapy in the treatment of snake phobias. 1967 (submitted for publication). (b)

Hunt, H. F., Jernberg, P., & Brady, J. V. The effect of electroconvulsive shock (E.C.S.) on a conditioned emotional response: The effects of post-E.C.S. extinction on the reappearance of the response. *Journal of Comparative and Physiological Psychology*, 1952, **45**, 589–599.

Kirchner, J. H., & Hogan, R. A. The therapist variable in the implosion of phobias. *Psychotherapy: Theory, Research and Practice*, 1966, **3**, 102–104.

Knapp, R. K. Acquisition and extinction of avoidance with similar and different shock and escape situations. *Journal of Comparative and Physiological Psychology*, 1965, **60**, 272–273.

Leonard, W. E. *The locomotive god.* New York: Appleton-Century-Crofts, 1927.

Levis, D. J. Implosive therapy. Part II. The subhuman analogue, the strategy, and the technique. In S. G. Armitage (Ed.), *Behavioral modification techniques in the treatment of emotional disorders.* Battle Creek, Mich.: V. A. Publication, 1967, 22–27.

Levis, D. J., & Carrera, R. N. Effects of 10 hours of implosive therapy in the treatment of outpatients: A preliminary report. *Journal of Abnormal Psychology*, 1967, **72**, 504–508.

Lowenfeld, J., Rubenfeld, S., & Guthrie, G. M. Verbal inhibition in subception. *Journal of General Psychology*, 1956, **54**, 171–176.

Mowrer, O. H. A stimulus-response analysis of anxiety and its role as a reinforcing agent. *Psychological Review*, 1939, **46**, 553–565.

Mowrer, O. H. *Learning theory and behavior.* New York: Wiley, 1960. (a)

Mowrer, O. H. *Learning theory and the symbolic processes.* New York: Wiley, 1960. (b)

Shoben, E. J. Psychotherapy as a problem in learning theory. *Psychological Bulletin*, 1949, **46**, 366–392.

Solomon, R. L. & Wynne, L. C. Traumatic avoidance learning:The principles of anxiety conservation and partial irreversibility. *Psychological Review*, 1954, **61**, 353–385.

Stampfl, T. G. Implosive therapy: A learning theory derived psychodynamic therapeutic technique, 1961. In Lebarba & Dent (Eds.), *Critical issues in clinical psychology.* New York: Academic Press, 1967.

Stampfl, T. G. Implosive therapy, Part I. The theory. In S. G. Armitage (Ed.), *Behavioral modification techniques in the treatment of emotional disorders.* Battle Creek, Mich.: V. A. Publication, 1967. Pp. 12–21.

Stampfl, T. G., & Levis, D. J. The essentials of implosive therapy: A learning theory based psychodynamic behavioral therapy. *Journal of Abnormal Psychology*, 1967, **72**, 496–503. (a)

Stampfl, T. G. & Levis, D. J. Implosive therapy. In R. M. Jurjevich (Ed.), *Handbook of direct and behavior psychotherapies.* Chapel Hill: University of North Carolina Press, 1967. (b)

Stampfl, T. G. & Levis, D. J. Learning theory, an aid to dynamic therapeutic practice. In L. D. Eron & R. Callahan (Eds.), *Relationship of theory to practice in psychotherapy.* Chicago: Aldine, 1968.

Wall, H. N., & Guthrie, G. M. Extinction of responses to subceived stimuli. *Journal of General Psychology,* 1959, 3, 1–14.

Weinberger, N. M. Effects of detainment on extinction of avoidance responses. *Journal of Comparative and Physiological Psychology,* 1965, **60**, 135–138.

30

A Theory of Therapy and Personality Change: As Developed in the Client-Centered Framework*

CARL R. ROGERS

... This theory is of the if-then variety. If certain conditions exist (independent variables), then a process (dependent variable) will occur which includes certain characteristic elements. If this process (now the independent variable) occurs, then certain personality and behavioral changes (dependent variables) will occur. This will be made specific.

In this and the following sections the formal statement of the theory is given briefly. ...

A. CONDITIONS OF THE THERAPEUTIC PROCESS

For therapy to occur it is necessary that these conditions exist.

1. That two persons are in *contact*.
2. That the first person, whom we shall term the client, is in a state of *incongruence*, being *vulnerable*, or *anxious*.
3. That the second person, whom we shall term the therapist, is *congruent* in the *relationship*.
4. That the therapist is *experiencing unconditional positive regard* toward the client.
5. That the therapist is *experiencing* an *emphatic* understanding of the client's *internal frame of reference*.
6. That the client *perceives*, at least to a minimal degree, conditions 4 and 5, the *unconditional positive regard* of the therapist for him, and the *empathic* understanding of the therapist.

Comment

These seem to be the necessary conditions of therapy, though other elements are often or usually present. The process is more likely to get under way if the client is anxious, rather than merely vulnerable. Often it is necessary for the contact or relationship to be of some duration before the therapeutic process begins. Usually the empathic understanding is to some degree expressed verbally, as well as experienced. But the process often commences with only these minimal conditions, and it is hypothesized that it never commences *without* these conditions being met.

The point which is most likely to be misunderstood is the omission of any statement that the therapist *communicates* his empathic understanding and his unconditional positive regard to the client. Such a statement has been omitted only after much consideration, for

---

these reasons. It is not enough for the therapist to communicate, since the communication must be received, as pointed out in condition 6, to be effective. It is not essential that the therapist *intend* such communication, since often it is by some casual remark, or involuntary facial expression, that the communication is actually achieved. However, if one wishes to stress the communicative aspect which is certainly a vital part of the living experience, then condition 6 might be worded in this fashion:

6. That the communication to the client of the therapist's empathic understanding and unconditional positive regard is, at least to a minimal degree, achieved.

The element which will be most surprising to conventional therapists is that the same conditions are regarded as sufficient for therapy, regardless of the particular characteristics of the client. It has been our experience to date that although the therapeutic relationship is used differently by different clients, it is not necessary nor helpful to manipulate the relationship in specific ways for specific kinds of clients. To do this damages, it seems to us, the most helpful and significant aspect of the experience, that it is a genuine relationship between two persons, each of whom is endeavoring, to the best of his ability, to be himself in the interaction.[1]

The "growing edge" of this portion of the theory has to do with point 3, the congruence or genuineness of the therapist in the relationship. This means that the therapist's symbolization of his own experience in the relationship must be accurate, if therapy is to be most effective. Thus if he is experiencing threat and discomfort in the relationship, and is aware only of an acceptance and understanding, then he is not congruent in the relationship and therapy will suffer. It seems important that he should accurately "be himself" in the relationship, whatever the self of that moment may be.

Should he also express or communicate to the client the accurate symbolization of his own experience? The answer to this question is still in an uncertain state. At present we would say that such feelings should be expressed, if the therapist finds himself persistently focused on his own feelings rather than those of the client, thus greatly reducing or eliminating any experience of empathic understanding, or if he finds himself persistently experiencing some feeling other than unconditional positive regard. To know whether this answer is correct demands further testing of the hypothesis it contains, and this is not simple since the courage to do this is often lacking, even in experienced therapists. When the therapist's real feelings are of this order: "I find myself fearful that you are slipping into a psychosis," or "I find myself frightened because you are touching on feelings I have never been able to resolve," then it is difficult to test the hypothesis, for it is very difficult for the therapist to express such feelings.

Another question which arises is this: is it the congruence, the wholeness, the integration of the therapist in the relationship which is important, or are the specific attitudes of empathic understanding and unconditional positive regard vital? Again the final answer is

---

[1]This paragraph may have to be rewritten if a recent study of Kirtner[23] is confirmed. Kirtner has found, in a group of 26 cases from the Counseling Center at the University of Chicago, that there are sharp differences in the client's mode of approach to the resolution of life difficulties and that these differences are related to success in therapy. Briefly, the client who sees his problem as involving his relationships, and who feels that he contributes to this problem and wants to change it, is likely to be successful. The client who externalizes his problem and feels little self-responsibility is much more likely to be a failure. Thus the implication is that different conditions of therapy may be necessary to make personality change possible in this latter group. If this is verified, then the theory will have to be revised accordingly.

unknown, but a conservative answer, the one we have embodied in the theory, is that for therapy to occur the wholeness of the therapist in the relationship is primary, but a part of the congruence of the therapist must be the experience of unconditional positive regard and the experience of empathic understanding.

Another point worth noting is that the stress is upon the experience *in the relationship.* It is not to be expected that the therapist is a completely congruent person at all times. Indeed if this were a necessary condition there would be no therapy. But it is enough if in this particular moment of this immediate relationship with this specific person he is completely and fully himself, with his experience of the moment being accurately symbolized and integrated into the picture he holds of himself. Thus it is that imperfect human beings can be of therapeutic assistance to other imperfect human beings.

The greatest flaw in the statement of these conditions is that they are stated as if they were all-or-none elements, whereas conditions 2 to 6 all exist on continua. At some later date we may be able to say that the therapist must be genuine or congruent to such and such a degree in the relationship, and similarly for the other items. At the present we can only point out that the more marked the presence of conditions 2 to 6, the more certain it is that the process of therapy will get under way, and the greater the degree of reorganization which will take place. This function can only be stated qualitatively at the present time.

Evidence

Confirmatory evidence, particularly of item 5, is found in the studies by Fiedler[9, 10] and Quinn[28]. Fiedler's study showed that experienced therapists of different orientations created relationships in which one of the most prominent characteristics was the ability to understand the client's communications with the meaning these communications had for the client. Quinn found that the quality of therapist communication was of crucial significance in therapy. These studies add weight to the importance of empathic understanding.

Seeman[36] found that increase in the counselor's liking for the client during therapy was significantly associated with therapeutic success. Both Seeman and Lipkin[24] found that clients who felt themselves to be liked by the therapist tended to be more successful. These studies tend to confirm condition 4 (unconditional positive regard) and condition 6 (perception of this by the client).

Though clinical experience would support condition 2, the client's vulnerability or anxiety, there is little research which has been done in terms of these constructs. The study by Gallagher[11] indicates that less anxious clients tend never to become involved in therapy, but drop out.

B. THE PROCESS OF THERAPY

When the preceding conditions exist and continue, a process is set in motion which has these characteristic directions:

1. The client is increasingly free in expressing his *feelings*, through verbal and/or motor channels.
2. His expressed feelings increasingly have reference to the *self*, rather than nonself.
3. He increasingly differentiates and discriminates the objects of his *feelings* and *perceptions*, including his environment, other persons, his *self*, his *experiences*, and the interrelationships of these. He becomes less *intensional* and more *extensional* in his

perceptions, or to put it in other terms, his experiences are more *accurately symbolized.*

4. His expressed *feelings* increasingly have reference to the *incongruity* between certain of his *experiences* and his *concept of self.*
5. He comes to experience in awareness the threat of such *incongruence.*
   (a) This *experience of threat* is possible only because of the continued *unconditional positive regard* of the therapist, which is extended to *incongruence* as much as to *congruence,* to *anxiety* as much as to absence of *anxiety.*
6. He *experiences* fully, in *awareness,* feelings which have in the past been *denied to awareness,* or *distorted in awareness.*
7. His *concept of self* becomes reorganized to assimilate and include these *experiences* which have previously been *distorted in* or *denied to awareness.*
8. As this reorganization of the *self-structure* continues, his *concept* of *self* becomes increasingly *congruent* with his *experience*; the *self* now including *experiences* which previously would have been too *threatening* to be in *awareness.*
   (a) A corollary tendency is toward fewer perceptual *distortions in awareness,* or *denials to awareness,* since there are fewer *experiences* which can be *threatening.* In other words, *defensiveness* is decreased.
9. He becomes increasingly able to *experience,* without a feeling of *threat,* the therapist's *unconditional positive regard.*
10. He increasingly feels *an unconditional positive self-regard.*
11. He increasingly *experiences* himself as the *locus of evaluation.*
12. He reacts to *experience* less in terms of his *conditions of worth* and more in terms of an *organismic valuing process.*

Comment

It cannot be stated with certainty that all of these are *necessary* elements of the process, though they are all characteristic. Both from the point of view of experience, and the logic of the theory, 3, 6, 7, 8, 10, 12, are necessary elements in the process. Item 5a is not a logical step in the theory but is put in as an explanatory note.

The element which will doubtless be most puzzling to the reader is the absence of explanatory mechanisms. It may be well to restate our scientific purpose in terms of an example. *If* one strokes a piece of steel with a magnet, and *if* one places the piece of steel so that it can rotate freely, *then* it will point to the north. This statement of the if-then variety has been proved thousands of times. Why does it happen? There have been various theoretical answers, and one would hesitate to say, even now, that we know with certitude *why* this occurs.

In the same way I have been saying in regard to therapy, "If these conditions exist, *then* these subsequent events will occur." Of course we have speculations as to *why* this relationship appears to exist, and those speculations will be increasingly spelled out as the presentation continues. Nevertheless the most basic element of our theory is that if the described conditions exist, then the process of therapy occurs, and the events which are called outcomes will be observed. We may be quite wrong as to *why* this sequence occurs. I believe there is an increasing body of evidence to show that it *does* occur.]

Evidence

There is confirming evidence of varying degrees of relevance for a number of these items describing the therapeutic process. Item 2 (increasing self-reference) is supported by our many recorded therapeutic cases, but has not been reduced to a statistical finding. Stock's study[40] supports item 3, indicating that client self-referent expressions become more objective, less strongly emotional. Mitchell[25] shows that clients become more extensional.

Objective clinical evidence supporting items 4, 5, and 6 is provided in the form of recordings from a case by Rogers[31].

The findings of Vargas[43] are relevant to item 7, indicating the way the self is reorganized in terms of emergent new self-perceptions. Hogan[19] and Haigh[14] have studied the decrease in defensiveness during the process, as described in item 8a, their findings being confirmatory. The increased congruence of self and experience is supported in an exhaustive single case investigation by Rogers[31]. That such congruence is associated with lack of defensiveness is found by Chodorkoff.

Item 10, the increase in the client's positive self-regard, is well attested by the studies of Snyder[39], Seeman[37], Raimy[29], Stock[40], Strom[41], Sheerer[38], Lipkin[24]. The client's trend toward experiencing himself as the locus of evaluation is most clearly shown by Raskin's research[30], but this is supported by evidence from Sheerer[38], Lipkin[24], Kessler[22].

C. OUTCOMES IN PERSONALITY AND BEHAVIOR

There is no clear distinction between process and outcome. Items of process are simply differentiated aspects of outcome. Hence the statements which follow could have been included under process. For reasons of convenience in understanding, there have been grouped here those changes which are customarily associated with the terms outcomes, or results, or are observed outside of the therapeutic relationship. These are the changes which are hypothesized as being relatively permanent:

1. The client is more *congruent*, more *open to his experience*, less *defensive*.
2. He is consequently more realistic, objective, *extensional* in his *perceptions*.
3. He is consequently more effective in problem solving.
4. His *psychological adjustment* is improved, being closer to the optimum.
   (a) This is owing to, and is a continuation of, the changes in *self-structure* described in *B*7 and *B*8.
5. As a result of the increased *congruence* of *self* and *experience* (*C*4 above) his *vulnerability* to *threat* is reduced.
6. As a consequence of *C*2 above, his perception of his *ideal self* is more realistic, more achievable.
7. As a consequence of the changes in *C*4 and *C*5 his *self* is more *congruent* with his *ideal self.*
8. As a consequence of the increased *congruence* of *self* and *ideal self* (*C*6) and the greater *congruence* of *self* and *experience*, tension of all types is reduced—physiological tension, psychological tension, and the specific type of psychological tension defined as *anxiety*.
9. He has an increased degree of *positive self-regard*.
10. He *perceives* the *locus of evaluation* and the locus of choice as residing within himself.
    (a) As a consequence of *C*9 and *C*10 he feels more confident and more self-directing, (b) As a consequence of *C*1 and *C*10, his values are determined by an *organismic valuing process.*
11. As a consequence of *C*1, and *C*2, he *perceives* others more realistically and accurately.

12. He *experiences* more *acceptance* of others, as a consequence of less need for distortion of his perceptions of them.
13. His behavior changes in various ways.
    (a) Since the proportion of *experience* assimilated into the *self-structure* is increased, the proportion of behaviors which can be "owned" as belonging to the *self* is increased.
    (b) Conversely, the proportion of behaviors which are disowned as *self-experiences*, felt to be "not myself," is decreased.
    (c) Hence his behavior is *perceived* as being more within his control.
14. His behavior is perceived by others as more socialized, more *mature*.
15. As a consequence of *C*1, 2, 3, his behavior is more creative, more uniquely adaptive to each new situation, and each new problem, more fully expressive of his own purposes and values.

Comment

The statement in part *C* which is essential is statement *C*1. Items 2 through 15 are actually a more explicit spelling out of the theoretical implications of statement 1. The only reason for including them is that though such implications follow readily enough from the logic of the theory, they are often not perceived unless they are pointed out.

Evidence

There is much confirmatory and some ambiguous or nonconfirming evidence of the theoretical statement of outcomes. Grummon and John[13] find a decrease in defensiveness, basing judgments on the TAT. Hogan[19] and Haigh[14] also supply some scanty evidence on this point. As to the greater extensionality of perceptions (item 2), Jonietz[20] finds these changes to be in the direction of extensionality.

Item 4, stating that adjustment is improved, is supported by evidence based upon TAT, Rorschach, counselor rating, and other indexes, in the studies of Dymond[7, 8], Grummon and John[13], Haimowitz[15], Muench[27], Mosak[26], Cowen and Combs[6]. Carr[4], however, found no evidence of change in the Rorschach in nine cases.

Rudikoff[35] found that the self-ideal becomes more achievable, as stated in item 6. The increased congruence of self and ideal has been confirmed by Butler and Haigh[3], Hartley[17], and its significance for adjustment supported by Hanlon, Hofstaetter, and O'Connor[16].

The decrease in physiological tension over therapy is attested by the studies of Thetford[42] and Anderson[1]. The reduction in psychological tension as evidenced by the Discomfort-Relief Quotient has been confirmed by many investigators: Assum and Levy[2], Cofer and Chance[5], Kaufman and Raimy[21], N. Rogers[34], Zimmerman[44].

The increase in positive self-regard is well attested, as indicated in *B*, Evidence. The shift in the locus of evaluation and choice is supported in the evidence provided by Raskin[30] and Sheerer[38]. Rudikoff[35] presents evidence which suggests that others may be perceived with greater realism. Sheerer[38], Stock[40], and Rudikoff[35] show that others are perceived in a more acceptant fashion as postulated in item 11. Gordon and Cartwright[12] provide evidence which is complex but in general nonconfirming on this point. Haimowitz[15] also has findings which seem to indicate that nonacceptance of minority groups may be more openly expressed.

The behavior changes specified in items 13 and 14 find support in the Rogers study[32] showing that in improved cases both the client and his friends observe greater maturity in his behavior. Hoffman[18] finds that the behavior the client describes in the interviews becomes more mature. Jonietz's study[20] of perception of ink blots might lend some support to the postulate of item 15.

Comments on the Theory of Therapy

It is to be noted that this theory of therapy involves, basically, no intervening variables. The conditions of therapy, given in A, are all operationally definable, and some have already been given rather crude operational definitions in research already conducted. The theory states that if A exists, then B and C will follow. B and C are measurable events, predicted by A.

It should also be pointed out that the logic of the theory is such that: if A, then B; if A, then B and C; if A, then C (omitting consideration of B), if B, then C (omitting consideration of A).

Specification of Functional Relationships

At this point, the functional relationships can only be stated in general and qualitative form. The greater the degree of the conditions specified in A, the more marked or more extensive will be the process changes in B, and the greater or more extensive the outcome changes specified in C. Putting this in more general terms, the greater the degree of anxiety in the client, congruence in the therapist in the relationship, acceptance and empathy experienced by the therapist, and recognition by the client of these elements, the deeper will be the process of therapy, and the greater the extent of personality and behavioral change. To revert now to the theoretical logic, all we can say at present is that

$$B = (f)A \qquad C = (f)A$$
$$B + C = (f)A \qquad C = (f)B$$

Obviously there are many functional interrelationships not yet specified by the theory. For example, if anxiety is high, is congruence on the part of the therapist less necessary? There is much work to be done in investigating the functional relationships more fully.

D. SOME CONCLUSIONS REGARDING THE NATURE OF THE INDIVIDUAL

From the theory of therapy as stated above, certain conclusions are implicit regarding the nature of man. To make them explicit involves little more than looking at the same hypotheses from a somewhat different vantage point. It is well to state them explicitly, however, since they constitute an important explanatory link of a kind which gives this theory whatever uniqueness it may possess. They also constitute the impelling reason for developing a theory of personality. If the individual is what he is revealed to be in therapy, then what theory would account for such an individual?

We present these conclusions about the characteristics of the human organism:

1. The individual possesses the capacity *to experience in awareness* the factors in his *psychological maladjustment*, namely, the *incongruences* between his *self-concept* and the totality of his *experience*.

2. The individual possesses the capacity and has the tendency to reorganize his *self-concept* in such a way as to make it more *congruent* with the totality of his *experience*, thus moving himself away from a state of *psychological maladjustment*, and toward a state of *psychological adjustment*.
3. These capacities and this tendency, when latent rather than evident, will be released in any interpersonal *relationship* in which the other person is *congruent* in the relationship, experiences *unconditional positive regard* toward, and *empathic* understanding of, the individual, and achieves some communication of these attitudes to the individual. (These are, of course, the characteristics already given under *A* 3, 4, 5, 6.)

It is this tendency which ... is elaborated into the tendency toward actualization.

I believe it is obvious that the basic capacity which is hypothesized is of very decided importance in its psychological and philosophical implications. It means that psychotherapy is the releasing of an already existing capacity in a potentially competent individual, not the expert manipulation of a more or less passive personality.[2] Philosophically it means that the individual has the capacity to guide, regulate, and control himself, providing only that certain definable conditions exist. Only in the absence of these conditions, and not in any basic sense, is it necessary to provide external control and regulation of the individual.

REFERENCES

1. Anderson, R. An investigation of the relationship between verbal and physiological behavior during client-centered therapy. Unpublished doctoral dissertation, University of Chicago, 1954.
2. Assum, A. L., & Levy, S. J. Analysis of a non-directive case with follow-up interview. *Journal of Abnormal and Social Psychology*, 1948, **43**, 78–89.
3. Butler, J. M., & Haigh, G. V. Changes in the relation between self concepts and ideal concepts consequent upon client-centered counseling. In C. R. Rogers & R. F. Dymond (Eds.), *Psychotherapy and personality change.* Chicago: University of Chicago Press, 1954. Chapter 4.
4. Carr, A. C. Evaluation of nine psychotherapy cases by the Rorschach *Journal of Consulting Psychology*, 1949, **13**(3), 196–205.
5. Cofer, C. N., & Chance, J. The discomfort-relief quotient in published cases of counseling and psychotherapy. *Journal of Psychology*, 1950, **29**, 219–224.
6. Cowen, E. L., & Combs, A. W. Follow-up study of 32 cases treated by nondirective psychotherapy. *Journal of Abnormal and Social Psychology*, 1950, **45**, 232–258.
7. Dymond, R. F. Adjustment changes over therapy from self-sorts. In C. R. Rogers & R. F. Dymond (Eds.), *Psychotherapy and personality change.* Chicago: University of Chicago Press, 1954. Chapter 5. (a)
8. Dymond, R. F. Adjustment changes over therapy from Thematic Apperception Test ratings. In C. R. Rogers & R. F. Dymond (Eds.), *Psychotherapy and personality change.* Chicago: University of Chicago Press, 1954. Chapter 8. (b)
9. Fiedler, F. E. A comparative investigation of early therapeutic relationships created by experts and non-experts of the psychoanalytic, non-directive and Adlerian schools. Unpublished doctoral dissertation, University of Chicago, 1949.
10. Fiedler, F. E. A comparison of therapeutic relationships in psychoanalytic, non-directive and Adlerian therapy. *Journal of Consulting Psychology*, 1950, **14**, 436–445.

---

[2]In order to correct a common misapprehension it should be stated that this tentative conclusion in regard to human capacity grew out of continuing work with clients in therapy. It was not an assumption or bias with which we started our therapeutic endeavors. A brief personal account of the way in which this conclusion was forced upon me is contained in an autobiographical paper.

11. Gallagher, J. J. The problem of escaping clients in non-directive counseling. In W. U. Synder (Ed.), *Group report of a program of research in psychotherapy.* Psychotherapy Research Group, Pennsylvania State University, 1953, Pp. 21–38.

12. Gordon, T., & Cartwright, D. The effects of psychotherapy upon certain attitudes toward others. In C. R. Rogers & R. F. Dymond (Eds.), *Psychotherapy and personality change.* Chicago: University of Chicago Press, 1954. Chapter 11.

13. Grummon, D. L., & John, E. S. Changes over client-centered therapy evaluated on psychoanalytically based Thematic Apperception Test scales. In C. R. Rogers & R. F. Dymond (Eds.), *Psychotherapy and personality change.* Chicago: University of Chicago Press, 1954. Chapter 11.

14. Haigh, G. V. Defensive behavior in client-centered therapy. *Journal of Consulting Psychology,* 1949, **13**(3), 181–189.

15. Haimowitz, N. R., & Morris, L. Personality changes in client-centered therapy. In W. Wolff (Ed.), *Success in psychotherapy.* New York: Grune & Stratton, 1952, Chapter 3.

16. Hanlon, T. E., Hofstaetter, P. R., & O'Connor, J. P. Congruence of self and ideal self in relation to personality adjustment. *Journal of Consulting Psychology,* 1954, **18**, 215–218.

17. Hartley, M. Changes in the self-concept during psychotherapy. Unpublished doctoral dissertation, University of Chicago, 1951.

18. Hoffman, A. E. A study of reported behavior changes in counseling. *Journal of Consulting Psychology,* 1949, **4**, 373–382.

19. Hogan, R. The development of a measure of client-defensiveness in the counseling relationship. Unpublished doctoral dissertation, University of Chicago, 1948.

20. Jonietz, A. A study of phenomenological changes in perception and psychotherapy as exhibited in the content of Rorschach percepts. Unpublished doctoral dissertation, University of Chicago, 1950.

21. Kaufman, P. E., & Raimy, V. C. Two methods of assessing therapeutic progress. *Journal of Abnormal and Social Psychology,* 1949, **44**, 379–385.

22. Kessler, C. Semantics and non-directive counseling. Unpublished master's thesis, University of Chicago, 1947.

23. Kirtner, W. L. Success and failure in client-centered therapy as a function of personality variables. Unpublished master's thesis, University of Chicago, 1955.

24. Lipkin, S. Clients' feelings and attitudes in relation to the outcome of client-centered therapy. *Psychological Monographs,* 1954, **68**(1, Whole No. 372).

25. Mitchell, F. H. A test of certain semantic hypotheses by application of client-centered counseling cases: Intensionality-extensionality of clients in therapy. Unpublished doctoral dissertation, University of Chicago, 1951.

26. Mosak, H. Evaluation in psychotherapy: A study of some current measures. Unpublished doctoral dissertation, University of Chicago, 1951.

27. Muench, G. A. An evaluation of non-directive psychotherapy by means of the Rorschach and other tests. *Applied Psychology Monographs,* 1947, No. 13, 1–163.

28. Quinn, R. D. Psychotherapists as an index to the quality of early therapeutic relationships established by representatives of the non-directive, Adlerian, and psychoanalytic schools. Unpublished doctoral dissertation, University of Chicago, 1950.

29. Raimy, V. C. Self reference in counseling interviews. *Journal of Consulting Psychology,* 1948, **12**, 153–163.

30. Raskin, N. J. An objective study of the locus of evaluation factor in psychotherapy. Unpublished doctoral dissertation, University of Chicago, 1949.

31. Rogers, C. R. The case of Mrs. Oak: A research analysis. In C. R. Rogers & R. F. Dymond (Eds.), *Psychotherapy and personality change.* Chicago: University of Chicago Press, 1954. Chapter 15. (a)

32. Rogers, C. R. Changes in the maturity of behavior as related to therapy. In C. R. Rogers & R. F. Dymond (Eds.), *Psychotherapy and personality change.* Chicago: University of Chicago Press, 1954. Chapter 13. (b)

33. Rogers, C. R., & Dymond, R. F. (Eds.), *Psychotherapy and personality change.* Chicago: University of Chicago Press, 1954.

34. Rogers, N. Measuring psychological tension in nondirective counseling. *Personal Counselor*, 1948, **3**, 237-264.
35. Rudikoff, E. C. A. A comparative study of the changes in the concept of the self, the ordinary person, and the ideal in eight cases. In C. R. Rogers & R. F. Dymond (Eds.), *Psychotherapy and personality change*. Chicago: University of Chicago Press, 1954, Chapter 11.
36. Seeman, J. A study of the process of non-directive therapy. *Journal of Consulting Psychology*, 1949, **13**, 157–168.
37. Seeman, J. Counselor judgments of therapeutic process and outcome. In C. R. Rogers & R. F. Dymond (Eds.), *Psychotherapy and personality change*. Chicago: University of Chicago Press, 1954. Chapter 11.
38. Sheerer, E. T. The relationship between acceptance of self and acceptance of others. *Journal of Consulting Psychology*, 1949, **13**(3), 169–175.
39. Snyder, W. U. An investigation of the nature of non-directive psychotherapy. *Journal of Genetic Psychology*, 1945, **33**, 193–223.
40. Stock, D. The self concept and feelings toward others. *Journal of Consulting Psychology*, 1949, **13**(3), 176–180.
41. Strom, K. A re-study of William U. Snyder's "An investigation of the nature of non-directive psychotherapy." Unpublished master's thesis, University of Chicago, 1948.
42. Thetford, W. N. An objective measure of frustration tolerance in evaluating psychotherapy. In W. Wolff (Ed.), *Success in psychotherapy*. New York: Grune & Stratton, 1952, Chapter 2.
43. Vargas, M. Changes in self-awareness during client-centered therapy. In C. R. Rogers & R. F. Dymond (Eds.), *Psychotherapy and personality change*. Chicago: University of Chicago Press, 1954, Chapter 10.
44. Zimmerman, J. Modification of the discomfort-relief quotient as a measure of progress in counseling. Unpublished master's thesis, University of Chicago, 1950.

Suggested Additional Readings

Allen, F. H. *Psychotherapy with children.* New York: Norton, 1942.

Axline, V. M. *Play therapy.* Boston: Houghton Mifflin, 1947.

Ayllon, T., & Azrin, N. H. *The token economy: A motivational system for therapy and rehabilitation.* New York: Appleton-Century-Crofts, 1968.

Bandura, A. *Principles of behavior modification.* New York: Holt, Rinehart & Winston, 1969.

Dollard, J., & Miller, N. E. *Personality and psychotherapy.* New York: McGraw Hill, 1950.

Ellis, A., & Harper, R. *A guide to rational living.* North Hollywood, Calif.: Wilshire Book Co., 1970.

Eysenck, H. J. New ways in psychotherapy. In *Readings in clinical psychology today.* Del Mar, Calif.: CRM Books, 1970. Pp. 65–75.

Ferster, C. B. Perspectives in psychology. XXV. Transition from animal laboratory to clinic. *Psychological Record,* 1967, **17**, 145–150.

Ford, D. H., & Urban, H. B. *Systems of psychotherapy: A comparative study.* New York: Wiley, 1963.

Frank, J. *Persuasion and healing.* Baltimore: Johns Hopkins Press, 1961.

Freud, S. *The interpretation of dreams.* New York: Random House, 1951.

Jones, E. (Ed.), *Collected papers of Sigmund Freud.* New York: Basic Books, 1959.

Patterson, C. H. *Theories of counseling and psychotherapy.* New York: Harper & Row, 1966.

Rogers, C. R. *Client-centered therapy.* Cambridge, Mass.: Riverside Press, 1951.

Schutz, W. C. *Joy.* New York: Grove Press, 1967.

Stampfl, T. G., & Levis, D. J. The essentials of implosive therapy: A learning-theory-based psychodynamic behavioral therapy. *Journal of Abnormal Psychology,* 1967, **72**, 496–503.

Sullivan, H. S. *The psychiatric interview.* New York: Norton, 1954.

Truax, C. B., & Carkhuff, R. R. *Toward effective counseling and psychotherapy: Training and practice.* Chicago: Aldine, 1967.

Wolf, M., Risley, T., & Mees, H. Application of operant conditioning procedures to the behavior problems of an autistic child. *Behavior, Research and Therapy,* 1964, **1**, 305–312.

Wolpe, J. *Behavior therapy.* 2nd. ed. New York: Pergamon Press, 1973.

Group Therapy Approaches

31

The Dynamics of Group Psychotherapy and its Application*

LOUIS WENDER

Group psychotherapy has been practiced at the Hastings Hillside Hospital for nearly six years. Initial experimentation with this method was prompted by the need for devising forms of therapy adapted to meeting the peculiar problems created by the segregation of mild mental patients and psychoneurotics under one roof. Carefully tested experience with this method has convinced the writer that this form of therapy is efficacious in selected situations and that it merits much wider application in hospitals where patients amenable to psychotherapy receive care.

In distinction to the method of extra-mural group analysis described by Trigant Burrows, which is psychoanalytic in technique and carries large sociological and philosophic implications, group psychotherapy is a method confined to the intra-mural treatment of certain types of mild mental disease.

In the ensuing material the writer will attempt to review some of the conditions that prompted the adoption of this approach, to define this method of therapy, to show its ideologic basis, to describe its application and scope and to evaluate its results.

In considering the treatment of patients within a hospital, one has to bear in mind that the choice between extra-mural and intra-mural care is not arbitrary. Hospitalization is the last resort, after efforts at extra-mural care have failed, and it is usually the severity of the patient's condition that precludes continued treatment on the outside. To the patient himself hospitalization is a crisis. His sporadic efforts in the direction of adjustment need no longer be maintained, since not only has his illness been acknowledged to himself, but there has been a corresponding certification to society and a meting out of "punishment." Hospitalization also deprives the patient of the attention he received from his family group and of the power he exercised over them because of his illness. He compensates for this loss by identifying the hospital with his family group (home) and proceeds to seek recognition in the new milieu. Since he no longer competes for supremacy with normal people who accede to his demands because of the illness which distinguishes him from the rest, he resorts to an intensification of his complaints, in order to focus attention on himself in the new setting, where he has to endure the competition of other sick people.

Another condition prevailing in hospitals, as in other assemblies, which requires recognition in considering approaches to therapy is the formation of friendships and cliques and the choice of "buddies." Problems are frequently analyzed and discussed among patients with greater candor than with the physician and it is a common occurrence to learn the problems and conflicts of a patient through his confidant.

*From Wender, L., *Journal of Nervous and Mental Disease*, 1939, **84**, 54–60. Copyright © 1939 by The Williams & Wilkins Company. Reprinted by permission of The Williams & Wilkins Company, and Dr. Wender.

McDougall's theory "that the gregarious impulse receives the highest degree of satisfaction from the presence of human beings who most closely resemble the individual, who behave in like manner and respond to the same situations with similar emotions" is amply demonstrated in hospital life. One encounters daily a group interaction, with its resultant infectiousness of symptoms and suggestibility of moods, that demands the diverting of these impulses and the utilization of group interaction into positive therapeutic channels, if we are not to promote "symptoms orgies."

In viewing intra-mural methods of therapy, one is impressed by the gap between the profound influence psychoanalytic thinking has exerted on our understanding of the individual patient and the barriers to the wide application of individual analysis to hospital patients. In this connection one must remember that as a therapeutic method psychoanalysis has a limited field of application. Hospitalization still further restricts the use of this method for the following reasons: (a) the difficulty of establishing transference where separation of patients cannot be maintained as in private practice and where patients have opportunities to compare physicians and to develop jealousies of one another while sharing a therapist; (b) the prohibitive financial cost; (c) the dearth of patients with a suitable intellectual and cultural equipment; (d) the practical barrier of extending the length of hospitalization to make possible the completion of an analysis.

The conditions enumerated, as well as many minor ones into a discussion of which we have not the time to enter, make clear the need for seeking and crystallizing methods of approach that are applicable to wider groups of patients, that are shorter in duration and that are realistically adapted to prevailing hospital conditions. To meet these requirements a proposed method of therapy would have to take cognizance not only of the individual through a psychoanalytic approach but also of the psychology of the group with its common reactions, its individual-to-individual identifications and its responses to the therapist.

Group psychotherapy is based on the assumption that the application of some of the hypotheses and methods of psychoanalysis, in combination with intellectualization, when applied to a group for the purposes of treatment under conditions of active therapeutic control, will lead to the release of certain emotional conflicts and a partial reorganization of the personality and ultimately to an increased capacity for social amalgamation. In distinction to individual psychoanalysis this method places greater emphasis on sociological factors (group interaction) and on intellectual comprehension of behavior. The material for this form of therapy is elicited through theoretical discussions with a group of patients, affording a natural tie-up with the individual participants' experiences and problems. The base, or meeting-ground, for these patients is established through what Giddings calls "consciousness of kind." He says "that this consciousness is the basis of alliance, of rules of intercourse, of peculiarities of policy and that our conduct toward those whom we feel to be most like ourselves is instinctively and rationally different from our conduct toward others who are different from ourselves." These patients are in the same predicament; they have diminished need for concealment; in a sense, they are temporarily in a different state of society, with different mores, and their resistance to a relatively intimate sharing of problems is reduced by prevailing attitudes in the new set-up. These comments are not hypothetical. They are deductions from extended observation of patients and the progressive changes in their perspective and attitudes during hospitalization. These changes are inevitable; the only question that arises is whether one is to permit them to lie fallow or whether they are to be utilized and released through some method such as this form of therapy.

Experience has shown that group psychotherapy is applicable only to disorders in which intellectual impairment is absent and in which some degree of affect is retained. It is believed that the following groups lend themselves to this type of treatment: (a) early schizophrenics where the delusional trends are not fully systematized and in which hallucinatory phenomena are completely absent; where the splitting of the personality is not marked and there is no blocking; (b) depressions without marked retardation and those who libidinize their ideation—depression sine depression; (c) psychoneuroses, with the exception of severe compulsion neuroses of long duration.

The application of this method does not preclude the continuance of individual treatment. As a matter of fact, individual interviews are undertaken in conjunction with the patient's participating in a group and in many instances it has been found that the group stimulated the patient's desire for individual treatment and that during these interviews such patients spoke readily of experiences the discussion of which they had avoided previously.

A group consists of six to eight patients of the same sex. Attendance is entirely voluntary. The procedure is elastic. No patient is introduced into a group immediately upon his arrival in the hospital, as some degree of adaptation to the hospital is considered essential. A new patient learns soon after his arrival that this form of therapy is an established procedure and that some of his fellow-patients participate in a group. Frequently requests for this form of treatment come from the patients and great tact and patience have to be exercised in explaining the exclusions. A group has two or three one-hour sessions each week and continues for a period which varies according to the needs of its members and the objectives of the therapist (usually four to five months). New patients are not admitted to a group already in session. At early meetings the group is instructed not to discuss the content of sessions with patients outside the group but they are encouraged to discuss the material freely with one another.

Sessions are begun with what is almost lecture material: a simple exposition of why we behave as we do, a description of primitive instinctual drives, conscious and unconscious elements, significance of dreams, early infantile traumata, reaction formations, repressions, rationalizations, etc. The material is presented in elementary form, with simple, everyday illustrations, the intellectual content and method of presentation being adapted to the general cultural and emotional tenor of the group, and varying accordingly. Presentations are planned with a view to arousing sincere interest in the background of everyday life without inculcating a " psychology hobby." This pitfall can be avoided by the therapist, and the response obtained from groups has always been on the level desired. The use of theoretical material in the beginning stimulates intellectual interest and serves to divert patients from their immediate problems. It also serves as an instrument of facilitating a kind of intimacy and social good will that is analogous to the reaction which we experience after spending an evening with a group in stimulating and vital conversation that gives us a feeling of closeness to people toward whom we have never felt this previously.

Even in the early period of the group's existence there are individual members who have established a transference to the therapist and there are others who have identified themselves with patients who have this transference. What occurs progressively is a common rapport, patient-to-patient transference and patient-to-therapist transference. A sense of intimacy within the group develops, greater freedom from inhibitions is observed in theoretical discussions and is followed by a spontaneous readiness on the part of some patients to discuss their own problems in relation to the theoretical material. Beginning with illustrations of individual incidents in their own lives which they regard as traumatic or significant, the patients go on to a discussion of their own and one another's symptoms and adjustments. They discuss dreams, which are interpreted on a superficial level with some of the patients participating in the interpretation. The therapist exercises no pressure and when the term "active control" is used, it is in the sense of active awareness, in distinction to any form of manipulation. Whenever resistances are observed in any particular patient, skillful guidance can divert the discussion into safe and still theoretical waters until such a time as the patients wish to resume the subject. Moreover, the use of this more generic approach minimizes resistance and trauma, since the patient is left free to accept as much as he is ready to accept as applying to him, and to the degree necessary for him is also able to project explanations painful to him onto other patients. Nevertheless, the most carefully gauged awareness as to the individual and collective reactions of the group is essential. Both the theoretical material and the guidance of the patients' own discussions have to be adapted to the changing attitudes and receptivity of the group, so that even the tempo of discussion and the duration of a group will be determined accordingly.

It is the writer's intention to make available at a later date the complete material of one group throughout its entire duration, so that the techniques may be more intensively scrutinized and evaluated. At the present time it seems expedient to summarize briefly some of the dynamics operating in group psychotherapy.

1. *Intellectualization*   In our awareness of how prominent and destructive a role the Conscious can play, we may have neglected it too completely as a factor in the healing process. While there may be no pure intellectual acceptance and everything that may seem like logical acceptance is accompanied by emotional tone, the fact remains that a synthesis of intellect and emotion dominates every phase of our lives and is the basis of all social adjustment. Nor can we overlook entirely the fact that there are intellectual disciplines like the Yogi philosophy, the application of which results in the regulation of emotional responses through a self-determined intellectual discipline. What we term "insight" or emotional acceptance may have similar components of self-discipline. While group therapy in no way professes or strives to be an intellectual discipline, it does tend to a comprehension of emotional reactions that enables the patient to meet new situations with greater awareness and skill. The writer is convinced that intellectual awareness is a therapeutic aid as indisputable as the fact that while we may be panic-stricken at an unexpected noise coming from behind, we accept such a noise calmly when we know its origin.

2. *Patient-to-Patient Transference*   The influence exerted by one individual on another may contain elements corresponding to the psychoanalytic transference. In group psychotherapy this patient-to-patient transference is made use of in several ways. It is used to facilitate transference to the therapist through the identification of one patient with another who has established such transference. This type of transference is encouraged, since it serves to meet the needs of the patients more permanently than the transference to the therapist which has to be abrogated for practical reasons as well as for the purpose of sustaining the patient's independence. It is also believed that the relationship which is established between patients in time takes an outward course, embracing a wider area of interests and activities (socialization).

3. *Catharsis-in-the-Family*   In the group there is undoubtedly a transference of tendencies originally directed toward the parents and siblings. There is a possibility that the entire group set-up provides a kind of "Catharsis-in-the-Family," with an accompanying resolvement of conflicts and the displacement of parent love onto new objects. The patient finds himself sitting on terms of equality with the therapist (symbolic of the parent) and the other patients (who represent the siblings). He experiences (it may be for the first time in his life) the receiving of understanding from the just parent whom he shares with siblings who are equal in the eyes of that parent. He is not only receiving understanding but is also

free to rebel openly, thus averting repression with its concomitant sense of guilt. In the writer's opinion this experience serves as a means of effecting a degree of emotional release, particularly in situations where the early traumata in child-parent relationships have remained unresolved. The fact that the actual set-up is on an adult level and that the patient is conscious of it only as a treatment process makes it acceptable to him.

4. *Group Interaction*   Group interaction is a phenomenon to which every patient was exposed prior to his hospitalization. His development, his ego ideal and his sense of values had their roots in his societal experience. In this method the patient's association with other patients, his new group experience, is made use of. Inevitably this association will influence his mode of thinking and his reactions , as manifested by the patients' competing with their respective complaints during their early sojourn. Under guidance this interaction results in the development of a changed perspective on behavior, which in turn gives rise to new ego ideals and strivings. In the group the patient develops criteria for evaluating his own problem against the problems of others in a way that is not feasible in individual treatment. An individual who prior to his hospitalization regarded his problems as unique and peculiar to himself learns through exchange with the group that many of his fellows have similarly predicated ego conflicts and begins to view his own problems with greater detachment. The individual experiences a resultant lessening of personal tensions, his attitudes undergo modification and his whole outlook on behavior changes. In this entire experience he is reinforced by the experience of his group.

The patient's drive to get well derives greater impetus through this method than when only individual treatment is undertaken. This drive is motivated in part by the new ego ideal which the individual has adopted and is strengthened by the apparent feasibility of attaining health, since the recovery of other members of the group presents convincing evidence.

It may be argued that suggestion is a major factor in the results gained through group interaction. If by suggestion we mean the concepts as defined by MacDougall or Freud, these types of suggestion play no greater role in this method than in any other technique. In no sense is there acceptance without logical basis or a continued infantile emotional dependence, implicit in suggestion. In the use of group psychotherapy, the patient derives an understanding of the nature and direction of his unconscious trends, experiencing simultaneously an emotional release. This is accompanied by his being exposed to observation and experience which involve himself and others, ultimately leading to a partial reorganization of his personality. In this unified process it is not an outside agent like suggestion which accomplishes the change but the saturation of the individual with the forces of his own experience.

The results yielded by this method which has been used in the treatment of about seventy-five patients over a period of six years, cannot be computed statistically. Interpretation on the basis of follow-up (in some cases for four to five years), since that is the only form of evaluation open to us in analyzing material of this nature, shows fairly conclusively that this form of therapy carries positive values for social adjustment. It has been observed repeatedly that friendships formed while groups were in session persist on the outside; that these patients retain a common bond of mutual interest, helpfulness and understanding which is a source of strength to them; and that their drive to remain well is more dynamic and characterized by a competitive quality. While the recovered patients' opinions cannot be interpreted as having scientific validity, it is significant that they attach importance to this form of therapy and attribute to the group experience their continued capacity to discuss their problems freely and their enhanced ability to deal successfully with new and difficult emotional material and experience.

32

Preliminary Report on the Application of Contingent Reinforcement Procedures (Token Economy) on a "Chronic" Psychiatric Ward*[1]

JOHN M. ATTHOWE, Jr. and LEONARD KRASNER

Although investigators may disagree as to what specific strategies or tactics to pursue, they would agree that current treatment programs in mental hospitals are in need of vast improvement. Release rates for patients hospitalized 5 or more years have not materially changed in this century (Kramer, Goldstein, Israel, & Johnson, 1956). After 5 years of hospitalization, the likelihood of release is approximately 6% (Kramer *et al.*, 1956; Morgan & Johnson, 1957; Odegard, 1961), and, as patients grow older and their length of hospitalization increases, the possibility of discharge approaches zero. Even for those chronic patients who do leave the hospital, more than two out of every three return within 6 months (Fairweather, Simon, Gebhard, Weingarten, Holland, Sanders, Stone & Reahl, 1960). There is certainly need for new programs of demonstrated efficiency in modifying the behavior of long-term hospitalized patients.

In September 1963 a research program in behavior modification was begun which was intimately woven into the hospital's ongoing service and training programs. The objective was to create and maintain a systematic ward program within the ongoing social system of the hospital. The program reported here involves the life of the entire ward, patients, and staff, plus others who come in contact with the patients. The purpose of the program was to change the chronic patients' aberrant behavior, especially that behavior judged to be apathetic, overly dependent, detrimental, or annoying to others. The goal was to foster more responsible, active, and interested individuals who would be able to perform the

*Atthowe, J. M., Jr., and Krasner, L., "Preliminary report on the application of contingent reinforcement procedures (token economy) on a "chronic" psychiatric ward," *Journal of Abnormal Psychology*, 1968, 73, 37–43. Copyright © 1968 by the American Psychological Association, and reproduced by permission.

[1]Parts of this paper were presented to the annual meeting of the American Psychological Association, Chicago, September 1965. Supported by the Psychology Research Associate Program of the Veterans Administration at the VA Hospital, Palo Alto, California and United States Public Health Service Grants MH 6191 and MH 11938 to Stanford University and The State University of New York at Stony Brook. The authors wish to acknowledge the following staff members and trainees who participated in the program: Dave Panek, Robert Houlihan, Ralph Sibley, Gordon Paul, Lois Brockhoff, Joseph McDonough, Loraine Ceaglske, Martha May, Rose Peter; psychiatric aides Ed Noseworthy, Donald Bradford, Herbert Bowles, Sam Asbury, Kay Key, Harriet Faggitt, Van Cliett, Calvin Johnson, Hope Wood, Wilbert Butler, Doris Hughley, and Alice Bruce; Arlene Stevens, ward secretary; Martha Smiley; W. G. Beckman, ward psychiatrist; J. J. Prusmack, and Thomas W. Kennelly.

routine activities associated with self-care, to make responsible decisions, and to delay immediate reinforcement in order to plan for the future.

THE WARD POPULATION

An 86-bed closed ward in the custodial section of the Veterans Administration Hospital in Palo Alto was selected. The median age of the patients was 57 years and more than one-third were over 65. Their overall length of hospitalization varied from 3 to 48 years with a median length of hospitalization of 22 years. Most of the patients had previously been labeled as chronic schizophrenics; the remainder were classified as having some organic involvement.

The patients fell into three general performance classes. The largest group, approximately 60% of the ward, required constant supervision. Whenever they left the ward, an aide had to accompany them. The second group, about 25%, had ground privileges and were able to leave the ward unescorted. The third group, 15% of the patients, required only minimal supervision and could probably function in a boarding home under proper conditions if the fear of leaving the hospital could be overcome.

In order to insure a stable research sample for the 2 years of the project, 60 patients were selected to remain on the ward for the duration of the study. The patients selected were older and had, for the most part, obvious and annoying behavioral deficits. This "core" sample served as the experimental population in studying the long-term effectiveness of the research program, the token economy.

THE TOKEN ECONOMY

Based on the work of Ayllon and his associates (Ayllon, 1963; Ayllon & Azrin, 1965; Ayllon & Houghton, 1962; Ayllon & Michael, 1959) and the principle of reinforcement as espoused by Skinner (1938, 1953), we have tried to incorporate every important phase of ward and hospital life within a systematic contingency program. The attainment of the "good things in life" was made contingent upon the patient's performance.

If a patient adequately cared for his personal needs, attended his scheduled activities, helped on the ward, interacted with other patients, or showed increased responsibility in any way, he was rewarded. The problem was to find rewards that were valued by everyone. Tokens, which could in turn be exchanged for the things a patient regards as important or necessary, were introduced. As stated in the manual distributed to patients (Atthowe, 1964):

> The token program is an incentive program in which each person can do as much or as little as he wants as long as he abides by the general rules of the hospital, *but*, in order to gain certain ends or do certain things, he must have tokens. . . . The more you do the more tokens you get [p. 2].

Cigarettes, money, passes, watching television, etc., were some of the more obvious reinforcers, but some of the most effective reinforcers were idiosyncratic, such as sitting on the ward or feeding kittens. For some patients, hoarding tokens became highly valued. This latter practice necessitated changing the tokens every 30 days. In addition, the tokens a patient still had left at the end of each month were devaluated 25%, hence the greater incentive for the patient to spend them quickly. The more tokens a patient earned or spent, the less likely he would be to remain apathetic.

In general, each patient was reinforced immediately after the completion of some "therapeutic" activity, but those patients who attended scheduled activities by themselves were paid their tokens only once a week on a regularly scheduled pay day. Consequently, the more independent and responsible patient had to learn "to punch a time card" and to receive his "pay" at a specified future date. He then had to "budget" his tokens so they covered his wants for the next 7 days.

In addition, a small group of 12 patients was in a position of receiving what might be considered as the ultimate in reinforcement. They were allowed to become independent of the token system. These patients carried a "carte blanche" which entitled them to all the privileges within the token economy plus a few added privileges and a greater status. For this special status, the patient had to work 25 hours per week in special vocational assignments. In order to become a member of the "elite group," patients had to accumulate 120 tokens which entailed a considerable delay in gratification.

The token economy was developed to cover all phases of a patient's life. This extension of contingencies to all of the patient's routine activities should bring about a greater generality and permanence of the behavior modified. One criticism of conditioning therapies has been that the behavior changed is specific with little evidence of carry-over to other situations. In this project plans were incorporated to program transfer of training as well as behavior change, per se. As a major step in this direction, token reinforcements were associated with social approval.

The attainment of goals which bring about greater independence should also result in strong sustaining reinforcement in and of itself. The aim of this study was to support more effective behavior and to weaken ineffective behavior by withdrawal of approval and attention and, if necessary, by penalties. Penalties comprised "fines" of specified numbers of tokens levied for especially undesirable behavior or for *not* paying the tokens required by the system. The fines can be seen as actually representing a high token payment to do something socially undesirable, for example, three tokens for cursing someone.

METHOD

The research program was initiated in September of 1963 when the senior author joined the ward as the ward psychologist and program administrator. The remainder of 1963 was a period of observation, pilot studies, and planning. Steps were taken to establish a research clinic and to modify the traditional service orientation of the nursing staff. In January 1964, the base-line measures were begun. The base-line or operant period lasted approximately 6 months and was followed by 3 months in which the patients were gradually prepared to participate in the token economy. In October 1964, the token economy was established and, at the time of writing, is still in operation. This report represents results based on the completion of the first year of the program.

The general design of the study was as follows: A 6 month base-line period, a 3-month shaping period, and an 11-month experimental period. During the base-line period, the frequency of particular behaviors was recorded daily, and ratings were carried out periodically. The shaping period was largely devoted to those patients requiring continual supervision. At first, the availability of canteen booklets, which served as money in the hospital canteen, was made contingent upon the amount of scheduled activities a patient attended. It soon became clear that almost one-half of the patients were not interested in money or canteen books. They did not know how to use the booklets, and they never bought things for themselves. Consequently, for 6 weeks patients were taken to the canteen and urged or "cajoled" into buying items which seemed to interest them (e.g., coffee, ice cream, pencils, handkerchiefs, etc.) Then all contingencies were temporarily abandoned, and patients were further encouraged to utilize the canteen books. Next, tokens were introduced but on a noncontingent basis. No one was allowed to purchase items in the ward canteen without first presenting tokens. Patients were instructed to pick up tokens from an office directly across the hall from the ward canteen and exchange them for the items they desired. After 2 weeks the tokens were made contingent upon performance and the experimental phase of the study began.

Within a reinforcement approach, the principles of successive approximation in gradually shaping the desired patient behavior were utilized. Once the tokens were introduced, shaping procedures were reduced. It would be impossible to hold reinforcement and shaping procedures constant throughout the experimental period or to match our ward or our patients with another ward or comparable group of patients. Consequently, a classical statistical design does not suit our paradigm. It is much more feasible, in addition to reducing sampling errors, to use the patients as their own controls. Therefore, we first established a base-line over an extended period of time. Any changes in behavior from that defined by the base-line must be taken into account. The effects of any type of experimental intervention become immediately obvious. We do not have to rely solely on the inferences teased out of statistical analyses.

Other than an automatic timer for the television set, the only major piece of equipment was the tokens. After a considerable search, a durable and physically safe token was constructed. This token was a $1\frac{3}{4} \times 3\frac{1}{2}$ in. plastic, nonlaminated, file card which came in seven colors varying from a bright red to a light tan. Different exchange values were assigned to the different colors. The token had the appearance of the usual credit card so prevalent in our society.

Whenever possible, the giving of the tokens was accompanied by some expression of social approval such as smiling, "good," "fine job," and a verbal description of the contingencies involved, for example, "Here's a token because of the good job of shaving you did this morning."

RESULTS

There has been a significant increase in those behaviors indicating responsibility and activity. Figure 32.1 shows the improvement in the frequency of attendance at group activities. During the base-line period, the average hourly rate of attendance per week was 5.85 hours per patient. With the introduction of tokens, this rate increased to 8.4 the first month and averaged 8.5 during the experimental period, except for a period of 3 months when the reinforcing value of the tokens was increased from one to two tokens per hour of attendance. Increasing the reinforcing value of the tokens increased the contingent behavior accordingly. With an increase in the amount of reinforcement, activity increased from 8.4 hours per week in the month before to 9.2 the first month under the new schedule. This gain was maintained throughout the period of greater reinforcement and for 1 month thereafter.

Thirty-two patients of the core sample comprised the group-activity sample. Nine patients were discharged or transferred during the project, and the remaining patients were on individual assignments and did not enter into these computations. Of the 32 patients, 18 increased their weekly attendance by at least 2 hours, while only 4 decreased their attendance by this amount. The probability that this is a significant difference is 0.004, using a

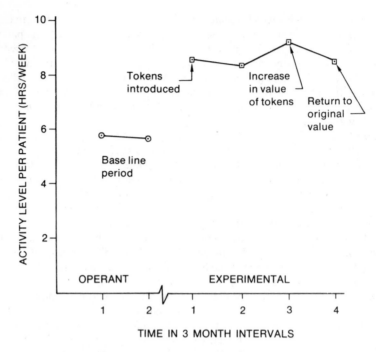

Fig. 32.1   Attendance at group activities.

sign test and a two-tailed estimate. Of those patients going to group activities, 18% changed to the more token-producing and more responsible individual assignments within 4 months of the onset of the token economy.

A widening of interest and a lessening of apathy were shown by a marked increase in the number of patients going on passes, drawing weekly cash, and utilizing the ward canteen. Of the core sample of 60 patients, 80% had never been off the hospital grounds on their own for a period of 8 hours since their hospitalization. During the experimental period, 19% went on overnight or longer passes, 17% went on day passes, and 12% went out on accompanied passes for the first time. In other words, approximately one-half of these who had been too apathetic to leave the hospital grounds increased their interest and commitment in the world outside. Furthermore, 13% of the core sample left on one or more trial visits of at least 30 days during the token program, although 6 out of every 10 returned to the hospital.

For the entire ward, the lessening of apathy was dramatic. The number of patients going on passes and drawing weekly cash tripled. Twenty-four patients were discharged and 8 were transferred to more active and discharge-oriented ward programs as compared to 11 discharges and no such transfers in the preceding 11-month period. Of the 24 patients released, 11 returned to the hospital within 9 months.

Independence and greater self-sufficiency were shown by an increase in the number of patients receiving tokens for shaving and appearing neatly dressed. Fewer patients missed their showers, and bed-wetting markedly diminished.

At the beginning of the study, there were 12 bed-wetters, 4 of whom were classified as "frequent" wetters and 2 were classified as "infrequent." All bed-wetters were awakened and taken to the bathroom at 11 p.m., 12:30 a.m., 2 a.m., and 4 a.m. regularly. As the program progressed, patients who did not wet during the night were paid tokens the following morning. In addition, they were only awakened at 11 p.m. the next night. After a week of no bed-wetting, patients were taken off the schedule altogether. At the end of the experimental period no one was wetting regularly and, for all practical purposes, there were no bed-wetters on the ward. The aversive schedule of being awakened during the night together with the receiving of tokens for a successful non-bed-wetting night seemed to instigate getting up on one's own and going to the bathroom, even in markedly deteriorated patients.

Another ward problem which had required extra aide coverage in the mornings was the lack of "cooperativeness" in getting out of bed, making one's bed, and leaving the bed area by a specified time. Just before the system of specific contingency tokens was introduced, the number of infractions in each of these areas was recorded for 3 weeks. This 3-week baseline period yielded an average of 75 "infractions" per week for the entire ward, varying from 71 to 77. A token given daily was then made contingent upon not having a recorded infraction in any of the three areas above. This token was given as the patients line up to go to breakfast each morning. In the week following the establishment of the contingency, the frequency of infractions dropped to 30 and then to 18. The next week the number of infractions rose to 39 but then declined steadily to 5 per week by the end of 9 weeks (see Fig. 32.2). During the last 6 months, the frequency of infractions varied between 6 and 13, averaging 9 per week.

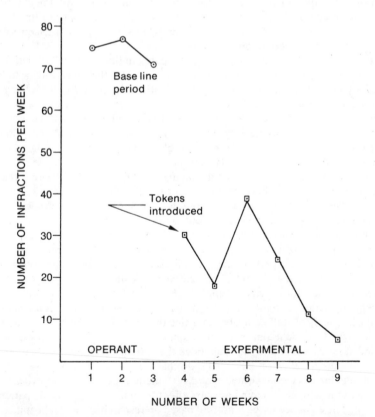

Fig. 32.2 Number of infractions in carrying out morning routines.

A significant increase was shown in measures of social interaction and communication. A brief version of the Palo Alto Group Psychotherapy scale (Finney, 1954) was used to measure social responsiveness in weekly group meetings. The change in ratings by one group of raters 1 month before the introduction of tokens compared with those of a second group of raters 4 months later was significant at the 0.001 level. A simple sign test based upon a two-tailed probability estimate was used. Neither set of raters knew which of their patients was included within the core sample. The rater reliability of the scale is 0.90 (Finney, 1954). Evidence of enhanced social interaction was dramatically shown by the appearance of card games using tokens as money among some of the more "disturbed" patients and an increased frequency in playing pool together.

DISCUSSION AND CONCLUSION

A detailed description of the entire procedures and results is in preparation. However, we wish to point out in this paper the usefulness of a systematic contingency program with chronic patients. The program has been quite successful in combating institutional behavior. Prior to the introduction of tokens most patients rarely left the ward. The ward and its surrounding grounds were dominated by sleeping patients. Little interest was shown in ward activities or parties. Before the tokens were introduced, the ward was cleaned and the clothing room operated by patients from "better" wards. During the experimental period the ward was cleaned and the clothing room operated by patients of this ward themselves. Now, no one stays on the ward without first earning tokens, and, in comparison to prior standards, the ward could be considered "jumping."

Over 90% of the patients have meaningfully participated in the program. All patients do take tokens, a few only infrequently. However, for about 10%, the tokens seem to be of little utility in effecting marked behavior change. With most patients, the changes in behavior have been quite dramatic; the changes in a few have been gradual and hardly noticeable. These instances of lack of responsiveness to the program seem to be evident in those patients who had previously been "catatonically" withdrawn and isolated. Although most of the patients in this category were favorably responsive to the program, what "failures" there were did come from this type of patient. Our program has been directed toward all patients; consequently, individual shaping has been limited. We feel that the results would be more dramatic if we could have dealt individually with the specific behavior of every patient. On the other hand, a total ward token program is needed both to maintain any behavioral gains and to bring about greater generality and permanence. Although it was not our initial objective to discharge patients, we are pleased that the general lessening of apathy has brought about a greater discharge rate. But, even more important, the greater discharge rate would point to the generalized effects of a total token economy.

The greater demands on the patient necessitated by dealing with future events and delaying immediate gratifications which were built into the program have been of value in lessening patients' isolation and withdrawal. The program's most notable contribution to patient life is the lessening of staff control and putting the burden of responsibility, and thus more self-respect, on the patient himself. In the administration of a ward, the program provides behavioral steps by which the staff can judge the patient's readiness to assume more responsibility and thus to leave on pass or be discharged.

The program thus far has demonstrated that a systematic procedure of applying contingent reinforcement via a token economy appears effective in modifying specific patient behaviors. However, the evidence in the literature based on research in mental hospitals indicates that many programs, different in theoretical orientation and design, appear to be successful for a period of time with hospitalized patients. The question which arises is whether the success in modifying behavior is a function of the specific procedures utilized in a given program or a function of the more general social influence process (Krasner, 1962). If it is the latter, whether it be termed "placebo effect" or "Hawthorne effect," then the specific procedures may be irrelevant. All that would matter is the interest, enthusiasm, attention, and hopeful expectancies of the staff. Advocates of behavior-modification procedures (of which the token economy is illustrative) argue that change in behavior is a function of the specific reinforcement procedures used. The study which most nearly involves the approach described in this paper is that of Ayllon and Azrin (1965) whose procedures were basic to the development of our own program. Their study was designed to demonstrate the relationship between contingency reinforcement and change in patient behavior. To do this they withdrew the tokens on a systematic basis for specific behaviors and, after a period of time, reinstated them. They concluded, based upon six specific experiments within the overall design, that

> the reinforcement procedure was effective in maintaining desired performance. In each experiment, the performance fell to a near-zero level when the established response-reinforcement relation was discontinued. On the other hand, reintroduction of the reinforcement procedure restored performance almost immediately and maintained it at a high level for as long as the reinforcement procedure was in effect [Ayllon & Azrin, 1965, p. 381].

They found that performance of desirable behaviors decreased when the response-reinforcement relation was disrupted by: delivering tokens independently of the response while still allowing exchange of tokens for the reinforcers; or by discontinuing the token system by providing continuing access to the reinforcers; or by discontinuing the delivery of tokens for a previously reinforced response while simultaneously providing tokens for a different, alternative response.

In the first year of our program we did not test the specific effects of the tokens by withdrawing them. Rather, we approached this problem in two ways. First, we incorporated within the base-line period of 9 months a 3-month period in which tokens were received on a noncontingent basis. During this period patients received tokens with concomitant attention, interest, and general social reinforcement. This resulted in slight but nonsignificant change in general ward behavior. The results of the experimental period were then compared with the base-line which included the nonspecific reinforcement. The results indicate that the more drastic changes in behavior were a function of the specific procedures involved. The other technique we used was to change the token value of certain specific activities. An increase in value (more tokens) was related to an increase in performance; return to the old value meant a decrement to the previous level of performance (see Fig. 32.1).

We should also point out that the situation in the hospital is such that the token economy did not mean that there were more of the "good things in life" available to these patients because they were in a special program. The patients in the program had access to these items, for example, extra food, beds, cigarettes, chairs, television, recreational activities, passes, before the program began, as had all patients in other wards, free of charge. Thus we cannot attribute change to the fact of more "good things" being available to these patients and not available to other patients.

Thus far, a contingent reinforcement program represented by a token economy has been successful in combating institutionalism, increasing initiative, responsibility, and social interaction, and in putting the control of patient behavior in the hands of the patient. The behavioral changes have generalized to other areas of performance. A token economy can be an important adjunct to any rehabilitation program for chronic or apathetic patients.

REFERENCES

Atthowe, J. M., Jr. *Ward* 113 *program: Incentives and costs—a manual for patients.* Palo Alto, Calif.: Veterans Administration Hospital, 1964.

Ayllon, T. Intensive treatment of psychotic behavior by stimulus satiation and food reinforcement. *Behavior Research and Therapy,* 1963, **1**, 53–61.

Ayllon, T., & Azrin, N. H. The measurement and reinforcement of behavior of psychotics. *Journal of the Experimental Analysis of Behavior,* 1965, **8**, 357–384.

Ayllon, T., & Houghton, E. Control of the behavior of schizophrenic patients by food. *Journal of the Experimental Analysis of Behavior,* 1962, **5**, 343–352.

Ayllon, T., & Michael, J. The psychiatric nurse as a behavioral engineer. *Journal of the Experimental Analysis of Behavior,* 1959, **2**, 323–334.

Fairweather, G. W., Simon, R., Gebhard, M. E., Weingarten, E., Holland, J. L., Sanders, R., Stone, G. B., & Reahl, J. E. Relative effectiveness of psychotherapeutic programs: A multi-criteria comparison of four programs for three different patient groups. *Psychological Monographs,* 1960, **74** (5, Whole No. 492).

Finney, B. C. A scale to measure interpersonal relationships in group psychotherapy. *Group Psychotherapy,* 1954, 52–66.

Kramer, M., Goldstein, H., Israel, R. H., & Johnson, N. A. Application of life table methodology to the study of mental hospital populations. *Psychiatric Research Reports,* 1956, **5**, 49–76.

Krasner, L. The therapist as a social reinforcement machine. In H. H. Strupp & L. Luborsky (Eds.), *Research in psychotherapy.* Washington, D. C.: American Psychological Association, 1962. Pp. 61–94.

Morgan, N. C., & Johnson, N. A. The chronic hospital patient. *American Journal of Psychiatry,* 1957, **113**, 824–830.

Odegard, O. Current studies of incidence and prevalence of hospitalized mental patients in Scandinavia. In P. H. Hoch & J. Zubin (Eds.), *Comparative epidemiology of the mental disorders.* New York: Grune & Stratton, 1961. Pp. 45–55.

Skinner, B. F. *The behavior of organisms.* New York: Appleton-Century-Crofts, 1938.

Skinner, B. F. *Science and human behavior.* New York: Macmillan, 1953.

33

The Process of the Basic Encounter Group*

CARL R. ROGERS

I would like to share with you some of my thinking and puzzlement regarding a potent new cultural development—the intensive group experience.[1] It has, in my judgment, significant implications for our society. It has come very suddenly over our cultural horizon, since in anything like its present form it is less than two decades old.

I should like briefly to describe the many different forms and different labels under which the intensive group experience has become a part of our modern life. It has involved different kinds of individuals, and is has spawned various theories to account for its effects.

As to labels, the intensive group experience has at times been called the *T-group* or *lab group*, "T" standing for training laboratory in group dynamics. It has been termed *sensitivity training* in human relationships. The experience has sometimes been called a *basic encounter group* or a *workshop*—a workshop in human relationships, in leadership, in counseling, in education, in research, in psychotherapy. In dealing with one particular type of person—the drug addict—it has been called a *synanon*.

The intensive group experience has functioned in various settings. It has operated in industries, in universities, in church groups, and in resort settings which provide a retreat from everyday life. It has functioned in various educational institutions and in penitentiaries.

An astonishing range of individuals have been involved in these intensive group experiences. There have been groups for presidents of large corporations. There have been groups for delinquent and predelinquent adolescents. There have been groups composed of college students and faculty members, of counselors and psychotherapists, of school dropouts, of married couples, of confirmed drug addicts, of criminals serving sentences, of nurses preparing for hospital service, and of educators, principals, and teachers.

The geographical spread attained by this rapidly expanding movement has reached in this country from Bethel, Maine (starting point of the National Training Laboratory movement), to Idyllwild, California. To my personal knowledge, such groups also exist in France, England, Holland, Japan, and Australia.

In their outward pattern these group experiences also show a great deal of diversity. There are T-groups and workshops which have extended over three to four weeks, meeting six to eight hours each day. There are some that have lasted only $2\frac{1}{2}$ days, crowding twenty or more hours of group sessions into this time. A recent innovation is the "marathon" weekend, which begins on Friday afternoon and ends on Sunday evening, with only a few hours out for sleep and snacks.

*From *Challenges of Humanistic Psychology* by J. F. T. Bugental. Copyright © 1967 by McGraw-Hill, Inc. Used by permission of McGraw-Hill Book Company, and Dr., Rogers.

[1]In the preparation of this paper I am deeply indebted to two people, experienced in work with groups, for their help: Jacques Hochmann, M.D., psychiatrist of Lyon, France, who has been working at WBSI on a U.S.P.H.S. International Post-doctoral Fellowship, and Ann Dreyfuss, M.A., my research assistant. I am grateful for their ideas, for their patient analysis of recorded group sessions, and for the opportunity to interact with two original and inquiring minds.

As to the conceptual underpinnings of this whole movement, one may almost select the theoretical flavor he prefers. Lewinian and client-centered theories have been most prominent, but gestalt therapy and various brands of psychoanalysis have all played contributing parts. The experience within the group may focus on specific training in human relations skills. It may be closely similar to group therapy, with much exploration of past experience and the dynamics of personal development. It may focus on creative expression through painting or expressive movement. It may be focused primarily upon a basic encounter and relationship between individuals.

Simply to describe the diversity which exists in this field raises very properly the question of why these various developments should be considered to belong together. Are there any threads of commonality which pervade all these widely divergent activities? To me it seems that they do belong together and can all be classed as focusing on the intensive group experience. They all have certain similar external characteristics. The group in almost every case is small (from eight to eighteen members), is relatively unstructured, and chooses its own goals and personal directions. The group experience usually, though not always, includes some cognitive input, some content material which is presented to the group. In almost all instances the leader's responsibility is primarily the facilitation of the expression of both feelings and thoughts on the part of the group members. Both in the leader and in the group members there is some focus on the process and the dynamics of the immediate personal interaction. These are, I think, some of the identifying characteristics which are rather easily recognized.

There are also certain practical hypotheses which tend to be held in common by all these groups. My own summary of these would be as follows: In an intensive group, with much freedom and little structure, the individual will gradually feel safe enough to drop some of his defenses and facades; he will relate more directly on a feeling basis (come into a basic encounter) with other members of the group; he will come to understand himself and his relationship to others more accurately; he will change in his personal attitudes and behavior; and he will subsequently relate more effectively to others in his everyday life situation. There are other hypotheses related more to the group than to the individual. One is that in this situation of minimal structure, the group will move from confusions, fractionation, and discontinuity to a climate of greater trust and coherence. These are some of the characteristics and hypotheses which, in my judgment, bind together this enormous cluster of activities which I wish to talk about as constituting the intensive group experience.

As for myself, I have been gradually moving into this field for the last twenty years. In experimenting with what I call *student-centered teaching*, involving the free expression of personal feelings, I came to recognize not only the cognitive learnings but also some of the personal changes which occurred. In brief intensive training courses for counselors for the Veterans Administration in 1946, during the postwar period, I and my staff focused more directly on providing an intensive group experience because of its impact in producing significant learning. In 1950, I served as leader of an intensive, full-time, one-week workshop, a postdoctoral training seminar in psychotherapy for the American Psychological Association. The impact of those six days was so great that for more than a dozen years afterward, I kept hearing from members of the group about the meaning it had had for them. Since that time I have been involved in more than forty ventures of what I would like to term—using the label most congenial to me—*basic encounter groups*. Most of these have involved for many of the members experiences of great intensity and considerable personal change. With two individuals, however, in these many groups, the experience contributed, I believe, to a psychotic break. A few other individuals have found the experience more unhelpful than helpful. So I have come to have a profound respect for the constructive potency of such group experiences and also a real concern over the fact that sometimes and in some ways this experience may do damage to individuals.

THE GROUP PROCESS

It is a matter of great interest to me to try to understand what appear to be common elements in the group process as I have come dimly to sense these. I am using this opportunity to think about this problem, not because I feel I have any final theory to give, but because I would like to formulate, as clearly as I am able, the elements which I can perceive at the present time. In doing so I am drawing upon my own experience, upon the experiences of others with whom I have worked, upon the written material in this field, upon the written reactions of many individuals who have participated in such groups, and to some extent upon the recordings of such group sessions, which we are only beginning to tap and analyze. I am sure that (though I have tried to draw on the experience of others) any formulation I make at the present time is unduly influenced by my own experience in groups and thus is lacking in the generality I wish it might have.

As I consider the terribly complex interactions which arise during twenty, forty, sixty, or more hours of intensive sessions, I believe that I see some threads which weave in and out of the pattern. Some of these trends or tendencies are likely to appear early and some later in the group sessions, but there is no clear-cut sequence in which one ends and another begins. The interaction is best thought of, I believe, as a varied tapestry, differing from group to group, yet with certain kinds of trends evident in most of these intensive encounters and with certain patterns tending to precede and others to follow. Here are some of the process patterns which I see developing, briefly described in simple terms, illustrated from tape recordings and personal reports, and presented in roughly sequential order. I am not aiming at a high-level theory of group process but rather at a naturalistic observation out of which, I hope, true theory can be built.[2]

Milling Around

As the leader or facilitator makes clear at the outset that this is a group with unusual freedom, that it is not one for which he will take directional responsibility, there tends to develop a period of initial confusion, awkward silence, polite surface interaction, "cocktail-party talk," frustration, and great lack of continuity. The individuals come face-to-face with the fact that "there is no structure here except what we provide. We do not know our purposes; we do not even know one another, and we are committed to remain together over a considerable period of time." In this situation, confusion and frustration are natural. Particularly striking to the observer is the lack of continuity between personal expressions. Individual A will present some proposal or concern, clearly looking for a response from the

---

[2]Jack and Lorraine Gibb have long been working on an analysis of trust development as the essential theory of group process. Others who have contributed significantly to the theory of group process are Chris Argyris, Kenneth Benne, Warren Bennis, Dorwin Cartwright, Matthew Miles, and Robert Blake. Samples of the thinking of all these and others may be found in three recent books: Bradford, Gibb, & Benne (1964); Bennis, Benne, & Chin (1961); and Bennis, Schein, Berlew, & Steele (1964). Thus, there are many promising leads for theory construction involving a considerable degree of abstraction. This chapter has a more elementary aim—a naturalistic descriptive account of the process.

group. Individual B has obviously been waiting for his turn and starts off on some completely different tangent as though he had never heard A. One member makes a simple suggestion such as, "I think we should introduce ourselves," and this may lead to several hours of highly involved discussion in which the underlying issues appear to be, "Who is the leader?" "Who is responsible for us?" "Who is a member of the group?" "What is the purpose of the group?"

Resistance to Personal Expression or Exploration

During the milling period, some individuals are likely to reveal some rather personal attitudes. This tends to foster a very ambivalent reaction among other members of the group. One member, writing of his experience, says:

> There is a self which I present to the world and another one which I know more intimately. With others I try to appear able, knowing, unruffled, problem-free. To substantiate this image I will act in a way which at the time or later seems false or artificial or "not the real me." Or I will keep to myself thoughts which if expressed would reveal an imperfect me.
>
> My inner self, by contrast with the image I present to the world, is characterized by many doubts. The worth I attach to this inner self is subject to much fluctuation and is very dependent on how others are reacting to me. At times this private self can feel worthless.

It is the public self which members tend to reveal to one another, and only gradually, fearfully, and ambivalently do they take steps to reveal something of their inner world.

Early in one intensive workshop, the members were asked to write anonymously a statement of some feeling or feelings which they had which they were not willing to tell in the group. One man wrote:

> I don't relate easily to people. I have an almost impenetrable facade. Nothing gets in to hurt me, but nothing gets out. I have repressed so many emotions that I am close to emotional sterility. This situation doesn't make me happy, but I don't know what to do about it.

This individual is clearly living inside a private dungeon, but he does not even dare, except in this disguised fashion, to send out a call for help.

In a recent workshop when one man started to express the concern he felt about an impasse he was experiencing with his wife, another member stopped him, saying essentially:

> Are you sure you want to go on with this, or are you being seduced by the group into going further than you want to go? How do you know the group can be trusted? How will you feel about it when you go home and tell your wife what you have revealed, or when you decide to keep it from her? It just isn't safe to go further.

It seemed quite clear that in his warning, this second member was also expressing his own fear of revealing *himself* and *his* lack of trust in the group.

Description of Past Feelings

In spite of ambivalence about the trustworthiness of the group and the risk of exposing oneself, expression of feelings does begin to assume a larger proportion of the discussion. The executive tells how frustrated he feels by certain situations in his industry, or the housewife relates problems she has experienced with her children. A tape-recorded exchange involving a Roman Catholic nun occurs early in a one-week workshop, when the discussion has turned to a rather intellectualized consideration of anger:

> **Bill:**   What happens when you get mad, Sister, or don't you?
> **Sister:**   Yes, I do—yes I do. And I find when I get mad, I, I almost get, well, the kind of

person that antagonizes me is the person who seems so unfeeling toward people—now I take our dean as a person in point because she is a very aggressive woman and has certain ideas about what the various rules in a college should be; and this woman can just send me into high "G"; in an angry mood. *I mean this.* But then I find, I . . . .

Facil.:[3]   But what, what do you do?

Sister: I find that when I'm in a situation like this, that I strike out in a very sharp, uh, *tone*, or else I just refuse to respond—"All right, this happens to be her way"—I don't think I've ever gone into a tantrum.

Joe: You just withdraw—no use to fight it.

Facil.:   You say you use a sharp tone. To *her,* or to other people you're dealing with?

Sister: Oh, no. To *her.*

This is a typical example of a *description* of feelings which are obviously current in her in a sense but which she is placing in the past and which she describes as being outside the group in time and place. It is an example of feelings existing "there and then."

Expression of Negative Feelings

Curiously enough, the first expression of genuinely significant "here-and-now" feeling is apt to come out in negative attitudes toward other group members or toward the group leader. In one group in which members introduced themselves at some length, one woman refused, saying that she preferred to be known for what she was in the group and not in terms of her status outside. Very shortly after this, one of the men in the group attacked her vigorously and angrily for this stand, accusing her of failing to cooperate, of keeping herself aloof from the group, and so forth. It was the first *personal current feeling* which had been brought into the open in the group.

Frequently the leader is attacked for his failure to give proper guidance to the group. One vivid example of this comes from a recorded account of an early session with a group of delinquents, where one member shouts at the leader (Gordon, 1955, p. 214):

> You will be licked if you don't control us right at the start. You have to keep order here because you are older than us. That's what a teacher is supposed to do. If he doesn't do it we will cause a lot of trouble and won't get anything done. [Then, referring to two boys in the group who were scuffling, he continues.] Throw 'em out, throw 'em out! You've just *got* to make us behave!

An adult expresses his disgust at the people who talk too much, but points his irritation at the leader (Gordon, 1955, p. 210):

> It is just that I don't understand why someone doesn't shut them up. I would have taken Gerald and shoved him out the window. I'm an authoritarian. I would have told him he was talking too much and he had to leave the room. I think the group discussion ought to be led by a person who simply will not recognize these people after they have interrupted about eight times.

Why are negatively toned expressions the first current feelings to be expressed? Some speculative answers might be the following: This is one of the best ways to test the freedom and trustworthiness of the group. "Is it really a place where I can be and express myself positively and negatively? Is this really a safe place, or will I be punished?" Another quite different reason is that deeply positive feelings are much more difficult and dangerous to express than negative ones. "If I say, 'I love you,' I am vulnerable and open to the most awful rejection. If I say, 'I hate you,' I am at best liable to attack, against which I can

---

[3]The term "facilitator" will be used throughout this paper, although sometimes he is referred to as "leader" or "trainer."

defend." Whatever the reasons, such negatively toned feelings tend to be the first here-and-now material to appear.

Expression and Exploration of Personally Meaningful Material

It may seem puzzling that following such negative experiences as the initial confusion, the resistance to personal expression, the focus on outside events, and the voicing of critical or angry feelings, the event most likely to occur next is for an individual to reveal himself to the group in a significant way. The reason for this no doubt is that the individual member has come to realize that this is in part *his group*. He can help to make of it what he wishes. He has also experienced the fact that negative feelings have been expressed and have usually been accepted or assimilated without any catastrophic results. He realizes there is freedom here, albeit a risky freedom. A climate of trust (Gibb, 1964, Chapter 10) is beginning to develop. So he begins to take the chance and the gamble of letting the group know some deeper facet of himself. One man tells of the trap in which he finds himself, feeling that communication between himself and his wife is hopeless. A priest tells of the anger which he has bottled up because of unreasonable treatment by one of his superiors. What should he have done? What might he do now? A scientist at the head of a large research department finds the courage to speak of his painful isolation, to tell the group that he has never had a single friend in his life. By the time he finishes telling of his situation, he is letting loose some of the tears of sorrow for himself which I am sure he has held in for many years. A psychiatrist tells of the guilt he feels because of the suicide of one of his patients. A woman of forty tells of her absolute inability to free herself from the grip of her controlling mother. A process which one workshop member has called a "journey to the center of self," often a very painful process, has begun.

Such exploration is not always an easy process, nor is the whole group always receptive to such self-revelation. In a group of institutionalized adolescents, all of whom had been in difficulty of one sort or another, one boy revealed an important fact about himself and immediately received both acceptance and sharp nonacceptance from members of the group:

> **George:** This is the thing. I've got too many problems at home—uhm, I think some of you know why I'm here, what I was charged with.
> **Mary:** I don't.
> **Facil.:** Do you want to tell us?
> **George:** Well, uh, it's sort of embarrassing.
> **Carol:** Come on, it won't be so bad.
> **George:** Well, I raped my sister. That's the only problem I have at home, and I've overcome that, I think. (*Rather long pause.*)
> **Freda:** Oooh, that's *weird*!
> **Mary:** People have problems, Freda, I mean ya know. . .
> **Freda:** Yeah, I know, but *yeOUW*!!!
> **Facil.:** (*to Freda*): You know about these problems, but they still are weird to you.
> **George:** You see what I mean; it's embarrassing to talk about it.
> **Mary:** Yeah, but it's O.K.
> **George:** It *hurts* to talk about it, but I know I've got to so I won't be guilt-ridden for the rest of my life.

Clearly Freda is completely shutting him out psychologically, while Mary in particular is showing a deep acceptance.

The Expression of Immediate Interpersonal Feelings in the Group

Entering into the process sometimes earlier, sometimes later, is the explicit bringing into the open of the feelings experienced in the immediate moment by one member about another. These are sometimes positive and sometimes negative. Examples would be: "I feel threatened by your silence." "You remind me of my mother, with whom I had a tough time." "I took an instant dislike to you the first moment I saw you." "To me you're like a breath of fresh air in the group." "I like your warmth and your smile." "I dislike you more every time you speak up." Each of these attitudes can be, and usually is, explored in the increasing climate of trust.

The Development of a Healing Capacity in the Group

One of the most fascinating aspects of any intensive group experience is the manner in which a number of the group members show a natural and spontaneous capacity for dealing in a helpful, facilitative, and therapeutic fashion with the pain and suffering of others. As one rather extreme example of this, I think of a man in charge of maintenance in a large plant who was one of the low-status members of an industrial executive group. As he informed us, he had not been "contaminated by education." In the initial phases the group tended to look down on him. As members delved more deeply into themselves and began to express their own attitudes more fully, this man came forth as, without doubt, the most sensitive member of the group. He knew intuitively how to be understanding and acceptant. He was alert to things which had not yet been expressed but which were just below the surface. When the rest of us were paying attention to a member who was speaking, he would frequently spot another individual who was suffering silently and in need of help. He had a deeply perceptive and facilitating attitude. This kind of ability shows up so commonly in groups that it has led me to feel that the ability to be healing or therapeutic is far more common in human life than we might suppose. Often it needs only the permission granted by a freely flowing group experience to become evident.

In a characteristic instance, the leader and several group members were trying to be of help to Joe, who was telling of the almost complete lack of communication between himself and his wife. In varied ways members endeavored to give help. John kept putting before Joe the feelings Joe's wife was almost certainly experiencing. The facilitator kept challenging Joe's facade of "carefulness." Marie tried to help him discover what he was feeling at the moment. Fred showed him the choice he had of alternative behaviors. All this was clearly done in a spirit of caring, as is even more evident in the recording itself. No miracles were achieved, but toward the end Joe did come to the realization that the only thing that might help would be to express his real feelings to his wife.

Self-acceptance and the Beginning of Change

Many people feel that self-acceptance must stand in the way of change. Actually, in these group experiences, as in psychotherapy, it is the *beginning* of change. Some examples of the kind of attitudes expressed would be these: "I *am* a dominating person who likes to control others. I do want to mold these individuals into the proper shape." Another person says, "I really have a hurt and overburdened little boy inside of me who feels very sorry for himself. I *am* that little boy, in addition to being a competent and responsible manager."

I think of one governmental executive in a group in which I participated, a man with high responsibility and excellent technical training as an engineer. At the first meeting of the group he impressed me, and I think others, as being cold, aloof, somewhat bitter, resentful, and cynical. When he spoke of how he ran his office it appeared that he administered it "by the book," without any warmth or human feeling entering in. In one of the early sessions, when he spoke of his wife, a group member asked him, "Do you love your wife?" He paused for a long time, and the questioner said, "OK, that's answer enough." The executive said, "No. Wait a minute. The reason I didn't respond was that I was wondering if I ever loved anyone. I don't think I *ever* really *loved* anyone." It seemed quite dramatically clear to those of us in the group that he had come to accept himself as an unloving person.

A few days later he listened with great intensity as one member of the group expressed profound personal feelings of isolation, loneliness, and pain, revealing the extent to which he had been living behind a mask, a facade. The next morning the engineer said, "Last night I thought and thought about what Bill told us. I even wept quite a bit by myself. I can't remember how long it has been since I have cried, and I really *felt* something. I think perhaps what I felt was love."

It is not surprising that before the week was over, he had thought through new ways of handling his growing son, on whom he had been placing extremely rigorous demands. He had also begun genuinely to appreciate the love which his wife had extended to him and which he now felt he could in some measure reciprocate.

In another group one man kept a diary of his reactions. Here is his account of an experience in which he came really to accept his almost abject desire for love, a self-acceptance which marked the beginning of a very significant experience of change. He says (Hall, 1965):

> During the break between the third and fourth sessions, I felt very droopy and tired. I had it in mind to take a nap, but instead I was almost compulsively going around to people starting a conversation. I had a begging kind of a feeling, like a very cowed little puppy hoping that he'll be patted but half afraid he'll be kicked. Finally, back in my room I lay down and began to know that I was sad. Several times I found myself wishing my roommate would come in and talk to me. Or, whenever someone walked by the door, I would come to attention inside, the way a dog pricks up his ears; and I would feel an immediate wish for that person to come in and talk to me. I realized my raw wish to receive kindness.

Another recorded excerpt, from an adolescent group, shows a combination of self-acceptance and self-exploration. Art had been talking about his "shell," and here he is beginning to work with the problem of accepting himself, and also the facade he ordinarily exhibits:

> **Art:** I'm so darn used to living with the shell; it doesn't even bother me. I don't even know the real me. I think I've uh, well, I've pushed the shell more away here. When I'm out of my shell—only twice—once just a few minutes ago—I'm really me, I guess. But then I just sort of pull in the [latch] cord after me when I'm in my shell, and that's almost all the time. And I leave the [false] front standing outside when I'm back in the shell.
>
> **Facil.:** And nobody's back in there with you?
>
> **Art** (*crying*): Nobody else is in there with me, just me. I just pull everything into the shell and roll the shell up and shove it in my pocket. I take the shell, and the real me, and put it in my pocket where it's safe. I guess that's really the way I do it—I go into my shell and turn off the real world. And here: that's what I want to do here in this group, ya know, come out of my shell and actually throw it away.
>
> **Lois:** You're making progress already. At least you can talk about it.
>
> **Facil.:** Yeah. The thing that's going to be hardest is to stay out of the shell.
>
> **Art** (*still crying*): Well, yeah, if I can keep talking about it, I can come out and stay out, but I'm gonna have to, ya know, protect me. It hurts; it's actually hurting to talk about it.

Still another person reporting shortly after his workshop experience said, "I came away from the workshop feeling much more deeply that 'It is all right to be me with all my strengths and weaknesses.' My wife has told me that I appear to be more authentic, more real, more genuine."

This feeling of greater realness and authenticity is a very common experience. It would appear that the individual is learning to accept and to *be* himself, and this is laying the foundation for change. He is closer to his own feelings, and hence they are no longer so rigidly organized and are more open to change.

The Cracking of Facades

As the sessions continue, so many things tend to occur together that it is difficult to know which to describe first. It should again be stressed that these different threads and stages interweave and overlap. One of these threads is the increasing impatience with defenses. As time goes on, the group finds it unbearable that any member should live behind a mask or a front. The polite words, the intellectual understanding of one another and of relationships, the smooth coin of tact and cover-up—amply satisfactory for interactions outside— are just not good enough. The expression of self by some members of the group has made it very clear that a deeper and more basic encounter is *possible*, and the group appears to strive, intuitively and unconsciously, toward this goal. Gently at times, almost savagely at others, the group *demands* that the individual be himself, that his current feelings not be hidden, that he remove the mask of ordinary social intercourse. In one group there was a highly intelligent and quite academic man who had been rather perceptive in his understanding of others but who had not revealed himself at all. The attitude of the group was finally expressed sharply by one member when he said, "Come out from behind that lectern, Doc. Stop giving us speeches. Take off your dark glasses. We want to know *you.*"

In Synanon, the fascinating group so successfully involved in making persons out of drug addicts, this ripping away of facades is often very drastic. An excerpt from one of the "synanons," or group sessions, makes this clear (Casriel, 1963, p. 81):

> **Joe** (*speaking to Gina*): I wonder when you're going to stop sounding so good in synanons. Every synanon that I'm in with you, someone asks you a question, and you've got a beautiful book written. All made out about what went down and how you were wrong and how you realized you were wrong and all that kind of bullshit. When are you going to stop doing that? How do you feel about Art?
>
> **Gina:** I have nothing against Art.
>
> **Will:** You're a nut. Art hasn't got any damn sense. He's been in there, yelling at you and Moe, and you've got everything so cool.
>
> **Gina:** No, I feel he's very insecure in a lot of ways but that has nothing to do with me....
>
> **Joe:** You act like you're so goddamn understanding.
>
> **Gina:** I was *told* to act as if I understand.
>
> **Joe:** Well, you're in a synanon now. You're not supposed to be acting like you're such a god-damn healthy person. Are you so *well*?
>
> **Gina:** No.
>
> **Joe:** Well why the hell don't you quit acting as if you were.

If I am indicating that the group at times is quite violent in tearing down a facade or a defense, this would be accurate. On the other hand, it can also be sensitive and gentle. The man who was accused of hiding behind a lectern was deeply hurt by this attack, and over the lunch hour looked very troubled, as though he might break into tears at any moment. When the group reconvened, the members sensed this and treated him very gently, enabling him to tell us his own tragic personal story, which accounted for his aloofness and his intellectual and academic approach to life.

The Individual Receives Feedback

In the process of this freely expressive interaction, the individual rapidly acquires a great deal of data as to how he appears to others. The "hail-fellow-well-met" discovers that others resent his exaggerated friendliness. The executive who weighs his words carefully and speaks with heavy precision may find that others regard him as stuffy. A woman who shows a somewhat excessive desire to be of help to others is told in no uncertain terms that some group members do not want her for a mother. All this can be decidedly upsetting, but as long as these various bits of information are fed back in the context of caring which is developing in the group, they seem highly constructive.

Feedback can at times be very warm and positive, as the following recorded excerpt indicates:

> **Leo** (*very softly and gently*):   I've been struck with this ever since she talked about her waking in the night, that she has a very delicate sensitivity. (*Turning to Mary and speaking almost caressingly.*) And somehow I perceive—even looking at you or in your eyes—a very—almost like a gentle touch and from this gentle touch you can tell many—things—you sense in—this manner.
> **Fred:**   Leo, when you said that, that she has this kind of delicate sensitivity, I just felt, *Lord yes*! Look at her eyes.
> **Leo:**   M-hm.

A much more extended instance of negative and positive feedback, triggering a significant new experience of self-understanding and encounter with the group, is taken from the diary of the young man mentioned before. He had been telling the group that he had no feeling for them, and felt they had no feeling for him (Hall, 1965):

> Then, a girl lost patience with me and said she didn't feel she could give any more. She said I looked like a bottomless well, and she wondered how many times I had to be told that I *was* cared for. By this time I was feeling panicky, and I was saying to myself, "My God, can it be true that I can't be satisfied and that I'm somehow compelled to pester people for attention until I drive them away?"
>
> At this point while I was really worried, a nun in the group spoke up. She said that I had not alienated her with some negative things I had said to her. She said she liked me, and she couldn't understand why I couldn't see that. She said she felt concerned for me and wanted to help me. With that, something began to really dawn on me, and I voiced it somewhat like the following. "You mean you are all sitting there, feeling for me what I say I want you to feel, and that somewhere down inside me I'm stopping it from touching me?" I relaxed appreciably and began really to wonder why I had shut their caring out so much. I couldn't find the answer, and one woman said: "It looks like you are trying to stay continuously as deep in your feelings as you were this afternoon. It would make sense to me for you to draw back and assimilate it. Maybe if you don't push so hard, you can rest awhile and then move back into your feelings more naturally."
>
> Her making the last suggestion really took effect. I saw the sense in it, and almost immediately I settled back very relaxed with something of a feeling of a bright, warm day dawning inside me. In addition to taking the pressure off myself, however, I was for the first time really warmed by the friendly feelings which I felt they had for me. It is difficult to say why I felt liked only just then, but, as opposed to the earlier sessions, I really *believed* they cared for me. I never have fully understood why I stood their affection off for so long, but at that point I almost abruptly began to trust that they did care. The measure of the effectiveness of this change lies in what I said next. I said, "Well, that really takes care of me. I'm really ready to listen to someone else now." I *meant* that, too.

Confrontation

There are times when the term "feedback" is far too mild to describe the interactions which take place, when it is better said that one individual *confronts* another, directly "leveling" with him. Such confrontations can be positive, but frequently they are decidedly negative, as the following example will make abundantly clear. In one of the last sessions of a group, Alice had made some quite vulgar and contemptuous remarks to John, who was entering religious work. The next morning, Norma, who had been a very quiet person in the group, took the floor:

> Norma (*loud sigh*): Well, I don't have *any* respect for you, Alice. *None!* (*Pause.*) There's about a hundred things going through my mind I want to say to you, and by God I hope I get through 'em all! First of all, if you wanted us to respect you, then why couldn't you respect *John's* feelings last night? Why have you been on him today? Hmm? Last night—couldn't you— couldn't you accept—*couldn't you* comprehend in any way at all that—that *he felt* his unworthiness in the service of God? Couldn't you accept this, or did you have to dig into it today to find something *else there*? And his respect for womanhood—he *loves* women—yes, he does, because he's a real person, but you—you're not a real woman—to me—and thank God, you're not my mother! ! ! ! I want to come over and beat the hell out of you ! ! ! I want to slap you across the mouth so hard and—oh, and you're so, you're many years above me—and I respect age, and I respect people who are older than me, *but I don't respect you, Alice. At all!* And I was so *hurt* and *confused* because you were making someone else feel *hurt* and *confused....*

It may relieve the reader to know that these two women came to accept each other, not completely, but much more understandingly, before the end of the session. But this *was* a confrontation!

The Helping Relationship Outside the Group Sessions

No account of the group process would, in my experience, be adequate if it did not make mention of the many ways in which group members are of assistance to one another. Not infrequently, one member of a group will spend hours listening and talking to another member who is undergoing a painful new perception of himself. Sometimes it is merely the offering of help which is therapeutic. I think of one man who was going through a very depressed period after having told us of the many tragedies in his life. He seemed quite clearly, from his remarks, to be contemplating suicide. I jotted down my room number (we were staying at a hotel) and told him to put it in his pocket and to call me anytime of day or night if he felt that it would help. He never called, but six months after the workshop was over he wrote to me telling how much that act had meant to him and that he still had the slip of paper to remind him of it.

Let me give an example of the healing effect of the attitudes of group members both outside and inside the group meetings. This is taken from a letter written by a workshop member to the group one month after the group sessions. He speaks of the difficulties and depressing circumstances he has encountered during that month and adds:

> I have come to the conclusion that my experiences with you have profoundly affected me. I am truly grateful. This is different than personal therapy. None of you *had* to care about me. None of you had to seek me out and let me know of things you thought would help me. None of you had to let me know I was of help to you. Yet you did, and as a result it has far more meaning than anything I have so far experienced. When I feel the need to hold back and not live spontaneously, for whatever reasons, I remember that twelve persons, just like those before me now, said to let

go and be congruent, to be myself, and, of all unbelievable things, they even loved me more for it. This has given me the *courage* to come out of myself many times since then. Often it seems my very doing of this helps the others to experience similar freedom.

The Basic Encounter

Running through some of the trends I have just been describing is the fact that individuals come into much closer and more direct contact with one another than is customary in ordinary life. This appears to be one of the most central, intense, and change-producing aspects of such a group experience. To illustrate what I mean, I would like to draw an example from a recent workshop group. A man tells, through his tears, of the very tragic loss of his child, a grief which he is experiencing *fully*, for the first time, not holding back his feelings in any way. Another says to him, also with tears in his eyes, "I've never felt so close to another human being. I've never before felt a real physical hurt in me from the pain of another. I feel *completely* with you." This is a basic encounter.

Such I-Thou relationships (to use Buber's term) occur with some frequency in these group sessions and nearly always bring a moistness to the eyes of the participants.

One member, trying to sort out his experiences immediately after a workshop, speaks of the "commitment to relationship" which often developed on the part of two individuals, not necessarily individuals who had liked each other initially. He goes on to say:

> The incredible fact experienced over and over by members of the group was that when a negative feeling was fully expressed to another, the relationship grew and the negative feeling was replaced by a deep acceptance for the other.... Thus real change seemed to occur when feelings were experienced and expressed in the context of the relationship. "I can't *stand* the way you talk!" turned into a real understanding and affection for you the *way* you talk.

This statement seems to capture some of the more complex meanings of the term "basic encounter."

The Expression of Positive Feelings and Closeness

As indicated in the last section, an inevitable part of the group process seems to be that when feelings are expressed and can be accepted in a relationship, a great deal of closeness and positive feelings results. Thus as the sessions proceed, there is an increasing feeling of warmth and group spirit and trust built, not out of positive attitude only, but out of a realness which includes both positive and negative feeling. One member tried to capture this in writing very shortly after the workshop by saying that if he were trying to sum it up, "... it would have to do with what I call confirmation—a kind of confirmation of myself, of the uniqueness and universal qualities of men, a confirmation that when we can be human together something positive can emerge."

A particularly poignant expression of these positive attitudes was shown in the group where Norma confronted Alice with her bitterly angry feelings. Joan, the facilitator, was deeply upset and began to weep. The positive and healing attitudes of the group, for their own *leader*, are an unusual example of the closeness and personal quality of the relationships.

> **Joan** (*crying*): I somehow feel that it's so *damned* easy for me to—to put myself *inside* of another person and I just guess I can feel that—for John and Alice and for you, Norma.
> **Alice:** And it's *you* that's hurt.
> **Joan:** Maybe I am taking some of that hurt. I guess I am. (*crying*.)

Alice: That's a wonderful gift. I wish I had it.

Joan: You have a lot of it.

Peter: In a way you bear the—I guess in a special way, because you're the—facilitator, ah, you've probably borne, ah, an extra heavy burden for all of us—and the burden that you, perhaps, you bear the heaviest is—we ask you—we ask one another; we grope to try to accept one another as we are, and —for each of us in various ways I guess we reach things and we say, *please* accept me. . . .

Some may be very critical of a "leader" so involved and so sensitive that she weeps at the tensions in the group which she has taken into herself. For me, it is simply another evidence that when people are real with each other, they have an astonishing ability to heal a person with a real and understanding love, whether that person is "participant" or "leader."

Behavior Changes in the Group

It would seem from observation that many changes in behavior occur in the group itself. Gestures change. The tone of voice changes, becoming sometimes stronger, sometimes softer, usually more spontaneous, less artificial, more feelingful. Individuals show an astonishing amount of thoughtfulness and helpfulness toward one another.

Our major concern, however, is with the behavior changes which occur following the group experience. It is this which constitutes the most significant question and on which we need much more study and research. One person gives a catalog of the changes which he sees in himself which may seem too "pat" but which is echoed in many other statements:

I am more open, spontaneous. I express myself more freely. I am more sympathetic, emphatic, and tolerant. I am more confident. I am more religious in my own way. My relations with my family, friends, and coworkers are more honest, and I express my likes and dislikes and true feelings more openly. I admit ignorance more readily. I am more cheerful. I want to help others more.

Another says:

Since the workshop there has been a new relationship with my parents. It has been trying and hard. However, I have found a greater freedom in talking with them, especially my father. Steps have been made toward being closer to my mother than I have ever been in the last five years.

Another says:

It helped clarify my feelings about my work, gave me more enthusiasm for it, and made me more honest and cheerful with my coworkers and also more open when I was hostile. It made my relationship with my wife more open, deeper. We felt freer to talk about anything, and we felt confident that anything we talked about we could work through.

Sometimes the changes which are described are very subtle. "The primary change is the more positive view of my ability to allow myself to *hear*, and to become involved with someone else's 'silent scream.'"

At the risk of making the outcomes sound too good, I will add one more statement written shortly after a workshop by a mother. She says:

The immediate impact on my children was of interest to both me and my husband. I feel that having been so accepted and loved by a group of strangers was so supportive that when I returned home my love for the people closest to me was much more spontaneous. Also, the practice I had in accepting and loving others during the workshop was evident in my relationships with my close friends.

DISADVANTAGES AND RISKS

Thus far one might think that every aspect of the group process was positive. As far as the evidence at hand indicates, it appears that it nearly always is a positive process for a majority of the participants. There are, nevertheless, failures which result. Let me try to describe briefly some of the negative aspects of the group process as they sometimes occur.

The most obvious deficiency of the intensive group experience is that frequently the behavior changes, if any, which occur, are not lasting. This is often recognized by the participants. One says, "I wish I had the ability to hold permanently the 'openness' I left the conference with." Another says, "I experienced a lot of acceptance, warmth, and love at the workshop. I find it hard to carry the ability to share this in the same way with people outside the workshop. I find it easier to slip back into my old unemotional role than to do the work necessary to open relationships."

Sometimes group members experience this phenomenon of "relapse" quite philosophically:

> The group experience is not a way of life but a reference point. My images of our group, even though I am unsure of some of their meanings, give me a comforting and useful perspective on my normal routine. They are like a mountain which I have climbed and enjoyed and to which I hope occasionally to return.

Some Data on Outcomes

What is the extent of this "slippage"? In the past year, I have administered follow-up questionaires to 481 individuals who have been in groups I have organized or conducted. The information has been obtained from two to twelve months following the group experience, but the greatest number were followed up after a three- to six-month period[4]. Of these individuals, two (i.e. less than one-half of 1 percent) felt it had changed their behavior in ways they did not like. Fourteen percent felt the experience had made no perceptible change in their behavior. Another 14 percent felt that it had changed their behavior but that this change had disappeared or left only a small residual positive effect. Fifty-seven percent felt it had made a continuing positive difference in their behavior, a few feeling that it had made some negative changes along with the positive.

A second potential risk involved in the intensive group experience and one which is often mentioned in public discussion is the risk that the individual may become deeply involved in revealing himself and then be left with problems which are not worked through. There have been a number of reports of people who have felt, following an intensive group experience, that they must go to a therapist to work through the feelings which were opened up in the intensive experience of the workshop and which were left unresolved. It is obvious that, without knowing more about each individual situation, it is difficult to say whether this was a negative outcome or a partially or entirely positive one. There are also very occasional accounts, and I can testify to two in my own experience, where an individual has had a psychotic episode during or immediately following an intensive group experience. On the other side of the picture is the fact that individuals have also lived through what were clearly psychotic episodes, and lived through them very constructively, in the context of a basic encounter group. My own tentative clinical judgment would be that the more positively the group process has been proceeding, the less likely it is that any

---

[4]The 481 respondents constituted 82 percent of those to whom the questionnaire had been sent.

individual would be psychologically damaged through membership in the group. It is obvious, however, that this is a serious issue and that much more needs to be known.

Some of the tension which exists in workshop members as a result of this potential for damage was very well described by one member when he said, "I feel the workshop had some very precious moments for me when I felt very close indeed to particular persons. It had some frightening moments when its potency was very evident and I realized a particular person might be deeply hurt or greatly helped but I could not predict which."

Out of the 481 participants followed up by questionnaires, two felt that the overall impact of their intensive group experience was "mostly damaging." Six more said that it had been "more unhelpful than helpful." Twenty-one, or 4 percent, stated that it had been "mostly frustrating, annoying, or confusing." Three and one-half percent said that it had been neutral in its impact. Nineteen percent checked that it had been "more helpful than unhelpful," indicating some degree of ambivalence. But 30 percent saw it as "constructive in its results," and 45 percent checked it as a "deeply meaningful, positive experience."[5] Thus for three-fourths of the group, it was *very* helpful. These figures should help to set the problem in perspective. It is obviously a very serious matter if an intensive group experience is psychologically damaging to *anyone*. It seems clear, however, that such damage occurs only rarely, if we are to judge by the reaction of the participants.

Other Hazards of the Group Experience

There is another risk or deficiency in the basic encounter group. Until very recent years it has been unusual for a workshop to include both husband and wife. This can be a real problem if significant change has taken place in one spouse during or as a result of the workshop experience. One individual felt this risk clearly after attending a workshop. He said, "I think there is a great danger to a marriage when one spouse attends a group. It is too hard for the other spouse to compete with the group individually and collectively." One of the frequent aftereffects of the intensive group experience is that it brings out into the open for discussion marital tensions which have been kept under cover.

Another risk which has sometimes been a cause of real concern in mixed intensive workshops is that very positive, warm, and loving feelings can develop between members of the encounter group, as has been evident from some of the preceding examples. Inevitably some of these feelings have a sexual component, and this can be a matter of great concern to the participants and a profound threat to their spouses if these feelings are not worked through satisfactorily in the workshop. Also the close and loving feelings which develop may become a source of threat and marital difficulty when a wife, for example, has not been present, but projects many fears about the loss of her spouse—whether well founded or not—onto the workshop experience.

A man who had been in a mixed group of men and women executives wrote to me a year later and mentioned the strain in his marriage which resulted from his association with Marge, a member of his basic encounter group:

> There was a problem about Marge. There had occurred a very warm feeling on my part for Marge, and great compassion, for I felt she was *very* lonely. I believe the warmth was sincerely reciprocal. At any rate she wrote me a long affectionate letter, which I let my wife read. I was *proud* that Marge could feel that way about *me*. [Because he had felt very worthless.] But my wife was

---

[5]These figures add up to more than 100 percent since quite a number of the respondents checked more than one answer.

alarmed, because she read a love affair into the words—at least a *potential* threat. I stopped writing to Marge, because I felt rather clandestine after that.

My wife has since participated in an "encounter group" herself, and she now understands. I have resumed writing to Marge.

Obviously, not all such episodes would have such a harmonious ending.

It is of interest in this connection that there has been increasing experimentation in recent years with "couples workshops" and with workshops for industrial executives and their spouses.

Still another negative potential growing out of these groups has become evident in recent years. Some individuals who have participated in previous encounter groups may exert a stultifying influence on new workshops which they attend. They sometimes exhibit what I think of as the "old pro" phenomenon. They feel they have learned the "rules of the game," and they subtly or openly try to impose these rules on newcomers. Thus, instead of promoting true expressiveness and spontaneity, they endeavor to substitute new rules for old—to make members feel guilty if they are not expressing feelings, are reluctant to voice criticism or hostility, are talking about situations outside the group relationship, or are fearful of revealing themselves. These old pros seem to be attempting to substitute a new tyranny in interpersonal relationships in the place of older, conventional restrictions. To me this is a perversion of the true group process. We need to ask ourselves how this travesty on spontaneity comes about.

IMPLICATIONS

I have tried to describe both the positive and the negative aspects of this burgeoning new cultural development. I would like now to touch on its implications for our society.

In the first place, it is a highly potent experience and hence clearly deserving of scientific study. As a phenomenon it has been both praised and criticized, but few people who have participated would doubt that *something* significant happens in these groups. People do not react in a neutral fashion toward the intensive group experience. They regard it as either strikingly worthwhile or deeply questionable. All would agree, however, that it is *potent*. This fact makes it of particular interest to the behavioral sciences since science is usually advanced by studying potent and dynamic phenomena. This is one of the reasons why I personally am devoting more and more of my time to this whole enterprise. I feel that we can learn much about the ways in which constructive personality change comes about as we study this group process more deeply.

In a different dimension, the intensive group experience appears to be one cultural attempt to meet the isolation of contemporary life. The person who has experienced an I-Thou relationship, who has entered into the basic encounter, is no longer an isolated individual. One workshop member stated this in a deeply expressive way:

Workshops seem to be at least a partial answer to the loneliness of modern man and his search for new meanings for his life. In short, workshops seem very quickly to allow the individual to become that person he wants to be. The first few steps are taken there, in uncertainty, in fear, and in anxiety. We may or may not continue the journey. It is a gutsy way to live. You trade many, many loose ends for one big knot in the middle of your stomach. It sure as hell isn't easy, but it is a *life* at least—not a hollow imitation of life. It has fear as well as hope, sorrow as well as joy, but I daily offer it to more people in the hope that they will join me. . . . Out from a no-man's land of *fog* into the more violent atmosphere of extremes of thunder, hail, rain, and sunshine. It is worth the trip.

Another implication which is partially expressed in the foregoing statement is that it is an avenue to fulfillment. In a day when more income, a larger car, and a better washing machine seem scarcely to be satisfying the deepest needs of man, individuals are turning to the psychological world, groping for a greater degree of authenticity and fulfillment. One workshop member expressed this extremely vividly:

> [It] has revealed a completely new dimension of life and has opened an infinite number of possibilities for me in my relationship to myself and to everyone dear to me. I feel truly alive and so grateful and joyful and hopeful and healthy and giddy and sparkly. I feel as though my eyes and ears and heart and guts have been opened to see and hear and love and feel more deeply, more widely, more intensely—this glorious, mixed-up, fabulous existence of ours. My whole body and each of its systems seems freer and healthier. I want to feel hot and cold, tired and rested, soft and hard, energetic and lazy. With persons everywhere, but especially my family, I have found a new freedom to explore and communicate. I know the change in me automatically brings a change in them. A whole new exciting relationship has started for me with my husband and with each of my children—a freedom to speak and to hear them speak.

Though one may wish to discount the enthusiasm of this statement, it describes an enrichment of life for which many are seeking.

Rehumanizing Human Relationships

This whole development seems to have special significance in a culture which appears to be bent upon dehumanizing the individual and dehumanizing our human relationships. Here is an important force in the opposite direction, working toward making relationships more meaningful and more personal, in the family, in education, in government, in administrative agencies, in industry.

An intensive group experience has an even more general philosophical implication. It is one expression of the existential point of view which is making itself so pervasively evident in art and literature and modern life. The implicit goal of the group process seems to be to live life fully in the here and now of the relationship. The parallel with an existential point of view is clear-cut. I believe this has been amply evident in the illustrative material.

There is one final issue which is raised by this whole phenomenon: What is our view of the optimal person? What is the goal of personality development? Different ages and different cultures have given different answers to this question. It seems evident from our review of the group process that in a climate of freedom, group members move toward becoming more spontaneous, flexible, closely related to their feelings, open to their experience, and closer and more expressively intimate in their interpersonal relationships. If we value this type of person and this type of behavior, then clearly the group process is a valuable process. If, on the other hand, we place a value on the individual who is effective in suppressing his feelings, who operates from a firm set of principles, who does not trust his own reactions and experience but relies on authority, and who remains aloof in his interpersonal relationships, then we would regard the group process, as I have tried to describe it, as a dangerous force. Clearly there is room for a difference of opinion on this value question, and not everyone in our culture would give the same answer.

CONCLUSION

I have tried to give a naturalistic, observational picture of one of the most significant modern social inventions, the so-called intensive group experience, or basic encounter group. I have tried to indicate some of the common elements of the process which occur in the climate of freedom that is present in such a group. I have pointed out some of the risks and shortcomings of the group experience. I have tried to indicate some of the reasons why it deserves serious consideration, not only from a personal point of view, but also from a scientific and philosophical point of view. I also hope I have made it clear that this is an area in which an enormous amount of deeply perceptive study and research is needed.

REFERENCES

Bennis, W. G., Benne, K. D., & Chin, R. (Eds.) *The planning of change.* New York: Holt, Rinehart & Winston, 1961.

Bennis, W. G., Schein, E. H., Berlew, D. E., & Steele, F. I. (Eds.) *Interpersonal dynamics.* Homewood, Ill.: Dorsey, 1964.

Bradford, L., Gibb, J. R., & Benne, K. D. (Eds.) *T-group theory and laboratory method.* New York: Wiley, 1964.

Casriel, D. *So fair a house.* Englewood Cliffs, N. J.: Prentice-Hall, 1963.

Gibb, J. R. Climate for trust formation. In L. Bradford, J. R. Gibb, & K. D. Benne (Eds.), *T-group theory and laboratory method.* New York: Wiley, 1964.

Gordon, T. *Group-centered leadership.* Boston: Houghton Mifflin, 1955.

Hall, G. F. A participant's experience in a basic encounter group. Mimeographed. Western Behavioral Sciences Institute, 1965.

34

Helping Disturbed Children: Psychological and Ecological Strategies*[1,2]

NICHOLAS HOBBS

... I wish to present a case study in institution building, an account of a planful effort at social invention to meet an acute national problem, the problem of emotional disturbance in children.

I should like to cast this account in large context as an example of the kind of responsibility psychologists must assume in order to respond to a major challenge of our time: to help increase the goodness of fit between social institutions and the people they serve. This commitment demands that we invent new social arrangements designed to improve the quality of human life, and, in doing so, to adhere to the exacting traditions of psychological science: that is, to be explicit about what we are doing, to assess outcomes as meticulously as possible, to relate practice and theory to the benefit of both, and to lay our work open to public and professional scrutiny.

Let me acknowledge here that the work I report is the product of a cooperative effort to which a number of psychologists have contributed, notably Lloyd M. Dunn, Wilbert W. Lewis, William C. Rhodes, Matthew J. Trippe, and Laura Weinstein. National Institute of Mental Health officials, mental health commissioners, consultants, and especially the teacher-counselors, have invented the social institution I shall describe. If on occasion I seem unduly enthusiastic, it springs from an admiration of the work of others.

THE PROBLEM

"Project Re-ED" stands for "a project for the reeducation of emotionally disturbed children." Re-ED was developed explicitly as a new way to meet a social need for which current institutional arrangements are conspicuously inadequate. It is estimated that there are some $1\frac{1}{2}$ million emotionally disturbed children in the United States today, children of average or superior intelligence whose behavior is such that they cannot be sustained with

*Hobbs, N., "Helping disturbed children: psychological and ecological strategies," *American Psychologist*, 1966, **21**, 1105–1115. Copyright © (1966) by the American Psychological Association, and reproduced by permission (Four figures have been omitted.)

[1]Address of the President to the Seventy-Fourth Annual Convention of the American Psychological Association, New York, September 3, 1966.

[2]The work here reported was made possible by Grant No. MH 929 of the United States Public Health Service, and by funds provided by Peabody College, the State of Tennessee, and the State of North Carolina. We are grateful for the support and wise counsel of Commissioner Joseph J. Baker and Commissioner Nat T. Winston, Jr., of Tennessee, Commissioner Eugene A. Hargrove and Sam O. Cornwell of North Carolina, Leonard J. Duhl and Raymond J. Balester of NIMH, and Paul W. Penningroth and Harold L. McPheeters of the Southern Regional Education Board.

normal family, school, and community arrangements. There is one generally endorsed institutional plan for the care of such children: the psychiatric treatment unit of a hospital. But this is not a feasible solution to the problem; the costs are too great, averaging $60 a day, and there are not enough psychiatrists, psychologists, social workers, and psychiatric nurses to staff needed facilities, even if the solution were a good one, an assumption open to question. There is a real possibility that hospitals make children sick. The antiseptic atmosphere, the crepe sole and white coat, the tension, the expectancy of illness may confirm a child's worst fears about himself, firmly setting his aberrant behavior.

But worse things can happen to children, and do. They may be sent to a state hospital to be confined on wards with psychotic adults. They may be put in a jail, euphemistically called a detention home, or committed to an institution for delinquents or for the mentally retarded; or they may be kept at home, hidden away, receiving no help at all, aggravating and being aggravated by what can become an impossible situation.

The problem is further complicated by the professional advocacy of psychotherapy as the only means of effecting changes in behavior and by the pervasive and seldom questioned assumption that it takes at least 2 years to give any substantial help to a disturbed child. Finally, the availability of locks and drugs makes children containable, and the lack of evaluative research effectively denies feedback on the adequacy of approved methods. We became convinced 8 years ago that the problem of the emotionally disturbed child cannot be solved by existing institutional arrangements. The Re-ED program was developed as one alternative, surely not the only one or even the most satisfactory one, but as a feasible alternative that deserved a test.

THE RE-ED SCHOOLS

The National Institute of Mental Health made a test possible by a demonstration grant in 1961 to Peabody College to develop residential schools for disturbed children in which concepts of reeducation could be formulated and tried out. The States of Tennessee and North Carolina, represented by their departments of mental health, joined with Peabody College to translate a general idea into an operational reality. The grant further provided for a training program to prepare a new kind of mental health worker, called a teacher-counselor, and for a research program to evaluate the effectiveness of the schools to be established.

Cumberland House Elementary School in Nashville received its first students in November of 1962, and Wright School of Durham in January of 1963. The schools are located in residential areas not far from the universities (Vanderbilt and Peabody, Duke and North Carolina) that provide personnel and consultation. They are pleasant places, open, friendly, homelike, where children can climb trees and play dodge ball, go to school, and, at night, have a good meal, and a relaxed, amiable evening.

Both schools have nearby camps that are used in the summer and on occasion throughout the year. The camps are simple, even primitive, with children erecting their own shelters, preparing their own meals, making their own schedules. For staff and children alike there is a contagious serenity about the experience. Cooking is a marvelously instructive enterprise; motivation is high, cooperation is necessary, and rewards are immediate. Children for whom failure has become an established expectation, at school and at home, can learn to do things successfully. Nature study is a source of unthreatening instruction. And there is nothing quite like a campfire, or a dark trail and a single flashlight, to promote a sense of community. In this simpler setting, where avoidant responses are few or weakly established, the child can take the first risky steps toward being a more adequate person.

At capacity each school will have 40 children, ages 6 to 12, grouped in five groups of 8 children each. Each group is the responsibility of a team of two teacher-counselors, carefully selected young people, most of whom are graduates of a 9-month training program at Peabody. The two teacher-counselors, assisted by college students and by instructors in arts and crafts and physical education, are responsible for the children around the clock. Each school has a principal and an assistant principal, both educators, a liaison department staffed by social workers and liaison teachers, and a secretarial and house-keeping staff, who are full partners in the reeducation effort. The principal of a Re-ED school has an exacting job of management, training, interpretation, and public relations. The two schools have developed under the leaderships of four able men: John R. Ball and Neal C. Buchanan at Wright School and James W. Cleary and Charles W. McDonald at Cumberland House.[3]

Of course, the teacher-counselors are the heart of Re-ED. They are young people, representing a large manpower pool, who have had experience in elementary school teaching, camping, or other work that demonstrates a long-standing commitment to children. After careful screening, in which self-selection plays an important part, they are given 9 months of training in a graduate program leading to the Master of Arts degree. The program includes instruction in the characteristics of disturbed children, in specialized methods of teaching, including evaluation and remediation of deficits in reading, arithmetic, and other school subjects, in the use of consultants from mental health and educational fields, and in arts and crafts and games and other skills useful on the playing field, on a canoe trip, in the living units after dinner at night. They get a thorough introduction to child-serving agencies in the community and to the operation of a Re-ED school through an extensive practicum. Finally they are challenged with the task of helping invent what Re-ED will become.

But most of all a teacher-counselor is a decent adult; educated, well trained; able to give and receive affection, to live relaxed, and to be firm; a person with private resources for the nourishment and refreshment of his own life; not an itinerant worker but a professional through and through; a person with a sense of the significance of time, of the usefulness of today and the promise of tomorrow; a person of hope, quiet confidence, and joy; one who has committed himself to children and to the proposition that children who are emotionally disturbed can be helped by the process of reeducation.

The total school staff, and especially the teacher-counselors who work directly with the children, are backed by a group of consultants from psychiatry, pediatrics, social work, psychology, and education, an arrangement that makes available to the schools the best professional talent in the community and that has the further attractive feature of multiplying the effectiveness of scarce and expensive mental health and educational personnel.[4]

---

[3]So many people have worked to make Re-ED a reality it is impossible even to record their names. They will have received recompense from seeing children flourish in their care. Yet Alma B. McLain and Letha B. Rowley deserve special recognition for long service and uncommon skill and grace in managing many problems.

[4]The consultants have meant much more to Project Re-ED than can be recorded in this brief account. We here inadequately recognize the invaluable contribution of our colleagues: Jenny L. Adams, MSW, Gus K. Bell, PhD, Lloyd J. Borstelmann, PhD, Eric M. Chazen, MD, Julius H. Corpening, BD., Jane Ann Eppinger, MSW, John A. Fowler, MD, Ihla H. Gehman, EdD, W. Scott Gehman, PhD, Maurice Hyman, MD, J. David Jones, MD, and Bailey Webb, MD.

THE CHILDREN

What kind of children do the teacher-counselors work with? It can be said, in general, that diagnostic classification has not been differentially related to a successful outcome; that the children are normal or superior in intelligence but are in serious trouble in school, often retarded 2 or 3 years in academic development; that they do not need continuing medical or nursing care, and that they can be managed in small groups in an open setting. Re-ED is not a substitute for a hospital. There are children too disturbed, too out of touch, too aggressive, too self-destructive to be worked with successfully in small groups in an open setting. However, Re-ED schools do take many children who would otherwise have to be hospitalized.

Susan was 11, with a diagnosis of childhood schizophrenia. She had attended school 1 day, the first day of the first grade, and had been in play therapy for 4 years. She was a pupil at Cumberland House for a year, staying longer than most children. She has been in a regular classroom for 3 years now, an odd child still but no longer a prospect for life-long institutionalization. Ron was a cruelly aggressive child, partly an expression of inner turmoil and partly an expression of class values and habits; he is much less destructive now, and is back in school. Danny was simply very immature, so that school was too much for him; his problem could be called school phobia if that would help. Dick was extremely effeminate, wearing mascara and painting his nails. Both boys responded to masculine activities guided by a trusted male counselor. Billy was a gasoline sniffer and an ingenious hypochondriac; he returned to a reunion recently much more mature though still having trouble with school work. Larry, age 12, was quite bright yet unable to read; nor were we able to teach him to read. So we failed with him. It is such children as these that we aspire to help. To call them all "emotionally disturbed" is clearly to use language to obscure rather than to clarify. Nonetheless, they are all children who are in serious trouble, for whom the Re-ED idea was developed.

During the past summer, under the direction of William and Dianne Bricker and Charles McDonald, we have been working at Cumberland House with six of the most severely disturbed children we could find, mostly custodial cases from state institutions. Regular Re-ED activities are supplemented by a 24-hour schedule of planned behaviors and contingent rewards, the staff being augmented to make such individualized programming possible, but still using inexpensive and available personnel, such as college students. While it is too early to assess the effectiveness of this effort, we are pleased with the progress that most of the children are making, and we are certain we are giving them more of a chance than they had when their principal challenge was to learn how to live in an institution.

ECOLOGICAL CONCEPTS

Let us turn now to an examination of the theoretical assumptions and operational procedures involved in the process of reeducation. We do not, of course, make use of the principles involved in traditional psychotherapy; transference, regression, the promotion of insight through an exploration of inner dynamics and their origins are not a part of the picture. The teacher-counselor is not a psychotherapist, nor does he aspire to be one.

We have become increasingly convinced that a major barrier to effective national planning for emotionally disturbed children is the professional's enchantment with psychotherapy. Everything in most model institutions revolves around getting the child to his therapist 1, 2, or maybe 3 hours a week. A few superb treatment centers combine psychotherapy with a program of daily activities conducive to personal growth and integration. But these are rare indeed. It is not uncommon to find children locked 15 stories high in steel and glass, with a caged roof to play on, drugged to keep them from doing too much damage to the light fixtures and air conditioning, while they await their precious hour, guarded by attendants who think disturbed children must scream, fight, climb walls, cower in a corner. Most frequently, of course, therapy is not available; most hospitals hold children hoping somehow they will get better.

An overcommitment to individual psychotherapy seems to us to stem from an uncritical acceptance of "cure" as the goal in working with a child, a consequence of defining the problem initially as one of "illness." That some disturbed children are "ill" in the usual sense may be accepted, but to define them all as such leads, we think, to a host of unvalidated and unquestioned assumptions; to a preoccupation with the intrapsychic life of the child, with what goes on inside his skull; to an easy use of drugs without knowledge of their long-term effects on character development; to the extended isolation of children from their families, the presumed source of contagion; to a limitation of professional roles; to the neglect of schools and of schooling; and so on. The preemptive character of a definition and the semantic sets that ensue are major barriers to innovation in working with disturbed children.

Of course we have our own ways of talking about the problem, and our metaphors are no less preemptive, making it all the more important for us to be explicit about definitions.We prefer to say that the children we work with have learned bad habits. They have acquired nonadaptive ways of relating to adults and to other children. They have learned to perceive themselves in limiting or destructive terms and to construe the world as an uncertain, rejecting, and hurtful place. We also recognize that the child lives in a real world that often falls short in giving him the affection, support, and guidance he needs. So we deal directly with social realities as well as with private perceptions.

This kind of thinking has led us gradually to a different way of defining our task, a definition of considerable heuristic merit (see Fig. 34.1). For want of a more felicitous phrase, we have been calling it a systems approach to the problem of working with a disturbed child. We assume that the child is an inseparable part of a small social system, of an ecological unit made up of the child, his family, his school, his neighborhood and

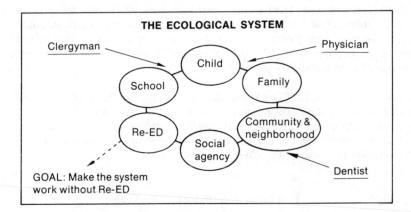

Fig. 34.1 Chart of ecological system, the smallest unit in a systems approach to working with a disturbed child.

community. A social agency is often a part of the picture when a child has been designated emotionally disturbed, and other people—a physician, a clergyman—may be brought in as needed. The system may become "go" as a result of marked improvement in any component (the father stops drinking and goes back to work, a superb teacher becomes available, the child improves dramatically), or it may work as a result of modest improvement in all components. The effort is to get each component of the system above threshold with respect to the requirements of the other components. The Re-ED school becomes a part of the ecological unit for as brief a period of time as possible, withdrawing when the probability that the system will function appears to exceed the probability that it will not. We used to speak of putting the child back into the system but we have come to recognize the erroneous assumptions involved; the child defines the system and all we can do is withdraw from it at a propitious moment.

Once we abandoned cure as a goal and defined our problem as doing what we can to make a small social system work in a reasonably satisfactory manner, there ensued a number of operational patterns that contrast sharply with the practices of existing residential treatment centers for children.

For one thing, parents are no longer viewed as sources of contagion but as responsible collaborators in making the system work. Parents are involved in discussion groups and are helped to get assistance from mental health centers. They actively participate in the ongoing program of the school. They organize an annual reunion, publish a parent's manual, sew for the children, and in many ways assume responsibility for reestablishing the child as quickly as possible in his own home, school, and community.

The children go home on weekends to keep families and children belonging to each other, to avoid the estrangement that can come from prolonged separation, and to give the child and his parents and brothers and sisters an opportunity to learn new and more effective ways of living together. Visitors ask, "Aren't your Mondays awful?" They are, indeed, but we cherish their chaos as a source of new instruction; we try to keep in mind that our goal is not to run a tranquil school but to return the child as quickly as possible to his own home and regular school.

The ecological model requires new strategies to involve home, neighborhood, school, agency, and community in a contract with us to help a child. It requires new patterns for the deployment of personnel, and it has led to the development of a new kind of mental health worker: the liaison teacher. The liaison teacher is responsible for maintaining communication with the child's regular school, again to prevent alienation and to arrange optimum conditions for the child's early return to a regular classroom. For example a liaison teacher may personally accompany a child to a new school to which he has been transferred in order to increase the probability that that component of the ecological system will function effectively.

The social worker in Re-ED honors an early heritage of his profession, before the lamentable sit-behind-the-desk-and-do-psychotherapy era got established. He reaches out to the family, to community agencies, and to individuals—to any reasonable source of help for a child in trouble. Again, the goal is to make the system work, not simply to adjust something inside the head of the child.

THE PROCESS OF REEDUCATION

Now, let us turn to the child himself, to our relationships with him, and to what is meant operationally by the process of reeducation. Here are an even dozen underlying concepts that have come to seem important to us as we try to talk about what goes on in a Re-ED school.

Item 1: Life Is to Be Lived Now

We start with the assumption that each day, that every hour in every day, is of great importance to a child, and that when an hour is neglected, allowed to pass without reason and intent, teaching and learning go on nonetheless and the child may be the loser. In Re-ED, no one waits for a special hour. We try, as best we can, to make all hours special. We strive for immediate and sustained involvement in purposive and consequential living. We constantly test the optimistic hypothesis that if children are challenged to live constructively, that if they are given an opportunity for a constructive encounter with other children and with decent adults, they will come off well—and they do, most of the time. They learn, here and now, that life can be lived on terms satisfactory to society and satisfying to themselves. Our task is to contrive each day so that the probability of success in this encounter clearly outweighs the probability of failure. I paraphrase Jessie Taft when I say, in the mastery of this day the child learns, in principle, the mastery of all days.

Item 2: Time Is an Ally

We became convinced, in the early stages of planning the project, that children are kept too long in most traditional treatment programs. The reasons for this are many. The abstract goal of cure through psychotherapy leads to expectations of extensive personality reorganization, of the achievement of adequacy in a wide array of possible life roles. It thus takes a long time either to succeed in this ambitious endeavor or to become aware that one has failed. Staff and children become fond of each other, making separation difficult. The widespread practice of removing the child from his home for extended periods of time causes a sometimes irreparable estrangement; the family closes ranks against the absent member. While everyone recognizes the importance of school in the life of the child, mental health programs have neither operational concepts nor specialized personnel necessary to effect an easy transition for the child from the institution back to his own school. Furthermore, the expectation of a prolonged stay in a treatment center becomes a self-validating hypothesis. A newly admitted child asks, "How long do kids stay here?" He is told "about 2 years," and he settles down to do what is expected of him, with full support of staff and parents who also "know" that it takes 2 years to help a disturbed child. Myriad other constraints get established; for example, the treatment center hires just enough secretaries to move children in and out of a 2-year cycle, and it is not possible to speed the process without hiring more secretaries, a restraint on therapeutic progress that is seldom identified. So before we admitted the first child, we set 6 months as the expected, average period of stay, a goal we have now achieved.

Time is an issue of importance in the process of reeducation in yet another way. We work with children during years when life has a tremendous forward thrust. Several studies suggest that therapeutic intervention is not demonstrably superior to the passage of time without treatment in the subsequent adjustment of children diagnosed as emotionally disturbed (Lewis, 1965). Treatment may simply speed up a process that would occur in an unknown percentage of children anyway. There is a real possibility that a long stay in a treatment center may actually slow down this process. Furthermore, in ecological perspective, it is clear that children tend to get ejected from families at low points in family organization and integrity. Most families get better after such periods; there is only one direction for them to go and that is up. The systems concept may entail simply observing when the family has regained sufficient stability to sustain a previously ejected child. The great tragedy is that children can get caught up in institutional arrangements that must inexorably run their course. In Re-ED we claim time is an ally and try to avoid getting in the way of the normal restorative processes of life.

Item 3: Trust Is Essential

The development of trust is the first step in reeducation of the emotionally disturbed child. The disturbed child is conspicuously impaired in his ability to learn from adults. The mediation process is blocked or distorted by the child's experience-based hypothesis that adults are deceptive, that they are an unpredictable source of hurt and help. He faces each adult with a predominant anticipation of punishment, rejection, derision, or withdrawal of love. He is acutely impaired in the very process by which more mature ways of living may be acquired. A first step, then, in the reeducation process, is the development of trust. Trust, coupled with understanding, is the beginning point of a new learning experience, an experience that helps a child know that he can use an adult to learn many things: how to read, how to be affectionate, how to be oneself without fear or guilt.

We are intrigued by the possibility, indeed are almost sure the thesis is true, that no amount of professional training can make an adult worthy of the trust of a child or capable of generating it. This ability is prior to technique, to theory, to technical knowledge. After seeing the difference that teacher-counselors in our two schools have made in the lives of children I am confident of the soundness of the idea that some adults know, without knowing how they know, the way to inspire trust in children and to teach them to begin to use adults as mediators of new learning.

Item 4: Competence Makes a Difference

The ability to do something well gives a child confidence and self-respect and gains for him acceptance by other children, by teachers, and, unnecessary as it might seem, even by his parents. In a society as achievement oriented as ours, a person's worth is established in substantial measure by his ability to produce or perform. Acceptance without productivity is a beginning point in the process of reeducation, but an early goal and a continuing challenge is to help the child get good at something.

What, then, in the process of reeducation, does the acquisition of competence mean? It means first and foremost the gaining of competence in school skills, in reading and arithmetic most frequently, and occasionally in other subjects as well. If a child feels that he is inadequate in school, inadequacy can become a pervasive theme in his life, leading to a consistent pattern of failure to work up to his level of ability. Underachievement in school is the single most common characteristic of emotionally disturbed children. We regard it as sound strategy to attack directly the problem of adequacy in school, for its intrinsic value as well as for its indirect effect on the child's perception of his worth and his acceptance by people who are important in his world. A direct attack on the problem of school skills does not mean a gross assault in some area of deficiency. On the contrary, it requires utmost skill and finesse on the part of the teacher-counselor to help a disturbed child move into an area where he has so often known defeat, where failure is a well-rooted expectancy, where a printed page can evoke flight or protest or crippling anxiety. The teacher-counselor need make no apologies to the psychotherapist with reference to the level of skill required to help a disturbed child learn.

So, in Re-ED, school keeps. It is not regarded, as it is in many mental health programs, as something that can wait until the child gets better, as though he were recovering from measles or a broken leg. School is the very stuff of a child's problems, and consequently, a primary source of instruction in living. Special therapy rooms are not needed; the classroom is a natural setting for a constructive relationship between a disturbed child and a competent, concerned adult.

Much of the teaching, incidentally, is through the unit or enterprise method. For example, a group of boys at Cumberland House was invited to go camping with some Cherokee Indian children on their reservation. The trip provided a unifying theme for 3 month's instruction in American History, geography, arithmetic, writing, and arts and crafts. At Wright School, rocketry has provided high motivation and an entrée to mathematics, aerodynamics, and politics. The groups are small enough to make individualized instruction possible, even to the point of preparing special programmed materials for an individual child, a method that has been remarkably effective with children with seemingly intractable learning disorders. The residential character of the Re-ED school means that the acquisition of competence does not have to be limited to increased skill in school subjects. It may mean learning to swim, to draw, to sing; it may mean learning to cook on a Dakota Hole, to lash together a table, to handle a canoe, to build a shelter in the woods; it may mean learning to talk at council ring, to assert one's rights, to give of one's possessions, to risk friendship, to see parents as people and teachers as friends.

Item 5: Symptoms Can and Should Be Controlled

It is standard doctrine in psychotherapeutic practice that symptoms should not be treated, that the one symptom removed will simply be replaced by another, and that the task of the therapist is to uncover underlying conflicts against which the symptom is a defense, thus eliminating the need for any symptom at all. In Re-ED we contend, on the other hand, that symptoms are important in their own right and deserve direct attention. We are impressed that some symptoms are better to have than other symptoms. The bad symptoms are those that alienate the child from other children or from the adults he needs as a source of security or a source of learning. There is much to be gained then from identifying symptoms that are standing in the way of normal development and working out specific plans for removing or altering the symptoms if possible. The problem is to help the child make effective contact with normal sources of affection, support, instruction, and discipline. We also work on a principle of parsimony that instructs us to give first preference to explanations involving the assumption of minimum pathology, as contrasted to professional preference for deep explanations and the derogation of all else as superficial.

Item 6: Cognitive Control Can Be Taught

Though little emphasis is placed on the acquisition of insight as a source of therapeutic gain, there is a lot of talking in Re-ED about personal problems and how they can be managed better. The teacher-counselor relies primarily on immediate experience, on the day-by-day, hour-by-hour, moment-by-moment relationship between himself and the child; he relies on specific events that can be discussed to increase the child's ability to manage his own life. The emotionally disturbed child has fewer degrees of freedom in behavior than the normal child, yet he is not without the ability to shape his own behavior by self-administered verbal instruction. He can signal to himself if he can learn what the useful signals are. The teacher-counselor works constantly to help a child learn the right signals.

The focus of this effort is on today and tomorrow, not on the past or the future, and on ways for the child to signal to himself to make each day a source of instruction for the living of the next. At the council ring at night, at a place set apart from the business of living, children in a group are helped to consider what was good about the day just past, what went wrong that might be handled better tomorrow, and what was learned, especially in successes and failures in relationships among themselves. Possibly more important than the solving of particular problems is the acquisition of the habit of talking things over for the purpose of getting better control over events, a habit that can frequently be carried over into the child's home and become a new source of strength for his family.

Item 7: Feelings Should Be Nurtured

We are very interested in the nurturance and expression of feeling, to help a child own all of himself without guilt. Children have a way of showing up with animals and we are glad for this. A child who has known the rejection of adults may find it safest, at first, to express affection to a dog. And a pet can be a source of pride and of sense of responsibility. Anger, resentment, hostility are commonplace, of course, and their expression is used in various ways: to help some children learn to control their violent impulses and to help others give vent to feelings too long repressed. In Re-ED Schools one finds the familiar ratio of four or five boys to one girl, a consequence in part, we believe, of a lack of masculine challenge in school and community today. Thus we contrive situations of controlled danger in which children can test themselves, can know fear and become the master of it. The simple joy of companionship is encouraged. We are impressed by the meaningfulness of friendships and how long they endure. The annual homecoming is anticipated by many youngsters as an opportunity to walk arm-in-arm with an old friend associated with a period of special significance in their lives. And we respect the need to be alone, to work things through without intrusion, and to have a private purpose. Feelings also get expressed through many kinds of creative activities that are woven into the fabric of life in a Re-ED school. Throwing clay on a potter's wheel gives a child a first sense of his potential for shaping his world. A puppet show written by the children may permit freer expression than is ordinarily tolerable. Drawing and painting can be fun for a whole group. And an object to mold gives something to do to make it safe for an adult and child to be close together.

Item 8: The Group Is Important to Children

Children are organized in groups of eight, with two teacher-counselors in charge. The group is kept intact for nearly all activities and becomes an important source of motivation, instruction, and control. When a group is functioning well, it is extremely difficult for an individual child to behave in a disturbed way. Even when the group is functioning poorly, the frictions and the failures can be used constructively. The council ring, or powwow, involving discussion of difficulties or planning of activities can be a most maturing experience. And the sharing of adventure, of vicissitudes, and of victories, provides an experience in human relatedness to which most of our children have been alien.

Item 9: Ceremony and Ritual Give Order, Stability, and Confidence

Many Re-ED children have lived chaotic lives, even in their brief compass. They may come from homes where interpersonal disarray is endemic. We have stumbled upon and been impressed by the beneficence of ceremony, ritual, and metaphor for children and have come to plan for their inclusion in the program.The nightly backrub is an established institution with the Whippoorwills, a time of important confidences. Being a Bobcat brings a special sense of camaraderie and has its own metaphorical obligations. And a Christmas pageant can effect angelic transformation of boys whose ordinary conduct is far from seraphic.

Item 10: The Body Is The Armature of the Self

We are intrigued by the idea that the physical self is the armature around which the psychological self is constructed and that a clearer experiencing of the potential and the boundaries of the body should lead to a clearer definition of the self, and thus to greater psychological fitness and more effective functioning. The Outward Bound schools in England, developed as an experience for young men to overcome the anomie that is the product of an industrial civilization, are built around the concept. Austin Des Lauriers' ideas about treatment of schizophrenia in children emphasize differentiating the body from the rest of the world. Programmatically, in Re-ED, the idea has been realized in such activities as swimming, climbing, dancing, tumbling, clay modelling, canoeing, building a tree house, and walking a monkey bridge.

Item 11: Communities Are Important

The systems concept in Re-ED leads to an examination of the relationship of the child to his home community. Many children who are referred to our schools come from families that are alienated or detached from community life or that are not sufficiently well organized or purposeful to help the child develop a sense of identity with his neighborhood, his town or city. He has little opportunity to discover that communities exist for people and, while the goodness of fit between the two may often leave much to be desired, an important part of a child's education is to learn that community agencies and institutions exist for his welfare and that he has an obligation as a citizen to contribute to their effective functioning. This is especially true for many of the boys referred to Re-ED, whose energy, aggressiveness, lack of control, and resentment of authority will predispose them to delinquent behavior when they are a few years older and gain in independence and mobility. This idea has a number of implications for program planning. Field trips to the fire, police, and health departments are useful. Memberships in the YMCA, a children's museum, a playground group, or a community center may be worked out for a child. Church attendance may be encouraged and a clergyman persuaded to take special interest in a family, and a library card can be a proud possession and a tangible community tie.

Item 12: Finally, a Child Should Know Joy

We have often speculated about our lack of a psychology of well-being. There is an extensive literature on anxiety, guilt, and dread, but little that is well developed on joy. Most psychological experiments rely for motivation on avoidance of pain or hunger or some other aversive stimuli; positive motivations are limited to the pleasure that comes from minute, discrete rewards. This poverty with respect to the most richly human of motivations leads to anaemic programming for children. We thus go beyond contemporary psychology to touch one of the most vital areas of human experiencing. We try to develop skill in developing joy in children. We believe that it is immensely important, that it is immediately therapeutic if further justification is required, for a child to know some joy in each day and to look forward with eagerness to at least some joy-giving event that is planned for tomorrow.

COSTS AND EFFECTIVENESS

Now, let us turn to the practical questions of cost and of effectiveness.

A Re-ED school costs about $20 to $25 per child per day to operate. Thus the per-day cost is about one-third the cost of the most widely accepted model and perhaps four times the cost of custodial care. Cost per day, however, is not the best index to use, for the purpose of a mental health program is not to keep children cheaply but to restore them to home, school, and community as economically as possible. In terms of cost per child served, the cost of a Re-ED program is equivalent to or less than the cost of custodial care. The cost per child served is approximately $4,000. If Re-ED can prevent longer periods of institutionalization, this is a modest investment indeed.

Appropriate to the systems analysis of the problem, most of our studies of effectiveness of Re-ED schools have employed ratings by concerned observers: mother, father, teacher, our own staff, and agency staffs, all important persons in the ecological space of the child. However, Laura Weinstein (1965) has been interested in the way normal and disturbed children construct interpersonal space.... She used two techniques. In the first (the replacement technique), each of two figure pairs—a pair of human figures and a pair of rectangles—is present on a different board and equally far apart.... The child is asked to replace the felt figures "exactly as far apart as they are now." Normal and disturbed children make systematic errors, but in opposite directions: normal children replace human figures closer together while Re-ED children replace human figures farther apart.... In the second technique (the free placement technique), human figures are used, representing mothers, fathers, and children. The children are asked to place the figures on the board "any way you like." Again systematic differences occur. Normal children place the child very close to the mother. Re-ED children place greater distance between the mother and the child than between any other human pair.... The mother-child relationship is clearly crucial in the life space of the 6- to 12-year-old children with whom we work. It is gratifying to report that children after the Re-ED experience put the child figure closer to the mother than they did before; that is, they structure interpersonal space as normal children do.

The basic design for evaluating the effectiveness of the Re-ED schools involves observations taken at time of enrollment and repeated 6 months after discharge. Preliminary results present an encouraging picture. A composite rating of improvement, based on follow-up information on 93 graduates provided by all evaluators, gives a success rate of approximately 80%. We are in process of obtaining comparison data from control groups to determine the extent to which the reeducation effort is superior to changes that occur with the passage of time.

Detailed analyses show that mothers and fathers independently report a decrease in symptoms such as bedwetting, tantrums, nightmares, and school fears, and an increase in social maturity on a Vineland type check list. School adjustment as rated by teachers shows the same favorable trends. On a semantic differential measure of discrepancy between how the child is seen and parental standards for him, there is an interesting and dynamically significant difference between fathers and mothers. Both see the child as having improved. For fathers the perceived improvement results in lower discrepancy scores between the child as seen and a standard held for him. For some mothers, however, improvement results in a raising of standards so that discrepancy scores frequently remain high. This is not true of all mothers but it is more frequently true of mothers than of fathers.

But *T* tests seldom determine the fate of institutions; public and professional acceptance is crucial.

To obtain an informed and mature professional appraisal of Re-ED, we have established a panel of visitors composed of men whose judgment is held in high esteem: Eli M. Bower, psychologist; Reginald S. Lourie, psychiatrist; Charles R. Strother, psychologist; and Robert L. Sutherland, sociologist. Members of the panel have been visiting the schools regularly since their inception and will make public their final appraisal at the end of the project period. It is enough to say now that they are all strong supporters of the Re-ED idea.

A test of public support of the Re-ED idea was adventitiously obtained when the Legislature of the State of North Carolina last June terminated state funds for the support of Wright School after July 1, 1966. Protest from all over the state was immediate and strong; in less than 3 years of operation the school had won impressive public support. Funds have been raised to continue Wright School in operation until the Legislature convenes again.[5] The Governor has assured the mental health officials of North Carolina that he will support legislative measures to restore state funds for the operation of Wright School. Fortunately the Tennessee school has not been put to such public test but professional and political endorsement is evident in the decision to build two new schools, one in Memphis and one in Chattanooga, that will be operated as reeducation centers. Finally, it is encouraging that several other states have committees working to establish Re-ED schools.

Our aspiration and our growing confidence are that the Re-ED model will be replicated in many states, that it will have its influence on the character of more traditional treatment programs, and that the beneficiaries will be the disturbed children of America.

We further think of Re-ED as an institution that exemplifies, in its development, the contemporary challenge to psychologists to concern themselves with the invention of social arrangements that put psychological knowledge to use to improve the quality of human life.

REFERENCES

Hobbs, N. Mental health's third revolution. *American Journal of Orthopsychiatry*, 1964, 34, 822–833.
Lewis, W. W. Continuity and intervention in emotional disturbance: A review. *Exceptional Children*, 1965, 31 (9), 465–475.
Weinstein, L. Social schemata of emotionally disturbed boys. *Journal of Abnormal Psychology*, 1965, 70, 457–461.

---

[5]Among the major contributors are the Wright Refuge Board, the Sarah Graham Kenan Fund, the Mary Duke Biddle Foundation, the Hillsdale Fund, and the Stanley County Mental Health Association. Many gifts have come from churches, mental health associations, civic organizations, and individuals. We gratefully acknowledge their help in keeping Wright School in operation.

Suggested Additional Readings

Ayllon, T. & Azrin, N. H. *The token economy: A motivational therapy.* New York: Appleton-Century-Crofts, 1968.

Bach, G. R. *Intensive group psychotherapy.* New York: Ronald Press, 1953.

Bindrim, P. A report on a nude marathon. In *Readings in clinical psychology today.* Del Mar, Calif.: CRM Books, 1970. Pp. 141–145.

Durkin, H. E. The theory and practice of group psychotherapy. *Annals of the New York Academy of Science,* 1949, **49,** 889–901.

Durkin, H. E. *The group in depth.* New York: International Universities Press, 1964.

Egan, G. *Encounter: Group processes for interpersonal growth.* Belmont, Calif.: Brooks/Cole, 1970.

Egan, G. *Encounter groups: Basic readings.* Belmont, Calif.: Brooks/Cole, 1971.

Foulkes, S. H., & Anthony, E. J. *Group psychotherapy.* Baltimore: Penguin Books, 1957.

Gazda, G. M. (Ed.) *Basic approaches to group psychotherapy and group counselling.* Springfield, Ill.: Charles C Thomas, 1968.

Gazda, G. M. *Innovations to group psychotherapy.* Springfield, Ill.: Charles C Thomas, 1968.

Johnson, J. A. *Group therapy: A practical approach.* New York: McGraw-Hill, 1963.

Luchins, A. S. *Group psychotherapy.* New York: Random House, 1964.

Mowrer, O. H. *The new group therapy.* New York: Van Nostrand, 1964.

Powdermaker, F. B., & Frank, J. O. *Group psychotherapy.* Cambridge, Mass.: Harvard University Press, 1953.

Yalom, I. D. *The theory and practice of group psychotherapy.* New York: Basic Books, 1970.

Therapy Approaches with Special Populations

35

Treatment of Alcoholism*

NATIONAL INSTITUTE OF MENTAL HEALTH

The alcoholic who needs or seeks help faces at the outset a number of vital questions.

Should he begin his search for help with a relative or a well-meaning family friend? With his family physician, a psychiatrist or a worker from Alcoholics Anonymous? With a clergyman or a social worker? Can he cure himself?

Should he be treated at home, in a sanitarium or in a hospital?

Should he try to taper off gradually or stop all drinking immediately? Should he look to drugs or psychotherapy? Will his treatment require a day, a month, a year or longer? What are his chances of recovery?

Many of the answers will be dictated by his personal prejudices, his fears, his finances and the pressures of his family. Other answers will be influenced subtly but powerfully by community attitudes toward alcohol and the alcoholic. Some may be influenced by knowledge of the new advances in alcoholism therapy—knowledge on his own part, and knowledge on the part of his therapist.

In any effective State or local alcoholism treatment program, it is clearly essential that alcoholics and their relatives—as well as physicians, clergymen, probation officers, personnel workers, social workers and various social agencies—be provided with sound, up-to-date information on the types of treatment available in their own communities, the precise locations where such therapy can be obtained, the probable costs, and the possible results.

PRELIMINARY TREATMENT

Some alcoholics will begin treatment during a stage of temporary sobriety, others during the throes of a severe hangover or during acute intoxication. For many it will be during the drying-out or withdrawal stage, marked by such conditions as delirium tremens. In some cases of acute intoxication, and in most with severe withdrawal symptoms, competent medical management directed by a physician is essential. Without such care, the patient may die[11, 13].

In the past, treatment of withdrawal symptoms was based largely on such alcohol substitutes as chloral hydrate or paraldehyde. In the last 15 years, these drugs have been replaced in part with new synthetic tranquilizers such as reserpine, chlorpromazine, meprobamate, promazine hydrochloride and chlordiazepoxide. The impact of these tranquilizing drugs on the treatment of the acute alcoholic stage has been described by some clinicians as revolutionary[3]. With appropriate use of tranquilizers and other therapeutic aids, and

*From Alcohol and alcoholism, Washington, D.C.: U.S. Government Printing Office, 1968. Reprinted by permission of the National Institute of Mental Health, Health Services and Mental Health Administration, U.S. Department of Health, Education, and Welfare. (References have been renumbered.)

especially the control of fluid and electrolyte balance, most patients recover promptly from delirium, hallucinations and tremors, and are ready to start other forms of treatment.

HOSPITAL ADMISSION

An acutely ill alcoholic—or the non-alcoholic who is acutely intoxicated —may be given satisfactory care at home, or in a special detoxification or drying-out center, but a general hospital ward is considered the best setting for preliminary treatment. A few American and Canadian general hospitals have long offered such care, but until the late 1950s nearly all hospitals were reluctant to accept alcoholics as patients.

The traditional position of most hospital officials has been attributed to hostile feelings evoked by the so-called typical alcoholic patient, who at admission was often dirty, disheveled, disturbing and demanding. If the patient was boisterous, it was difficult to think of him as sick. Often he was viewed as weak-willed and immoral, offensive to other patients, upsetting to hospital routine, and likely to assault attendants and nurses.

A wealthy or prominent patient might be admitted—often under a camouflaged diagnosis—but only if he paid for a private room and 24-hour-a-day private nursing care. Most patients, unable to afford such care, were sent to the "drunk tank" of the local jail, the psychiatric ward of a State hospital, or the emergency ward of a local hospital. In most emergency wards, attendants concerned themselves primarily with sobering the patient, treating obvious wounds or contusions, and discharging him as quickly as possible. Often, a few days or weeks later, the same patient would reappear for the same type of temporary patching-up.

Probably the most eloquent demonstration that this technique was out-moded and needless came in 1957 at San Francisco's Mount Zion Hospital[2], after officials decided to accept alcoholics simply as sick people needing hospital care. These patients were placed in regular open wards and treated by physicians, nurses and other personnel who had been carefully trained in the use of new drugs and oriented to treat them as patients who were ill and not necessarily immoral.

It quickly became evident that other patients were not disturbed, hospital routines were not upset, and most of the alcoholics were willing to undertake follow-up therapy.

"The advent of the tranquilizing drugs has made sedation safer, simpler and more effective, and has greatly facilitated the nursing and medical care of the detoxification and withdrawal period," reported Dr. Jack D. Gordon, the director of the study. "In addition, our increased understanding of the psychological aspects of illness has prompted us to treat alcoholics in a routine, nonpunitive atmosphere with understanding and without discrimination. The alcoholic has responded both to drugs and the atmosphere, and has become manageable."

The experiment demonstrated, first, that modern hospitals can meet their community responsibilities in alcoholism therapy, and second, that hospitalized alcoholic patients usually require no more attention than do patients with diabetes, fractured hips, or coronary attacks.

Although the success at Mount Zion has been duplicated at other hospitals, and leaders of the American Medical Association and the American Hospital Association have urged hospitals throughout the country to follow this lead, many are still unwilling to accept alcoholics as ordinary patients.

The strategic importance of the therapist's attitude during these early phases of treatment has recently been emphasized by the results of a research project undertaken by Dr.

Morris E. Chafetz and his associates at Massachusetts General Hospital [5, 6]. Studying alcoholic patients admitted to the emergency ward services of the hospital, they found that meeting the patients from the outset with understanding, sympathy, and attention to expressed needs could assure higher rates of follow-through on treatment recommendations.

DRUG THERAPY

Once over the acute stages of intoxication or withdrawal, the alcoholic starting long-range treatment may require a kind of pharmacological bridge over the difficult early days or weeks. For this, physicians may prescribe a variety of treatments.

Tranquilizers are often used to produce relaxation and to reduce the tensions which many alcoholics believe to have triggered their drinking bouts [3, 10]. They are highly effective, but some alcoholics eventually become addicted to the very tranquilizers which helped them break away from their dependency on alcohol.

Other physicians use what is sometimes called conditioned-response or aversion therapy, administering an alcoholic beverage and at the same time a powerful nausea-producing agent like emetine or apomorphine. Repeated treatments with such a combination are intended to develop a conditioned reflex loathing for alcohol in any form. Because of the risk of severe physical reactions, this method of treatment requires close medical supervision [13].

More widely known and used are so-called deterrent agents such as disulfiram (Antabuse) and citrated calcium carbimide (Temposil). A patient regularly taking one of these compounds finds that ingestion of alcohol in any form quickly produces pounding headache, flushing, and usually violent nausea, vomiting, and other unpleasant symptoms [8].

Probably the greatest value of these and similar drugs is that they provide real if only temporary relief for many patients. For most patients, however, they can produce lasting benefit only as part of a program of psychotherapy which attempts to get at the emotional factors underlying the drinking of the alcoholic.

PSYCHOTHERAPY

In the past, alcoholics have been admonished, scolded, denounced, jailed, beaten, ducked, lashed and threatened with eternal damnation. There is no evidence that any of these measures has had significant therapeutic value for more than an occasional alcoholic. Available evidence seems to demonstrate that long-lasting results can be achieved primarily by a technique known generally as psychotherapy.

Broadly, psychotherapy is a label covering various kinds of self-examination, counseling and guidance, in which a trained professional works with (rather than on) a patient—alone or in groups—to help him change his feelings, attitudes and behavior in order to live more effectively.

Although there are variations, the psychotherapeutic approach in the case of alcoholism usually involves an attempt to bring about complete acceptance of the alcoholic—by himself and by the therapist—as a person who is sick but not evil, immoral or weak, and an equally complete acceptance by the patient of the idea that he needs help. Once some progress has been made, an effort is made to achieve understanding of the patient's underlying tensions as well as his more obvious problems, to alleviate or solve those problems that can be readily handled, and to find a means—other than drinking—which will enable the patient to live with those problems that cannot be solved.

Most successful therapists—however they may differ on details of treatment—indicate that pleadings, exhortations, telling the patient how to live his life, or urging him to use more willpower, are usually useless and may be destructive[17].

Many therapists stress the frequent need for including members of the patient's family in the therapy program. Research by some investigators has disclosed that the family may include another member who is even more emotionally disturbed than the alcoholic, and who may be partly responsible for the alcoholic's drinking[11].

Usually patients find that the termination of their excessive drinking means they must face accumulated internal and external problems. Treatment for alcoholics, many therapists hold, cannot be conducted on a hit-or-miss, intermittent basis, or restricted mainly to the management of occasional drinking episodes. Many believe the best schedule calls for very frequent sessions during the first weeks or months, and then sessions at longer intervals as the patient progresses. The patient and his family usually may expect the treatment to continue for at least a year, with the possibility that he may require occasional temporary psychotherapeutic support for many years more.

On the other hand, doctors at the Cleveland Center on Alcoholism [12] have claimed after five years of experience with nearly 2,000 patients that a substantial proportion can be given significant help in from one to five therapeutic sessions. Clearly not advocated for all alcoholics, this short-term psychotherapy was found to be most effective with patients having what were termed reasonably intact emotional and environmental resources—those with good family ties and a determination to get well—and who could, with help, face the reality of their situation quickly.

THE THERAPIST

In the early stages of excessive drinking, many individuals are able to reduce their intake or even stop drinking on their own for periods of time. If they resume drinking and addiction becomes evident, self-treatment is ineffective. Competent professional help is essential, and usually the earlier it is obtained, the better the long-term results. Many types of help are now available.

The Clergy

Traditionally, addictive drinking was considered a sin and its treatment, therefore, a responsibility of the clergy. Until recently, the goal of most religious workers in treating alcoholics was essentially moral reform, to induce the sinner to see the error of his ways and, with Divine aid, to mend them.

This situation has now changed considerably. After deep re-appraisal, many clergymen of various faiths have taken a different approach, utilizing modern psychological and psychiatric knowledge, and are following the pattern of pastoral counseling provided generally for people in trouble.

Alcoholics Anonymous

AA has been described as a loosely knit, voluntary fellowship of alcoholics gathered together for the sole purpose of helping themselves and each other to get sober and stay sober. It has also been pictured as serving its members first as a way back to life and then as a design for living. Widely publicized since the early 1940s, it has more than 7,000 local chapters, with one in almost every sizeable town.

Important to the AA approach is an admission by the alcoholic of his lack of power over alcohol. He must have hit what is termed "rock bottom," finding himself in a desperate and totally intolerable situation. For some this realization may come when they have lost everything and everybody. For others, it may occur when they are first arrested by the police or warned by their employer. At this point, the individual must decide to turn over his life and his will to a power greater than his own. Much of the program has a spiritual but non-sectarian basis[1].

During the early years of AA, some members rigidly insisted that "only an alcoholic can understand an alcoholic," and there was minimal cooperation between AA workers on the one hand and physicians, clergymen and social workers on the other. With the accumulation of more experience and knowledge, however, most AA members no longer hold these concepts, and cooperation with therapists in other professions has been increasing.

Many physicians emphasize that, valuable and widely accessible as it is, AA should not be considered as a complete form of treatment for all alcoholics, but should be viewed for most as an adjunct to and not a substitute for various forms of professional therapy[19].

Physicians

If alcoholism is by definition a disease, treatment should logically begin under the direction of a physician. But at least in the past, many physicians have been reluctant to accept alcoholic patients. A 1946 study in New York, for example, showed that 60 percent of 1,609 doctors reporting did not treat alcohol addiction, and alcoholics made up only one percent of the practices of the other 40 percent[18].

"The situation has improved markedly since then," says Dr. Marvin A. Block, chairman of the American Medical Association's former Committee on Alcoholism, "but it is not improving quickly enough." At least partly responsible, he claims, is the teaching program of most medical schools. "With only a few exceptions, most schools devote less than two hours out of a four-year curriculum to the study of normal and abnormal drinking and the treatment of alcoholics." The students spend far more time learning about rare diseases which they may never encounter in their practice, he says.

In general, the techniques of psychotherapy used in the treatment of alcoholism are no more complex than those used in other conditions, and can be learned and utilized effectively by family physicians, internists and other medical specialists.

Other Specialists

With special training, clinical psychologists and psychiatric social workers in many communities have undertaken responsibility for the long-term care of alcoholics and their families, usually working as members of a therapeutic team. Vocational rehabilitation workers, public welfare caseworkers, visiting nurses, and probation and parole officers have also been trained to help alcoholics, as have many personnel workers in industry, who have often been the first to detect the heavy drinking of employees and start them on the way to treatment[14].

Special Family Aid

Because the drinking of an alcoholic may seriously affect other members of his family— or be affected by them—increasing attention has been directed toward treatment of the family as a whole. This has sometimes meant the inclusion of the patient's immediate family in the therapy group. One organization, *Al-Anon*, has been established to help the wives and husbands of alcoholics, using techniques similar to those of AA. Another, *Al-Ateen*, is devoted to aiding the children of alcoholics to understand their parents' problems and to develop more effective ways to handle whatever social and emotional difficulties they themselves may be experiencing.

INDIVIDUAL VS. GROUP THERAPY

Some experienced therapists claim that individual treatment on a one-to-one basis is the most successful. Others prefer group therapy, especially when a group of patients is treated simultaneously by a team of therapists.

An outstanding example of the latter approach is the State of Georgia's Georgian Clinic in Atlanta. "Our conviction from the beginning," says Dr. Vernelle Fox, director of the clinic, "was that these patients were sick in mind, body and soul. If they went to a single therapist, they would get one attitude from the psychiatrist, one from the internist and one from the clergyman. We felt we needed a consolidated attitude from all three."

With a staff of specially trained internists, psychiatrists, nurses, social workers, psychologists, vocational rehabilitation counselors, occupational therapists and clergymen of many faiths, the clinic opened in 1953. It now treats voluntary patients from all over the State, either as inpatients, outpatients, day hospital patients, night hospital patients, or some combination of these. If possible, each patient begins therapy by living in the center for from seven to ten days while undergoing an intensive diagnostic and treatment design process. The program has been described as follows[9]:

> After physical evaluation, the patient undergoes psychiatric, social and vocational screening in an attempt to determine his recovery potential. Medical management and treatment prescription is begun immediately and continued throughout the contact. A series of orientation procedures follows: the patient sees appropriate films, attends personal interviews and counseling sessions, and participates in group meetings. Each week, there are 69 group meetings, together with 16 staff group meetings. A network of occupational, recreational and vocational activities designed to aid self-expression is woven into the program. The patients themselves form a therapeutic community, earlier members sponsoring the newer and more frightened. This "acceptance attitude therapy" is an important factor in orienting and strengthening the new patient. After leaving the clinic, all patients are urged to attend group meetings regularly for at least two years in the outpatient clinic, or at a local chapter of Alcoholics Anonymous or a community-based clinic, and to continue indefinitely if possible.

In 1964, the Atlanta clinic was capable of treating 237 inpatients a year, at an average cost of about $14.53 a day, each. Together with a smaller clinic at Savannah, it could provide day hospital or outpatient care for about 1,500 patients a year.

CHANCES OF RECOVERY

In evaluating the future outlook of alcoholics, many therapists divide patients into three broad groups.

1. *The Psychotic Alcoholics*   These are patients, usually in State mental hospitals, with a severe chronic psychosis. They may account for five to ten percent of all alcoholics.

2. *The Skid Row Alcoholics*   These are the impoverished "homeless men" who usually

no longer have—or never did have—family ties, jobs, or an accepted place in the community. They may account for three to eight percent.

3. *The "Average" Alcoholics* These are men and women who are usually still married and living with their families, still holding a job—often an important one—and still are accepted and reasonably respected members of their community. They account for more than 70 percent of the alcoholics.

From the scanty information available, it would appear that the prognosis for chronic psychotic and Skid Row alcoholics is poor, and that less than 10 to 12 percent can obtain substantial aid from ordinary therapy. For the average alcoholic, the outlook is far more optimistic. Here, three different yardsticks of control have been utilized.

1. *Complete Cure* By strict definition, this would mean that the alcoholic would become able to drink normally or socially, using alcohol moderately and under complete control. Most specialists hold that no alcoholic can ever learn to drink moderately and regard statements to the contrary[4, 7, 15] as unwise or dangerous.

2. *Permanent Abstinence* For most therapists, the goal of treatment is complete abstinence from alcohol, in any form and under any condition, for the rest of the patient's life. According to available information, only a small percentage—perhaps less than 20 percent of all treated patients—have been able to maintain absolute abstinence for more than three to five years. In certain highly selective industrial and business groups, the rate of abstinence may be as high as 50 percent[16].

3. *Rehabilitation* Recently, some leading therapists have been using a different basis of measurement in which success is considered achieved when the patient maintains or re-establishes a good family life, a good work record and a respectable position in the community, and is able to control his drinking *most of the time.*

Depending on the motivation and intelligence of the patient, and his determination to get well; the competence of the therapist; the availability of whatever hospital or clinic facilities, tranquilizers and other drugs which may be needed; and the strong support of family, employer and community—a successful outcome can be expected in at least 60 percent, and some therapists have reported success in 70 or 80 percent.

"It is doubtful that any specific percentage figure has much meaning in itself," says Dr. Selden D. Bacon, director of the Center of Alcohol Studies at Rutgers. "What has a great deal of meaning is the fact that tens of thousands of such cases have shown striking improvement over many years."

There is no evidence that any particular type of therapist—physician, clergyman, AA worker, psychologist or social worker—will achieve better results than another. The chances for a successful outcome apparently depend more on the motivation of the patient and the competence of the therapist than on the type of psychotherapy employed. The earlier that treatment is begun, the better are the prospects for success, although some patients have been treated successfully after many years of excessive drinking....

REFERENCES

1. Alcoholics Anonymous. *Alcoholics Anonymous.* New York: Alcoholics Publishers, 1955.
2. Berke, M., Gordon, J. D., Levy, R. I., & Perrow, C. B. *A Study on the Nonsegregated hospitalization and Alcoholic Patients in a General Hospital.* (Hospital Monograph Series No. 7). Chicago: American Hospital Association, 1959.
3. Block, M. A. Medical treatment of alcoholism. In American Medical Association. *A manual on alcoholism.*

4. Cain, A. H. *The cured alcoholic.* New York: John Day, 1964.
5. Chafetz, M. E., Blane, H. T., Abram, H. S., Golner, J., Lacy, E., McCourt, W. F., Clark, E., & Meyers, W. Establishing treatment relations with alcoholics. *J. Nerv. Ment. Dis.*, 1962, **134**, 395.
6. Chafetz, M. E., Blane, H. T., Abram, H. S., Clark, E., Golner, J. H., Hastie, E. L., & McCourt, W. F. Establishing treatment relations with alcoholics: A supplementary report. *J. Nerv. Ment. Dis.*, 1964, **138**, 390.
7. Davies, D. L. Normal drinking in recovered alcohol addicts. *Quart. J. Stud. Alcohol*, 1962, **23**, 94.
8. Fox, R. Antabuse as an adjunct to psychotherapy in alcoholism. *New York J. Med.*, 1958, **58**, 1540.
9. Fox, V., & Smith, M. A. Evaluation of a chemopsychotherapeutic program for the rehabilitation of alcoholics. *Quart. J. Stud. Alcohol*, 1959, **20**, 767.
10. Hoff, E. C. The use of pharmacological adjuncts in the psychotherapy of alcoholics. *Quart. J. Stud. Alcohol*, 1961, **138** (Suppl. 1).
11. Hoff, E. C. Comprehensive rehabilitation program for alcoholics. *Arch. Environm. Health*, 1963, **7**, 460.
12. Krimmel, H. E. & Falkey, D. B. Short-term treatment of alcoholics. *Social Work*, 1962, **7**, 102.
13. Lolli, G. Alcoholism, 1941–51: A survey of activities in research, education and therapy. V. The treatment of alcohol addiction. *Quart. J. Stud. Alcohol*, 1952, **13**, 461.
14. Mann, M. *New primer on alcoholism.* New York: Holt, Rinehart & Winston, 1958.
15. Pfeffer, A. Z. *Alcoholism.* New York: Grune & Stratton, 1958.
16. Rouse, K. A. *What to do about the employee with a drinking problem.* Chicago: Kemper Insurance Group, 1964.
17. Smith, J. A. Psychiatric treatment of the alcoholic. *JAMA*, 1957, **163**, 734.
18. Straus, R. Medical practice and the alcoholic. *Am. Acad. Polit. Soc. Sci. Ann.*, 1958, **315**, 117.
19. Willard, W. R., & Straus, R. Community approaches to the problems of alcoholism. *New York J. Med.*, 1958, **58**, 2256.

36

Daytop Lodge—A New Treatment
Approach for Drug Addicts*

JOSEPH A. SHELLY and ALEXANDER BASSIN

It hardly seems necessary to beat kettledrums of alarm about the seriousness of the drug addiction problem. Let it suffice to note that at the White House Conference on Narcotic and Drug Abuse, Mayor Wagner of New York startled the gathering by estimating that the city's addicts steal up to a billion dollars worth of merchandise a year to support their habit. In other words, an addict constitutes a one-man crime wave, committing burglaries, larcenies, frauds and/or prostitution to acquire the wherewithal to engage in a strictly cash-on-the-barrelhead business transaction, the purchase of narcotics.)

Addicts fill about half the cells of the New York Penitentiary on Riker's Island. They constitute a sizable percentage of the population of the state prisons. They pillage and plunder the community. Their activities deteriorate neighborhoods, impoverish families and demoralize parents, wives and children.

Thus far, efforts to treat this disorder by conventional means have been consistently and grossly ineffective. Riverside Hospital, a New York facility for adolescent addicts, in operation for a decade, has been able to report only a handful of abstainers over a five-year period, leading some wag to estimate that each cure cost close to a million dollars. Statistics emanating from the U.S. Public Health Service hospitals at Lexington, Kentucky, and Fort Worth, Texas, are equally discouraging. Follow-up studies indicate that many addicts do not display the simple decency—merely out of respect for the $40-a-day treatment taxpayers provide for them at these excellent medical facilities, if nothing else—of at least waiting 48 hours after their release before taking an initial shot of heroin.

Nevertheless, probation departments have a reality problem in this area. Despite the fearfully poor prognosis, men are placed on probation and they almost invariably start "chipping" (occasional usage) on weekends, gradually building up an increased dependence on drugs until they are fully hooked and thoroughly committed to the whirlwind of crime and depredation to support their habit.

Several years ago we heard of the use of Nalline by the correction authorities on the West Coast to provide early detection of the use of heroin, and we reasoned that perhaps such a system of examination of probationers would enable us to determine at an early stage of usage what the situation was so that remedial steps could be taken to nip the habit before it devastated the user. Furthermore, we reasoned that, if the probationer became aware that our department had a surefire means of detection, he would be less inclined to start experimenting with the use of drugs.)

To obtain funds for such an experiment we proposed to the National Institute of Mental Health that a program of Nalline testing be initiated. Dr. Carl Anderson replied with the

*From Shelly, J. A., and Bassin, A., *Corrective Psychiatry and Journal of Social Therapy*, 1965, **11**, 186–193. Copyright © 1965 by the Martin Psychiatric Research Foundation, Inc. Reprinted by permission of the Martin Psychiatric Research Foundation, Inc., and Mr. Shelly and Dr. Bassin.

suggestion that (a) there might be a better detection procedure than Nalline; thin-layer chromatography, for example, and (b) perhaps we should consider the use of a halfway house as a therapeutic community to alter the addict's value system.

At Dr. Anderson's suggestion, we made a study of the treatment and detection procedures throughout the United States. In the company of the eminent criminologist, Dr. Herbert A. Bloch of Brooklyn College, and a psychiatrist with many years' experience in attempting to treat drug addicts, Dr. Daniel Casriel, we visited facilities in different parts of the country but found nothing particularly impressive. Nothing at all, that is, until we came upon the somewhat down-at-the-heel, offbeat operation on the West Coast called Synanon, which made a deep impression on us. We examined the procedures employed at that institution and decided that some of the features could be incorporated into a small facility operated under the auspices of a court bureaucracy.

A number of the free-flowing, spontaneous aspects of Synanon could not be grafted into the somewhat rigid corpus of a court structure. We finally hammered out a research proposal which we trusted would enable us (a) to establish a halfway house for the treatment of drug addicts on probation, (b) to evaluate the rehabilitative effects of such an institution in comparison with results of supervising drug addicts on probation in a small specialized caseload and a large general caseload, (c) to formulate and operate a program of activity designed to provide the addict in the halfway house with a value system and status organization leading to his eventual and reasonably speedy integration into normal society, (d) to employ a testing procedure, thin-layer chromatography, to quantify the progress of an abstinence program among the subjects involved in this experiment and to determine if this chemical procedure may perhaps of itself be an inhibitory mechanism in keeping the addict from returning to the use of narcotics.

NIMH, on the heels of the White House conference, provided a grant of $390,000 to be expended over a five-year period for this purpose. As many before us involved in demonstration research have discovered, we found that there is many a slip between the neat promulgation of a program within the safe covers of a document and its eventual execution in the tough world of reality. Real estate was our first problem. We finally located a white elephant millionaire's mansion consisting of 20 rooms in a suburban section of the New York area on a seven-acre wooded lot overlooking Raritan Bay. But our difficulties with real estate paled to insignificance when we began to wrestle with the problem of management.

During the first year we went through some four managers, all of whom were well-meaning but who simply expired under the strain of attempting to cope with the population of the most skillful manipulators, liars and con-men our civilization seems to be able to produce. Nevertheless, despite ups and downs and a daily crisis situation, the project seemed to be doing well. In contrast with most prison and hospital situations, our men impressed all, including even their closest relatives, as having become remarkably friendly, outgoing, self-possessed. We administered thin-layer chromatography examinations regularly and, although occasionally we obtained a positive or questionable test finding, we were able to resolve most of the situations without difficulty. Because of "splits" (unauthorized departures) we were unable during the first year of operation to obtain the 25 residents the program permitted. As a new probationer was admitted, another resident would depart for one reason or another.

But our overall evaluation of the situation, the undeniable spirit of hope and confidence that we observed at every visit, gave us the confident spirit that we were on the road to pioneering a new and significant treatment methodology for the addict.

Last October we were finally able to obtain the services of a Synanon graduate, David

Deitch, who had a history of some 14 years of heroin addiction. Deitch installed two assistants, fellow drug addicts he had trained at Synanon, and with his bride of a few months, Sue, a wonderfully warm-hearted girl of 24, a graduate of Brandeis University, who became acquainted with Deitch when he was director of the Westport facility of Synanon, moved in as the new manager of Daytop Lodge.

INTAKE INTERVIEW

All features of our treatment approach were described in the original proposal to NIMH, but seemed to take on new meaning and direction under the supervision of Deitch. The first step in the basic process occurs when it is established that a particular defendant meets the basic eligibility requirements for admission to Daytop Lodge. He is presented to the judge on the basis of a presentence investigation with a recommendation that he be given an opportunity to attempt to enter our research facility. We explain to the judge that we have no control over the operation; it is entirely up to the man to prove to the management of the halfway house that he sincerely wishes to give up the habit and reform. The man is released from jail, makes his way across the street to our office, where he receives a short interview, a hand-written copy of directions for reaching Daytop and a dollar bill to cover his expenses on the way.

When the man arrives at Daytop, after a ferry and bus ride, he is usually told to sit on a chair in a veranda, and he usually remains there with no one speaking to him for as long as two hours. He finds himself in the midst of the easy-going camaraderie of men, but he observes that the atmosphere is completely different from what he has experienced in the past in hospitals, prisons and other institutions. What shakes him the most, however, is to see former associates with whom he might have shot up in alleyways, perhaps sharing the same spike, who seem not to see him, who look through him as if he were not there. He remains sitting before an open, unlocked door, but somehow does not get up to leave. He thus passes successfully the first step in the initiation procedure to enter the Daytop fraternity.

Finally, the applicant is called into the office for an interview. The office is comfortably furnished but without a desk or other appurtenances of status. Instead, there is only a large coffee table with books and papers on it, a couch and soft chairs around it. Three clean-cut, conventionally dressed young men start questioning him in a kindly, sympathetic manner. Within a few minutes, the addict feels that he is at long last in control of the situation. These are obviously social worker types whom he can con out of their back teeth. They let him continue without interruption for several minutes before one of them brings him up short.

"Hey, stop this garbage. Who do you think you're talking to!"

The two interviewers speak to each other: "Did you ever hear such s—t in your life!"

"This dope fiend thinks he's inside another joint."

"He didn't get enough affection and love from his mudder and fodder, I bet."

They continue to ridicule the now devastated addict before beginning a "cleanup" operation. They explain they are not social workers, as he had obviously thought, who can be fooled, bamboozled and conned. On the contrary, they are reformed addicts who only a short time before would have behaved exactly as he did. But now they are living in an environment where honesty, reliability and responsibility are the watchwords. Here one gets nothing for nothing. You have to earn everything. You can lie and cheat no more.

During the early orientation interviews, the addict will repeatedly be advised that, despite his physical stature and chronological age, he is a child in terms of maturity, responsibility and ability to think ahead. He will be regarded as a 3-year-old who must be told what to do with the expectation that if he disobeys he will be punished promptly. The whole design of the program is to help him grow from a child of 3 to an adult. We have only one year available for this progress, so he'll have to work hard if he wants to make it. On the other hand, if he wishes to return to chasing the bag, to be a childish addict, to die in some gutter from an o.d., that would be his decision.

Finally, the newcomer is advised that we have little confidence in the usual preoccupation of social workers, psychologists and psychiatrists with the finding of the essential *cause* of his addiction. The addict uses the professional to slough off responsibility for his behavior. The personnel at Daytop does not permit the addict to blame for his behavior his parents, the school, the neighborhood, associates or society. The only cause recognized at Daytop for being an addict is STUPIDITY.

In other words, the concept of the drug addict as an ill person and therefore automatically entitled to the recognized prerogatives of the role of the ill in our society in terms of sympathetic understanding, special concern, leniency and forgiveness is vehemently fought as an ideology.

"Did anybody force you to stick a dirty needle into your arm and infect yourself with milk sugar?" the addict is challenged. "Was it your father or mother who insisted you shoot up? Was it the tough cop on the beat? Was it your girl friend or school teacher?"

If the addict attempts to extricate himself from his tendency to throw blame in all directions, the resident and staff bring him to the reality of his behavior: that he alone is to blame and the only tenable explanation for his behavior is simple, unadulterated stupidity on his part.

THE RESOCIALIZATION PROCESS CONTINUES

After his initial interview, the defendant is introduced to some senior members of the house who shake him down from head to toenails with the thoroughness of experts. He is advised that from this point onward, so long as he wishes to remain in the Lodge, he may not make any phone calls, write any letters, receive mail or possess money without specific permission. All these steps are necessary to help him be reformed and become a man. On the other hand, he is not held in the Lodge by force. He can leave any time he wants to. There are no bars on the windows or locks on the doors. "We don't need you, you need us!" he is told over and over.

At the same time the newcomer receives this orientation, his family obtains some astonishing advice: For the time being, they are to become as cold, rejecting and hostile to the defendant as they possibly can. If he telephones, they are not to answer; if he sneaks out a letter, they should return it unopened to Daytop Lodge; if he appears at their home with the pitiful, woebegone, contrite attitude the addict knows so well how to assume and starts to make excuses for leaving the Lodge, they are to say: "Go back to Daytop. Get lost. We have nothing to say to you," and slam the door in his face.

GROUP THERAPY BY AUTHENTIC ENCOUNTERS

The principal formal medium for effecting value and behavioral changes is a variety of group therapy sessions called group encounters. These are compulsory for all residents and are held three times a week in the evening from 8 to 9:30. The population of the house is divided in groups of three with an approximately even number of no more than 10 at each session. The composition of the group is changed for every session and any house member may request he be included in an encounter with any specific other residents. Or, if the member demands it, an emergency encounter may be scheduled on only a few minutes' notice.

How do these sessions materially differ from conventional group therapy? In the first place, there is no formal leader, but each group includes at least one member trained and experienced in this form of group interaction. Second, the search for elusive primary causes for addiction based on some alleged childhood trauma or deprivation is hooted down as a waste of time and a maneuver on the part of the participant to avoid facing his problems. Third, the resident's behavior in specific terms become the subject of discussion and criticism rather than events of decades ago. Finally, every member is expected to react spontaneously on a visceral level employing, if he feels the need for it, the crudest terminology and vehement verbal expression. The group concentrates on reaching a "gut level" with the intent of having participants react at a rock bottom emotional level rather than on the intellectual plane that is so frequently characteristic of conventional group therapy.

The vehemence of these interchanges is hard to believe. Four-letter epithets and gutter language bounce off the walls as the participants engage in the process of "ungluing" a man to make him open to the possibility of basic change. The members examine each other and are critical about the extent to which they are adhering to the basic precepts of the house for remaking themselves into honest, decent, conscientious human beings. They remind each other that they are trying to become worthwhile people free of the criminal code of the street and prepared to accept the square values about the primary goodness of hard work, decent relations with one's fellows, concern about the welfare of his brothers. The primary rules of the house are: 1. No drugs or alcohol of any type. 2. No physical violence. 3. No shirking of responsibility. These are repeated so that no newcomer has the excuse that he didn't know the law. If a dispute develops during the day, the contenders are expected to maintain their decorum until the opportunity to square off at a group encounter arrives. The group meeting is repeatedly presented to the residents as a "pressure cooker" for fast personality change, as well as the safety valve for house arguments.

The process of indoctrination started during the admission procedure continues throughout the residence of the addict. At least a dozen times a day the newcomer hears someone tell him that the group is antidrug, antialcohol and anticrime. He is reminded that, like a 3-year-old child, he may not be permitted outside the building alone because he could get killed. He must check in and out at the desk and leave only with the permission of a coordinator in the company of a senior resident. He is not to speak to newcomers and at the beginning he must realize that, as an addict, the only thing he really knows how to do is to shoot dope and to go to prison.

The newcomer is forbidden to engage in the type of conversation that constitutes 90% of the verbal intercourse that takes place in the usual institutional setting of drug addicts. He may not express any sympathy for the code of the street, which calls on a criminal to remain silent about the antisocial activities of his peers. He is expected to apply an honor code that is stricter in many respects than the one imposed at West Point. The law of the street, which forbids squealing, finking and bearing tales, the resident is advised, may be appropriate for dope-shooting addicts and criminals, but here at the Lodge we are involved in saving lives, and any member who fails to assume responsibility for straightening out a tottering brother is endangering that man's salvation as well as the fate of the entire enterprise. On this score, it is not sufficient for a resident to abstain from violating any of the tenets of the organization himself. On the contrary, he is expected to bring up at the thrice-weekly encounter meetings a critique of a fellow member who may be careless about such a triviality as washing his coffee cup in order to gain practice in informing the environment when a fellow resident is thinking of leaving to return to the use of drugs. A man may be censured for not calling an emergency fireplace meeting to discuss the waywardness of a buddy who seems to be "in a bag," involved in morbid self-analysis instead of working for the welfare of all.

THE SEMINAR MEETINGS

Residents at Daytop Lodge are provided an opportunity to deal with abstract and sometimes highly philosophical material in the course of the daily seminar sessions, which take place after lunch. A passage from Ralph Waldo Emerson, for example, may be written on the blackboard and members in turn get up and react to the material on an extemporaneous level.

To continue the resocialization process, every Saturday night a party is held to which outsiders are invited. The residents mingle with the guests and practice their newly acquired skills in social relations. Students from colleges and universities within a radius of 50 miles are frequent visitors at these get-togethers.

THE STATUS LADDER

The management of Daytop Lodge is involved in the operation of a carefully formulated status system in which ascendancy is gained by displaying the virtues of old-fashioned hard work, integrity, honesty and concern for the well-being of one's fellow men. The length of time in which a resident has remained "clean" is a primary factor in moving up the status ladder. The resident manager, with the help of his two assistants, is on a constant lookout for developing the potential of each member and the prospects for moving up are constantly discussed at the group encounters and even during casual conversations during the day.

SPECIAL MEETINGS AND PROCEDURES

Probe sessions are held from time to time to analyze some particular problem or difficulty that might have been developing. For example, since the composition of the house is almost equally divided between white, Negro and Puerto Ricans, meetings of the various ethnic groups may be held under the leadership of the resident manager to discuss any stresses that may be related to matters of bias and discrimination.

Formal role-training sessions, at which members are provided with a chance to try out various situations they may encounter in the community, constitute a favorite form of teaching.

Promotion to the procurement team, which has the duty of visiting community merchants in an effort to obtain donations of items not available under terms of the grant, is another form of therapeutic endeavor.

The house is now experimenting with the most intensive form of group therapy, a *Marathon Encounter*, which is planned to last for 24 hours, during which members will continue in constant interaction to reach, as Deitch expresses it, "the most fundamental of gut levels."

We have been approached by the city administration to assist in the establishment of a Daytop Lodge type of program involving a minimum of 300 addicts, with the possibility of reaching a maximum of 1,000, to be housed within a complex to be called Daytop Village. We are inclined to feel that the larger number of residents will provide a richer environment, including the presence of females, for the dynamics leading to personality change and speedier maturation to occur. We trust that this confidence will be supported by objective data when we report on this matter a year from now.

37

Geriatric Behavioral Prosthetics*†

OGDEN R. LINDSLEY

Human behavior is a functional relationship between a person and a specific social or mechanical environment. If the behavior is deficient, we can alter either the individual or the environment in order to produce effective behavior. Most previous attempts to restore behavioral efficiency by retraining, punishment, or physiological treatment have focused on only one side of this relation, the deficient individual. This approach implies that normal individuals can function in all currently existing social environments, that deficient individuals can be normalized, and that there are ordinarily no deficient environments. Scientists have only recently directly focused on the environmental side of deficient behavior functions and on the design of specialized or *prosthetic environments* to restore competent performance.

Prosthetic environments are not new, however. For centuries specialized environments have supported or reinforced the behavior of infants and children. Special foods, feeding devices, bedding, furniture and clothing for infants are commonplace. Special entertainments—toys, primary colors, simple books, music, games—have been less clearly recognized in their behavioral role of reinforcers designed particularly for children. All of these are provided by society in expectation of the services the child will provide as an adult.

More recently, prosthetic environments have been extended to the physically handicapped. Blind persons use Braille books, noise-making canes, seeing-eye dogs, and specially designed houses. Paraplegic veterans of war have specially designed homes provided by a grateful public for relatively brief service to society.

But what of the aged, veterans of an entire lifetime of social service? Are they provided with special environments designed to support their behavior at its maximum? Are we using their behavior most efficiently?

To prolong health, physicians offer aging persons a wide range of physiological prosthetics, from vitamins and hormones to increased oxygen utilization, for their internal

*From *New thoughts on old age*, edited by R. Kastenbaum. Copyright © 1964 by Springer Publishing Company. Reprinted by permission of Springer Publishing Company, and Dr. Lindsley.

†Read at Second Annual Symposium on Old Age, Cushing Hospital, Framingham, Mass., May 21, 1963, and dedicated to my grandmother, Mrs. James Ogden Lindsley, who lived well beyond her environment and died in an institution at age 89.

Research was conducted in the Behavior Research Laboratory, Department of Psychiatry, Harvard Medical School, located at Metropolitan State Hospital, Waltham, Mass., and was supported by research grant MH-05054 from the Psychopharmacology Service Center, National Institute of Mental Health, U.S. Public Health Service.

The cooperation of the Department of Psychiatry (Jack R. Ewalt, M.D., Chairman) and the staff of Metropolitan State Hospital (William F. McLaughlin, M.D., Superintendent), the able assistance of our laboratory staff, and, most especially, the participation of our patients has greatly facilitated our research.

environment[8, 10, 17]. Beyond providing eyeglasses, hearing aids, dentures, cribs, and crutches, however, science has done little to modify the external mechanical and social environments of the aged. The skills of current behavioral science, and free-operant conditioning in particular, can provide more than compound lenses, audio amplifiers, and mechanical restraint and support. Behavioral engineers can design prosthetic environments to support the behavior of the aged as crutches support their weight.

In this chapter, I will offer suggestions, developed from the methods and discoveries of free-operant conditioning, for developing geriatric prosthetic environments.[1]

In *free-operant conditioning* the frequency of performance of an act is altered by locating and arranging suitable consequences (reinforcement). The person being conditioned is at all times free to make the response and receive the arranged consequences, or to make other responses. By isolating the individual within an appropriate enclosure, the behavior specialist can empirically—rather than merely statistically —control all environmental events which can affect the behavior he is studying. The behavioral response and any environmental manipulations whose effects on the response are being studied can be automatically and continuously recorded. This environmental control and automatic, continuous recording mark the method as a laboratory natural science, comparable to modern chemistry, physics and biology.

Free-operant methods are suited to behavioral geriatrics for several reasons.[2] Concentrating on *motivational aspects*, or consequences, of behavior, free-operant conditioning alters the *immediate environment* to generate and maintain behavior. The sensitivity of the methods to subtle changes in such aspects of the person's performance as response rate, efficiency and perseverance makes these methods appropriate to the study of *single individuals*. Because the sensitivity does not decrease with very long periods of application with the same individual, reliable *longitudinal studies* are possible. Free-operant conditioning methods for the analysis of functional and dynamic relationships between individuals and both their *social and nonsocial environments* can produce separate measures of mechanical dexterity, intellectual functioning, and social adjustment.

Free-operant principles and techniques may provide behavioral geriatrics with (1) a fresh theoretical approach; (2) laboratory description, prognosis, and evaluation; (3) design of prosthetic environments; and (4) individualized prosthetic prescriptions. Although I know of no free-operant experiments on the aged, and research in our laboratory with senile psychotics has not been extensive, preliminary suggestions can be well supported by the results of extensive experiments on the behavior of psychotic, neurotic, and mentally retarded individuals, whose behavioral deficits are usually as debilitating and challenging as those of aged persons.[3]

A FRESH THEORETICAL APPROACH

Free-operant conditioning principles can provide a highly relevant approach for increasing the efficiency of ward management and patient care routines. In this new approach,

---

[1]Suggestions for designing prosthetic environments for the behavior of retarded persons have also been made recently[29].

[2]These reasons also make free-operant methods especially appropriate to a wide range of clinical behavioral problems. For a discussion of applications of the method to psychotherapy see Lindsley[30].

[3]For an excellent review of these experiments see Rachman, S.[34].

ward attendants do not perform custodial tasks. They are instead trained to act as behavioral engineers in arranging appropriate behavioral programs and reinforcements, so that the patients themselves maintain their ward and their persons.[4] Most important in this application of free-operant methods are (1) precise behavioral description; (2) functional definition of stimulus, response, and reinforcement; and (3) attention to behavioral processes.

Precise behavioral description facilitates communication between behavioral engineer and ward supervisor. It not only focuses attention on the actual behavioral movement which is occurring at either too high or too low a rate, but also permits observing and counting the response and directly reinforcing it with suitable consequences.

Functional definition of stimulus, response, and reinforcement focuses the attention of the nurse or attendant on the relationship between the behavior she is attempting to manage and her management procedures. When she realizes that an event may be a stimulus for one patient but not for another, and that a second event may be reinforcing to one patient but punishing to still another, then she recognizes the full complexity of human behavior, and in behavioral management no longer makes errors based upon misplaced empathy and generalization. For example, the socially deprived patients found in large hospitals may be rewarded by any attention from the nurse, even scolding for misbehavior. Consequently, a patient will continue to do the thing for which he was scolded in attempts to obtain the social contacts from the nurse, even though the nurse designed the topography of these contacts as punishment for what the patient was doing.

Attention to the behavioral processes of positive reinforcement, extinction, satiation, and mild punishment has proven extremely useful in engineering a ward for maximal behavioral accomplishment. Ayllon and Michael[3] successfully trained ward nurses to increase patients' self-feeding by talking to patients only when they fed themselves. Ayllon[2] also trained nurses to satiate a towel hoarder by filling her room with towels, and to punish the wearing of extra clothing by letting a patient eat only when she was below a certain weight with her clothes on.

Important for generating maximal behavior on a geriatric ward is the early establishment of a conditioned general reinforcer, or token, which must be used to purchase all items and opportunities of importance and reinforcing value to the patients. The ward tokens are used by the attendants and the nurses to reinforce appropriate behavior. The patients can then use the tokens to purchase personal articles, cigarettes, afternoon naps, television and record playing time, talks with chaplains and volunteers, and all other events of value and importance to them. The patients will readily perform custodial duties on their ward in order to earn the tokens. Ayllon has successfully used tokens in this way in managing a ward of chronic psychotic patients[5].

High on the list of types of behavior that it is desirable to generate in a geriatric patient are very mild physical exercise and sun-bathing. The patient is immediately reinforced with a token for each exercise period and for small daily gains in his exercise achievement. Such

---

[4]Research scientists suggesting new approaches for managing patients often overlook the crucial administrative problem of recruiting and training personnel. It is a good idea, but if it works who will put it into practice? An excellent source of behavioral engineers who could train and supervise attendants and nurses in these new prosthetic procedures would be Special Educators. Their current training, motivation, and philosophy are ideal for operant prosthetic methods. A few graduate courses and some ward experience under the supervision of an expert should make Special Educators into excellent Prosthetic Behavioral Engineers.

[5]Personal communication from T. Ayllon, State Hospital, Anna, Ill., 1963.

exercise, shaped very gradually and watched carefully by the ward physician, can do much to restore physical health and well-being to a geriatric patient.

LABORATORY DESCRIPTION, PROGNOSIS, AND EVALUATION

Free-operant conditioning methods can be used to develop a behavior research laboratory for the accurate measurement and description of behavior deficits found in the aged. Inglis[19] has found that psychometric tests are almost useless in these applications and recommends that experimental methods be applied to geriatric problems.

Over the past 10 years, we have clearly demonstrated that a free-operant conditioning laboratory is useful in describing, prognosticating and evaluating psychoses[24, 28]. In brief, our laboratory consists of several small experimental rooms which provide controlled environments for automatically recording behavioral deficits. Patients are brought to the rooms by a technician and permitted to behave freely in them for a period of time long enough to determine accurately the presence and degree of certain behavioral deficits.

The rooms differ from one another only in the equipment necessary for measuring different behavioral deficits. One room, for example, may have a chair and a wall panel with a single knob on it. Pulling the knob is reinforced by the illumination of a television screen mounted in the panel. The rate at which a patient pulls the knob indicates the reinforcing power of the narrative material presented to him via the television system. The material televised can be standard commercial broadcasts, specialized programs recorded on audiovisual tape, or a family visitor seated in front of a closed-circuit television camera in another part of the laboratory. In this room, the differential reinforcing value of audiovisual narrative reinforcers can be objectively determined by the continuous, automatic, cumulative records of knob-pulling. Similar rooms have been developed for recording behaviors as disparate as hallucinating and pacing in chronic psychotics, social deficits, and a patient's interest in his psychotherapist or visitor[11, 26, 27, 28].

Fully automatic programming of stimuli and recording of responses insures completely objective measurement. Technicians who do not differentially involve themselves with the data handle the patients and equipment and therefore do not introduce complicating observer bias. Furthermore, longitudinal studies are not disrupted when technicians are changed. Because there is no observer bias, cross-hospital and cross-cultural comparisons can be made. Because a fully controlled environment and automatic recording dispense with observer ratings, longitudinal studies can be conducted without the loss of observer sensitivity which occurs with repeated measurement[21]. With automatic programming and recording, verbal instructions can be used or not. This opportunity to dispense with verbal instructions permits analysis of their effects and consequently more specific behavioral analysis, as well as the study of nonverbal patients. Free-operant methods thus provide prognostic data and reliable, valid behavioral measures which can be included in case histories even more confidently than blood pressure and blood cell count, which usually involve observer bias.

Long-term laboratory measures of the type and degree of behavioral deficits of individual patients permit exact evaluation of the effects of therapeutic variables on each patient's behavior. The behavioral effects of medications, as well as the effects of such social variables as ward reassignments, home visits and deaths in the family, can be readily determined.

Since records are available on each patient, objective, high quality behavioral research can be conducted by physicians in charge of medication by occasionally referring a patient to the behavior laboratory for a current evaluation. Therapeutic dosage can be accurately adjusted to the deficit and drug-response of each patient. Individualized behavioral treatment can then be conducted with the same precision with which individualized physiological treatment is now conducted in well-staffed general hospitals.

DESIGN OF PROSTHETIC ENVIRONMENTS

There is little hope of retarding the aging process at this time, but we can reduce its behavioral debilitation by designing environments which compensate for or support the specific behavioral deficits of each aged person.[6] Because we will not actually alter the deficits, but merely provide an environment in which the deficits are less debilitating, these environments cannot be considered purely therapeutic. Therapeutic environments generate some behavior which is maintained when the patient is returned to the normal or general social environment. Therapeutic environments are essentially training or retraining centers for the generation of behavioral skills which maintain themselves once the patient has left the therapeutic environment. Prosthetic environments, however, must operate continually in order to decrease the debilitation resulting from the behavioral deficit. Eyeglasses are prosthetic devices for deficient vision, hearing aids for deficient hearing, and crutches and wheel chairs for deficient locomotion.

To describe suggestions for geriatric prosthetic environments as accurately as possible, I will use the analytical categories of the laboratory behavioral scientist: (1) discriminative stimuli; (2) response devices; (3) reinforcers; and (4) reinforcement schedules. The number of different types of special stimuli and devices required for prosthesis in each of these categories must be determined by the analysis of each aged individual. The types of environmental alteration required to support aged behavior cannot be determined until the number, degree, and range of behavioral deficits are determined. It may be that a given prosthetic device can be used to prosthetize more than one type of behavioral deficit. Adequately detailed analysis may also show that a single behavioral deficit can be prosthetized by more than one device. In these cases, the most economic and most general devices would be selected first.

My suggestions for the design of specific prosthetic environments for aged individuals are certainly not exhaustive. They are only suggestions for the direction of future research, examples of the kinds of things we should try in searching for new prosthetic devices. The range of prosthetic devices is limited only by the creativity and ingenuity of the investigator and the time and funds at his disposal. His time and funds are, in turn, limited only by society's interest in providing devices for restoring effective behavior to its older citizens.

Geriatric Discriminative Stimuli

The environmental events which signal when a response is appropriate and when it should not be made are extremely important in controlling behavior. Traffic lights are a

---

[6]The American Psychiatric Association (1959) conducted a survey on the care of patients over 65 in public mental hospitals and gleaned the following suggestions for improving the design of geriatric facilities: tilted bathroom mirrors for wheelchair patients; better lighting with no glare; ramps and short stair risers; guardrails, hold-bars, and non-skid floors; draft-free radiant heat; higher chairs to eliminate stooping to sit; facilities for daytime naps; and work, recreational, and social activities geared to the physical abilities of the patients.

familiar example. These colored lights are useful discriminative stimuli to a person with normal color vision, much less useful to a color-blind person, and of no use to a totally blind person. The geriatric patient may well have behavioral deficits which, like blindness, limit the range of discriminative stimuli in the normal environment which can control his behavior. The full and exact nature of geriatric behavioral deficits has not yet been determined.

The *intensity and size of discriminative stimuli* for the aged has received some prosthetic attention. Eyeglasses have been developed for amplifying and correcting visual responses. Hearing aids have been developed for amplifying sounds to serve as discriminative stimuli for people whose hearing is deficient. Touch, smell, and taste amplifiers have not yet been developed, probably because our basic knowledge of these senses is more limited.

Simple and dramatic patterns, long durations and higher intensities of stimulation should be investigated, for we can increase the intensity of the environmental stimulus when prosthetic amplifiers are not available.[7] It is amazing, for example, that although we give children books with large type, we force elderly people with deficient vision to use heavy eyeglasses or hand magnifying lenses to read normal-size type. We might find that even with large type, certain aged persons with deficient vision develop headaches or become nervous while reading. If we provided Braille or "talking books" for these individuals, we might find an increase in their usefulness to us and to themselves.

Multiple sense displays should be investigated in attempts to design geriatric discriminative stimuli. While an older person might not respond appropriately to a loud sound alone or to a bright light alone, he might respond appropriately to a simultaneous combination of loud sound and bright light. A normal person under the high control of a small portion of his environment is much more likely to respond to a multiple sense display than to a single sense display in the rest of his environment. Similarly, an aged person with generally weakened attention might respond more appropriately to a multiple sense display.

Expanded auditory and visual narrative stimuli should also be investigated. Melrose [32] has found that many aged persons who cannot hear normal speech can hear expanded speech. Expanded speech does not differ in intensity or tone from normal speech. It is just spread out more in time, being truly slower. Melrose's finding suggests that old people cannot integrate rapidly presented information. It is the frequency of the *words*, not the frequency of the sounds, which they cannot integrate. This suggests that the visual discriminative response to a pictorial drama might also be deficient when the drama is presented at the normal rate. By using video-tape recording systems to expand visual materials, we might restore understanding of and interest in visual narration to many aged people. The possibility of using expanded auditory and visual materials as reinforcing stimuli is discussed below.

Response-controlled discriminative stimulation should be tried as a prosthetic device for geriatric patients who appear to have intermittent attention. If a patient is periodically unresponsive to stimulation, the stimuli which occur during these "dead" periods in his attention may as well not be presented. To him the world has missing portions, as if a normal person were watching a movie and periodically the projector lens was covered for brief periods of time while the narration continued. There would be many important portions of the movie narration to which he would have no opportunity to respond.

---

[7] I have been told that Lord Amulree of University College Hospital, London, arranged for stronger odors to be added to utility gas so that aged persons with decreased senses of smell would know when the gas heaters had blown out and would not be asphyxiated.

Response-controlled stimulation permits the narration to move along in time only when the patient is responding to it. If the patient does not respond to a given stimulus, the next stimulus is not presented. Rather, it is stored until the patient responds again. The stimulus can be stored either by stopping the tape or film or by running a small continuous loop in which the last narrative event responded to is repeated. When the patient becomes attentive again and the next response is made, the narration continues. With this technique, the "dead" portions in the patient's attention would merely increase the total presentation time without removing portions of the narration.

Response-controlled stimulation could, of course, be used for non-narrative discriminative stimuli such as signal lights, as well as for more complicated and more socially relevant narrative forms of stimulation. Many other modifications of discriminative stimuli should be tried in attempts to prosthetize discrimination deficits in the aged. The examples given are merely suggestions of what can be done in this field.

Geriatric Response Devices

The design of prosthetic response devices for geriatric patients is a wide-open field. Innumerable response force amplifiers are available for normal persons. Most hand tools, for example, amplify response force. Hammers increase the force of manual pounding by extending the leverage of the arm; wrenches, the force of finger grip. In a sense, most modern machinery is designed to increase the force or accuracy of normal human action.

Response force amplifiers should be provided for old people with extremely weak motor responses. Geriatric environments should contain a much wider range of response force amplifiers than the fully automated factory or fully electrified home. Why, for example, must the aged open their own doors in hospitals when supermarket and garage doors are opened electronically?

For elderly people with feeble voices, the force of speech could be amplified by throat microphones and transistorized amplifiers. Such a simple device might greatly facilitate communication between older persons.

Wide response topographies should be provided so that palsied movements and inaccurate placement of hands and fingers would not be disabling. An individual with extreme palsy, for example, could operate a telephone with push buttons, instead of the normal dial arrangement, if the buttons were far enough apart and required enough pressure so they could not be accidentally pushed by a shaking hand. The voice-operated telephones in the Bell system design will, of course, completely prosthetize dialing deficits.

The standard electrical typewriter, sensitive to the slightest touch, is an example of a device which maximizes the efficiency of a normal person for whom accuracy and placement is no problem, but which is probably the most poorly designed typewriter for operation by an older person. The older person would make many errors of placement, and in trembling would jam the sensitive machine by depressing two keys simultaneously.

Rate switches, which operate only when repeatedly pressed above a certain rate, would be useful in maintaining high constant attention from aged persons with intermittent or weak attention. Most complicated and dangerous manufacturing machinery previously was operated by single-throw hand switches. The machine operated as long as the switch stayed in the "down" position. An inattentive operator could mash his fingers or cut off his arm. Stationary switches of this sort were found to be too dangerous even for normal individuals. They were replaced with spring-loaded switches which require continuous force in order for the machine to operate. Foot switches which must be continually depressed by the operator have greatly reduced industrial accidents, because when the operator turns away or leaves the machine, he takes his foot off the control switch and the machine stops.

An even higher degree of attention could be demanded by using a switch which had to be pressed repeatedly at a high rate in order for the machine to operate. A high rate of pressing demands closer attention than does continual depression of a switch. Impulse shorteners in the circuits of operant conditioning response levers are used for this purpose. Remember that a sleeping, dozing or even dead person could operate a spring-loaded switch and its connected machinery by the weight of his inactive body. A switch that must be continually pressed should reduce the accident hazards of machine operation for many older persons with mild attention disorders. When their attention drifted so that they failed to press the switch at the required rate, the machine would automatically stop.

Response feedback systems should be developed so that response location errors can be corrected before they actually occur. For example, if an older person could not always control his fingers, he could be prevented from pushing a wrong button or placing his finger at the edge of a saw by a loud tone which sounded whenever his finger was moving away from the appropriate response location. Such response feedback systems could greatly compensate for a reduced kinesthetic ability. In effect, they would substitute for the deficient afferent input from the aged limbs which once guided the hands so accurately.

If a little time, money, and thought were applied to the problem, I am sure that a wide range of imaginative and successful devices could be developed for helping aged persons overcome their fairly obvious response deficits.

Geriatric Reinforcers

The generally low interest or motivation of the aged is very familiar. The elderly person appears capable of behaving but has lost his "will to live." We assume that he is able to respond, because on occasional brief instants he "lights up" and behaves appropriately. Rather than interpreting brief periods of appropriate behavior as normal episodes or phases in the aging process, we usually attribute them to special circumstances which temporarily increase motivation.

In precise behavioral terms, this means either that the reinforcers currently programmed in his immediate environment are no longer adequate or that the old person has simply lost the ability to be reinforced. The difference is of great importance and should be tested experimentally by attempting to reinforce his behavior with a wide range of events.

Individualized historical reinforcers. We should look closely at a geriatric patient's rare moments of high behavioral rate. Is some unusual, more appropriate reinforcer operating—something from the past—an old song, an old food, an old friend? If parts of such individualized historical reinforcers were recorded and presented on audio tape or closed-circuit television, an old person might perform regularly at high rates to hear and see them.

Expanded narrative reinforcers. Melrose's[32] recent research suggests another possibility. If an aged person can comprehend expanded speech but not speech presented at a normal rate, he might be reinforced by expanded music and narrative themes, when the same themes presented at the normal rates would not be reinforcing. In seeking more adequate reinforcers for aged persons, we should explore music, movies, and video tapes expanded in both the audio and visual dimensions; for example, video tapes could be used to expand visits from family and friends.

Casual observation of music preferences of different generations supports this notion. Today's oldster, who prefers the waltz, did the turkey trot as a youth. Today's middle-ager prefers ballads and ballroom tempos, but did the Charleston or big-apple in high school and college. Today's teenage twister may also be waltzing a few decades from now. The perennial reinforcing value of the waltz to older persons may be due to their need for a slower, more expanded auditory reinforcer. Conversely, the high interest of youngsters in the chipmunk-singing, sound-effects records suggests that very young children might be more reinforced by compressed music presented at extremely high rates.

If appropriate historical or expanded reinforcers could be located for each aged individual, newer and more generally available events might even be conditioned to the idiosyncratic reinforcers—that is, the adequate but idiosyncratic reinforcers might be used to develop or restore value to the general conditioned reinforcers currently used in society. By gradual shaping and conditioning, an old person could be given a new interest in contemporary life.

Long-range personal reinforcers, such as education, development of a skill, or the building of a reputation, would have little value for an old person. Each step in the development of skill or reputation would have little conditioned reinforcement value, since it would merely be a step on a stairway which an old person could hardly hope to scale completely. He might reasonably ask, "Build a skill for what? To die tomorrow?"

A child is almost completely under the control of the immediate environment because he has not yet acquired long-range personal reinforcers. An old person may be solely at the mercy of the immediate environment, not only because of severe recent memory loss, but because long-range personal reinforcers are made impotent by brief and uncertain life expectancy. This dependence of both old people and children on immediate personal reinforcers may be why aged persons are often described as "childish."

Long-range social reinforcers which would be of value to society no matter when the older person died might be more useful with the aged. The conditioned reinforcement would be the contribution to the next generation. However, the development of this type of reinforcer would be extremely complicated, would require the participation of the members of society at large, and would still have to be conditioned to immediate personal reinforcers.

Extremely powerful, immediate personal reinforcers might be located. We should try highly compelling expanded musical and visual narrations, exciting foods, costly and beautiful clothing, and so forth. Reinforcers of this nature are costly, but they might generate such high rates of behavior in aged persons that their high dollar cost would be compensated by savings in medical care and ward management.

Geriatric Reinforcement Schedules

In most social situations, reinforcement occurs intermittently [14]. Not all responses are immediately reinforced; only a small portion are followed by a reinforcing episode. Nevertheless, in normal individuals, responding continues at high, predictable rates which are presumably maintained by conditioned reinforcement from the occasionally reinforced responses. In our long-term experiments with psychotic children and adults, however, we have found many patients who are unable to maintain high rates of responding on intermittent schedules of reinforcement, even when adequate reinforcers are used [24]. These deficits in responding for intermittent reinforcement are probably attributable to deficits in recent memory and in formation of conditioned reinforcement.

It is very possible that many geriatric patients will prove unable to maintain high rates of responding on intermittent schedules and will have to be kept on regular reinforcement contingencies in which every response is immediately followed with a reinforcing episode. Other patients may have to be reinforced on conjugate programs in which the intensity of a continuously available reinforcer is a direct function of the response rate. Conjugate reinforcement permits the use of narrative social reinforcers and appears to go deeper into sleep, anesthesia, infancy and psychosis than does episodic reinforcement [22, 25, 31]. Conjugate reinforcement may also go deeper into aging and generate behavior in geriatric patients who would not behave on any episodic schedule of reinforcement.

INDIVIDUALIZED PROSTHETIC PRESCRIPTIONS

If a geriatric hospital were equipped with a behavior laboratory, each aged patient could visit the laboratory upon admission. His specific behavioral deficits would be measured, and prosthetic stimuli, responses, reinforcers and reinforcement schedules prescribed. The laboratory would determine the patient's current learning ability and assess the extent to which his current behavioral repertoire could be used in place of newly acquired responses.[8]

In our own laboratory, we found that 90% of our involutional psychotics, 85% of our chronic psychotics, and only 65% of our retarded children had deficits in acquiring new discrimination and differentiations [6, 23].[9] The severe deficits in current learning ability in involutional and chronic psychotic patients were surprising, since many of these patients had large repertoires of complex behavior which they could emit at a moment's notice. Laboratory measurements proved, however, that their current learning abilities in a novel situation were extremely deficient. These patients had apparently acquired their complicated behavioral repertoires prior to developing their severe learning deficits.

Clearly, the fact that a complicated response can be emitted appropriately is no indication that a new response of equal complexity can be acquired. Retarded children with learning deficits since birth have had no opportunity to acquire complicated repertoires. Therefore, since they never exhibit complex behaviors, casual observation of their behavior is not as misleading in predicting current learning ability as it is with psychotics or the aged. Furthermore, some involutional psychotics are very skillful at "covering up" their severe current learning deficits. In brain damaged patients, less skillful attempts at "covering up" are well known.

These data suggest that we may find severe current learning deficits more frequent among older people than in retarded individuals. These data also suggest that current learning deficits will be very difficult to ascertain by sampling current behavioral repertoires or by ward observations. Moreover, with geriatric patients we should expect general reinforcers to be less adequate because of the historical aging of appropriate reinforcers and because of the need for reinforcer expansion.

There is little doubt that each aged individual can and should have his current behavioral abilities and deficits measured in the laboratory so that an individualized prosthetic environment could be prescribed to support his particular behavioral deficits. Possibly, the patient could be assigned to a ward specializing in patients with similar, but not necessarily the same, patterns of behavioral deficits. On the other hand, we may find wards that are more efficiently designed to cover a wide range of deficits. On these vertically organized

---

[8]Barrett [5] has recently stressed the need for individualized prosthetic prescriptions based upon laboratory behavioral measurement for use in designing and selecting different programs of instruction for retarded children.

[9]For a conclusive review of the experimental literature on learning deficits in elderly patients, see Inglis [18].

wards, the more skillful patients could act as leaders and programmers for their more deficient peers. In hospitals with a vertical ward design, patients with similar deficits could be assigned similar roles about the hospital, but on different wards.

THEORIES OF AGING

It is my opinion that theories of behavioral deviation in the grand or inclusive sense are academic luxuries unless they help us prevent or reduce the behavior pathology, or make it less debilitating. Nevertheless, there are people who insist that theories are not only useful but necessary. To validate their own position, they attribute theories to those researchers who actively state that they have none. The important points seem to be how inclusive and general theories are, how strongly they are held, and whether they are descriptive or explanatory.

The developmental theory of aging presented by Kastenbaum[20] is an explanatory theory. It attempts to explain how and why aging develops as a small part of a larger general process in the behavior of man. This general developmental process is assumed to be found in both the ontogenetic development of the infant and in perception. The same process is found reversed or in regression in the delusions of the psychotic and in the deterioration of the aged. In this sense, the inclusive property of this explanatory theory is historically related to the schools of philosophy which attempted to describe all things by the simplest possible set of laws or statements.

In contrast, I find the disengagement theory presented by Cumming[12] more descriptive than explanatory. She describes the process of aging as disengagement with society and the dilemma of the aged whose behavior is no longer supported by society. In my terms, disengagement means mostly the abrupt cessation of reinforcement, or extinction.

My own approach to aging is even more finely descriptive than Cumming's disengagement theory and might be described as a descriptive multiple cause-deficit-repair theory of aging. In other words, the aged person has an accumulation of behavioral deficits in all areas, each patient with his own pattern of multiple deficits. In physiological deterioration of the aged, there is rarely a single cause of organic debility, although one specific debility may be more outstanding at a given moment in time than the others. Similarly, we may locate syndromes or patterns of specific behavioral deficits which later will be related to deterioration of specific behavioral function, and most older people have suffered so many traumas, periods of disease, abuse and poor environments, that most will have several measurable deficits in differing degrees, and each specific deficit will undoubtedly have multiple causes.

Also, as with organic illness, there undoubtedly is more than one way of treating a specific behavioral deficit. Therefore, we face not only multiple causation and multiple deficit, but multiple treatment, in both organic and behavioral medicine. In general, we now use the term *old age* whenever performance becomes less efficient without any known disruptive factor other than time and practice.

When specific geriatric behavioral deficits have been accurately measured and prosthetized, a fuller experimental analysis may permit the development of explanatory theories of specific deficit syndromes. Involved in the development of these explanatory or etiologic theories will be the experimental induction or catalysis of geriatric deficits and symptoms. I know of only one experiment of this sort which has been conducted to date. Cameron[9] placed senile patients in dark rooms and was able to catalyze or induce senile nocturnal delirium. This experiment showed that senile nocturnal delirium was not due to fatigue at the end of the day as had been previously supposed, but was due to the darkness which also came at the end of the day. Further research in which the environmental variables which precipitate and control geriatric behavioral deficits are isolated will do much to produce useful explanatory sub-theories of aging.

CONTINUITY OF AGING

Even though the severe deficits characteristic of aging do not show up until very late in life, the process of aging might develop much earlier. The behavioral debilities produced by this continuous process of aging may not appear because there are ample devices available for middle-aged persons to use in prosthetizing their milder behavioral deficits. For example, our recent memory may become poorer either because our ability to remember simply decreases with age or because our storage system becomes filled or overloaded. The older we become, however, the more we use prosthetic devices such as notebooks, address books, the telephone information operator and mnemonic devices. The young executive relies on his accurate recent memory, but the older and still highly productive executive relies heavily on his young secretary. It may be that it is only when he loses his secretary that he loses his "recent memory."

In other words, the age at which we see marked, severe behavioral deficits in older persons may only be the point at which appropriate prosthetic devices are no longer available. In this sense, forced retirement or "disengagement" may not only deprive a man of necessary reinforcement, but rob him of his prosthetic devices at the time they are most needed. A justification of retirement by comparing his productive efficiency before and after retirement would therefore erroneously self-validate itself unless reinforcement and prosthetic devices were equated in each condition.

SOCIAL NEGLECT OF THE AGED

The problem of the aged has only recently become a major one. This is not only because more people are living to an older age because of the marked success of organic medicine, but because our more urban and complicated society provides situations in which the deficits of the aged are more debilitating. The increased complexity of the behavioral tasks required of modern society members is displacing not only the less skillful aged, but also the less skillful middle-aged person.

Since our aged citizens are less able to produce in this more complicated society, they have fewer reinforcers for the rest of society and will suffer greater social neglect. They have nothing with which to reinforce social attention from either their peers or the rest of society.

Even patients with organic illnesses may have social responses with which to reinforce their attendants, nurses, physicians and family visitors. The plucky words and weak smile of the organically ill patient are extremely strong reinforcement to a nurse or visitor.

An infant has little behavior with which to acquire reinforcing objects to distribute among his family, but people are so constituted that the gurgle, smile and primitive movements of an infant are strong social reinforcers for adults. The infant also promises genetic and cultural immortality to the adults who contribute to his genetic constitution or cultural education and training. These genetic and cultural immortality factors are also strong social reinforcers.

The retarded individual, although he has little future and does not promise much genetic or cultural immortality, has much behavior which is very similar to the infant's and therefore provides society with social reinforcers to satisfy what might be called "maternal instinct." The smile or caress of a retarded child is a strong social reinforcer for those who attend him or visit him. This is probably why the retarded have always been fairly well treated by society and considered the "children of God" or the "holy innocents."

The psychotic, of course, has fared less well. And this may be because his behavior is not only less rewarding to normal adults, but in many cases is socially aversive. It is a strong attendant who can withstand the verbal onslaught of a sensitive paranoid who criticizes and verbally attacks the attendant's weakest spot. This aversive behavior of the psychotic, coupled with his inability to be a productive member of society, may be why the psychotic has been for centuries maligned, rejected, and considered "possessed by the devil." Family visits to chronic psychotics are much less frequent than visits to the mentally retarded. It is much more difficult to maintain volunteer groups to assist in the care of psychotics than it is to maintain those to care for the retarded. And again, among a group of chronic psychotics it is the laughing, joking, pleasant patient—the classic hebephrenic—who receives the most attention on the ward and is the most welcome at hospital parties and home visits.

And so with the aged, the patient with laugh wrinkles, a full head of white hair, and clean white dentures receives more attention and is more reinforcing to attendants and family than the tragic oldster with a scowl, vertical worry wrinkles, a toothless smile and skin lesions. The aged person whose countenance and behavior present aversive stimuli to other individuals is bound to be avoided and neglected. When he also has behavioral deficiencies, so that he no longer can produce in society or reinforce us with pleasant conversation, he becomes extremely aversive and subject to severe social neglect.

A realistic approach to the social neglect of the psychotic and the aged would accept the fact that they are just too aversive for us to expect highly motivated social response to them from normal middle-aged individuals. Rather than spend a great deal of time and money trying to talk people into overcoming this aversion in charitable attempts to help the psychotic and aged, it may be more economical to remove the source of aversion.

Psychotic and aged patients could be made less aversive by cosmetic attention. Also, if prosthetic devices were developed which would permit them to communicate with normal people and produce positive, though limited, products for the use of society, they would become much more reinforcing to normal individuals and suffer much less neglect. By permanently removing the aversive causes of social neglect, this approach would be more lasting than the current attempts to reduce social neglect by repeated compensatory verbal appeals and the generation of guilt in others.

CONCLUSION

Since 1953, more than 100 applications of free-operant methods to human behavioral pathology have been published. Continuing, systematic investigations are being conducted in psychoses [15, 21, 24, 28], mental retardation [6, 13, 33, 35], neurological disorders [4], and neuroses [7, 16]. These experiments have demonstrated that free-operant principles and methods have wide applicability in social and behavioral research.

The method shows promise for analyzing and prosthetizing geriatric behavioral deficits. The time and money spent in developing behavioral prosthetics should be more than compensated by reduced management costs as more aged patients are made capable of caring for themselves and their peers. A properly engineered geriatric hospital, maximally utilizing the behavior of the patients, should require little more than supervisory non-geriatric labor.

At this time, no systematic applications of operant methods to geriatric behavior have been made. However, the method is ready and the hour is late. Organic medicine has shown great progress in keeping our bodies alive well past the point where behavioral medicine is able to keep our bodies behaving appropriately.

Until we can halt the process of aging, we owe our grandparents, our parents, and eventually ourselves, the right not only to live, but to behave happily and maximally. Until behavioral medicine catches up with organic medicine, terminal boredom will fall to those unfortunates who live beyond their environment.

REFERENCES

1. American Psychiatric Association. Report of patients over 65 in public mental hospitals. 1959.
2. Ayllon, T. Intensive treatment of psychotic behavior by stimulus satiation and food reinforcement. To be published.
3. Ayllon, T., & Michael, J. The psychiatric nurse as a behavioral engineer. *J. Exp. Anal. Behav.*, 1959, **2**, 323–334.
4. Barrett, B. H. Reduction in rate of multiple tics by free operant conditioning methods. *J. Nerv. Ment. Dis.*, 1962, **135**, 187–195.
5. Barrett, B. H. Programmed instruction and retarded behavior. Paper read at American Association of Mental Deficiency, Portland, Ore., May 1963.
6. Barrett, B. H., & Lindsley, O. R. Deficits in acquisition of operant discrimination and differentiation shown by institutionalized retarded children. *Amer. J. Ment. Defic.*, 1962, **67**, 424–426.
7. Brady, J. P., & Lind, D. L. Experimental analysis of hysterical blindness. *Arch. Gen. Psychiat.*, 1961, **4**, 331–339.
8. Caldwell, B. McD. An evaluation of psychological effects of sex hormone administration in aged women. 2. Results of therapy after eighteen months. *J. Gerontol.*, 1954, **9**, 168–174.
9. Cameron, D. E. Studies in senile nocturnal delirium. *Psychiat. Quart.*, 1941, **15**, 47–53.
10. Cameron, D. E. Impairment of the retention phase of remembering. *Psychiat. Quart.*, 1943, **17**, 395–404.
11. Cohen, D. J. Justin and his peers: An experimental analysis of a child's social world. *Child Developm.*, 1962, **33**, 697–717.
12. Cumming, E. Further thoughts on the theory of disengagement. In R. Kastenbaum (Ed.), *New thoughts on old age.* New York: Springer, 1964.
13. Ellis, N. R., Barnett, C. D., & Pryer, M. W. Operant behavior in mental defectives: Exploratory studies. *J. Exp. Anal. Behav.*, 1960, **3**, 63–69.
14. Ferster, C. B. Reinforcement and punishment in the control of human behavior by social agencies. *Psychiat. Res. Rep.*, 1958, **10**, 101–118.
15. Ferster, C. B., & DeMyer, M. K. The development of performances in autistic children in an automatically controlled environment. *J. Chron. Dis.*, 1961, **13**, 312–345.
16. Flanagan, B., Goldiamond, I., & Azrin, N. Operant stuttering: The control of stuttering behavior through response-contingent consequences. *J. Exp. Anal. Behav.*, 1958, **1**, 173–177.
17. Garnett, R. W., & Klingman, W. O. Cytochrome C: Effects of intravenous administration on presenile, senile and arteriosclerotic cerebral states. *Amer. J. Psychiat.*, 1949, **106**, 697–702.
18. Inglis, J. Psychological investigations of cognitive deficit in elderly psychiatric patients. *Psychol. Bull.*, 1958, **54**, 197–214.
19. Inglis, J. Psychological practice in geriatric problems. *J. Ment. Sci.*, 1962, **108**, 669–674.
20. Kastenbaum, R. Is old age the end of development? In R. Kastenbaum (Ed.), *New thoughts on old age.* New York: Springer, 1964.

21. Lindsley, O. R. Operant conditioning methods applied to research in chronic schizophrenia. *Psychiat. Res. Rep.*, 1956, **5**, 118–139.
22. Lindsley, O. R. Operant behavior during sleep: A measure of depth of sleep. *Science*, 1957, **126**, 1290–1291.
23. Lindsley, O. R. Analysis of operant discrimination and differentiation in chronic psychotics. Paper read at Eastern Psychological Association, Atlantic City, April 1958.
24. Lindsley, O. R. Characteristics of the behavior of chronic psychotics as revealed by free-operant conditioning methods. *Dis. Nerv. Sys.*, 1960, **21** (Suppl.), 66–78.
25. Lindsley, O. R. Conjugate reinforcement. Paper read at American Psychological Association, New York, September 1961.
26. Lindsley, O. R. Experimental analysis of cooperation and competition. Paper read at Eastern Psychological Association, Philadelphia, April 1962.
27. Lindsley, O. R. Direct behavioral analysis of psychotherapy sessions by conjugately programed closed-circuit television. Paper read at American Psychological Association, St. Louis, September 1962.
28. Lindsley, O. R. Operant conditioning methods in diagnosis. In J. H. Nodine & J. H. Moyer (Eds.), *Psychosomatic medicine: The first Hahnemann Symposium*. Philadelphia: Lea & Febiger, 1962. Pp. 41–54.
29. Lindsley, O. R. Direct measurement and prosthesis of retarded behavior. Paper read at Boston University, Department of Special Education, March 1963.
30. Lindsley, O. R. Free-operant conditioning and psychotherapy. In J. H. Masserman (Ed.), *Current psychiatric therapies*. Vol. III. New York: Grune & Stratton, 1963. Pp. 47–56.
31. Lindsley, O. R., Hobika, J. H., & Etsten, B. E. Operant behavior during anesthesia recovery: A continuous and objective method. *Anesthesiology*, 1961, **22**, 937–946.
32. Melrose, J. Research in the hearing of the aged. Paper read at National Association of Music Therapy, Cambridge, Mass., October 1962.
33. Orlando, R., & Bijou, S. W. Single and multiple schedules of reinforcement in developmentally retarded children. *J. Exp. Anal. Behav.*, 1960, **3**, 339–348.
34. Rachman, S. Learning theory and child psychology: Therapeutic possibilities. *J. Child Psychol. Psychiat.*, 1962, **3**, 149–163.
35. Spradlin, J. E. Effects of reinforcement schedules on extinction in severely mentally retarded children. *Amer. J. Ment. Defic.*, 1962, **66**, 634–640.

38

Behavior Modification in Rehabilitation:
The Rehabilitation of Special Children*[1]

LEE MEYERSON, NANCY KERR, and JACK L. MICHAEL

The treatment of handicapped persons in rehabilitation centers often requires them to engage in activities that are difficult, effortful, or unpleasant to perform. It is not surprising, in view of this factor alone and without consideration of other possible influential variables, that many rehabilitation clients resist rehabilitative efforts. Nor is it surprising that rehabilitation personnel complain frequently of "lack of motivation" in their clients or that the proportion of cases discharged from rehabilitation centers for this reason is relatively high.

Characteristically, the patient whose behavior fails to conform to the expectations of the rehabilitation staff is referred to the psychologist for "evaluation." Much of the work of the psychologist in rehabilitation is at present devoted to the routine evaluation of client intelligence, personality, and achievement, in the belief that these data are "good things" to know and that they may help the staff do better work. Most of the data obtained, however, seem strikingly unrelated to the behavior required in the rehabilitation center. They may lead the psychologist to believe that he "understands" better why a client acts as he does, but the data lend little aid in changing unacceptable behavior to more-acceptable behavior. Most often the psychologist confirms the observation of others that the client is unmotivated, and he assigns a reason for it. This reason is usually some inaccessible trait of the client: "He hasn't accepted his disability." "He isn't bright enough or mature enough to understand what is best for him." "He is overly dependent." "His super-ego is weak."

Sometimes such evaluations are accompanied by vague directions to give the client "psychological support," to coax him more, or counsel him so that he will understand himself better. More often they seem to result in a decision to discharge the client as unmotivated or as having reached the maximum medical benefit that is possible without long-term psychotherapy which may or may not change the underlying or "real" personality problems.

This kind of approach to rehabilitation not only places an overwhelming, needless, and often unfulfillable responsibility on the client to be the architect of his own rehabilitation,

*From *Child development: Readings in experimental analysis*, edited by S. W. Bijou and D. M. Baer. Copyright © 1967 by Appelton-Century-Crofts. Reprinted by permission of Appleton-Century-Crofts Educational Division, and Dr. Meyerson.

[1]Edward Hanley, William Heard, Brian Jacobson, Karl Minke, Albert Neal, and Larry Sayre, graduate students at Arizona State University, were the experimenters in the studies reported in this paper. Their collaboration is acknowledged with appreciation and thanks.

The research training program of which this work was a part was supported by National Institute of Mental Health Grant MH-7818 and by Vocational Rehabilitation Administration Grant 344-T.

We are grateful to our colleagues at the Valley of the Sun School and the Gompers Memorial Rehabilitation Center for their many courtesies.

but also neglects two other basic variables that can be manipulated for the client's benefit: his environment and, as a result of the manipulation of his environment, his behavior.

Most rehabilitation psychologists will accept the formula $B=f(P, E)$, or behavior is a function of a person's interaction with his environment. In concentrating on the P term in the formula, however, it is easy to neglect the fact that the formula has three terms and that B and E can be independent variables also. Among psychologists who strive to do more than measure and categorize the traits of disabled persons, present practice is to attempt direct changes in the person by counseling and verbal psychotherapeutic procedures. It is not generally perceived that equally indirect changes of the psychological situation by manipulation of the environment may be equally valuable and far more feasible. It may be better, for example, to assist a physical therapist in achieving his goal of restoring functional use of an arm or leg than to attempt to deal with the inferiority feelings or dependency status that may be engendered in a person because he lacks such functional use. Counseling and psychotherapy were developed in an attempt to modify abnormal reactions to normal situations. It is by no means clear that they are the treatments of choice for normal reactions to abnormal situations.

Following the pattern of previous experimentation (Meyerson & Kerr, in press,) in which operant conditioning techniques were used to obtain striking behavioral changes in rehabilitation clients, we accepted at face value the behavioral problems referred to us by other members of a rehabilitation-center team. We gave no tests; we made no evaluations; we held no interviews; we took no history. In fact, we generally knew nothing at all about the person referred to us except that he was not engaging in some behavior that was desirable for his rehabilitation. In addition, almost all of the experimental work was conducted by first-year graduate students who had had no previous experience in clinical psychology or rehabilitation, but who did know learning theory.

We were guided in this work by the theoretical formulations of the Workgroup on Learning of the Miami Conference on Psychological Research and Rehabilitation (Meyerson, Michael, Mowrer, Osgood, & Staats, 1963). In particular, we took seriously the following statements:

> Motivation may be considered the task of specifying adequate reinforcers (p. 91).
>
> If an individual "should" do something . . . you must provide strong reinforcers contingent upon his behavior . . . (p. 92).
>
> One of the most important things that we can offer . . . is a frame of reference which induces (psychologists in rehabilitation) to look for adequate reinforcers and to apply them correctly, skillfully and subtly . . . if this approach were followed, many presently difficult problems might become readily amenable to solution (p. 101).
>
> Psychologists in rehabilitation (should) look for causal, manipulable variables in a situation which they would then use to facilitate the generally accepted goals of rehabilitation workers (p. 78).

Some of the problems referred to us were remarkably simple ones that could be solved immediately by the application of a single behavioral principle. Others were much more complex, and the results reported here can be considered only a beginning in the application of behavioral principles to some rehabilitation problems. As in other beginnings, our initial experiments have been crude, lacking in the precision and elegance of design, the data collecting, and the reporting that are desirable, but a start has been made, and the fruitfulness of the approach may be apparent. . . . .

CASE 1 : INABILITY TO WALK IN A MENTALLY RETARDED CHILD

Background

Mary was a nine-year-old girl who, in addition to having other behavioral deficits, didn't walk, didn't talk, and wasn't toilet trained. She was classified by the residential institution in which she lived as "congenitally mentally retarded." She was reported to have crawled when she was two years old, but she never walked. At the time of first observation, she would not stand on her feet unless someone lifted her by the hands or arms and supported most of her weight.

It wasn't clear why Mary didn't walk. She was somewhat bow-legged, as if she had had rickets at the age when most children begin to walk, but there were no other physical abnormalities now that would tend to interfere with walking or standing unsupported.

To the institution, however, it was an old and familiar story. Many mentally retarded children do not walk. It is believed to be one of the "characteristics" of severely mentally retarded children that is related not to their muscular strength but to their not being smart enough or sufficiently coordinated to learn to walk. An inquiry sometimes follows this pattern:

> "Why doesn't Mary walk?"
> "Well, she's severely mentally retarded, and it is not uncommon among the severely mentally retarded that they don't walk."
> "I see, but what is the reason for it?"
> "She's slow in development."
> "I see. And what is it that is responsible for her slow development?"
> "It is the fact that she is mentally retarded."
> "I see. And how do you know that she is mentally retarded?"
> "Why you can see for yourself. She doesn't walk, she doesn't talk, she isn't toilet trained and doesn't do many other things like a mentally normal child."

There may be many reasons for the impoverished behavioral repertory of long-institutionalized children. Not the least of these variables are the impoverished environmental contingencies to which the child must respond appropriately either to receive reinforcement or to avoid punishment. A diagnosis of mental retardation, however, which by definition is an "incurable" disorder, tends to lead to the easy acceptance of the inevitability of behavioral deviance and behavioral deficits and to choke off some simple rearrangements of the environment which might lead to the generation of more adequate behavior.

Observation

Mary, except for her very thin, bowed legs and lack of muscular development in the calf, seemed physically capable of walking. Her primary mode of locomotion, however, was scooting across the floor on her buttocks by pushing with her feet and hands. She could be pulled to a standing position if the experimenter supported most of her weight, but she could not be induced to move her legs, and she would drop to the floor as soon as support was removed or relaxed.

Behavioral Analysis

For physical reasons, Mary may not have had the capacity to walk when she was younger. The acceptance of her as "a child who doesn't walk," however, led to neglect in providing environmental contingencies which would shape up and maintain walking. At present there were no important positive consequences contingent upon walking, or aversive consequences contingent upon not walking. She was carried or wheeled in a chair wherever it was necessary for her to go.

The behavior desired from Mary was that she should stand unsupported and walk independently; first, upon request of the experimenter in the experimental room and, later, in response to the naturally reinforcing contingencies of the ward. The task here . . . was to get her over the hump of initiating the strange and strenuous effort of walking so that this ultimately less effortful mode of locomotion could be experienced and so that the naturally reinforcing contingencies in the environment that are available to one who walks could exert their effects. No attempt was to be made to induce the ward attendants not to carry Mary or not to push her in a wheelchair, since these efforts would introduce uncontrolled variables. Since Mary was highly reinforceable with edibles such as popcorn, raisins, crackers, nuts, and ice cream, it was believed that these reinforcers would be sufficient to generate walking behavior and that the reinforcing effects of walking itself would maintain the behavior on the ward.

Behavioral Treatment

Mary was seen twice a week in experimental sessions usually lasting 20 to 45 minutes. In the initial sessions, resting periods of 5 to 15 minutes were as long as or longer than working periods; but later, as her muscles became stronger, the walking periods were about twice as long as the resting periods.

In Phase 1, lasting one session, Mary was lifted to her feet and given a reinforcer while she was standing. Gradually the experimenter released his support. In the beginning, when the child supported on her own legs even a small portion of her weight for a fraction of a second, she was reinforced with an edible. Later, the contingencies were modified to require higher degrees of weight-bearing over longer periods of time, until at the end of the first session she would stand unsupported for 5 to 15 seconds at a time. Detailed records were not kept of this session.

In Phase 2, two folding chairs were placed approximately 30 inches apart, back to back. Mary was placed on the floor between the chairs while an experimenter stood behind each chair. She was told and shown how to pull herself to her feet by grasping the back of one chair, then turn around and grasp the back of the other chair first with one hand and then with both hands. When Mary was standing, the experimenter behind her would say, "Mary, come over here." If the command was followed, she was reinforced with an edible. If it was not followed, or if she dropped to the floor and scooted on her buttocks to the other chair, a reinforcer was not dispensed.

When Mary was effectively making the transfer from chair to chair upon command, the distance between the chairs was very gradually increased until it was impossible for her to move from one chair to the other while holding on to either of them. Initially she was able to release one chair with one hand and, standing unsupported, lean over until she could grasp the second chair with the other hand. As the distance between the chairs increased, however, it was necessary for her at first to take one unsupported step and later several, before she was reinforced. In the seven sessions of Phase 2, the greatest distance between the chairs was 45 inches.

In Phase 3, the chairs were removed and the procedure was as follows: One experimenter would hold Mary's hand while the other experimenter, a few feet away, would hold out a reinforcer. When she had taken a few steps toward the reinforcer, the first experimenter would release her hand while the second experimenter walked backwards away from

her. Initially, Mary was given a reinforcer after taking three or four steps, but this requirement was gradually increased at each session. By Session 12, for example, reinforcement
was contingent upon taking at least 25 steps. The number of steps taken was recorded as
"Steps from Supported Start." In addition, an attempt was made to keep Mary walking for
additional reinforcements as the experimenter moved away from her. The steps taken
under this contingency were recorded as "Steps from Unsupported Start." These
categories were not really meaningful after Session 11, as by that time it was Mary who
released her hand from the experimenter's hand rather than vice versa.

In Sessions 13, 14 and 15, the procedure was modified further by placing the second
experimenter across the room rather than having him lead the child by a few steps. If, when
she was called, Mary walked across the room without sinking to the floor, she received a
reinforcer. If she sat down, no reinforcement was given, she was walked back to the
starting point, and the command was given again. The same attempt was made as before to
keep Mary walking for additional reinforcements as the experimenter moved across the
room.

Results

The results are shown in Tables 38.1 and 38.2 and in Figs. 38.1 and 38.2. It will be seen in
Table 38.1 that there was a gradual but consistent shift from transferring from one chair
while holding on to the other, to standing unsupported between the chairs, to taking unsupported steps between the chairs. By the end of Session 8 of Phase 2, and after the
expenditure of less than 200 minutes of experimental time, Mary had taken 28 unsupported
steps in one session. The cumulative performances under the Phase 2 contingency are
shown in Fig. 38.1

Table 38.2 shows that a gradually increasing total number of steps was obtained in each
succeeding 45-minute session. Session 11 lasted for more than an hour and resulted in an

Table 38.1 Progression in Alternating Between Chairs During Phase 2
Training.

Session	Commands*	Reinforced Transfers Between Chairs	Standing Unsupported Between Chairs	No. of Un- supported Steps Be- tween Chairs
1†				
2	66	34	6	
3	64	39	18	
4	23	18	1	
5	57	32	24	
6	68	32	25	17
7	20	7	3	3
8	39	9	0‡	28

*The number of commands given provides a rough index to the length of a
working session. Sessions 4, 7, and 8 were shorter than others.

†Session 1 was part of Phase 1 and consisted only of reinforcement for
standing unsupported for a short time. Records were not kept.

‡The chairs were separated by a distance that required one or more steps for
completion of the task.

Table 38.2 Steps Reinforced with Supported and Unsupported Starts in Phase 3 of Training.

Cumula-tive Session*	Steps from Supported Start	Steps from Unsup-ported Start	Total Steps	Rein-force-ments	Steps/Reinf.
9	190		190	31	6.1
10	560		560	36	15.5
11*	790	223	1013	61	16.6
12	414	249	663	20	33.1
13	422	391	813	29	28.0
14	806	111	917	22	41.7
15*	445	40	485	10	48.5

*Each session was 45 minutes long except Session 11, which ran for 70 minutes, and Session 15, which was interrupted after 30 minutes.

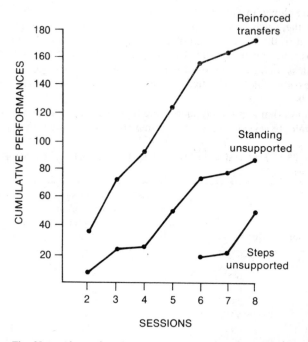

Fig. 38.1 Alternations between chairs by Mary in Phase 2.

unusually large number of steps, while Session 15 was terminated after 30 minutes. The table also shows the gradually increasing number of steps obtained per reinforcer as the reinforcement contingency was raised, from six steps in Session 9 to 40 consecutive steps in Session 15. Figure 38.2 presents the same data in cumulative record form.

By the end of the last session, the institutional attendants reported that Mary was taking

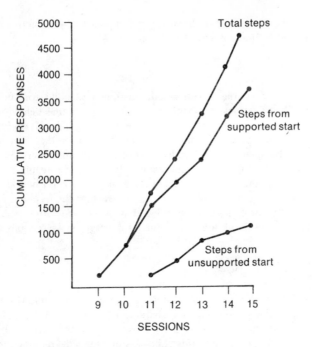

Fig. 38.2   Walking by Mary in Phase 3.

unsupported steps in the ward. No attempt was made, as would ordinarily be desirable, to generalize the walking behavior to the ward or to fade out gradually the food reinforcers and replace them with other reinforcers. At the present writing, however, six months after the training sessions were completed, Mary is walking freely and frequently throughout the institution. Less than 9 hours of experimental effort had removed a behavioral deficit of 9 years' standing.

CASE 2:   SELF-DESTRUCTIVE BEHAVIOR IN AN AUTISTIC CHILD

Background

Phil was a 4-year-old child, physically small for his age, who was confined to a crib in an institution for the mentally retarded. He attracted the attention of visitors, when he was not restrained, by the forcefulness with which he slapped and punched himself on his cheeks and mouth, banged his head, and scratched his body. These behaviors, which left visible injuries, were part of his almost ceaseless motor and tactual activity during most of his waking hours.

Problem

Physical assault on one's own body, sometimes to the point of injury, is not uncommon among autistic children. Such children are often confined in strait-jackets or restrained in other ways. It would be desirable to extinguish or alter such self-destructive behavior, but the variables that control it are not well understood.

Observation

Systematic observation of the unrestrained, unstimulated child for three 10-minute periods led to the identification of 20 different motor and tactual behaviors. These included hitting, slapping, kicking, scratching, biting, and rocking himself; sucking on thumb, finger, hand, arm; rubbing or flipping fingers against teeth and other parts of the body, chewing on bedsheet, banging head against the bars of the crib, and others. Several of these behaviors were sometimes manifested simultaneously, and once begun, a particular behavior such as finger-flipping or rocking might continue for several hours.

Simultaneous observation by four observers, each recording the frequency and duration in seconds of five different behaviors, revealed that during three 10-minute periods the child was stimulating himself in some way for an average of 44 seconds out of every minute.

Behavioral Analysis

Phil's behavior did not appear to be a socially reinforced operant. His behavior was accepted by the institution's attendants as "characteristic of that kind of child," and little attention was paid to it except for periodic imposition of mechanical restraints. It was speculated that sensory deprivation in this child was of such a degree that tactual stimulation, even of a painful kind, was reinforcing in itself; and self-destructive behavior might be reduced if an external source of tactual stimulation were available.

It was desirable in this case to reduce the frequency of self-destructive behaviors and to determine the functional relationship between such a reduction, if it occurred, and two kinds of tactile stimulation which would be applied for brief periods. As in other behavioral alteration experiments in which the stimuli controlling the undesired behavior are not known and extinction procedures, therefore, are not possible, the intent here was to generate a behavior that was incompatible with self-destruction—namely, lying quietly.

Experimentation, Phase 1

Four observers gathered around the child's crib. Each observer was responsible for recording the frequency and duration of five of the 20 self-destructive behaviors that the child had exhibited in the past. A 50-minute experimental period consisting of alternating 10-minute periods of stimulation with 10-minute periods of nonstimulation had the following format: 1. No stimulation. 2. Vibrating pillow applied to child's back. 3. No stimulation. 4. The experimenter scratched the child's back gently. 5. No stimulation. There were two such 50-minute sessions spaced one week apart.

Results, Phase 1

The results of alternate periods of stimulation and no stimulation are shown in Fig. 38.3. It is evident from inspection that applying stimulation from an external source was an effective means of reducing the behaviors that were classified as self-destructive in various degrees. The kind of stimulation appears to have been less important than its ordinal position within the series. Back-scratching was more effective than vibration in reducing self-

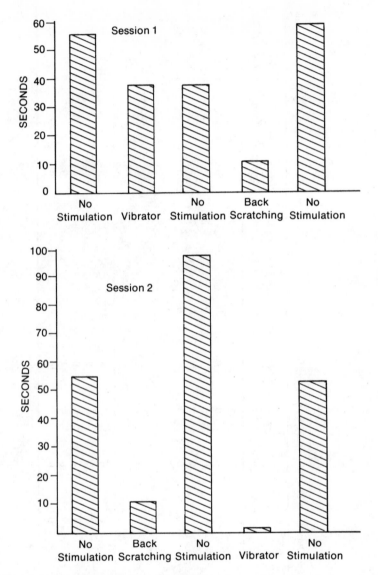

Fig. 38.3 Average duration of self-destructive behaviors per minute* under natural and tactually stimulating conditions.

destructive behaviors when vibration came second in the series and back-scratching came fourth, but vibration was more effective than back-scratching when the order of the stimuli was reversed. This phenomenon, when combined with the striking reductions in the duration of self-destructive behaviors during periods of stimulation in Session 2 as compared to

---

*Subject engaged in several temporally overlapping, self-destructive behaviors. Bars show sum of duration of all observed behaviors divided by minutes of observation.

Table 38.3 Distribution and Duration in Seconds of Self-Destructive Behaviors Observed Under Two Conditions in Alternating Ten Minute Trials.

Condition	Finger Flipping	Ear Pulling	Slapping Hitting	Kicking	Scratching	Chewing on Sheet	Rocking	Sucking	Tooth Rubbing	Fingers in Mouth	Total Secs.	Average Per Min
Session 1												
No Stim.	7	0	0	12	90	0	392	45	5	0	551	55.1
Vibrator	0	0	0	0	0	0	0	0	0	385	385	38.5
No Stim.	9	0	40	96	19	0	82	120	22	0	388	38.8
Back Scratch	15	0	0	8	20	0	0	20	0	52	115	11.5
No Stim.	0	0	0	5	0	0	520	18	0	0	543	54.3
Session 2												
No Stim.	41	0	76	37	34	32	97	215	9	0	541	54.1
Back Scratch	0	0	0	0	0	0	0	0	0	106	108	10.8
No Stim.	0	133	0	34	0	0	390	407	0	0	964	96.4
Vibrator	0	0	0	0	1	1	0	0	0	2	3	.3
No Stim.	0	0	0	0	20	20	511	5	0	0	536	53.6

Session 1 (which did not occur during periods of no stimulation) lent support to the belief that external stimulation was intrinsically reinforcing, in the sense that it reduced some and eliminated other self-stimulating activities. The distributions of the durations of the several behaviors during periods of no stimulation and stimulation show quite clearly the shift from more self-destructive classes of behavior to less self-destructive classes of behavior. The distributions for Sessions 1 and 2 are shown in Table 38.3. It will be seen that during periods of stimulation, almost the entire activity time was accounted for by the minimally self-destructive behavior of keeping fingers in mouth. This was a behavior that did not occur at all during the periods of no stimulation, although other, more self-destructive behaviors were manifested.

Experimentation, Phase 2

If a stimulus is reinforcing, it increases the frequency of the behavior that was emitted immediately prior to its presentation. It seemed important, for two reasons, to know if external tactual stimulation was intrinsically reinforcing. First, tactual stimulation is not presently included in the list of known primary reinforcers, although some reports of sensory-deprivation phenomena indicate that it might well be one. Second, if tactual stimulation is a primary reinforcer, it offers a powerful tool for altering the self-destructive behaviors of children like Phil, and it becomes potentially possible to modify and improve a tremendous range of behaviors in children for whom tactual deprivation may be a naturally occurring phenomenon.

Back-scratching does not lend itself very well to precise programming or automation, but a vibratory stimulus does. Inasmuch as the results of Phase 1 did not indicate compelling reasons for preferring one kind of tactual stimulation to the other, experimentation was continued with vibration.

To assess the reinforcing properties of vibratory stimuli, a vibrator imbedded in a pillow (Sears catalogue #2858) was sewn immediately beneath the surface of the mattress in the child's crib. The vibrator was controlled by automated programming equipment which turned it on for 10 seconds of vibratory stimulation after each light pressing of a foam-rubber-padded, leather-covered, oblong lever, $8\frac{1}{2}$ inches by $5\frac{1}{2}$ inches in size, that was mounted on the side of the child's crib. The lever was mounted a few inches away from one of Phil's arms so that he would be likely to hit it by chance while engaging in the gross motor activity that he frequently exhibited, but his hand would have to turn at a sharp angle in order to strike the lever with his fingers or palm.

The vibration was contingent on pressing the lever; so if vibratory stimulation was reinforcing, after a few reinforcements resulting from adventitious lever pressing, Phil would be expected to strike the lever with increasing frequency. Two one-hour sessions, spaced one week apart, were run.

Results, Phase 2

The cumulative records are shown in Figure 38.4. It will be seen that the results of Session 1 were strikingly successful. It appeared evident that vibratory stimulation was reinforcing. Temporary satiation seemed to occur after 5 to 10 minutes of stimulation, but recovery was rapid. Records of the topography of the lever-pressing response showed that all except the first few presses were made by hand and fingers and were clearly not accidental.

Figure 38.4 also shows the cumulative record of the first 20 minutes of Session 2. The

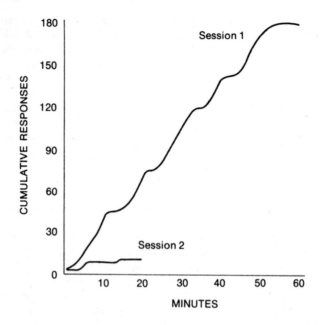

Fig. 38.4   Cumulative record of lever-pressing for vibratory stimulation by an autistic child.

lever-pressing behavior that was so evident in Session 1 was no longer present. Moreover, attempts to hand-shape the response by delivering vibratory stimulation for successive approximations to lever pressing were unsuccessful. No progress toward reinstating the lever-pressing response was evident after 60 minutes of experimental effort.

DISCUSSION

Case 2 was included in this paper to indicate that behavioral experimentation is not always, or even usually, a hop, skip, and jump from isolating a problem, to devising a procedure, to successful outcome. In every case reported, there were some false starts and some difficulties of greater or lesser degree that had to be solved. In Case 2, we may or may not be on the track of important phenomena. It is clearly evident, however, that the problem has not been solved; nor is there a clear interpretation for the data obtained. Additional experimentation is necessary. It is now planned to place the lever and the automatically recording vibratory apparatus in Phil's crib on a 24-hour-per-day basis over a period of several weeks to determine if a longer period of experimentation will yield more interpretable data. The reader may conceive of other procedures that would be equally promising or better.

The responses of behavioral scientists, medical personnel, parents, and others to the kind of experimentation and applied psychology that is exemplified by the cases reported have been very encouraging. The psychologist in rehabilitation who tests, evaluates, classifies, and describes the strengths and weaknesses of candidates for rehabilitation services is not uniformly valued by his colleagues or those he serves. There appears to be an increasing demand for psychologists who have the knowledge and the ability to modify behavior—to generate desirable behavior when it is not present, to maintain good behavior in strength, and to extinguish or alter undesirable behavior. The role of the psychologist in rehabilitation of the future clearly requires a specialist in behavioral engineering who by open, clearly specifiable, non-esoteric, and non-subjective procedures can alter human behavior and thereby contribute more fully to the improved functioning of disabled persons.

Helping a child learn to work productively in activities that will improve his hand-eye coordination, to fall safely, and to walk, when these behaviors were not present previously, is surely beneficial. Some individuals, however, appear to have strong emotional reactions to the procedures that are used in the experimentation that was described and doubts about the value of what was done. It may be of value to discuss two spontaneous, but perhaps unthinking, objections that are most frequently made:

1. "I don't believe in bribing children." Critics who make this comment appear to be expressing the belief that children should "voluntarily" engage in certain behaviors because "it is for their own good," or "it is the right thing to do," and that it is somehow dishonest, evil, ineffective, or contrary to some immutable moral law to offer them extrinsic inducements to behave as they "should" behave.

Such critics appear to forget that infants and children learn to behave in ways that the significant others in their lives consider right and good—they are not born with such behaviors. The learning is accomplished as a consequence of thousands and thousands of materially and socially reinforced responses and exposure to the naturally reinforcing or punishing contingencies of the environment.

For various reasons, some children do not receive the kind or frequency of reinforcement that shapes the behavior of most children to the ordinary demands of the social environment. Other children, because of the physical or social effects of disabilities, or other fortuitous circumstances that are presently relatively unexplored, do not come under the control of the naturally occurring contingencies in the environment. The critical choice for those who work with children whose behavior is maladaptive is whether to view the problem as a scientific, valuatively neutral task of facilitating the learning of more adaptive behavior—even though the behavior "should have" been learned earlier—or to view it as a moral problem of the childrens' own making which requires that they be consigned to limbo in preference to "bribing" them to behave more adaptively. The scientifically oriented psychologist should experience no conflict in making this choice.

The student-psychologist, perhaps because of his own moral training, may sympathize initially with the rehabilitation therapist who resolutely refuses to permit extrinsic reinforcement to be given in his clinic on the grounds that "these children are here to work and to improve themselves. If they won't work, we'll discharge them." The sympathy is considerably diluted when, on further inquiry, it becomes clear that the therapist himself would not show up for work if *his* reinforcements (money, social approval, accomplishment) were terminated; and he apparently expects that the behavior of his clients "should be" controlled by principles of behavior that are markedly different from those that control his own.

Some further clarification may be obtained by considering the appropriateness of an emotionally loaded term such as "bribe." To bribe means to influence dishonestly, to pervert the judgment or to corrupt the conduct of a person in a position of trust by means of some reward. It refers to inducing a person by some payment or promised action to violate a trust, and sometimes it is extended metaphorically to include payment for some *undesirable* behavior that the person would not engage in were it not for the payment.

The therapeutic effort is not of this nature. It is aimed at generating, maintaining, or strengthening desirable behavior and altering undesirable behavior. It is the same kind of social control that is exerted by the employer who says, "I will pay you $2 an hour to come to work in my pickle factory," by the professor who indicates that if you learn the material in his course, he will give you a good grade, or by the parent who praises a child for polite and unselfish behavior. We do not designate such reinforcements as "bribery."

One may attempt to distinguish the behavior required of rehabilitation clients from these examples on the grounds that rehabilitative therapy is for the client's own good and "should be" engaged in without payment, but this is not tenable. It is for their own good that college students "should" acquire as much knowledge as possible, and children "should be" polite and unselfish without the aid of symbolic or social payment. But these behaviors must be learned, and it is necessary in the learning process to reinforce them.

One real difference between college students, children, and rehabilitation clients who behave appropriately and those who do not may be that the desirable behaviors of the former have already come under the control of a wide variety of secondary reinforcers. A good grade, for example, is simply a mark on paper which has acquired significance because in the past it has repeatedly been closely followed by more powerful, primary reinforcers. The individuals who are not under the control of the secondary reinforcers that our culture values as "good" become school dropouts, delinquents, and "unmotivated" rehabilitation clients. Effective rehabilitative therapy in such cases may require the use of primary reinforcement or relatively crude extrinsic reinforcement such as is common with infants and young children. It may be that it is this necessary use of overtly seductive rather than more subtle reinforcement that leads to the unwarranted judgment of "bribery." However, as Michael (1964) has remarked, "If behavior which 'should' be engaged in without extrinsic reinforcement is not, in fact, occurring, a program of extrinsic reinforcement must be evaluated, not in an absolute sense, but in comparison with the common alternative approaches: increased aversive control, or simply accepting failure."

On a similarly practical level, some professional persons are not so much concerned with the moral implications of dispensing extrinsic reinforcements as they are with the likelihood that the behavior obtained will be temporary or cease abruptly when the reinforcement is discontinued.

It is not possible here to describe the processes by which behavior comes under the control of secondary and so-called intrinsic reinforcement, but the transition to secondary reinforcement is often necessary for long-term persistence of behavior under natural conditions. If such additional learning does not occur, and the behavior does not come under the control of naturally occurring reinforcement in the environment, it is true that the behavior developed and maintained by experimentally manipulated, extrinsic reinforcement will cease. We deceive ourselves if we believe that any behavior that is without consequences will be maintained indefinitely. "All experimental evidence indicates that when behavior is no longer followed by positive reinforcement and when it no longer escapes or avoids aversive consequences, it ceases" (Michael, 1964). It is probably to our advantage that it does, for otherwise we would be greatly impeded in learning new and more-adaptive behavior that environmental changes may require. The transience of much behavior is both inevitable and desirable.

When long-term persistence is desired for some behavior that does not receive primary reinforcement from the environment, it is necessary for the behavioral engineer to ensure that the behavior comes under the control of readily available secondary reinforcement. To ensure the maintenance of some behaviors in handicapped persons, it may be necessary to construct prosthetic environments. There are no approaches to learning that are free of these requirements, although the terminology employed may be different.

2. "What is the value of changing one or two discrete bits of behavior? The children are still physically handicapped or mentally retarded, aren't they?" It would be delightful if varied, complex, and poorly understood disorders could be put completely right at one blow, but that process is called a miracle, and people who believe in it generally resort to prayer. The scientific process tends to proceed by slow accretion and the step-by-step solution of discrete problems.

From an immediate, practical standpoint, when one compares the time, effort, and resources that are necessary to care for ambulant and non-ambulant, toilet-trained and non-toilet-trained, self-destructive and non-self-destructive, or hyperactive and non-hyperactive children, it seems clear that changing one or two bits of discrete behavior should not be despised.

In addition, the objection quoted neglects the fact that no learned behavior appears in full bloom. It is learned bit by bit from the moment of birth, or earlier, and refined by thousands and thousands of repetitions. The learning of congenitally physically handicapped or retarded persons may be obstructed or impeded by insuperable physical barriers, chance exposure to conditions that are detrimental to learning, lack of knowledge of how to facilitate learning under unusual conditions, or perhaps more frequently, lack of skilled application of the learning principles that are already known.

In the rehabilitation setting, one or more behavioral deficits of a sensory, motor, or discriminative nature may be evident in handicapped persons when comparison is made with non-handicapped individuals of similar age. There is presently no alternative to treating such deficits one by one; and the outcome, in terms of the total person or total behavior, depends on how many and how severe the deficits are and the degree to which generalization of newly learned behavior may be possible. As progress is made in overcoming behavioral deficits that are presently beyond rehabilitative knowledge, and as increased behavioral engineering skill is gained in reducing or removing other deficits, we may expect that the behavioral deficits that are presently associated with some physical disabilities will disappear, and some kinds of so-called mental retardation will be remediable.

REFERENCES

Meyerson, L., & Kerr, Nancy. *Learning theory and rehabilitation.* New York: Random House. In press.

Meyerson, L., Michael, J. L., Mowrer, O. H. Osgood, C. E., & Staats, A. W. Learning, behavior, and rehabilitation, In *Psychological research and rehabilitation.* Washington D.C.: American Psychological Association, 1963.

Michael, J. L. Guidance and counseling as the control of behavior. In *Guidance in American education: backgrounds and prospects.* Cambridge: Harvard Graduate School of Education, 1964. (Distributed by Harvard University Press.)

Suggested Additional Readings

Anant, S. S. Treatment of alcoholics and drug addicts by verbal aversion techniques. *Canadian Psychologist*, 1967, **80**, 19–22.

Bassin, A. Daytop village. In *Readings in clinical psychology today*. Del Mar, Calif.: CRM Books, 1970, Pp. 127–133.

Birnbauer, J. C., Wolf, M. M., Kedder, J. D., & Tague, C. E. Classroom behavior of retarded pupils with token reinforcement. *Journal of Experimental Child Psychology*, 1965, **2**, 219–235.

Blake, B. G. The application of behavior therapy to the treatment of alcoholism. *Behavior Research and Therapy*, 1965, **3**, 75–85.

Blake, B. G. A follow-up of alcoholics treated by behavior therapy. *Behavior Research and Therapy*, 1967, **5**, 89–94.

Caldwell, W. V. *LSD psychotherapy*. New York: Grove Press, 1968.

Cameron, D. E., Sved, S., Solyom, L., Wainrib, B., & Barik, H. Effects of ribonucleic acid on memory defect in the aged. *American Journal of Psychiatry*, 1963, **120**, 320–325.

Chafetz, M. E. A procedure for establishing therapeutic contact with the alcoholic. *Quarterly Journal of Studies on Alcohol*, 1961, **22**, 325–328.

Enesco, H. E. RNA and memory: A re-evaluation of present data. *Canadian Psychiatric Association Journal*, 1967, **12**, 29–34.

Fox, R. (Ed.) *Alcoholism—behavioral research, therapeutic approaches.* New York: Springer, 1967.

Franks, C. M. Behavior modification and the treatment of the alcoholic. In R. Fox (Ed.), *Alcoholism—behavioral research, therapeutic approaches.* New York: Springer, 1967. Pp. 186–203.

Hill, M. J. & Blane, H. T. Evaluation of psychotherapy with alcoholics: A critical review. *Quarterly Journal of Studies on Alcohol*, 1967, **28**, 76–104.

Kastenbaum, R. (Ed.) *New thoughts on old age.* New York: Springer, 1964.

Kerr, N., Meyerson, L., & Michael, J. A procedure for shaping vocalizations in a mute child. In L. Ullmann & L. Krasner (Ed.), *Case studies in behavior modification.* New York: Holt, Rinehart & Winston, 1965.

Mental health care and the elderly: Shortcomings in public policy. Washington, D. C.: United States Government Printing Office, 1971.

Milmore, S., Rosenthal, R., Blaine, H. T., Chafetz, M. E., & Wolf, I. The doctor's voice: Posdictor of successful referral of alcoholic patients. *Journal of Abnormal Psychology*, 1967, **72**, 78–84.

Rimland, B. *Infantile autism.* New York: Appleton-Century-Crofts, 1964. Saronson, S. B., Doris, J. *Psychological problems in mental deficiency.* (4th ed.) New York: Harper & Row, 1969.

Thompson, T., Grabowski, J., Erickson, E. & Johnson, R. Development and maintenance of a behavior modification program for institutionalized profoundly retarded adult males. *Psychological Aspects of Disability* 1970, **17**, 117–124.

Volpe, A. & Kastenbaum, R. Beer and TLC. *American Journal of Nursing*, 1967, **67**, 100–103.

Wilner, D. M., & Kassebaum, G. G. (Eds), *Narcotics.* New York: McGraw-Hill, 1965.

Yablonsky, L. *Synanon: The tunnel back.* Baltimore: Penguin, 1967.

Zigler, E. Mental retardation: Current issues and approaches. In L. W. Hoffman & M. L. Hoffman (Eds.), *Review of child development research.* Vol. 2. New York: Russell Sage Foundation, 1966. Pp. 107–168.

UNIT V

Perspectives in Prevention

INTRODUCTION

Until the mid-1950s, the care and treatment afforded the vast majority of our society's mentally ill was centered in the mental hospital. Many of these hospitals, approximately 300 of which were state-funded institutions, were located in areas near large cities, occupying tens of acres of land, and housing 5,000 to 10,000 patients. The professional staff was typically not very large, and only a small percentage were psychologists and psychiatrists.

It is of no great surprise, therefore, that the *primary* function of these hospitals was to provide custodial and nursing care rather than intensive psychotherapy. Individual, group, and other forms of psychological therapy were practiced at these institutions, but because of the rather large patient-to-professional-staff ratio, it was virtually impossible to offer each patient the amount of therapy that he or she needed. This state of affairs was one of the reasons chemotherapy became so popular. It gave the clinician a means by which he could provide the majority of patients with something other than custodial care.

In the mid-1950s, the public became more aware of the overcrowded and understaffed conditions in mental hospitals as well as the type of treatment which patients received. This awareness resulted not only from information conveyed by the news media, but also from such books as Mary Jane Ward's *The Snake Pit* (1955). In 1955, in response to public dissatisfaction, the federal government appointed a Joint Commission on Mental Illness and Mental Health to investigate the treatment and care given the mentally ill, and to perform a thorough, nationwide analysis of the problems associated with mental illness. The final report of the joint commission, published in 1961, supported what had been reported earlier—that mental hospitals were understaffed, that there was a steady increase in the number of chronic patients in mental hospitals, and that patients primarily were receiving custodial care. The commission also emphasized the need for basic research over a long period of time, for mental health professionals to broaden their definition of who can provide treatment and what treatment consists of, and for the development of community-based mental health services.

Recognizing the findings and recommendations of this commission, President John F. Kennedy, in his mental health message to Congress in 1963, called for a "bold new approach" to the problem of mental illness. He advocated the establishment of community mental health centers in an attempt to combat mental health problems in our society. Legislation followed this proposal, and federal funds became available for the construction of community-based mental health centers.

This legislation, as well as the dissatisfaction with the medical model and discontent over previous mental health practices, led to the development of the *community mental health approach.* With this approach the emphasis is on helping people before their problems become so serious that hospitalization is necessary and on intervening in crises which place a person's mental health in jeopardy. The underlying assumption regarding the nature of abnormal behavior is very similar to Szasz's position (discussed in Unit I), namely, that it represents nothing more than problems in living. Advocates of this approach state that if the development of maladaptive behavior is to be prevented, intervention must be an active process. For example, the clinician should go into a home and talk with each member of a family in order to straighten out a family feud, call a person's boss to explain why he is always late to work, or meet with a child every day after school to help him with his reading.

This view necessitates a reorganization of the mental health professional's thinking with respect to his function and self-image. According to this position, the clinician becomes an active member of the community, is involved in neighborhood meetings as well as social functions, and tries to keep in touch with all that is going on in the community. His role is not that of an expert who waits in his office to treat maladaptive behavior, but that of a member of the community who attempts to help people having problems, undergoing a crisis, or who need information.

With a model such as this, the clinician may also have to move his office from the hospital setting or the city's major business section to a vacant store or apartment in the center of the community so that he can keep in close contact with the members of the community.

Article 39 is by Mike Gorman who discusses the history and goals of the community mental health movement in this country. He points out that this approach has brought professional help to people who were never reached previously or who were reached only after they were placed in a mental hospital. He also discusses some of the issues concerning community mental health and some of the current problems facing these centers, such as community control over the mental health center, funding from governmental sources, and criticisms from mental health professionals.

Article 40 by Emory L. Cowen is directed toward a specific aspect of the community mental health movement, namely, the identification of those children who show signs of mental health problems or show the potential for developing such problems. One place particularly well suited for identifying these children is the school classroom because of the various activities in which children are typically required to engage. Cowen describes a long-range project, started in 1958, for the early detection and prevention of maladaptation in school. The project was directed at the primary level, where children who were maladaptive or showed signs of becoming maladaptive were "red-tagged." The next step was to develop a means of helping these children. Since there were not enough clinicians available to deal with the demand for mental health services. Cowen and his associates began training nonprofessionals (e.g., housewives, undergraduate students, and neighborhood teenagers) as child-aides to work with these children under the supervision of a professional. Cowen discusses the results of this project as well as recent developments in the program and some of the problems associated with carrying out a research project of this magnitude.

Article 41 by Richard Schmuck and Mark Chesler discusses the opposition of some "superpatriots" to community mental health programs. Superpatriotism, according to these authors, is characterized by a patriotic or nationalistic conservatism, a vigorous anticommunism, and a commitment to action regarding the nation's condition. They point out that the superpatriot's concern is related to the belief that psychological testing constitutes an invasion of privacy; that mental health programs represent extensions of the federal bureaucracy; that mental health workers encourage immorality, sin, and social disorganization; that mental health programs are politically and ideologically biased; and that mental health programs are part of a communist plot in America. An analysis also is presented of some of the personal characteristics and the recruitment tactics of these people.

REFERENCE

Ward, M. J. *The snake pit*. New York: New American Library, 1955.

39

Community Mental Health: The Search for Identity*[1]

MIKE GORMAN

The timing of this plenary session on community mental health at so distinguished an international gathering is most fortunate, since in various parts of the world there is considerable debate going on about the future of community psychiatry generally, and of the community mental health center in particular. As a representative of the United States on this panel, I am delighted that we have a future to talk about—up until very recently in this country, we could really only venture tangential references to some limited experimentation in the heart of the community.

In the admittedly constricted perspective which six years of operation on a national scale bestows upon us, we are beginning to comprehend the truly revolutionary nature of what we have wrought in altering radically the profile of American psychiatry.

The distinguished Boston revolutionary and abolitionist, Wendell Phillips, noted more than a century ago that:"Revolutions are not made; they come. A revolution is as natural a growth as an oak. It comes out of the past. Its foundations are laid far back."

For almost two centuries here in America, the psychiatric landscape was grim and forbidding. The large mental hospitals—secular cloisters of the mad—grew to such outlandish size that as recently as the mid-1950s, a number of them were in the ten to fifteen thousand bed range.

The cumbrous custodial institution had its fair share of critics over a span of many years, but the voices of discontent became a loud chorus after World War II. During the Second World War, we in this country—and those of you representing other countries around the globe—were quite shocked at the number of young men whom we had to reject for the armed services because of psychiatric disabilities. On the other hand, the American public got its first glimpse of what non-institutional psychiatry could do in restoring men with psychological breakdowns to active duty.

There were other elements contributing to a revolt against the warehousing of the mentally ill in remote institutions. In certain parts of our land, newspapers began to probe into the inhumane level of custody in state hospitals. The internal criticism was accelerated by American professionals who travelled abroad and brought back reports of the beginnings of a new and exciting community-based psychiatry in Amsterdam, in Scotland, in England, and in the Scandinavian countries. Always eager to discover history—for the first time—our scientific journals printed stories of the glories of the care and treatment of the mentally ill in the community going back to the 11th century in Gheel, Belgium.

It is difficult to delineate the exact ingredients which, when properly simmered over a stove, produce a revolution. But there is little doubt that many of our hospital superinten-

---

*From Gorman, M., *Community Mental Health Journal*, 1970, **6**, 347–355. Copyright © 1970 by Behavioral Publications, Inc. Reprinted by permission of Behavioral Publications, Inc., and Mr. Gorman.

[1]This paper was originally given at the Inaugural Plenary Session, World Mental Health Assembly in Washington, D.C., November 1969.

dents, in the great tradition of Marie Antoinette, rattled their keys in defiance at those who were trying to smuggle a breath of the community beyond the feudal walls. Secondly, although our professional jurisdictions were beginning to deal antiseptically with the idea of community mental health, progress was slow. In the period 1945 to 1955 alone, 130,000 *additional* mental patients were jammed into the already over-crowded wards of our 300 state hospitals.

I am in full agreement with Dr. Arne Querido on the one common factor which has generated community mental health services in a number of countries: "A certain urgency, a certain must, a certain pressure requiring action. The theory comes much later."

The various rumblings of discontent finally coalesced into a consensus leading to the establishment of a Congressionally supported Joint Commission on Mental Illness and Health in 1955. Its final report, released six years later, sounded the death knell of the isolated cities of the mad. President John F. Kennedy endorsed the major recommendations of the Commission's report; in his historic 1963 mental health message to Congress, he called for a network of community mental health centers to replace eventually the backwater, insulated institutions of the past.

I suppose it is not surprising that neither the Joint Commission report nor President Kennedy's 1963 message were greeted with universal acclaim. Neither, for that matter, was our own Declaration of Independence in 1776. As the very perceptive French social critic, Maurice Maeterlinck, observed many years ago: "At every crossway on the road that leads to the future, each progressive spirit is opposed by a thousand men appointed to guard the past."

... how are we faring with the centers program in relation to President Kennedy's goal of 2,000 centers by 1980? We made a strong beginning, but the fiscal limitations dictated by the war in Vietnam ... hurt us badly .... There are approximately 250 centers open at the present time, and another 150 which have pulled together varying amounts of local, state, and federal matching monies and will open in the next year or two. In the face of admonitions to the contrary, we still hold fast to the goal of 2,000 centers by 1980.

What are we trying to achieve in the community mental health center concept? Our goal is simple and clear: It was expressed quite well in a recent publication of the Group for Advancement of Psychiatry, a coterie of some of our nation's most progressive psychiatrists: "We are no longer content to banish the mentally ill to a world that we shun and deny. Instead, with all the unpleasantness, difficulties and trials that accompany professional role changes, we seek ways to bring the mentally ill into the life of the community."

Viewed in context, the community mental health center is part and parcel of a healthy revolt against the impersonal colossi of our age—big government, the vast military-industrial complex, enormous universities which have become insensitive diploma mills, and social welfare institutions of all kinds whose bureaucratic procedures violate and offend the dignity of the individual.

The better mental health centers—many of them concentrated in the ghetto areas of our large cities—seek out the disturbed individual formerly lost in the chaos and confusion of urban life. Mental health professionals join with specially trained community residents and move into homes, schools, police stations, churches, and onto the streets themselves. Mental health services are now as close to the people as the store front clinic down the block or around the corner.

Many walk in off the street and through the open door. One such was a middle-aged man who told the receptionist at a center in one of our largest cities: "My son is 15. He is a smart boy but he is afraid to go to school. He gets nervous. The same thing with my missus; she is nervous, she aggravates him. The whole house is upset."

In a few days, the whole family was attending a two-hour family therapy session jointly conducted by one of the center's psychiatrists and a social worker. A number of these sessions followed, each costing the family the sum of one dollar.

These centers learn quickly that a patient coming out of a severely denuded environment cannot be helped significantly until the noxious milieu in which the illness festers is tackled. This has resulted in a number of our centers becoming involved in housing committees and tenant councils which force slumlords to improve living conditions; in efforts to improve the low level of medical services in an area, with particular emphasis upon good prenatal care leading to a reduction in the high rate of premature babies born with brain damage and other sequelae of the ghetto; in establishing remedial educational courses, many of them staffed by the older children in the neighborhood and, yes, even encouraging these previously alienated people to register and to vote so that they can truly participate in electing officials pledged to improve conditions which presently generate so much mental illness and mental disturbance. As the director of one of these centers put it recently: "Mental illness is really a social problem. It is not exclusively a psychological or a biological one. We frankly have to help people change their communities if necessary."

Engaging the people who are the consumers, the supposed raison d'être of the center's activities, in its decision-making processes is not without its problems. In several recent instances, the newly liberated people revolted against the professional overlords of the center and demanded a major say in the promulgation of policy and personnel decisions. It is too early in the history of community psychiatry here in this country to hazard any definitive pronouncements as to the best possible mix of professional stewardship and consumer involvement, but it is incumbent upon those who now tell us they knew we were headed for trouble to remember that any sharp and revolutionary break with heavily encrusted tradition involves a good deal of disturbance and controversy. Many of these hand-wringing critics embraced the idea of community psychiatry within the safe confines of pallid essays in their jurisdictional journals; they now look askance at the physical implementation of the archtype. Most revolutions start off with lofty pronouncements; they threaten the existing order only when the cobblestones begin to fly and the barricades are stormed.

At this point in time, what are the pluses and minuses in drawing up a balance sheet of the performance and potential of the community mental health center movement?

On the positive side, I think even the most vociferous critics of the center program will agree that it has brought psychiatric care to hundreds of thousands of our citizens who were never reached before. Furthermore, it has added a fresh and attractive dimension to mental health services by visualizing the patient in the totality of his fantastically diverse inter-relationships as a member of the family, of the world of work and of an alien society. There is a new thrust toward understanding, and helping the patient grapple with, the fierce external pressures which cascade in upon him. Until very recently in this country, therapists seemed to be treating endogenous, carefully isolated symptoms within a narrowly defined spectrum of "acceptable and manageable" maladies. In our public institutions, these symptoms served to define the very identity of the patient; he was quickly and conveniently labeled, put on the ward which handled that kind of disorder, and expected to act up or out in strict conformity with his prescribed diagnostic status. If he was affluent enough to afford private psychiatric care, he quietly slipped into a darkly furnished office and regurgitated symptoms from the approved lexicon upon cue from the omnipotent therapist.

The better centers in this country treat the patient as both enmeshed in, and a product of, a complex and stressful world. Their efforts are tailored toward supportive measures so that he may function, in however limited a way, in this society; they reach for positive strengths which can be capitalized upon to bring him into a degree of adaptation with his environment. For almost 200 years, we wrongfully stripped him of this individuality so that he could conform to the requirements of our massive, understaffed public mental hospitals.

He shuffled in endless lines; he sat in rocking chairs; he had no individual clothing or belongings, and he ate from a tin plate in a grimy mess hall with several thousand robotized brethren.

This—the affirmation of the dignity of the individual suffering from an illness—is the most positive contribution of the community mental health center movement.

I could dwell at much greater length upon additional achievements of the center in the area of community psychiatry, but I think it would be much more helpful and illuminating to those of you representing other countries to discuss some of the nagging obstacles to the fulfillment of our dream.

There are centers in this country which are little more than the traditional closed-door psychiatric units in general hospitals. They have just changed the lettering on the entrance to the ward. There are other centers which are suffering from shortages of mental health manpower, although I am happy to note that these are definitely in the minority. We have engaged in this country, over the past 20 years, in a training effort in the field of mental health manpower which has no parallel in the annals of modern medicine. The younger products of this training pipeline are now gravitating in increasing numbers toward our centers.

A major obstacle to the development of centers which truly guarantee continuity of care for the patient is the pluralistic nature of our democratic society. We have a plethora of health and welfare agencies of all kinds in our communities; most of them seem to have a proprietary interest in some defined segment of the patient. In order to lead the patient through this thicket of predatory agencies, we are developing a new breed of guides, variously known as expediters, facilitators, indigenous workers, and so on. In visiting community mental health services in a number of countries in Western Europe and Russia, I got the distinct impression that continuity of care and constant evaluation of a patient was possible without a traffic cop to help the patient through a maze of conflicting jurisdictions....

...I have tried to give you an honest picture of the community mental health center movement in America at this very early stage in its development. If the report leans a bit too heavily upon the agony rather than the ecstasy, it is done thusly because there are major issues which must still be resolved. A decade or so from now maybe some of us can come back and give you a more balanced view of community psychiatry, somewhat similar to the following summary of the successes and failures of the National Health Service in Great Britain which Dr. David H. Clark gave to the American Psychiatric Association last year:

> The National Health Service was a wonderful vision in 1948, born of the excitements of mighty victory, a belief that proper national organization could solve the problems of peace as well as it had those of war, and a determination to solve the manifest problems of the 1930s—parents too poor to pay for necessary treatment for their children, hospitals shabby, disorganized, and forever in debt, doctors flocking to wealthy middle-class areas and neglecting the sick poor of the industrial cities. It was based on a great ideal—that no individual or family should have to bear unaided the cost of illness. Like all revolutionary schemes for solving human ills, it has had both successes and failures. In general, it has solved the problems it set out to remedy, but created others which it cannot cure.

In like manner, community psychiatry is a great ideal which is being tested daily in the crucible of experience. For those of us who have had the privilege of tilting a lance or two against man's inhumanity to the mentally ill, the future of the community mental health center is bright and clear, for our effort is directed toward bringing mental health services to all segments of our society in a troubled age when the individual is increasingly lost in the impersonalities of mass technology and dehumanized services.

Our credo is akin to that of the distinguished American novelist William Faulkner who, on receiving the Nobel Prize in 1950, proclaimed: "I believe that man will not merely endure; he will prevail."

40

Emergent Directions in School Mental Health: The Development and Evaluation of a Program for Early Detection and Prevention of Ineffective School Behavior*[1]

EMORY L. COWEN

More so than ever before, society today is appalled by precipitous awarenesses of serious social and human-adaptive problems such as explosive inner-city riots, antisocial behaviors in high school dropouts, the rampant, destructive problems of addiction, the shocking conditions of many of our institutions (e.g. mental hospitals, detention settings, and prisons), and the bombing of public buildings. Nowadays such events and circumstances are all too evident because of the immediacy and drama of reports in the public media. Profound social eruptions polarize reactions from the entirely repressive, at one extreme, to well-meaning, humanitarian surges to develop crash programs to overpower these social blights, at the other. However well conceived these programs may be, they are subject to the dangers of being crisis-motivated, palliative counter-measures rather than planned, reasoned, long-term approaches.

The obvious and vexing presence of social eyesores also generates political pressure for immediate solutions. Proposals that grow out of such an atmosphere often lead to heavily invested crash programs, characteristically directed to manifest current symptoms and designed to solve these problems by "overwhelming" them. There are, however, hidden assumptions behind even the best designed and executed of such programs. They start, for example, with at least two strikes against them by being directed to conditions that are already florid, entrenched, and basic to the individual's life economy.

Even if that were not so, programs targeted specifically to advanced, well-developed, adverse "end states" (e.g. addiction) rest on the tenuous assumption that such conditions have specific determinants and can be treated effectively by specific interventions. They overlook the strong possibility that many personally or socially unfortunate outcomes—the

---

*From Cowen, E. L., *American Scientist*, 1971, **59**, 723–733. Copyright © 1971 by the Society of the Sigma Xi. Reprinted by permission of the Society of the Sigma Xi, and Dr. Cowen.

[1]The author acknowledges, with gratitude, the significant contributions of Mary Ann Trost, Chief Project Social Worker; Louis D. Izzo, Chief Project Psychologist; Darwin A. Dorr, Research Coordinator; and Angelo L. Madonia, Psychiatric Consultant; and our four senior aides, Mesdames Frieda Behrmann, Ruth Isaacson, Norma Finzer, and Dina Zwick, to the work reported in this paper. The author also thanks The Pilot and Experimental Training Branch of NIMH; the Monroe County Youth Board; the N.Y.S. Urban Education Program; the School Districts of Rochester, Fairport, Rush Henrietta, and West Irondequoit, New York; the John F. Wegman, Max A. Adler, Davenport-Hatch, and Wilmot-V. Castel Foundations; Rochester Jobs, Inc.; and several anonymous donors, whose generous support has made this work possible.

2 strikes against program
① — many are entrenched in mid life summary
② — already are adverse "end solutions" to similar life problem
Therefore must concentrate on prevention
Schools are place for it

Perspectives in Prevention   **457**

psychoses, alcoholism, addiction, crime and delinquency, the neuroses—merely reflect alternative, adverse "end solutions" to earlier life problems. Otherwise stated, it is more than admissible that effective generalized programs in early detection and prevention could cut down the flow of *many* different types of maladaptive end states—indeed most of those that fall under the umbrella of human disordered behavior.

If this argument has merit, it is not only appropriate but essential that society allocate a far greater share of its mental health resources to before-the-fact prevention rather than to costly, ineffective attempts at after-the-fact repair (which, in the last analysis, can be viewed analogically as applying undersized, frayed Band-Aids to profusely bleeding psyches). This point of view is well reflected in the recent report of the President's Task Force on the Mentally Handicapped (1970) which states on page 18: "By proverbial wisdom and common sense, prevention of disability is greatly to be preferred to treatment and rehabilitation." Schools, as social institutions that significantly shape the development of all human beings in modern society, are potentially ideal settings for preventive interventions.

Since the beginning of the current century, mental health professionals have been performing a variety of clinical services in American schools, reflecting two basic assumptions: (1) that schools have both the responsibility, and the potential, for promoting the child's psychological as well as his educational well-being and (2) that these two spheres of development are intimately intertwined—i.e. psychological maladaptation encourages educational failure and vice versa.

The day-to-day activities of school mental health professionals have long been guided by prevailing conceptions of pathological behavior and by a *reactive* orientation to deficit. Psychologists and social workers in the schools have been cast in the role of "experts" or "trouble-shooters," called on to do their magic in the face of significant educational or interpersonal failure. Striking and understandable parallels exist between the specific problems of school mental health today and the broader ones confronting society in this area: Professionals are in woefully short supply. Demand for assistance, and certainly latent need, far exceeds resources. Established helping techniques are limited in value and their distribution across social strata is inequitable. Thus, the meager firepower generated from scarce mental health resources is directed to a relatively small percent of florid, rooted dysfunctions, which, unfortunately, are precisely the ones with the poorest prognoses.

Recent surveys (Glidewell & Swallow, 1969) indicate that roughly 30 percent of all children have school maladaptation problems ranging from mild to severe. In some quarters, that figure is as high as 70 percent. The absolute numbers thus implicated are staggering, and our present resource system cannot provide effective help for them. The magnitude of the mismatch between school-failure data and resource data dictates consideration of alternative conceptualizations and stratagems to guide future school mental health approaches. Greater attention must be directed to engineering school environments that potentiate adaptation, developing delivery systems that feature widespread early identification of ineffective school function, and creating interventions designed to short-circuit maladaptation. Such efforts must pay heed to the realities of current manpower shortages if they are to be successful. They must meet the twin challenges of identifying effective new manpower deployments and more socially utilitarian uses of scarce professional time.

We shall describe here the development and evaluation of a long-range program for early detection and prevention of school maladaptation which offers a logically attractive alternative to past after-the-fact, crisis-oriented school mental health delivery systems. Although the foregoing views were present in germinal form when our program started more than a decade ago, they were far less clearly articulated. At that time we were more

early identification & intervention of
chronic & current maladaptation

impressed by several earthy, "battle-line" observations hinting at weaknesses in the school mental health delivery system. The first, a point frequently made by teachers, was that 40 to 60 percent of class time was preempted by three or four children who were unable, for any of several reasons, to meet the challenge of school. This condition was unhealthy for the affected few, seriously undermined the educational environment of the many, and threatened the teacher's equanimity and well-being.

A second perturbing problem was the rash of referrals, some complicated and serious, in children about to move from elementary to high school. Typically, resources for dealing with such problems were not available. Study of these children's cumulative dossiers often indicated that prodromal signs had been present in fifth, or third, grade or even at the very start of the child's school career. Either appropriate services for the child had not been available earlier or people had hoped that, if they closed their eyes long enough, the difficulties would go away. Far from vanishing, in most cases they "picked up steam" over time, became rooted, and assumed even more serious proportions during the later elementary period.

Faced with many such serious chronic problems, we decided to allocate existing mental health resources to early detection and prevention at the primary level, even at the risk of losing traditional clinical services at the upper levels. Our hope was that this emphasis might sharply reduce the incidence of chronic school maladaptation and, with it, heavy later service demands. In a world of finite resources, such as the world of mental health today, critical decisions have less to do with whether a given objective (i.e. program) is "good" absolutely and more with which of many "goods" have the *greatest* prospective social value. Merely to perpetuate known programs without considering other possible allocations of the scarce resources restricts innovation by default. The value clearly reflected in our decision is that prevention is preferable to repair—indeed it is essential if truly effective school mental health programs are to develop.   0 *early ident + secondary prevention develop*

THE EARLY YEARS, 1958-1969

Our work on the Primary Mental Health Project (PMHP), spanning 13 years, falls into three periods. In the first, 1958 to 1963, new techniques for early identification of school maladaptation and a primitive program in early secondary prevention were developed. A school psychologist and a school social worker were assigned, full-time, to promote these ends in the primary grades of a single elementary school in Rochester, N.Y. Children in this school were largely from the upper-lower and lower-middle socioeconomic strata and were ethnically representative of the city of Rochester at large, except for an underweighting of Negro and Jewish children.

Estimates of actual, or incipient, school maladaptation were formulated for first-grade children based on an amalgam of four sources: group psychological screening of intellectual and personality status, social work interviews with mothers, direct classroom observation, and teachers' reports of the child's behavior and educational status. Based on these data a dichotomous clinical judgment—red-tag vs. non-red-tag—was rendered for each child. This was a private research diagnosis, to avoid labeling the child or promoting self-fulfilling prophecies. Red-taggers were those who had already manifested dysfunction or in whom such dysfunction seemed imminent; the non-red-taggers were children who had adapted adequately to school. Later research clarified the basis for this initially dichotomous clinical judgment, particularly the contribution of the social worker's interview, and established a framework for rendering continuous judgments of school adaptation (Beach,

Cowen, Zax, Laird, Trost, & Izzo, 1968). The red-tag judgment has been shown to relate to other salient facets of the child's behavior and performance, including school record and achievement data, and teacher and parent judgments (Zax, Cowen, Izzo, & Trost, 1964; Liem, Yellott, Cowen, Trost, & Izzo, 1969; Cowen, Huser, Beach, & Rappaport, 1970).

About a third of the primary graders were classified red-tag, a figure that compares closely to Glidewell and Swallow's 30 percent school maladjustment datum (Cowen, Izzo, Miles, Tolschow, Trost, & Zax, 1963; Cowen, Zax, Izzo, & Trost, 1966). These children were found to be functioning significantly more poorly than non-red-taggers on a variety of measures taken at the end of the third school year: school record indices, such as attendance and nurse-referrals; performance criteria, including report-card grades, standard, system-wide achievement tests, and achievement-aptitude discrepancy scores; behavioral and adjustive indices, including behavior ratings made by teachers and mental health professionals; and peer ratings of sociometric status.

Figure 40.1 graphically depicts significant differences between red-tag and non-red-tag groups on 14 criterion measures, at the end of third grade. In all instances the observed differences favor the non-red-tag group. Follow-up evaluation at seventh grade level (Zax, Cowen, Rappaport, Beach, & Laird, 1968) indicated that, without special intervention during the elementary period, the red-tag child's dysfunction and inability to achieve continued. Thus in seventh grade, red-taggers were less well accepted by peers, were judged as more maladjusted by teachers, and had poorer health records, lower grades, and lower scores on standard achievement tests than non-red-taggers.

Initial secondary preventive efforts, over a three-year period, were built around recasting the professional's role away from traditional one-to-one clinical services for acute flare-ups or crises toward educative, resource, and consultative functions (Cowen, Zax, Izzo, & Trost, 1966; Zax & Cowen, 1969). At the end of the third school year, children in the prevention program (*E*'s) were compared with peers from demographically similar, geographically contiguous control schools (*C*'s) with traditional school mental health services. The *E*'s significantly exceeded *C*'s on seven measures, including fewer nurse referrals, higher grades and achievement test scores, superior achievement relative to aptitude, lower self-rated anxiety, and teacher behavior ratings indicating superior adjustment (Cowen, Zax, Izzo, & Trost, 1966). Figure 40.2 depicts significant differences between experimental and control children.

The two key conclusions emerging from our initial work were that (1) ineffective function can be accurately identified early in the child's school career and, without intervention, it has serious later consequences, and (2) there are significant positive effects, along several important dimensions, of an early secondary prevention program. These findings established a base for pursuing related objectives within a common conceptual net.

NONPROFESSIONAL AIDES

However accurate and efficient programs for early detection may be, their social value to date has been limited by an inability to follow through with appropriate remediation. This failing has been due both to the way society's interpersonal helping resources have been defined and to current acute shortages in professional mental health manpower. At the time we had to face this dilemma, important new explorations of the use of nonprofessionals in human service were getting under way. A central issue underlying such usage is whether the attributes required to help another person are those of I.Q., advanced specialty education, and professional degrees, or whether they are found in the spheres of personality, life

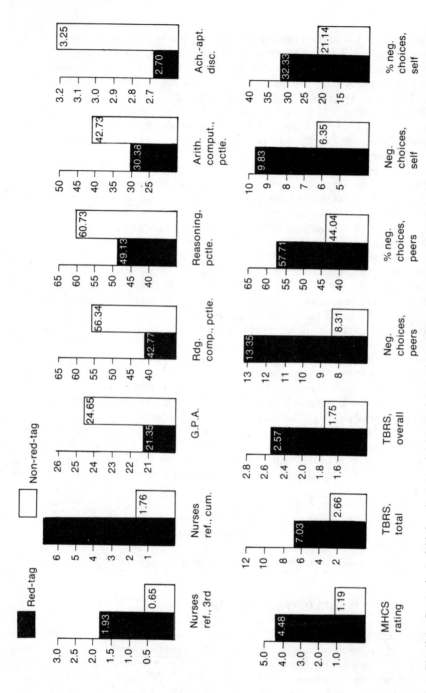

Fig. 40.1 Comparison of third grade status of red-tag and non-red-tag children shows superior adjustment or academic achievement on all measures for the non-red-tag group. *Nurses ref., 3rd:* Mean, number of referrals to nurse, 3rd grade. *Nurses ref., cum.:* Mean, number of referrals to nurse, 1st–3rd grades. *G.P.A.:* Mean, sum of end-of-year report card grades. *Rdg. comp., pctle.:* Mean, percentile score, SRA reading comprehension. *Reasoning, pctle.:* Mean, percentile score, SRA reasoning. *Arith. comput., pctle.:* Mean, percentile score, SRA arithmetic computation. *Ach.-apt. disc.:* Mean, discrepancy between achievement and aptitude. *MHCS rating:* Mean, maladjustment rating by mental-health professionals. *TBRS, total:* Mean, sum of teachers' behavior ratings. *TBRS, overall:* Mean, teachers' overall behavior rating for maladjustment. *Neg. choices, peers:* Mean, number of negative peer sociometric nominations. *% neg. choices, peers:* Mean, percent negative peer sociometric nominations. *Neg. choices, self:* Mean, number of negative role, self-nominations.

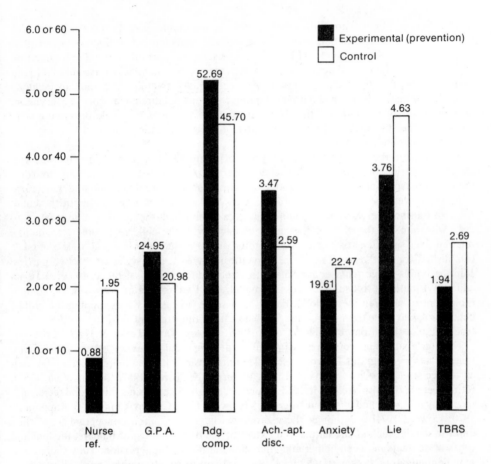

Fig. 40.2 Comparison of third grade status of experimental (prevention) and control groups on seven criterion measures shows superior adjustment or academic achievement on each for prevention group. *Nurse ref.*: Mean, number of referrals to nurse, 3rd grade. *G.P.A.*: Mean, sum of end-of-year report card grades. *Rdg. comp.*: Mean, percentile score, SRA reading comprehension. *Ach.-apt. disc.*: Mean, discrepancy between aptitude and achievement. *Anxiety*: Mean, anxiety scale score (Childrens Manifest Anxiety Scale). *Lie*: Mean, lie scale score (Childrens Manifest Anxiety Scale). *TBRS*: Mean, teachers' overall behavior rating for maladjustment.

experience, and stylistic variables. Given the shortage of resources, however, the choice we faced was either to repress identified problems or to develop new nonprofessional helping-services "checked and balanced" by alternative new professional roles.

Accordingly, we recruited a small group of six housewives, judged to be warm, natural, interpersonally adept, themselves effective mothers, with a strong interest in working with children, to serve as child-aides with maladapting primary-graders (Zax & Cowen, 1967). These women came from middle-class backgrounds, had a median high school education, and were on the average in their early forties. Since we counted heavily on the aides' styles and reflexes, rather than on mastery of the content of a Ph.D. curriculum, training was focused and brief (6 weeks). Its two major purposes were to develop an understanding and way of thinking about school adjustment problems and to minimize the anxiety some aides felt about prospective human service contacts with maladapting children—a heretofore sacrosanct professional function. The didactic-discussion portion of training touched on aspects of early childhood development, behavior problems in children, parent-child relations, and, briefly, on teaching methods and techniques. Its clinical component included case-history materials, films about maladapting children, and direct classroom observation, each followed by discussion of the observed behavior. Frequency of child-observations increased as the start of actual service activities neared, facilitating a natural transition between training and on-the-job activities.

Aides were hired as half-time employees to permit regular, planful interactions with children experiencing difficulties. Teachers referred youngsters to the aide program for a variety of reasons: aggressive, disruptive behaviors; shyness, timidity, and undersocialization; and more classic learning disorders. After background information about the child, from various sources, was shared and objectives established, the aide began to meet regularly with him. At the core of the aide's contacts with the child is a committed human relation. Her specific activities vary depending on the child's problem and, thus, the goals established for him, as well as the personalities, interests, and styles of the two parties. Joint activities range from conversation to direct educational assistance, to recreational and play functions, to use of expressive media, etc. Evaluations of aide-seen vs. comparable control children (see below), based on a series of rating scales tapping the child's behavioral and educational progress, indicated that the program is seen as effective by teachers, aides, and parents alike (Cowen, 1968; Cowen, Dorr, Trost, & Izzo, in press).

The housewife-aide program gave impetus to development of several other, conceptually related, service programs for young school children using different helping personnel such as college students (Cowen, Zax, & Laird, 1966; Zax & Cowen, 1967; Cowen, et al., 1969), retired people (Cowen, Leibowitz, & Leibowitz, 1968), indigenous neighborhood teenagers, inner-city mothers, and even fourth-graders (Cowen, 1970; Cowen, Chinsky, & Rappaport, 1970; Cowen, 1971b). Although these programs have a common conceptual base, they differ in details such as the nature and extent of the prior training of helpers, the loci and types of contacts between helper and child, and methods of supervision. They share common denominators, however, which, additively, point to an alternative approach to school dysfunction. All the programs focus on *young*, maladapting school children. They pivot around the strong commitment of the helping person to a child who needs assistance. They implicate key role-shifts by the school mental health professional in which traditional one-to-one clinical services are, in good measure, supplanted by educative, liaison, supervisory, consultative, and resource functions.

This redefined approach seems to have potential for expanding the reach of mental health helping activities in sorely needed geometric ways. To illustrate, a group of five half-time child-aides can see about 50 youngsters during the school year, for an average of thirty-five 40-minute sessions each. Not only are 50 children far more than the professional can see this intensively but they also represent a substantial proportion of the maladapting primary graders in any given school. While using nonprofessionals started as an expedient to meet professional manpower and fiscal problems, Sobey (1970) recently presented data suggesting that this development now stands on its own merits. Her survey of several hundred human service programs using nonprofessionals indicates that 85 percent report faster service, 89 percent, more extensive service, 84 percent, the ability to add new services, 76 percent, freeing up professional time, and 84 percent, gaining new viewpoints as a result of using nonprofessionals. In our program, ingredients such as the aides' strong motivation, their intrinsic "common sense," and the exciting challenge offered by the work combine to make this group a prospectively valuable asset in human service for maladapting children.

RECENT DEVELOPMENTS

The project's first decade developed methods for early detection of ineffective school function, studied its incidence, and assessed the efficacy of early secondary interventions. Research indicated that the model was workable and merited expansion from its initial experimental-demonstration base to one of broader system impact. Accordingly, in the late stages of the second project-period, after establishing a support base with responsible mental health planning groups in the community, discussions of how it might be extended were undertaken with Rochester City School District and several nearby county school districts. This period was marked by countless meetings, with school boards, superintendents, principals, and pupil personnel co-ordinators, around issues of feasibility and cost.

Ultimately a plan evolved to extend the project to six Rochester and five county schools in three adjacent districts. These eleven settings represented a wide range, including large ($N = 1,100$) and small ($N = 140$) schools; exclusively primary (kgn–3rd grade) and traditional elementary (kgn–7th grade) schools; locales ranging from the inner-city ghetto (97 percent nonwhite enrollment) to relatively affluent suburbia. While there were structural commonalities in *how* participating schools were staffed (i.e. portions of the time of a social worker and psychologist plus x child-aides for each pair of schools), specifics varied as a function of resources. Thus, whereas one full-time psychologist, one full-time social worker, and 10 aides staffed each two Rochester city schools, county schools averaged one-quarter to two-fifths of a psychologist and social worker and fewer (e.g. 6–8) aides per pair of schools. Most aides work half-time except in inner-city schools, where need and job realities dictated full-time employment.

While different saturations, particularly in professional time, in the several settings detract from program uniformity, they accurately mirror the reality of the current resource scene. The challenge they present is: "Given fixed and less than ideal resources in a setting, what programs and personnel deployments are most promising?" The project as it now exists is hardly a series of eleven identical models from a Sears Roebuck catalogue; it is far more a federation of philosophically linked, like-minded, but highly individualistic programs. Its specific implementation and detail necessarily vary across schools because needs, problems, and, particularly, resources vary. The linking orientations that bring programs together under a single umbrella are their shared emphasis on early detection and prevention of school maladaptation; their use of professionals as consultants and resource people, and building direct child-helping services around nonprofessional child-aides. Whatever its resource limits are, each setting thus seeks, realistically, to extend its individual and social impact.

THE PROGRAM IN ACTION

For the 1969–70 school year, the expanded PMHP had a six-month "build-up" period in the eleven participating schools during which professionals, many newly assigned, became known to school personnel, oriented them to project workings, made necessary space arrangements, and established referral systems. Training professionals and recruiting and training child-aides, each described more fully elsewhere (Cowen, in press), also took place during the build-up period.

The program's actual child-serving operations began in March 1970. By then schools had generated ample slates of child-referrals. Roughly 330 children were seen during the three month "debugging" period in the spring of 1970. During the 1970–71 academic year, 531 children were referred to the program, including about 150 carry-overs from the preceding spring. PMHP has thus seen about 700 youngsters in its first year. This total, roughly 17 percent of the primary grade enrollment of participating schools, includes most youngsters with serious maladaptive problems who otherwise would have gone without help.

Most often, aides see children two times a week for relatively brief (30–40 minute) sessions. At peak, the aide group renders about 800 child-serving contacts weekly, suggesting by extrapolation that a program of this magnitude can generate at least 20,000 child-contacts annually. To cite two hypothetical extremes in resource allocation, one could choose to see 4,000 children five times each or 200 children 100 times each. Neither extreme makes sense as a uniform prescription. Interventions with children must necessarily reflect their individual needs and problems. Some children can profit from a brief contact every other week; others will need to be seen three times a week. Since specific empirical relations among types of maladaptation, frequency of contact, and outcome are not yet established, diverse allocations of aide resources are being explored.

For example, aides during the 1970–71 school year were trained in group approaches, for children who might particularly be helped by a sheltered group socialization experience. This development has two potential values: expanding the number of children who can be seen, and as an intervention-modality of choice for children with specific types of school maladaptation (e.g. the timid and the withdrawn). In inner-city settings, which are frequently characterized by sharp communication barriers between home and school that subvert the child's educational growth, aides have been used effectively as home visitors to open doors between families and a school establishment often seen as alien. The aides, themselves neighborhood people, offer "know-how" and a "style match" (Reiff & Riessman, 1965) that help to gain entrance into heretofore impenetrable homes—a crucial first step in opening lines of communication.

How children get referred to PMHP and what, concretely, happens to them in their project experience bear further consideration. In their day-to-day contacts with children, teachers frame standards for behavior and educational development. They differ considerably in their reactions to departures from these expectancies. Children who show minor deviations are often effectively handled within the teacher's well-established repertoire of classroom-management techniques. However, when a problem defies "normal" handling or assumes "serious" proportions in her eyes, the teacher solicits help. PMHP stands as a potential resource in such instances. The principal difficulties that elicit the call for help are learning disabilities (e.g. the child who does not read), problems of withdrawal and under-socialization, and those of hyperactivity, aggressiveness, and distractibility. When the teacher determines that a more serious failing is present, or well along in process, she submits a referral to the mental health professionals indicating briefly the nature of the difficulty. Occasionally referrals come from other school personnel or from parents; in each case, however, formal recognition of a serious school adaptation problem energizes the helping process.

Available sources of information about the child are pooled at the time of referral. These include the referral statement itself; prior screening information (e.g. group intellectual, personality, and behavior measures) obtained routinely for all children early in the school year; and data from the social worker's contact with the mother. A staff conference is held, including mental health professionals serving as consultants, the teacher, prospective aide, and involved "others" (e.g. principal, nurse, lunchroom monitor) who interact with the child, to piece together available information, arrive at a preliminary understanding of his difficulties, and establish a set of working goals. Though on occasion another approach is recommended (e.g. social work contact with mother or a set of procedures for more effective classroom management), most often the child is assigned to meet regularly with an aide, with a particular set of objectives in mind.

CASE HISTORY

A résumé of a composite case may give a clearer picture of the modus operandi.

Bobby, a second-grader, was brought to the team's attention by his teacher. He was extremely disruptive in the classroom and aggressive to peers in the school corridors, gymnasium, and lunchroom. "Unless given complete attention and constant praise," said his teacher, "he strikes out at anyone near him and has tantrums." Although evidencing above-average potential in earlier intellectual screening, Bobby had already been left back once and now was identified as the *bête noire* of the primary grades. He was on the threshold of suspension from school.

Social work contact with his mother indicated an unstable family history. The oldest of four children, Bobby was the product of a stormy marriage that ended in divorce when he was four. His mother remarried and came to Rochester where, in the next four years, the family moved six times, and Bobby attended four schools with assignment to seven different classrooms.

At an initial staff conference, the boy's teacher, the mental health professionals, school principal, lunchroom monitor, and prospective aide pieced together a view of Bobby as a child who had spent his first years in an uncertain, ever-changing, menacing psychological world, who had learned to expect misfortune, and whose behavior was designed to probe and confirm his belief that his environment was hostile and people untrustworthy. On the positive side, Bobby had established interests in arts and model-making, his family situation was now more stable, and his mother showed genuine concern for his well-being.

Objectives and guidelines were established for those who would have frequent contact with Bobby. Most important were: trying to stabilize a positive, trusting view of his world; shoring up his battered self-concept; offering praise and support only for real achievement; and setting realistic limits firmly. He was assigned to see an aide twice weekly.

Thereafter, when Bobby challenged his teacher with his overt provocations, she unswervingly dealt with each transgression in a way that clearly labeled the action—but not the child—as unacceptable. After some time, this damped his need to act out; in fact, one day he said to his mother that his teacher "was really fair and I deserved to be punished!"

Bobby's initial approach to his aide was marked more by aloofness and disinterest than by the heralded pattern of aggressive provocation. The aide accepted his style and pacing without pushing him. When, after this early fencing, Bobby ventured several half-hearted, almost transparent attempts at provocation, the aide's response was again firm but accepting. His relation with the aide became more enthusiastic, and he became involved in high-level artistic and creative activities that won him deserved approval and support.

The teacher, aide, and mental health consultants conferred several times during the year to compare notes. It was clear within six weeks that the boy had "turned the corner." The frequency and intensity of his environmental testing had diminished sharply, and his formerly deficient academic work had improved markedly. Apparently, two relations of trust and security had been established, with a resultant change in Bobby's view of the world. This was helped along by further stabilization in his home situation, by his mother's clearer understanding, with the help of the social worker, of Bobby's perceptions, and by his mother's development of more effective ways to interact with him in critical choice-point situations.

The boy met with his aide 57 times during the eight-month school year. Two years later, he was showing above-average academic progress and was well accepted by his classmates. Virtually all signs of his prior Dennis-the-Menace behavior had disappeared.

FURTHER TRAINING AND NEW ROLES

Training for all project personnel is seen as on-going and open-ended. Professionals continue to have regular biweekly training sessions, as a "committee of the whole," to consider current problems of project conduct and management. They provide on-the-job supervision and case-review sessions for aides. Supervision, though regularized, varies in format across schools and includes both individual and group contacts. Teacher involvement is facilitated through extensive use of substitute teachers, which allows regular teachers to participate with professionals and aides in conferences concerning the children during school hours. Several principals regard the teachers' continuing growth in understanding and sensitivity, gained through participation in discussions of problem instances with teams and consultants and then translated to more effective, direct battle-line handling of classroom situations, as the principal project benefit. If the teacher learns to cope with budding dysfunction more effectively in the classroom, an important step toward primary prevention has been achieved.

Project staff provide extensive consultation to participating schools, with a broad range of objectives. Among the most basic is to strengthen the hand of program participants so that they can come to function more independently. ("Modeling" the consultant's role for school professionals and professionals-in-training furthers this end. Another consulting objective is to clarify project aims and roles continually so that they can be carried out most effectively. When difficulties come up (e.g. misuse of project resources, inadequate supervision, disagreements between team members), the consultant fulfills important information-finding and trouble-shooting roles. The format of consultation varies. There are individual meetings with school personnel, group conferences with child-aides and/or with teachers, and frequent case-centered consultations on specific problem children, with teachers, aides, and professionals.

Currently, to extend the project's consulting arm, four senior aides have assumed consultative responsibilities. These women, each with six years of prior supervised experience with children, serve as resource-persons for new aides. The decision to use senior aides as consultants was not a manpower expedient; rather, it grew out of our experience in training nonprofessionals, where we discovered that contact with seasoned aides was among the most useful, informative, and reassuring of all possible experiences for aides-in-training. While use of senior aides as consultants is new and still in the process of "finding its own level," initial reactions to it have been positive. The consulting aide brings experience and perspective to the beginner re specific problems that develop in contacts with children, "models" the aide role, and participates in individual and group supervision by professionals, representing another vantage point and set of experiences. Project staff supervise these senior aide activities.

The delivery system described, aiming as it does for geometric expansion of helping services, requires, in addition to new manpower uses, changing professional roles. The professional abandons a substantial portion of traditional, direct clinical service functions in favor of activities elsewhere described as mental health "quarterbacking" (Cowen, 1967; Cowen, 1971; Zax & Cowen, 1972). The cadre of nonprofessionals brought into line-contact roles extends the mental health helping arm significantly by bringing service to a substantial segment of maladapting school children who might otherwise become casualties of the system. The ultimate proof of the model rests in the empirical, rather than philosophical, arena. Way-station empirical indicants have been encouraging (see Fig. 40.2).

Reality, logic, and cost economics favor this new approach. For example, five half-time aides, at a total cost of about 50 percent of one full-time mental health professional, bring service to perhaps ten times as many children. If the initial relatively minor cost-increment of hiring aides averts personally disastrous and socially costly outcomes, such as institutional placement for mental disability, addiction, delinquent and criminal behavior, or less drastic ones, such as foster-home or special-class placement, then the model holds promise for important long-term financial as well as human gain. The professional in this new program in no sense becomes obsolescent; rather he assumes new, more socially utilitarian roles that significantly extend the reach of needed services.

RESEARCH COMPONENTS

From the start, the project has heavily emphasized research. Some of its early findings were described in the preceding text. Current project research is extensive; however, anchored as it is in a real, sometimes volatile world, the research is often hampered by extraneous external "noise" that detracts from a theoretical ideal of antiseptically pure laboratory work. Our research net touches, directly or indirectly, roughly 20,000 people, including children, teachers, parents, school personnel, and mental health professionals and nonprofessionals. Thus, sheer problems of numbers are overwhelming. Moreover, many of our "responders" understandably feel distant, or removed, from the research operation. They do not clearly perceive how marks on a piece of paper today can have much to do with effective education tomorrow. Consequently we expect, and get, a certain amount of careless responding, overt noncooperation, and passive aggression. The entire research operation is far less clean than the tightly controlled laboratory investigation. Impure data, weakened experimental designs, and absence of ideal controls are, for us, chronic hazards.

Another order of research problem stems from the rapid flux of the current urban educational scene. New programs are continually being introduced. School structures and compositions are changing. In Rochester, for example, there has been much interest in, and at times acrimonious debate about, redistricting schools to achieve racial balance. The Rochester School Board voted in the spring of 1970 to establish two such racially balanced zones, including, as it happened, two project schools. An immediate consequence of this decision was that these schools became kgn–3 structures rather than kgn–6. Because of the considerable investment in the redistricting plan, the shift in structure was understandably accompanied by other, hopefully salutary, changes (e.g. smaller classes, introduction of teacher-aide personnel, special reading programs, "voluntary" teachers).

While such drastic change can, in part, be neutralized experimentally by using comparably "zoned-but-nonproject" control schools, rapid change in school structures breeds a host of additional problems for the researcher. Some schools—and it is their autonomous right to do so—have, for example, eliminated grading completely or have introduced prose reports as substitutes. Others have abandoned the one-teacher/one-class notion that has long pervaded primary education, and now rotate children to several class groupings and teachers, for different subject areas or pursuits. Without arguing the merits of these changes, the fact that grades and teacher judgments, heretofore bellwether evaluation criteria, are simply unavailable or no longer comparable across schools renders the already complex challenge of long-term project evaluation extraordinarily difficult. An incidental irony is added when educational change, which an experimenter may favor as a professional or as a citizen, undercuts long years of heavily invested program development and carefully evolved experimental design.

Nor are the foregoing problems static, "one-shot" concerns. To the contrary, today's social sands shift with ever-accelerating speed. In Rochester, for example, the school board, the city's basic education policy-making and planning body, is a partisan group. Each November thus holds a potential for change that can seriously affect programs and research evaluations. All this makes for very real, built-in research risk, since basic change in school organization or programs becomes experimental noise confounding the supposed "main effect" of concern—the project itself. We have little control over the powerful social forces underlying educational change. The project sits in a real and, at the moment, thoroughly mercurial urban world. Unquestionably its research findings will be affected and limited by this fact.

Such realistic limitations notwithstanding, research on all facets of the project proceeds energetically. Past studies and those underway include methodological and substantive investigations, outcome evaluations, process analyses, selection and prediction studies, and examination of the complex interrelations among these classes of variables.

We are, of course, centrally concerned with the effectiveness of the program and its components (i.e. outcome). In the immediate sense, this calls for specific evaluation of the aide program, based on comparison of the behavioral and educational development of youngsters exposed to it and otherwise comparable controls. Over longer periods our evaluation framework will be broadened to allow comparison of *all* children in project vs. control schools on relevant measures of educational and personal development. Subtler aspects of the overall outcome question are also of concern, as for example: Do children with particular types of referral problems (e.g. undersocialization) profit more, or less, from the program than others (e.g. children referred for hyperactivity and aggression)? Are there relations between aide attributes and effectiveness with one or another type of child?

In a retrospective study of program outcomes (Cowen, Dorr, & Pokracki, 1972), mothers of 36 children seen by child-aides, an average of two years earlier, for an average of 55 sessions, were asked to judge the child's *current* status on a series of 7-point "change"-rating scales reflecting specific dimensions, such as getting along at home, getting along in school, peer relations, and attitude to school. Mothers and interviewers independently judged that significant growth had occurred in the child's subsequent educational and interpersonal development. Some of the findings of this study are depicted in Figure 40.3. Thus, relatively stable intermediate as well as short-term gain may be assumed to result from the aide program. The target children in question, almost without exception, had also made normal academic progress in the intervening period.

More microscopic study of the aide-child interaction is of interest to us both absolutely (i.e. descriptive accounts of what takes place during such contacts) and in terms of relations between process elements and many other variables, including outcome indices, aide characteristics, and structural aspects of program (professional and resource characteristics, nature of referrals, etc.). Accordingly, we have developed a comprehensive process-analysis form, including characterizations of both aide goals and actual aide activities with children (McWilliams, 1971). This form (shown in Fig. 40.4) is completed biweekly by each aide for each child she is seeing, a procedure that yielded about 4,500 completed process forms for the 1970–71 school year.

Data such as these permit study of a number of significant questions, as for example: What is the overall nature of the aide-child interaction process and how does it change over time? Are there overall, or time-period, differences in process for different types of referrals (e.g. acting out vs. withdrawn vs. children with learning disabilities)? Do settings differ in emphases and contact procedures as evidenced by different process reports? Are there relations between specific goals established for a child and the use of particular process activity categories? What relations exist between goals and/or process activities and

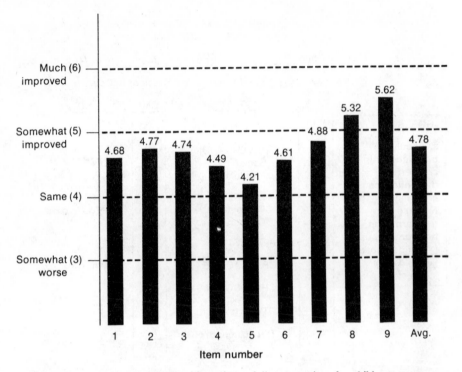

Fig. 40.3 Mean pooled parent and interviewer follow-up ratings for children seen two years earlier by child-aides. Each, except variable 5, indicates statistically significant improvement. *1:* Actual educational performance. *2:* Getting along with teachers. *3:* Getting along with schoolmates. *4:* Getting along with parents. *5:* Getting along with siblings. *6:* Getting along with neighborhood kids. *7:* Degree of happiness. *8:* Attitude toward school. *9:* Extent of project's responsibility for observed changes (from complete to none). *Avg.:* Average improvement scores based on items 1–9.

outcomes? Is there a relation between aide characteristics (e.g. personality factors, interest, attitudes, etc.) and how aides interact either with children in general or with specific groups?

Development of process information, particularly as it relates to outcome and aide-characteristics data, is essential. In addition to the theoretical value of establishing functional relations among these classes of variables, such information has considerable practical utility when fed back to participating schools (e.g. for optimizing assignment of children to aides and identifying maximally useful ways of interacting with them).

Considerable progress has already been made in identifying characteristics of child-aides. An interview study (Cowen, Dorr, & Pokracki, 1972) showed that school mental health professionals agreed well in assessing 18 job-relevant personal characteristics of the overall child-aide applicant sample. Furthermore, interviewing professionals discriminated reliably, along all 18 dimensions, between those accepted and those turned down for aide positions, even though the applicant group, as a whole, was homogeneously "select." A further study (Sandler, 1970) demonstrated that the selected aide sample differed from demographically comparable controls in terms of their greater empathy, higher affiliative and nurturant qualities, lesser aggression, stronger teaching and social service interests,

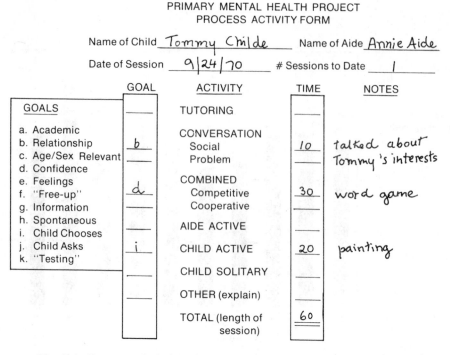

PRIMARY MENTAL HEALTH PROJECT
PROCESS ACTIVITY FORM

Name of Child Tommy Childe   Name of Aide Annie Aide

Date of Session   9/24/70   # Sessions to Date   1

	GOAL	ACTIVITY	TIME	NOTES
GOALS	___	TUTORING	___	
a. Academic		CONVERSATION		
b. Relationship	*b*	Social	10	talked about
c. Age/Sex Relevant	___	Problem	___	Tommy's interests
d. Confidence				
e. Feelings		COMBINED		
f. "Free-up"	*d*	Competitive	30	word game
g. Information	___	Cooperative		
h. Spontaneous		AIDE ACTIVE	___	
i. Child Chooses				
j. Child Asks	*i*	CHILD ACTIVE	20	painting
k. "Testing"				
	___	CHILD SOLITARY	___	
		OTHER (explain)	___	
		TOTAL (length of session)	60	

Fig. 40.4 Process-analysis form for aide goals and aide activities with children.

and more positive attitudes to schools and school-related concepts. The extensive three-hour test battery used to evaluate aides and controls is being factor-analyzed. We hope to examine more closely relations between derivative factor scores and both process and outcome measures based on aides' actual work with referred children.

As a project that heavily emphasizes early detection of ineffective school function, we are necessarily concerned with developing and refining screening procedures. Given the fact that our early identification programs now extend to many thousands of school children, we require techniques that are simple (i.e. easily responded to by the neophyte), brief, reliable, valid, and easy to score. To this end we have done a methodological study comparing several brief and lengthier teacher-screening measures for detecting early school maladaptation (Cowen, Dorr, & Orgel, 1971). A device shown by this research to be well-suited for mass screening of primary-graders is the AML Behavioral Rating Scale (Brownbridge & Van Vleet, 1969), an 11-item scale reflecting the factors of aggressiveness (A), moodiness (M), and learning disability (L). Teachers complete this form for all children early in the school year. Forms are scored and the data summarized within 24 to 48 hours. Test norms have been prepared and distributed to school mental health professionals. When test data are returned, summaries are prepared for school use, identifying children whose A, M, or L or sum AML scores exceed given percentiles. Readministration of the AML at the end of the school year permits comparison of children seen by aides to otherwise comparable controls.

Further AML research is in progress, as for example more refined norming studies, factor-analytic studies, and validation studies (e.g. comparing AML scores of project-referred and nonreferred children, and relating referral statements about children to AML profiles). We are also experimenting with variations in the AML test format (e.g. in item-wording, rating-point descriptions, number of rating points). Other specific studies using this measure are also underway, as for example studies of sex and developmental differences and comparisons of AML profiles of promoted vs. nonpromoted children.

While the project's research emphasis is on outcome, process, and aide-characteristics data and their interrelations, additional work is in progress that does not neatly fit these pigeonholes. For example, we are vitally concerned with developing information on utilization of project resources (Cowen, Dorr, Sandler, & McWilliams, 1971). Such work, while "unglamorous," provides two important classes of information: establishing the scope and "power" of the model used and developing concrete facts about specific utilization patterns for individual schools. The former information, combined with effectiveness data, makes possible cost/benefit analyses that facilitate comparison of the present approach both to traditional school mental health programs and other interventions (e.g. foster-home care, residential treatment, etc.) which stand as likely alternatives to this program. Preliminary cost/benefit analyses suggest that while the project involves a relatively small immediate cost increment, particularly for aide salaries, long-range savings accrued by averting more drastic and costly interventions are considerable. Providing concrete utilization data to individual schools allows each to see graphically how it has deployed its own (finite) resources, whether such use gives an optimal "needs/resources" match, and, if not, to correct course so as better to approach that balance.

School mental health consultation is central to the project's operation at two levels: consultation provided by project staff to schools; and that provided by school mental health professionals, within schools, to principals, teachers, aides, and other school personnel. The term consultation has had ever-increasing usage in the past decade and is defined in so many ways that it has assumed a catch-all quality. We hope, by using a largely naturalistic approach (i.e. recording consulting sessions and categorizing their component events), to identify more operationally the nature of consultation (i.e. what consultants actually *do* and how varied these interventions are) and its consequences (i.e. which consultative actions produce positive or negative outcomes and under what circumstances).

Project evaluation has heretofore been limited to relatively short-term effects. However, through the availability in this community of the comprehensive, cumulative Psychiatric Register of hospital, clinic, and private contacts with mental health practitioners, the temporal scope of follow-up evaluation is being extended. Together with the Register group we are conducting a follow-up study of the subsequent psychiatric history of 600 children who were seen through PMHP as first-graders between 1958–1963 and screened (red-tag vs. non-red-tag) for early school maladaptation. For this group—now ages 13–19—seven to twelve years have elapsed since the initial screening. The study thus seeks to establish whether children identified as maladapting at age six, and their families, have had different psychiatric histories than nonidentified peers.

The preceding examples illustrate, without exhausting, the category "project-related" studies. The project's nature and scope are such that it offers broad opportunities to explore a variety of questions pertaining specifically to early detection and prevention of dysfunction; adaptation to school; selection, training, and use of nonprofessionals; new roles for mental health professionals; and, more generally, issues of child development.

OVERVIEW

The foregoing account indicates that the project rests on a particular set of assumptions from which new programming and manpower uses logically derive. Key assumptions include the following: (1) Much of our mental health effort must be directed to the very young and to the institutions that shape their development. (2) There is need for greater emphasis on mental health programs that help the many to adapt effectively rather than on programs that react to marked adaptive failure in the few. Schools offer unique opportunities for the former type of programming. (3) Early detection and prevention of dysfunction are preferable to after-the-fact patchwork. The older, more entrenched the maladaptation, the more difficult and costly it is to cope with, and the greater the danger of irreparable personal consequences.

Given these assumptions, the following are our most important program emphases: (1) Introduction of widespread, early screening techniques for detection of school maladaptation. (2) Use of nonprofessional child-aides, selected for their warmth, facility in interpersonal relations, and interest in children, to bring immediate assistance to children identified as functioning ineffectively. (3) Development of preventive interventions designed to strengthen the hand of school personnel to deal with problems before they become negatively labeled, and to forestall the dire, cumulative consequences of educational failure. (4) Redefining the role of the school mental health professional as a consultant, trainer, and resource person for the many, rather than as a person largely restricted to one-to-one clinical services, on a crisis basis, for the severely malfunctioning few.

Whatever the satisfactions of the project experience, however much one may be persuaded that its delivery system is both logical and effective, there is a growing conviction on our part that it is insufficient. It has thus far been a program for early secondary prevention, and has not engaged the critical challenges of primary prevention. There are several reasons why this is so. First, primary prevention requires knowledge and skills that far transcend those of the mental health professional. Second, it has an ethereal quality because its pay-off criteria are abstract and futuristic. Schools by contrast, are heavily oriented to concrete, immediate problems that must be solved, if not instantly, then five minutes hence. In periods of fiscal austerity, school mental health priorities, like those in the emergency room of a hospital, are given to glaring here-and-now difficulties. That such an approach often guarantees future stultification rarely concerns those who must meet today's crises.

It is sure that no matter how a school is set up, it is an institution that profoundly influences child development. The choice we face is whether that influence is to be random or informed. Accordingly, the most important future role we can envision for the school mental health professional is as a social system analyst and social engineer. His challenge—and opportunity—must be measured in terms of how he can help to build health rather than how he can combat pathology. Optimally conceived, the school environment should potentiate adaptation for all children.

REFERENCES

Beach, D. R., Cowen, E. L., Zax, M., Laird, J. D., Trost, M. A., & Izzo, L. D. Objectification of the screening procedure for early detection of emotional disorder. *Child Development,* 1968, **39,** 1177–1188.

Brownbridge, R., & Van Vleet, P. *Investments in prevention: The prevention of learning and behavior problems in children: evaluation report.* San Francisco: Pace I. D. Center, 1969.

Cowen, E. L. Emergent approaches to mental health problems: An overview and directions for future work. In E. L. Cowen, E. A. Gardner, & M. Zax (Eds.), *Emergent approaches to mental health problems.* New York: Appleton-Century-Crofts, 1967. Pp. 389–455.

Cowen, E. L. The effectiveness of secondary prevention programs using nonprofessionals in the school setting. *Proceedings of the 76th Annual Convention, APA,* 1968, **2,** 705–706.

Cowen, E. L. Training clinical psychologists for community mental health functions: Description of a practicum experience. In I. Iscoe & C. D. Spielberger (Eds.), *Training and research in community mental health.* New York: Appleton-Century-Crofts, 1970. Pp. 99–124.

Cowen, E. L. On broadening community mental health practicum training for clinical psychologists. *Professional Psychology,* 1971, **3,** 159–168.

Cowen, E. L. A new approach to school mental health services. Chapter in NIMHOED Manual for Community Mental health Centers, in press.

Cowen, E. L., Carlisle, R. L., & Kaufman, G. Evaluation of a college student volunteer program with primary graders experiencing school adjustment problems. *Psychology in the Schools,* 1969, **6,** 371–375.

Cowen, E. L., Chinsky, J. M., & Rappaport, J. An undergraduate practicum in community mental health. *Community Mental Health Journal,* 1970, **6,** 91–100.

Cowen, E. L., Dorr, D. A., & Orgel, A. R. Interrelations among screening measures for early detection of school dysfunction. *Psychology in the Schools,* 1971, **8,** 135–139.

Cowen, E. L., Dorr, D. A., & Pokracki, F. Selection of nonprofessional child-aides for a school mental health project. *Community Mental Health Journal,* 1972, **8,** 220–226.

Cowen, E. L., Dorr, D. A., Sandler, I. N., & McWilliams, S. A. Utilization of a nonprofessional child-aide, school mental health program. *Journal of School Psychology,* 1971, **9,** 131–136.

Cowen, E. L., Dorr, D. A., Trost, M. A., & Izzo, L. D. A follow-up study of maladapting school children seen by nonprofessionals. *Journal of Consulting and Clinical Psychology,* **36,** in press.

Cowen, E. L., Huser, J., Beach, D. R., & Rappaport, J. Parental perceptions of young children and their relation to indices of adjustment. *Journal of Consulting and Clinical Psychology,* 1970, **34,** 97–103.

Cowen, E. L., Izzo, L. D., Miles, H., Telschow, E. F., Trost, M. A., & Zax, M. A mental health program in the school setting: Description and evaluation. *Journal of Psychology,* 1963, **56,** 307–356.

Cowen, E. L., Leibowitz, E., & Leibowitz, G. The utilization of retired people as mental health aides in the schools. *American Journal of Orthopsychiatry,* 1968, **38,** 900–901.

Cowen, E. L., Zax, M., Izzo, L. D., & Trost, M. A. The prevention of emotional disorders in the school setting: A further investigation. *Journal of Consulting Psychology,* 1966, **30,** 381–387.

Cowen, E. L., Zax, M., & Laird, J. D. A college student volunteer program in the elementary school setting. *Community Mental Health Journal,* 1966, **2,** 319–328.

Glidwell, J. C., & Swallow, C. S. *The prevalence of maladjustment in elementary schools.* (Report prepared for the Joint Commission on Mental Illness and Health of Children) Chicago: University of Chicago Press, 1969.

Liem, G. R., Yellott, A. W., Cowen, E. L., Trost, M. A., & Izzo, L. D. Some correlates of early detected emotional dysfunction in the schools. *American Journal of Orthopsychiatry,* 1969, **39,** 619–626.

McWilliams, S. A. Process analysis of a school-based mental health program. Unpublished doctoral dissertation, University of Rochester, 1971.

President's Task Force on the Mentally Handicapped. *Action against mental disability.* Washington, D.C.: United States Government Printing Office, 1970.

Reiff, R., & Riessman, F. The indigenous nonprofessional: A strategy of change in community action and community mental health programs. *Community Mental Health Journal,* 1965, Monograph No. 1.

Sandler, I. N. Characteristics of women working as child-aides in a school-based preventive mental health program. Unpublished doctoral dissertation, University of Rochester, 1970.

Sobey, F. *The nonprofessional revolution in mental health.* New York: Columbia University Press, 1970.

Zax, M., & Cowen, E. L. Early identification and prevention of emotional disturbance in a public school. In E. L. Cowen, E. A. Gardner, & M. Zax (Eds.), *Emergent approaches to mental health problems.* New York: Appleton-Century-Crofts, 1967. Pp. 331–351.

Zax, M., & Cowen, E. L. Research on early detection and prevention of emotional dysfunction in young school children. In C. D. Spielberger (Ed.), *Current topics in clinical and community psychology.* Vol. 1. New York: Academic Press, 1969. Pp. 67–108.

Zax, M., & Cowen, E. L. *Abnormal psychology: Changing conceptions.* New York: Holt, Rinehart & Winston, 1972.

Zax, M., Cowen, E. L., Izzo, L. D., & Trost, M. A. Identifying emotional disturbance in the school setting. *American Journal of Orthopsychiatry,* 1964, **34,** 447–454.

Zax, M., Cowen, E. L., Rappaport, J., Beach, D. R. & Laird, J. D. Follow-up study of children identified early as emotionally disturbed. *Journal of Consulting and Clinical Psychology,* 1968, **32,** 369-374.

41

Superpatriot Opposition To Community Mental Health Programs*

RICHARD SCHMUCK and MARK CHESLER

While most Americans support the growing national concern for mental health and the application of the behavioral sciences to community problems, some people are opposed to these developments. A wide variety of people object to mental health programs for many different reasons. One particular group of "opposers" is superpatriots. For them, anti-mental health attitudes are part of an embracing ideology and activism directed toward many contemporary trends. Not all superpatriots are opposed to mental health programs, however. It is the content and tenor of some typical superpatriot concerns about mental health programs that are explored in this report. Other data or insights into the psychology of superpatriotism as it relates to mental health may be found in Marmor, Bernard, and Ottenberg (1960), Auerback (1963), and Schiff (1964).

A DEFINITION OF SUPERPATRIOTISM

Several major dimensions of belief and activity define superpatriotism. One dimension is a *patriotic or nationalistic conservatism*. The investigators measured this dimension by asking respondents about their political affiliation, their identification with liberal or conservative elements of each major party, and their reaction to the statement "Whereas some people feel they are citizens of the world, that they belong to mankind and not to any one nation, I, for my part, feel that I am first, last, and always an American."

A second major dimension is a vigorous *anticommunism*, not only with regard to international affairs, but especially to the internal danger of subversion. Many superpatriots attribute great power to the communists, who are seen as the "agent provocateur" of most of the world's and nation's ills. This dimension was measured by asking respondents how many communists there were and how much danger they represented in the American government and in both major political parties. A third defining dimension of superpatriots is their clear *commitment to action*. Lecture audiences, magazine or newspaper subscribers, and group members are urged "to do something" about their nation's condition. Action may involve becoming educated, educating others, protesting, or politicizing, but the commitment to some action is a critical part of superpatriotism. This dimension was measured by asking respondents how many partisan, sociopolitical organizations they belonged to that had regular meetings, and what they did to act upon their attitudes and values. Individuals who share the first two characteristics of the superpatriot ideology but do not act

*From Schmuck, R., and Chesler, M., *Community Mental Health Journal*, 1967, **3**, 382–388. Copyright © 1967 by Behavioral Publications, Inc. Reprinted by permission of Behavioral Publications and Dr. Schmuck.

upon it are an important segment of the American population, perhaps even greater in number than the superpatriots. But precisely because they are not active opposers or resisters to change and are more passive, they are not the concern of this study.

In studying superpatriots' views, the authors first performed a content analysis of the literature published by extremist individuals and groups regarding mental health programs. Further, in order to ascertain whether such ideas were reflected in the beliefs of persons participating in superpatriot groups 62 superpatriots were interviewed and their views compared with those of 38 conservatives and 34 moderates. These three groups were defined by their positions on an index composed of the three dimensions described above. Conservatives were defined as politically conservative and fairly nationalistic, but not particularly active, certainly not active in extremist organizations, and not believing that communists have a strong influence in government and in both political parties. Moderates ranged from traditionally moderate Republicans to moderate Democrats; they saw little communist influence in government, none in the political parties, and were not active in political organizations.

SUPERPATRIOTS' CONCERNS REGARDING MENTAL HEALTH PROGRAMS

Mental health programs have been scrutinized and criticized by many people for many different reasons. The reactions range from scientific studies through literary critiques to ideological and political attacks. Much of this opposition does not come from superpatriot organizations and individuals. However, some virulent opposition is presented in the writings and activities of superpatriots that can be summarized into five issues.

1. Psychological Testing Often Constitutes an Invasion of Privacy and "Brainpicking."

Superpatriots are especially concerned with the use of psychological tests that assess personality characteristics. The concern for the use of such tests in the schools has been widely debated and some extreme criticisms have been entered into *The Congressional Record* (Ashbrook, 1962):

> A school would be in serious trouble if it would undress students for examination or inoculate them with some serum without parental permission. Yet virtually the same thing is being done all the time through these brain picking tests which literally undress young people and interfere in private areas which would be better left alone.

Psychological testing and invasions of private beliefs are seen sometimes as dangerous extensions of "adjustment theories of education." In a special issue of *The National Health Federation Bulletin* devoted to "Counselors and the Schools" (1962), it was argued that the purpose of the Minnesota Multiphasic Personality Inventory, the Blacky Test, and other psychological inventories was to destroy the child's moral and spiritual foundations. The resultant moral vacuum was seen as the ideal condition for the further promulgation and acceptance of the doctrine of the "welfare-police-slave state." It was also seen as providing:

> ...an opportunity for a vicious attack upon the children of the nation. Parents should not rest easy until they know exactly what is being done with their children and with others in the guidance counseling program in the school attended by their own children. Only united public action can stop this program of harm to children and of government control reaching into private thoughts and feelings.

In the interviews respondents were asked how they felt about psychological counseling in the public schools. Responses indicated that the superpatriots were much more opposed to psychological services in the school than were the conservatives and moderates. The results are presented in Table 41.1.

Table 41.1 Reactions of Superpatriots and Others to Psychological Counseling Services in the Schools. (Problems of adjustment and emotional problems have become an increasing concern of public schools in recent years. Many schools have hired professional psychologists and social workers to deal with these problems. Some people feel that such persons are beneficial in schools; others feel that they are more harmful to the children than good. Do you think that there should be such services in the elementary and high schools?)

	% Yes	% Ambivalent	% No
Superpatriots	37	15	48
Conservatives	63	8	29
Moderates	80	7	13

2. Community Mental Health Programs Are Extensions of the Federal Bureaucracy

In general, the superpatriots are concerned with increasing federal control of health and welfare programs. Further, they are generally opposed to further federal expansion, aid to education, or urban renewal programs and fear the end of local and private initiative in the face of a vast federal bureaucracy. Some critics have interpreted federal mental health efforts as attempts to secure "dictatorial powers" (Brengel, 1963). In addition to a concern about centralized power, others feared that many state and community mental health programs provide for aliens and intellectuals to take charge of individual citizens in every

Table 41.2 Reactions of Superpatriots, Others, and the General Public to the Inadequacy of Current Mental Health Facilities.

	% Inadequate	% Adequate
General public		
Roper, 1950	73	27
Jaco, 1955	79	21
Crawford,* 1959	85	15
Current study, 1964		
Conservatives and moderates	79	21
Superpatriots	50	50

*See Crawford, Rollins, and Southerland (1961).

phase of their lives. To be taken charge of, to lose personal and local independence, seems to be a major theme in superpatriot opposition to most federally financed programs.

The answers to one question in the interview also suggested that superpatriots would resist greater federal funds for mental health. The investigators asked for agreement or disagreement with the statement "Local medical facilities are inadequate." Table 41.2 suggests that whereas most citizens agree with this statement, superpatriots were more satisfied with current facilities.

3. Mental Health Practitioners Encourage Immorality, Sin, and Social Disorganization

One aspect of this view is that psychodynamic analysis de-emphasizes personal responsibility and encourages free expression and moral license. An example of these views of mental health was presented by Stormer in a widely distributed book, *None Dare Call It Treason* (1964). In discussing the psychiatric theories of Chisholm, Overstreet, and others, Stormer stated that:

> The Chisholms faced by a patient overcome with guilt because of extramarital relations, homosexual practices, or other antisocial tendencies will devote their efforts to convincing the patient that such actions are perfectly normal, that no guilt should be experienced. This is an outgrowth of the materialistic, psychodynamic approach to understanding human behavior. This school holds that when an individual feels a drive that the drive must be satisfied or resulting tensions will produce insanity.... Not relying on free will, morals or conscience for guidance, such amoral criminal minds are typical of the man Marx envisioned [pp. 162–163].

In addition, such a psychodynamic position has been seen as helping to identify "society" as the culprit when man errs. By finding root causes for deviant behavior in the character of the social system, mental health workers are seen as absolving man of moral culpability. Attempts to change or reorganize aspects of the society are seen as threatening personal adherence to established norms.

Perhaps one reason superpatriots are concerned about the assumptions and implications of mental health programs is their general emphasis on morality and moral principles. In discussing the things about modern America that most disturb or worry them, the superpatriots who were interviewed concentrated upon "moral decay," "a loss of morality," or "not sticking up for American principles." The investigators also asked the respondents: "What are some of the names of the three greatest contemporary Americans? What is it about him or her that is great?" The most frequent person named by the superpatriots was General Douglas MacArthur. Superpatriots differed from conservatives and moderates in that they more often attributed greatness to him on the basis of "his strong moral character," or "fighting for his principles." Conservatives and moderates who suggested MacArthur most often did so on the basis of his "service to his country," "great intellect," or "brilliant generalship." This perspective on traditional moral values is also evident in the finding that superpatriots were more strongly antihedonistic as compared to others. The investigators asked for agreement or disagreement with the statement: "Since life is so short, we might as well eat, drink and be merry and not worry too much about what happens to the world." Most interviewees disagreed with that statement, but 72% of the superpatriots, compared with 31% of the conservatives and 26% of the moderates, strongly disagreed with the statement.

4. Mental Health Programs Are Politically and Ideologically Biased

Often, mental health programs are seen as masking political policies of internationalism and racial integration. Brengal (1963) and McClay (1964) expressed this concern in interpretations of materials of the World Federation of Mental Health. The WFMH discusses some of the psychological and social problems created by prejudice, hostility, and excessive nationalism and was seen by these commentators as being committed to political positions rather than to health concerns. Another writer (Matthews, 1958) has criticized the World Health Organization, which is seen as an attempt to "internationalize" and "one-worldize" the American citizenry. WHO's concern for worldwide mental health has been interpreted as a plan to change the political, social, and economic institutions of society as well as to cure individual health problems.

One of the John Birch Society's directors expressed a similar fear about the partisanship inherent in current mental health policies. He noted that General Walker was forced to undergo a psychiatric examination but that the Freedom Riders were not (Anderson, 1962). Recently, news reports indicated that a southern mental health society was picketed by the Ku Klux Klan. The Klan distributed literature claiming that the purpose of the society was to brainwash Southerners into accepting integration and that lobotomies would be performed, making them submissive to communism and integration (Robinson, 1965).

Mental health program directors are sometimes seen as ideologically committed to liberal political ends. They are also seen as having power to refer or confine people to mental institutions. Consequently, mental health practitioners may be viewed as using their power for insidious purposes of controlling the thoughts and actions of the citizenry. In one view, people have been put into mental institutions because they are opposed to the "established liberal order."

One of the most dramatic case studies of this concern about mental health programs and political thought control revolved around a federal bill originally intended to finance a mental hospital in Alaska. Superpatriots interpreted this as the beginning of "Siberia, USA." A concise summary of this superpatriot concern was presented in Stormer's book:

> For the rare citizen who escapes indoctrination in the new social order in progressive schools, for the Bible believing Christian who rejects theologians who teach that socialism is the new kingdom of God on earth, for all the sturdy souls who hold to age-old concepts of right and wrong and are vocal about it; the collectivists have one final, ultimate weapon. Declare them insane!... The new leaders in the psychiatric field . . . hold the weapon of commitment to a mental institution over the heads of those reactionaries who rebel at accepting the new social order [p. 155].

5. Finally, There Is the Concern That Mental Health and Mental Health Practitioners Are Part of the Communist Plot to Destroy America

Several superpatriot attacks in this vein were documented in the article "Is Mental Health a Communist Plot?" in the *S. K. and F. Psychiatric Reporter* (1962). One description of the psychiatrist Chisholm that subtly presented this theme was delivered in a speech by a prominent superpatriot:

> While I do not contend he is a member of the Communist party, his philosophy calls for, freely and in sophisticated terms, the main key points of Communism, namely: an amoral society, ridicule of the family, of religion, and of patriotism, ruthless world-wide police force, and redistribution of wealth. Mental health enthusiasts decry as preposterous the many documented charges of Communists being active in the movement; in fact, they don't want to discuss such irresponsible criticisms. But there are plenty such connections.

The Russian leader, Beria, is said to have extolled the virtue of psychopolitics, skilled psychological manipulations for political ends. He is reported to have set out to train American psychopoliticians to take over our nation. Many American psychiatrists are viewed as foreigners who were educated in Russia. A spokesman for the Public Relations Forum also elaborated upon the perceived extent of such communist infiltration:

> If you are an officer in any club that wields some power, you doubtless have your psychopolitician. . . . If he or she is not a real psychopolitician and is really working in your best interests, then there are others who will eventually turn you against her and have her fired so that a psychopolitician can replace her. Now more than ever before, it is necessary to keep your wits about you. When confusion reigns supreme, the Communists make their greatest inroads.

PERSONAL CHARACTERISTICS AND RECRUITMENT PATTERNS OF SOME SUPERPATRIOTS

Although some of these views of mental health programs may seem extreme, the interviews suggested that superpatriots opposed to mental health programs were not typically psychotic, irrational, or disturbed; rather, they appeared to be socially effective and hospitable. For the most part, they seemed to be pleasant, considerate, and law abiding. Generally, they appeared to be comfortable and happy with their familial relations. Furthermore, they were not particularly dissatisfied or frustrated with their jobs or bureaucratic roles. In fact, within the present sample of superpatriots, little sense of personal anomie or demoralization was found. They were very much in touch with the world and were quite well informed and active in public affairs. The sample included people of all ages and social statuses. There were college students, young adults, middle-aged and older persons. They held all kinds of jobs and ranged from lower or lower-middle class to upper-middle or upper class.

Superpatriots were originally defined in part by their active involvement in public affairs. However, they also indicated more optimistic feelings of political effectiveness compared with the conservatives and moderates. Over 90% of the superpatriots either agreed or strongly agreed with the statement that "Working in groups is one way people like me can influence the government." Compared with others, these people did not feel politically alienated or helpless. They felt involved in, although in disagreement with, the process of local and federal government.

Another pervasive characteristic of superpatriots was their religious fundamentalism. Respondents were asked about their beliefs in God, in an afterlife, in punishment and rewards in the afterlife, and in the literal interpretation of the Bible. Those people who agreed strongly with all of these items were identified as religious fundamentalists. So-called religious modernists were those who had a belief in God and immortality but who minimized the idea of punishment in the afterlife and who disagreed that the entire Bible should be taken as literal truth. Nonbelievers were those who disagreed with all of the questions. Seventy-two percent of the superpatriots, compared with 49% of the conservatives and 32% of the moderates, were classified as fundamentalists.

In addition to this religious perspective, the superpatriots, in contrast to conservatives and moderates, scored higher on items to measure dogmatism (Rokeach, 1960). It appeared that they tended to reduce differences in the environment, especially when they viewed the objects of consideration to be evil. Other results of the interviews that showed the superpatriots reducing differences were that they engaged in stereotypic thinking about Jews. However, they showed little emotional fervor and hatred of Jews. Oversimplification of thought, involving reduction of information rather than hatred, characterized these superpatriots' views.

Many people with similar characteristics never express them through political means and never endorse superpatriot views. Moreover, such personal characteristics alone would not lead one to become an active member in superpatriot organizations. Some organizational means and supports must exist to channel and recruit these persons into existing groups and activities. In building local chapters, superpatriots often rely on neighborhood contacts and friendships. Members usually probe one another about their interested friends and are encouraged to invite newcomers. The approach is one of inclusion rather than exclusion: so long as a person shares an ideology and attitudes close to that of the superpatriot, he is recruited and readily accepted. Membership in religious or ethnic minorities does not typically disqualify or discourage a person from active membership. In this open search for new recruits, members are trained to inform others about the work of the organization and are taught that all good Americans, whoever they are, are likely to agree with the patriots once they are informed.

In some places, organizations such as the John Birch Society execute a subtle and well-planned introduction into the society. Typically, induction first involves convincing a new participant of the expertise of the chapter leader and other members, then interesting him in reading some of the society's literature, and finally getting him to recruit other members. In one of the interviews this story about Mr. X (superpatriot) and Mr. Y (John Birch Chapter leader) was told to the interviewer.

> X told me he has been feeling quite helpless about the world situation and had little information about it until he ran into the Birch Society. His first contact was going with neighborhood friends to Mr. Y's house in another town for a meeting. He had little to say about the meeting but was very impressed with the Birch library which he claimed had books and information you couldn't get anywhere else. The library is a lending library. He showed me a book, *Nine Men Against America*, which he had borrowed. He told me that the Birch Society teaches people that things don't have to keep going this way and that they can influence events as individuals. They must start work in the community—in the PTA—the local political parties and local government, then work up to the state and finally the national level. He started talking to the other employees where he works. At first, he claimed, they didn't know much about what was going on. But he told them things gradually, and now they can talk about a lot of things together. He has given them some pamphlets and lent them some books, but hasn't identified these as from the Birch Society. "Eventually, I will," he says, and hopes at least one or two will join.

In addition to neighborhood contacts and friendships, many superpatriot groups use the technique known as "popular fronting," i.e., identifying one's cause with a popular public issue while at the same time working out a more broadly based ideology. For instance, superpatriot-sponsored antifluoridation programs may sometimes have the effect of bringing Christian Scientists into a multifaceted group. Right wing campaigns against urban renewal attract some urban landowners, while anti-Negro organizations in the cities, such as the National Association for the Advancement of White People, may attract urban whites. Protests at PTA meetings over curriculum materials or the recommendations of counselors may recruit some disgruntled parents into an anti-school or anti-mental health campaign. Once in any of these specific-type campaigns, the new participants receive literature, make new friends, gain new satisfactions, and may gradually be brought into broader activities. Sometimes they may be persuaded to form new opinions against community mental health programs.

One particularly salient topic for recruitment recently involved the Supreme Court's decision regarding praying in the schools. The investigators asked the interviewees: "How do you feel about the Supreme Court decision against praying in the school?" Most of them, including a large number of moderates, were opposed to the decision. Ninety-two percent of the superpatriots, 73% of the conservatives and 60% of moderates disagreed with the ruling.

Since a large number of people opposed the Supreme Court decision, many of them were probably receptive to attempts to protest that decision. One can understand the broad public appeal of Project America, a product of the "20th Century Reformation Hour." This project organized mass rallies and petitions that asked for a constitutional amendment to overturn the Supreme Court's decision. Many conservatives and moderates were active in this superpatriot-organized protest. Under such circumstances, persons with a generally conservative to moderate outlook, or dogmatic fundamentalists who have been apolitical, may be recruited into other superpatriot activities, such as anti-mental health campaigns.

In all of these activities, involvement and commitment in superpatriot organizations have the effect of raising participants' feelings of esteem, status, and political effectiveness. This cycle of gratification serves to encourage members to be active and to seek continually new recruits to their organizations and ideology.

REFERENCES

Anderson, T. Mental health. *The Independent American*, 1962, **8**(7), 4.

Ashbrook, J. Brainpicking in school: A study of psychiatric testing. *Hum Events*, 1962, **19**(46), 883–886.

Auerback, A. The anti-mental health movement. *Amer. J. Psychiat.*, 1963, **120**, 105–111.

Brengel, M. H. Mental health bill—a new weapon for the Kennedy brothers? *The Independent American*, 1963, **9**(1), 3.

Counselors and the schools, *Nat. Hlth Fed. Bull.*, 1962, **8**.

Crawford, F., Rollins, G., & Southerland, R. Variations in the evaluation of the mentally ill. *J. Hlth hum. Behav.*, 1960, **1**, 211–219, **2**, 267–275.

Gurin, G., Veroff, J., & Feld, S. *Americans view their mental health.* New York: Basic Books, 1961.

Is mental health a Communist plot? *S. K. & F. psychiat. Reptr.*, 1962.

Marmor, J., Bernard, V., & Ottenberg, P. Psychodynamics of group opposition to health programs. *Amer. J. Orthopsychiat.*, 1960, **30**, 330–345.

Matthews, J. B. The World Health Organization. *American Opinion*, May 1958, 7–12, 31–35.

McClay, Ellen. *Bats in the belfry.* Los Angeles: Rosewood, 1964.

Robinson, C. The far right's fight against mental health. *Look*, January 26, 1965, 30–32.

Rokeach, M. *The open and closed mind.* New York: Basic Books, 1960.

Schiff, L. *The campus conservative movement.* Unpublished Doctoral Dissertation, Harvard University, 1964.

Stormer, J. *None dare call it treason.* Florissant, Mo.: Liberty Bell Press, 1964.

Suggested Additional Readings

Adelson, D., & Kalis, B. L. (Eds.) *Community psychology and mental health.* Scranton, Pa.: Chandler, 1970.

Bloom, B. L. The "medical model," miasma theory, and community mental health. *Community Mental Health Journal,* 1965, **1**, 333–338.

Cowen, E. L., Chinsky, J. M., & Rappaport, J. An undergraduate practicum in community mental health. *Community Mental Health Journal,* 1970, **6**, 91–100.

Cowen, E. L., Gardner, E. A., & Zax, M. *Emergent approaches to mental health problems.* New York: Appleton-Century-Crofts, 1967.

Cowen, E., Zax, M., & Laird, J. D. A college student volunteer program in the elementary school setting. *Community Mental Health Journal,* 1966, **2**, 319–328.

Guerney, B. G. (Ed.) *Psychotherapeutic agents: New roles for non-professionals, parents and teachers.* New York: Holt, Rinehart & Winston, 1969.

Hobbs, N. Mental health's third revolution. *American Journal of Orthopsychiatry,* 1964, **34**, 822–833.

Holder, H. D., & Dixon, R. T. Delivery of mental health services in the city of the future. *American Behavioral Scientist,* 1971, **14**, 893–908.

Lambert, N. Early identification of youth with potential mental health problems. *High School Journal,* 1968, **51**, 288–293.

Lewis, W. W. Child advocacy and ecological planning. *Mental Hygiene,* 1970, **54**, 475–483.

Riessman, F., Chen, J., & Pearl, A. (Eds.) *Mental health of the poor.* New York: Free Press, 1964.

Smith, M. B., & Hobbs, N. The community and the community mental health center. *American Psychologist,* 1966, **21**, 499–509.

Zax, M., & Cowen, E. L. Research on early detection and prevention of emotional dysfunction in young school children. In C. D. Speilberger (Ed.), *Current topics in clinical and community psychology,* Vol. 1. New York: Academic Press, 1969, 67–108.

UNIT VI

Reactions to Abnormal Behavior

INTRODUCTION

Though we have seen tremendous changes since the 1950s in the treatment and care of the mentally ill, as well as in our understanding of the factors which contribute to the development of abnormal behavior, we still see a generally unfavorable attitude toward the mentally ill in our society. This attitude has the potential not only of influencing the amount of federal, state, and private funds granted to various facets of the mental health field, but also of deterring people from seeking treatment because of their fear of stigmatization and the fear that knowledge of such treatment will affect their present and/or future employment opportunities. This attitude has been reported as influencing an individual's admission to a professional school (Dershowitz, 1970), and was a major factor in Senator Thomas Eagleton's withdrawal as the Democratic Party's 1972 nominee for Vice-President of the United States (*Time*, 1972).

In order to assess our society's reactions to abnormal behavior, a number of studies have been carried out. The first three articles in this unit are concerned with different aspects of these reactions. Article 42 by John Cumming and Elaine Cumming is addressed to the issue of stigma. These authors define stigma in terms of the loss of a valued attribute. In the case of hospitalization for mental illness, that loss is social competence in general and of predictability and reliability, in particular. Discussion is focused on the factors that affect the degree of stigma an ex-patient feels and the conditions which contribute to the undoing of stigmatization. The discussion is based on two pilot studies of patients recently discharged from a state mental hospital.

Article 43 by Thomas J. Scheff describes a study of the methods used to screen patients who have allegedly behaved in a deviant manner and who are to be involuntarily committed to a public mental hospital in a midwestern state. The results of Scheff's study show that screening procedures are generally perfunctory and that the decision to keep patients in the hospital is, to a large extent, based on the examiner's presumption of illness. This presumption was found to be based on three factors: financial, ideological, and political. Scheff's findings suggest further that once members of a community bring someone who appears deviant to the attention of officials, the reaction to this person by the officials performing the screening process will be one of presumed mental illness.

A variation of this reaction on the part of mental health professionals is discussed in a very interesting article by D. L. Rosenhan. He is concerned with studying whether psychiatric labels describe the characteristics of the individual being diagnosed or the environments and contexts in which the person is being diagnosed. To determine this, Rosenhan and seven other "pseudopatients" gained secret admission to different psychiatric hospitals across the United States. Despite the fact that they behaved in a sane manner while in the hospital, Rosenhan found that their sanity went largely unnoticed by the professional staff of the hospital ward. He concludes that once a person is diagnosed as abnormal, his behavior (though sane) is colored by this label as well as the environment in which he is found.

Some mental health professionals have voiced another type of reaction to abnormal behavior—that all involuntary commitment of persons to a psychiatric hospital is unfair and unjustified. A corollary to this view is the position that the law does not have the right to impose psychiatric treatment on a person who refuses it.

One of the foremost advocates of these viewpoints is Thomas S. Szasz, author of Article 45. He considers involuntary commitment to be a deprivation of liberty as well as a crime against humanity and likens this procedure to the enslavement of black men by white men. Moreover, he feels that such commitment practices represent a means of social control of those individuals whose behavior threatens established social values but does not violate any criminal statute. Szasz does not see any defensible reason for imposing treatment on someone who opposes such treatment. If this person, whom society has labeled mentally ill, threatens others or places their lives in danger, Szasz feels that he should be dealt with as someone who breaks the law. The article ends with Szasz's comparing the slave owner and the psychiatrist, pointing out that there appear to be many similarities between them. Szasz's position has sparked many interesting discussions in abnormal psychology as well as in law, and has laid the groundwork for the formation of various groups concerned with protecting the rights of mental patients (one such group being the American Association for the Abolition of Involuntary Mental Hospitalization).

REFERENCES

Dershowitz, A. M. Brief of the American Orthopsychiatric Association as *amicus curiae*. Submitted January, 1970, to the Supreme Court of the State of New York, County of New York.

Rosenhan, D. L. On being sane in insane places. *Science*, 1973, **179**, 250–258.

Time. McGovern's first crisis: The Eagleton affair. Chicago: Time, Inc., 1972.

42

On The Stigma Of Mental Illness*[1]

JOHN CUMMING and ELAINE CUMMING

The concept of stigma presented here was developed in the course of a series of studies directed toward illuminating the kinds of social environments most likely to promote ego reintegration after a psychotic illness. Briefly, we propose that the stigma associated with hospitalization for mental illness is a form of ego damage—the loss of a valued attribute; that stigma, unlike some ego-damaging losses, is reversible; and that the circumstances necessary for its reversal can eventually be specified.

STIGMA AS LOSS

The word "stigma" is often used to describe the way in which society stamps those who have been mentally ill. Its literal meaning is "a stain on one's good name," or a "loss of reputation." Originally, the word referred to a mark placed on a slave or a prisoner as a sign of his status. Whether it is a visible mark or an invisible stain, stigma acquires its meaning through the emotion it generates within the person bearing it and the feeling and behavior toward him of those affirming it. These two aspects of stigma are indivisible since they can each act as a cause or effect of the other. For example, the patient may have an inner feeling of shame or inferiority because he has been in a mental hospital, and this may lead him to act in a manner that induces others to respond in ways appropriate to his inner feeling. On the other hand, people may indicate their appraisal of a patient as a stigmatized person by their actions, and he in turn may accept and internalize their estimates. Either way, stigma, like other social definitions, is generated and reinforced in interaction. In a family, or any group tied together by ascriptive bonds, it would not be possible for one member to feel stigmatized, in our sense, without the others being affected.

The stigma that is said to be associated with hospitalization for a mental illness may be similar to the "feeling of unfortunateness" that Dembo attributes to amputatees (Dembo, 1956). She believes that the process by which a person becomes defined as "unfortunate" involves the loss, or absence, of something valuable. "Unfortunateness" is most likely to

*From the *Community Mental Health Journal*, 1965, **1**, 135–143. Copyright © 1967 by Behavioral Publications, Inc. Reprinted by permission of Behavioral Publications, Inc. and Dr. Cumming.

[1]The data for this analysis were collected under Research Grant Number 6911 Nursing Division, Department of Health, Education and Welfare. We wish to thank Drs. Newton Bigelow and Donald Graves of Marcy State Hospital and Drs. Marc Hollender and Philip Steckler of Syracuse Psychiatric Hospital for helping us to locate our groups of patients. We thank the students of the School of Public Health Nursing of the Upstate Medical Center and their faculty advisors for their collection of the data reported here.

As this research report was completed before the appearance of Erving Goffman's *Stigma* (Goffman, 1963), no attempt will be made to relate the two different, but probably not incompatible, approaches to the problem.

result when that which is lost is an intrinsic attribute of the person, such as health, honor, or reputation; it is less likely to occur when it is merely a possession such as money. Dembo argues that devaluation is unlikely to occur when the loss cannot be evaluated by ordinary normative standards. For example, as only the minority value absolute pitch, to be tone deaf, except perhaps in the families of musicians, is *not* to be unfortunate.

The process of "becoming unfortunate," like the process of becoming stigmatized, occurs in interaction. If something generally recognized as valuable is lacking or lost, the person who loses it is expected to suffer and to define himself as unfortunate. If he does not do so, sanctions will be brought to bear upon him automatically because the loser's disregard for his own loss is a direct challenge to the value system of the observer. If he cannot force the loser to an awareness of his loss, he must be prepared to revise his own values. Concretely, a widow must mourn, even if she has been unhappily married; and a spinster, no matter how comfortable, must feel a little disappointed, or the value of marriage is held in question. Some losses, like amputations, are totally irreversible. Some, like spinsterhood, are totally reversible. Some losses seem to require considerable work for reversal.

What can be said to have been lost when a person goes to a mental hospital? We propose, in the light of our own previous work and that of others (Cumming & Cumming, 1957; Clausen & Yarrow, 1955) that, in general, social competence and, in particular, predictability or reliability are lost. Because it is the loss of a *behavioral* attribute, the stigma of mental hospitalization should be reversible through a demonstration of competent and predictable behavior. Nevertheless, many lay people regard mental illness as essentially incurable, and thereby, inadvertently, build into its definition the necessary conditions for irreversible stigmatization. What, then, can be done to clear the reputation of the mentally-ill patient?

THE UNDOING-OF-THE-LOSS

When a patient returns from a mental hospital, he must enter into social interactions that automatically require him to understand the expectations of others and to make his own known. If he can do this, he belies the label "incurable" and is no longer appropriately labeled either incompetent or "unfortunate." It therefore becomes necessary to relabel him in such a way as to restore him to the world of competent, predictable people. However, a redefining of *all* mental illness as curable may be difficult because it would require a shift in a complex set of attitudes toward some grave forms of deviant behavior. One resolution of the paradox of recognizing both a cured patient and the incurability of his illness is to redefine his hospitalization as a mistake. We often hear relatives of patients explaining, "He wasn't like the others in there—the serious cases. It was only a "nervous breakdown." Thus they establish that this "cured" person was never "really crazy," that he was at no time socially incompetent or unpredictable and therefore cannot be now. This reversibility of the process of stigmatization we might call undoing-of-the-loss. Such mechanisms for restoring people to membership in normal society may underlie the reported discrepancies (Olshansky, 1959) between the generally poor *attitudes* people express toward the mentally ill and the fair and generous *treatment* that they so often mete out to them.

On the other hand, there appear to be cases in which those around the patient are apprehensive—both of him and for him—and the patient himself is openly ashamed of his illness and hospitalization. In such cases, where stigma remains, the hospitalization may have brought into focus secondary losses or inadequacies, present before, but now defined as "causes" of hospitalization. For example, a heavy drinker, after he has been hospitalized for schizophrenia, may be defined as "alcoholic." In other words, his stigma "spreads" so that the stain on his character becomes almost the total coloration. In general, we propose that when patients or their families cannot redefine the hospitalization so as to exempt the patient from the imputation of loss of a valued attribute, then stigma is likely to be felt.

These considerations suggest the following question: what kinds of environment favor undoing-of-the-loss, and what kinds favor continued stigmatization?

It seems clear that in any group apprehension about a member's social competence or predictability will create tension. Furthermore, other members of a primary group are implicated in the incompetence of their representative. The undoing mechanism, in a group in which an ex-patient is a participating member, can be expected to be part of that ongoing flow of integrative activity that prevents it from breaking up under the strain of inner tensions (Cumming & Henry, 1961). The task of lowering tension is usually allocated to specific members in stable groups; and it has been noted that in the ordinary division of labor between men and women, this integrative role is allocated to women (Parsons & Bales, 1955; Strodtbeck & Mann, 1956). These findings suggest that the women closely connected with the former mental patient may undertake the main burden of the undoing-of-the-loss.

Studies have shown, however, that when *male schizophrenics* live with their wives or mothers, they are more prone to relapse than when they live with more distant relatives (Brown, Carstairs & Topping, 1958; Freeman & Simmons, 1963). We might guess that conditions promoting relapse might also promote stigmatization as both are forms of ego damage. Relationships with close female relatives often require a division of labor based on a high level of competence and a clear division of authority, and this may generate too much ambivalence because of the demands of mutual obligation and emotional involvement. The undoing-of-the-loss for this group may best be accomplished by more distant female relatives who can provide sociability and solidarity without the burden of a complex and close relationship. There is some evidence from the work of Brown, Carstairs, and Topping (1958) that the presence of siblings protects schizophrenic men from relapse; studies of our own have shown that the presence of sisters is associated, for schizophrenic men, with a long delay between the onset of the illness and hospitalization (Cumming & Miller, 1961).

There is evidence, however, that nonschizophrenic male patients, living with their mothers or wives, relapse less often than a comparable group in other living arrangements. For these men and for female patients, it might be reasonable to expect that *all* adult female kin would, through the exercise of integrative skills, help the patient to redefine the hospitalization in such ways as to negate the loss of a valued attribute.

This argument is oversimplified but to set it forth in detail would require an excursion into the psychodynamics of sexual relations and the nature of the ego failure in the various mental illnesses. The results of relevant studies have been hard to integrate; for example, Brown *et al.* (1958) showed that having a wife improves the chance of discharge from hospital, but for chronic schizophrenics it also increases the relapse rate, and all male schizophrenics who live with their mothers have high relapse rates. For women, there are no comparable figures, although theory and general observation would suggest that the mother-daughter relationship should be protective. Among women, marriage raises the incidence of schizophrenia, but does not appear to affect the relapse rate. Manic-depressives, a small group, appear to be uniformly benefited by the availability of close female relatives of all kinds, and thus are different from schizophrenics in an important way.

ILLUSTRATIVE STUDY NO. 1

A cohort of 22 patients consecutively discharged from a state mental hospital was studied. They ranged from 16 to 77 years of age; the median age was 50. There were ten men and twelve women, including seven schizophrenics, two manic-depressives, one involutional psychotic, five arteriosclerotics, six neurotics, and one alcoholic. The unit of analysis was the family. Each patient was interviewed twice; and for the eighteen living in a family setting, a relative who lived in the house with him was also interviewed twice. These relatives included ten spouses, three mothers, three siblings, a daughter and an aunt. We lack comparable information from the families of the four remaining patients, two of whom lived alone, one in a nursing home, and one in a hostel. Interviews took place about eight months after discharge; the first was open-ended and the second structured. The interviewers tried to elicit the problems encountered while the patient was readjusting to the community. No direct questions about stigma were asked; its presence was inferred from the interview material.

Interviews were rated by the authors and an assistant independently. Differences were discussed and a composite rating developed. Instructions for recognizing stigma were worked out, and two raters scored the interviews independently. The authors' composite rating had 86.5% agreement with Rater 2, and 86.5% with Rater 3. Raters 2 and 3 agreed in 72.7% of cases. In the seven cases where there was not total agreement, the opinion of the two agreeing raters was used.

We found two basic evidences of stigmatization: the first an outright expression of shame or inferiority because of the hospitalization, and the second an expectation of discrimination or inferior treatment from others. Shame sometimes permeates an interview; for example, one patient's wife says of him, "My children think he is just lazy. Of course, because of the kind of hospital he was in, the union probably didn't think it was a proper thing to help him financially." His daughter interjects, "It was hard when he came home because there was all those stories in the paper about crimes and they always turned out to be done by former mental patients."

Expectation of inferior treatment because of having been in a mental hospital shows up in remarks like, "I didn't want anyone to know that I was at a mental hospital and call me crazy." "The fellows I work with didn't know I was there." Of the 22 patients, nine, or 41% felt stigma; of these, four expressed shame and five had a generalized expectation of discrimination. Some complaints of this general sort show a good assessment of reality, however. A sixteen-year-old boy wondered if he would have difficulty getting a driver's license because he had been hospitalized; according to New York state law he will have to have a psychiatric certificate of fitness next time he applies for licensing. A woman newly moved to her neighborhood says that she has not told her next door neighbor that she has been in a hospital since, "I don't want everybody knowing I was there—you know what they might think." Such cases may not really constitute stigma in our sense and their inclusion may inflate the number. Where there was doubt of this kind, the respondent was judged to be feeling stigma.

The patients were asked directly whom they visited and how frequently. A person was counted as a significant contact if he was visited once a week or oftener. The reason for hospitalization was not inquired after directly, but almost all of the respondents volunteered at least one. Such reasons as physical illness, overwork, and the stress associated with pregnancy were counted as socially acceptable. The commonest unacceptable reason given was excessive drinking, although two relatives said that hospitalization resulted from generalized incompetence. There is a hint in our material that drinking may be used deliberately to stigmatize some male patients because it may be easier to control them if they are ashamed of their behavior.

The remarks used for establishing the respondent's reasons for hospitalization were in every case different from the remarks used as evidence of the presence of stigma.

As Table 42.1 shows, an unacceptable reason for hospitalization is always accompanied by stigma, but no one who visits regularly with female kin fails to give an acceptable reason for the hospitalization. Furthermore, redefinitions are usually accompanied by freedom from stigma, and in three of the four cases where there is stigma in spite of there being a redefinition, there is no visiting with female kin. No differences were found by age, sex, work status, education, or household composition.

Table 42.1   Number of Former Mental Patients By Stigmatization and by Visiting with Female Kin Other Than Mother and Giving Acceptable Reasons for Hospitalization.

	Total	Acceptable Reasons Given		No Acceptable Reason Given	
	Interviewed	Visits Kin	Does Not	Visits Kin	Does Not
Total interviewed	22	11	6	0	5
Stigmatized	9	1	3	0	5
Not stigmatized	13	10	3	0	0

Fisher's Exact Test
$P = 0·008$
$P = 0·005$
$P = 0·036$

Not visiting kin is associated with stigma.
No acceptable reason for hospitalization is associated with stigma.
Acceptable reason for hospitalization is associated with visiting with female kin.

Because of the small numbers involved in this pilot study, it was planned to repeat it with new populations of patients. The following hypotheses were to be tested:

1. Stigma is related inversely to the rate of interaction with female kin. For schizophrenic men, the presence of mothers and spouses will be expected to be a countervailing force.

2. Destigmatization will be accompanied by reasons for exempting the patient from the label "mentally ill."

3. There may be additional differences between men and women arising from the differences in role demands made of them. Men should be able to prevent the spread of stigmatization by working successfully at an occupation, thus displaying competence. Women can help the undoing process by reassuming the spouse role and by caring adequately for children. Women, however, do not always have to reach a certain minimum of effectiveness in their core roles because others can help them in such matters as caring for children. Some women may only have to refrain from raising tension in the home, and from representing the family in a devalued way outside, in order to begin the undoing process. Men probably do not have as much leeway in the occupational world. It is therefore hypothesized that an adequate work situation, as well as interaction with female kin, will be

necessary for the destigmatization of men; and a supportive social system, presumably of female kin, will in itself be sufficient for women.

ILLUSTRATIVE STUDY NO. 2

The second study involves a group of 87 women between 18 and 65 with a median age of 36, who had been consecutively discharged from a mental hospital between 12 and 24 months before the interview. Circumstances made it impossible to include men in this study, and the hypotheses regarding work are still untested. Thirty-two were diagnosed as schizophrenic, 14 as depressed, 11 as having other psychoses and 30 as neurotic.

The 87 women were interviewed with a structured instrument designed to assess the level of stigma and the intensity of interaction. The degree of stigma is indicated in this preliminary analysis by the combined score on two separate Guttman Scales of 4 and 5 items each. One scale includes items reflecting the sense of shame or inadequacy identified in the first study and is called self-stigma; the other set reflects expectation of discrimination and is called situation-stigma. Items adapted from a stigma scale developed by Freeman and Simmons (1961) for use with the relatives of patients were also included, and a comparison with their results will be reported elsewhere.

Analysis of these data shows that although our hypotheses about women appear to be generally upheld, they are too simple and too specific. First, the redefinition of the reasons for hospitalization appears to be only one alternative expression of a more general psychological mechanism for undoing-the-loss. Besides having an acceptable reason for hospitalization, the patient can be redefined as changed or transformed through learning or conversion in such a way that she is no longer the person who became mentally ill. "I got sick worrying about my housework; now I have learned not to care if it doesn't get done."

A different type of mechanism is redefinition of the situation so that the "public" is held to be ignorant and prejudiced about those who must go to mental hospitals. In this mechanism, only the initiated know that such people are not crazy at all, but only temporarily ill, or in need of a rest. The relationship between these mechanisms and the two expressions of stigma is still to be explored.

Our prediction concerning the role of female kin appears to have been overspecific. Although it seems to be true that women must be available to play integrative roles if stigma is to be reversed, more generally, it appears, as Table 42.2 shows, that the integrative role must be embedded in a normatively-governed, consensually-validated social system in which there are both instrumental and integrative roles. Furthermore, the situation seems most propitious if the woman does not have to play a leadership role—that is, assume a role of high power in the family. As Table 42.2 shows, single women who do not have access, either in the same household or in weekly visits, to a complete nuclear family, including a sibling, are all stigmatized. Separated and divorced women are usually stigmatized no matter whom they interact with. Single women who have at least weekly access to a mother, father, and sibling, that is, a situation permitting role differentiation but not requiring the patient to assume a leadership role, are less often stigmatized. The stigma scores of the married women fall in between these groups, and whether or not they have children seems immaterial.

Table 42.2 also suggests that not only role differentiation but also position in the system makes a difference: the women in the least stigmatized group are in fully differentiated systems, either daughters in the parental home or widows in the homes of a married daughter; but they are not in high power positions. At first glance, it may appear that a position of

Table 42.2 Number of Female Former Mental Patients by Role Position and by Stigma Score.

Role Position	Total	Stigma Score Low (0–3)	High (4–9)
All women	87	40	47
Full role complement, dependent	12	10	2
Single	10	8	2
Widowed	2	2	0
Full role complement, leader	61	28	33
With children	47	19	28
Without children	14	9	5
Incomplete role complement	14	2	12
Separated and divorced	6	2	4
Single	8	0	8

$\chi^2 = 12.38$ d.f. = 2 $P < 0.01$

dependency is all that is required; but the most stigmatized group contains young women who live with their mothers and fathers but lack siblings. In other words, the peer role seems to be crucial for the undoing process. The most stigmatized group also includes separated and divorced women. Here the issue is difficult to clarify because of the lack of uniformity in the situations of these women. Among this small group, all lost the spouse role and hence presumably the role of integrative leader in a complete system. Beyond this, some have returned home, some live with one other family member, others with nonrelatives. Three of the four women with high stigma scores have had to place children in foster homes, while one of the two with low scores lives alone with her four children. The numbers are unfortunately too small for us to reach any conclusions although they suggest that stigma is associated with failure in both the spouse and mother role.

It appears from these findings that the kind of interaction system to which the patient returns is importantly associated with destigmatization, as is the position available in the system for the patient upon her return. As in the first study, no differences were found by

Table 42.3 Number of Female Former Mental Patients by Diagnosis and by Stigma Score.

Diagnosis	Total	Stigma Score Low (0–3)	High (4–9)
All women	87	40	47
Neuroses	30	7	23
Schizophrenias	32	14	18
Depressions	14	10	4
Remainder	11	9	2
Toxic psychoses	4	3	1
Psychopathic personality	3	3	0
Psychoses in physical illness	2	1	1
Undiagnosed	2	2	0

$\chi^2 = 15.56$ d.f. = 3 $P < 0.01$

age, work status, or education. In this second study, integrative status calculated in terms of the education and occupation of the head of the household is unrelated to stigma and so is the type of treatment received by the patient. Diagnosis, however, is related to stigma as Table 42.3 shows, with the neurotic group having the highest scores, the schizophrenic group next highest, the depressions next to lowest, and the residual group lowest of all. An adequate discussion of the psychiatric implications of these differences would take us beyond the scope of this paper.

When we combine diagnosis with role context, we see (Table 42.4) that in spite of the small numbers, the women with diagnoses of neurosis, schizophrenia, or "other" follow the same pattern of stigmatization that we saw in Table 42.2. Those in a low-power or dependent position in a full role complement have the lowest stigma, those in situations with an incomplete role complement have the highest, and the married group (full role complement, high-power) are intermediary. All of the depressive illnesses except one, however, are among the married women. Nevertheless, with the depressed women removed, the differences by role complement that we saw in Table 42.2 remain.

Finally, returning to our hypothesis that women are not required to perform at such

Table 42.4 Number of Female Former Mental Patients by Diagnosis and Role Position and by Stigma Score.

Diagnosis and Role Position	Stigma Score		
	Total	Low (0–3)	High (4–9)
All women	87	40	47
Full role complement, low power	12	10	2
Without depressive illness	12	10*	2*
Neurosis	4	3	1
Schizophrenia	4	3	1
Other	4	4	0
Depression	—	—	—
Full role complement, high power	61	28	33
Without depressive illness	48	18*	30*
Neurosis	20	4	16
Schizophrenia	21	9	12
Other	7	5	2
Depression	13	10	3
Incomplete role complement	14	2	12
Without depressive illness	13	2*	11*
Neurosis	6	0	6
Schizophrenia	7	2	5
Other	—	—	—
Depression	1	0	1

*For those women without depressive illness, $\chi^2 = 12.68$, d.f. = 2, $P < 0.01$

clearly specified levels as men, and therefore can make more use of the help of others in the undoing-of-the-loss, we found that the presence of other adult females made no difference to this group. For the married women, however, time out of hospital does make a difference to stigma score. The longer they have been out, the less likely they are to be stigmatized. It is possible that, apart from simply forgetting a disruptive episode, it takes some time for a married woman to reassemble all the parts of her role after hospitalization because some of her duties as integrative leader have fallen to others. Full role participation is, in a sense, necessary for a differentiated system.

This reasoning is supported by the fact that the other groups of women show no association between time out of hospital and stigma score. The unstigmatized may have returned to roles not filled in their absence, and the stigmatized are, as we have shown, in incomplete systems.

When we look at Table 42.5, however, we see that among the group of married women, diagnoses are not evenly distributed; those with depressive disorders are all among the group longest out of hospital. All of these women but one have been out of hospital between 15 and 22 months; when they are arrayed by the number of months out of the hospital, a Runs Test shows no significant difference. Once again, when this group is removed, the effect of time out of hospital remains significant.

Table 42.5 Number of Married, Female Former Mental Patients by Diagnosis and Length of Time Out of Hospital and by Stigma Score.

Diagnosis and Time Out of Hospital	Total	Stigma Score	
		Low (0–3)	High (4–9)
All married women	61	28	33
Out less than 15 months	20	4	16
Without depressive illness	19	3*	16*
Neurosis	9	0	9
Schizophrenia	8	2	6
Other	2	1	1
Depression	1	1	0
Out more than 15 months	41	24	17
Without depressive illness	29	15*	14*
Neurosis	11	4	6
Schizophrenia	13	7	7
Other	5	4	1
Depression	12	9	3

*Those without depressive illness and out of the hospital more than 15 months are less stigmatized than those more recently discharged.
χ^2 (corrected) = 4.88   d.f. = 1   .05 > P > .02

In summary, it appears from these women that some illnesses produce more stigma than others and that the type of role undertaken by the woman upon her return from hospital and the structure in which it is embedded are important in permitting the undoing-of-the-loss of reputation that hospitalization causes. Furthermore, for some women—those in role positions normally defined in terms of integrative leadership—time assists the process.

Finally, if our hypotheses regarding men were to be upheld, it would add credence to these findings because they were generated from the same theoretical base.

REFERENCES

Brown, G. W., Carstairs, G. M., & Topping, G. G. The post-hospital adjustment of chronic mental patients. *Lancet*, 1958, **2**, 685–689.

Clausen, J., & Yarrow, M. R. The impact of mental illness on the family. *J. soc. Issues*, 1955, **11**(4), whole issue.

Cumming, E., & Cumming, J. *Closed ranks.* Cambridge, Mass: Harvard University Press, 1957.

Cumming, E., & Henry, W. E. *Growing old.* New York: Basic Books, 1961. Chapter 8.

Cumming, J., & Miller, L. Isolation, family structure, and schizophrenia. In *Proc. of the Third world Cong. of Psychiat.* Toronto: University of Toronto Press, 1961.

Dembo, T. Leviton, G. L., & Wright, B. A. Adjustment to misfortune—A problem of social-psychological rehabilitation. *Artificial Limbs*, 1956, **3**(2), 4–62.

Freeman, H. E., & Simmons, O. G. Feelings of stigma among relatives of former mental patients. *Social Problems*, 1961, **8**, 312–321.

Freeman, H. E., & Simmons, O. G. *The mental patient comes home.* New York: Wiley, 1963.

Goffman, E. *Stigma: notes on the management of a spoiled identity.* Englewood Cliffs, N.J.: Prentice Hall, 1963.

Olshansky, S. Community aspects of rehabilitation, employer receptivity. In M. Greenblatt & B. Simon (Eds.), *The rehabilitation of the mentally ill.* (Publication No. 58) Washington, D.C.: American Association for the Advancement of Science, 1959. Pp. 213–222.

Parsons, T., & Bales, R. F. *Family, socialization, and interaction process.* New York: Free Press, 1955.

Strodtbeck, F., & Mann, R. D. Sex role differentiation in Jury deliberations. *Sociometry*, 1956, **19**, 3–11.

43

The Societal Reaction to Deviance: Ascriptive Elements in the Psychiatric Screening of Mental Patients in a Midwestern State*†

THOMAS J. SCHEFF
(with the assistance of DANIEL M. CULVER)

The case for making the societal reaction to deviance a major independent variable in studies of deviant behavior has been succinctly stated by Kitsuse (1962):

> A sociological theory of deviance must focus specifically upon the interactions which not only define behaviors as deviant but also organize and activate the application of sanctions by individuals, groups, or agencies. For in modern society, the socially significant differentiation of deviants from the non-deviant population is increasingly contingent upon circumstances of situation, place, social and personal biography, and the bureaucratically organized activities of agencies of control.

In the case of mental disorder, psychiatric diagnosis is one of the crucial steps which "organizes and activates" the societal reaction, since the state is legally empowered to segregate and isolate those persons whom psychiatrists find to be committable because of mental illness.

Recently, however, it has been argued that mental illness may be more usefully considered to be a social status than a disease, since the symptoms of mental illness are vaguely defined and widely distributed, and the definition of behavior as symptomatic of mental illness is usually dependent upon social rather than medical contingencies (Lemert, 1951; Goffman, 1962). Furthermore, the argument continues, the status of the mental patient is more often an ascribed status, with conditions for status entry external to the patient, than an achieved status with conditions for status entry dependent upon the patient's own behavior. According to this argument, the societal reaction is a fundamentally important variable in all stages of a deviant career.

The actual usefulness of a theory of mental disorder based on the societal reaction is largely an empirical question: to what extent is entry to the status of mental patient independent of the behavior or "condition" of the patient? The present paper will explore this question for one phase of the societal reaction: the legal screening of persons alleged to be mentally ill. This screening represents the official phase of the societal reaction, which occurs after the alleged deviance has been called to the attention of the community by a

*From Scheff, T. J., *Social Problems*, 1964, **11**, 401–413. Copyright © 1964 by the Society for the Study of Social Problems. Reprinted by permission of the Society for the Study of Social Problems, and Dr. Scheff.

†This report is part of a larger study, made possible by a grant from The Advisory Mental Health Committee of Midwestern State. By prior agreement, the state in which the study was conducted is not identified in publications.

496

complainant(This report will make no reference to the initial deviance or other situation which resulted in the complaint, but will deal entirely with procedures used by the courts after the complaint has occurred.)

The purpose of the description that follows is to determine the extent of uncertainty that exists concerning new patients' qualifications for involuntary confinement in a mental hospital, and the reactions of the courts to this type of uncertainty. The data presented here indicate that, in the face of uncertainty, there is a strong presumption of illness by the court and the court psychiatrists.[1] In the discussion that follows the presentation of findings, some of the causes, consequences and implications of the presumption of illness are suggested.

The data upon which this report is based were drawn from psychiatrists' ratings of a sample of patients newly admitted to the public mental hospitals in a Midwestern state, official court records, interviews with court officials and psychiatrists, and our observations of psychiatric examinations in four courts. The psychiatrists' ratings of new patients will be considered first.

In order to obtain a rough measure of the incoming patient's qualifications for involuntary confinement, a survey of newly admitted patients was conducted with the cooperation of the hospital psychiatrists. All psychiatrists who made admission examinations in the three large mental hospitals in the state filled out a questionnaire for the first ten consecutive patients they examined in the month of June, 1962. A total of 223 questionnaires were returned by the 25 admission psychiatrists. Although these returns do not constitute a probability sample of all new patients admitted during the year, there were no obvious biases in the drawing of the sample. For this reason, this group of patients will be taken to be typical of the newly admitted patients in Midwestern State.

The two principal legal grounds for involuntary confinement in the United States are the police power of the state (the state's right to protect itself from dangerous persons) and *parens patriae* (the State's right to assist those persons who, because of their own incapacity, may not be able to assist themselves) (Ross, 1959). As a measure of the first ground, the potential dangerousness of the patient, the questionnaire contained this item: " In your opinion, if this patient were released at the present time, is it likely he would harm himself or others?" The psychiatrists were given six options, ranging from Very Likely to Very Unlikely. Their responses were: Very Likely, 5%; Likely, 4%; Somewhat Likely, 14%; Somewhat Unlikely, 20%; Unlikely, 37%; Very Unlikely, 18%. (Three patients were not rated, 1%.)

As a measure of the second ground, *parens patriae*, the questionnaire contained the item: "Based on your observations of the patient's behavior, his present degree of mental impairment is: None _____ Minimal _____ Mild _____ Moderate _____ Severe _____ " The psychiatrists' responses were: None, 2%; Minimal, 12%; Mild, 25%; Moderate, 42%; Severe, 17%. (Three patients were not rated, 1%.)

To be clearly qualified for involuntary confinement, a patient should be rated as likely to harm self or others (Very Likely, Likely, or Somewhat Likely) and/or as Severely Mentally Impaired. However, voluntary patients should be excluded from this analysis, since the court is not required to assess their qualifications for confinement. Excluding the 59 voluntary admissions (26% of the sample) leaves a sample of 164 involuntary confined patients. Of these patients,(10)were rated as meeting both qualifications for involuntary confinement, 21 were rated as being severely mentally impaired, but not dangerous, 28 were

---

[1]For a more general discussion of the presumption of illness in medicine and some of its possible causes and consequences, see, Scheff (1963a).

rated as dangerous but not severely mentally impaired, and 102 were rated as not dangerous nor as severely mentally impaired. (Three patients were not rated.)

According to these ratings, there is considerable uncertainty connected with the screening of newly admitted involuntary patients in the state, since a substantial majority (63%) of the patients did not clearly meet the statutory requirements for involuntary confinement. How does the agency responsible for assessing the qualifications for confinement, the court, react in the large number of cases involving uncertainty?

On the one hand, the legal rulings on this point by higher courts are quite clear. They have repeatedly held that there should be a presumption of sanity. The burden of proof of insanity is to be on the petitioners, there must be a preponderance of evidence, and the evidence should be of a "clear and unexceptionable" nature.[2]

On the other hand, existing studies suggest that there is a presumption of illness by mental health officials. In a discussion of the "discrediting" of patients by the hospital staff, based on observations at St. Elizabeth's Hospital, Washington, D.C., Goffman (1962) states:

> [The patient's case record] is apparently not regularly used to record occasions when the patient showed capacity to cope honorably and effectively with difficult life situations. Nor is the case record typically used to provide a rough average or sampling of his past conduct. [Rather, it extracts] from his whole life course a list of those incidents that have or might have had "symptomatic" significance. . . . I think that most of the information gathered in case records is quite true, although it might seem also to be true that almost anyone's life course could yield up enough denigrating facts to provide grounds for the record's justification of commitment [pp. 155, 159].

Mechanic (1962) makes a similar statement in his discussion of two large mental hospitals located in an urban area in California:

> In the crowded state or county hospitals, which is the most typical situation, the psychiatrist does not have sufficient time to make a very complete psychiatric diagnosis, nor do his psychiatric tools provide him with the equipment for an expeditious screening of the patient. . .
>
> In the two mental hospitals studied over a period of three months, the investigator never observed a case where the psychiatrist advised the patient that he did not need treatment. Rather, all persons who appeared at the hospital were absorbed into the patient population regardless of their ability to function adequately outside the hospital.

A comment by Brown (1961, p. 60, fn.) suggests that it is a fairly general understanding among mental health workers that state mental hospitals in the U.S. accept all comers.

Kutner (1962), describing commitment procedures in Chicago in 1962, also reports a strong presumption of illness by the staff of the Cook County Mental Health Clinic:

> Certificates are signed as a matter of course by staff physicians after little or no examination . . . The so-called examinations are made on an assembly line basis, often being completed in two or three minutes, and never taking more than ten minutes. Although psychiatrists agree that it is practically impossible to determine a person's sanity on the basis of such a short and hurried interview, the doctors recommend confinement in 77% of the cases. It appears in practice that the alleged-mentally-ill is presumed to be insane and bears the burden of proving his sanity in the few minutes allotted to him . . .

These citations suggest that mental health officials handle uncertainty by presuming illness. To ascertain if the presumption of illness occurred in Midwestern State, intensive ob-

---

[2] This is the typical phrasing in cases in the *Dicennial Legal Digest*, found under the heading "Mental Illness."

servations of screening procedures were conducted in the four courts with the largest volume of mental cases in the state. These courts were located in the two most populous cities in the state. Before giving the results of these observations, it is necessary to describe the steps in the legal procedures for hospitalization and commitment.

STEPS IN THE SCREENING OF PERSONS ALLEGED TO BE MENTALLY ILL

The process of screening can be visualized as containing five steps in Midwestern State:

1. The application for judicial inquiry, made by three citizens. This application is heard by deputy clerks in two of the courts (C and D), by a court reporter in the third court, and by a court commissioner in the fourth court.
2. The intake examination, conducted by a hospital psychiatrist.
3. The psychiatric examination, conducted by two psychiatrists appointed by the court.
4. The interview of the patient by the guardian *ad litem*, a lawyer appointed in three of the courts to represent the patient. (Court A did not use guardians *ad litem*.)
5. The judicial hearing, conducted by a judge.

These five steps take place roughly in the order listed, although in many cases (those cases designated as emergencies) step No. 2, the intake examination, may occur before step No. 1. Steps No. 1 and No. 2 usually take place on the same day or the day after hospitalization. Steps No. 3, No. 4, and No. 5 usually take place within a week of hospitalization. (In courts C and D, however, the judicial hearing is held only once a month.)

This series of steps would seem to provide ample opportunity for the presumption of health, and a thorough assessment, therefore, of the patient's qualifications for involuntary confinement, since there are five separate points at which discharge could occur. According to our findings, however, these procedures usually do not serve the function of screening out persons who do not meet statutory requirements. At most of these decision points, in most of the courts, retention of the patient in the hospital was virtually automatic. A notable exception to this pattern was found in one of the three state hospitals; this hospital attempted to use step No. 2, the intake examination, as a screening point to discharge patients that the superintendent described as "illegitimate," i.e., patients who do not qualify for involuntary confinement.[3] In the other two hospitals, however, this examination was perfunctory and virtually never resulted in a finding of health and a recommendation of discharge. In a similar manner, the other steps were largely ceremonial in character. For example, in court B, we observed twenty-two judicial hearings, all of which were conducted perfunctorily and with lightning rapidity. (The mean time of these hearings was 1.6 minutes.) The judge asked each patient two or three routine questions. Whatever the patient answered, however, the judge always ended the hearings and retained the patient in the hospital.

What appeared to be the key role in justifying these procedures was played by step No. 3, the examination by the court-appointed psychiatrists. In our informal discussions of screening with the judges and other court officials, these officials made it clear that although the statutes give the court the responsibility for the decision to confine or release persons

---

[3]Other exceptions occurred as follows: the deputy clerks in courts C and D appeared to exercise some discretion in turning away applications they considered improper or incomplete, at step No. 1; the judge in Court D appeared also to perform some screening at step No. 5. For further description of these exceptions see Scheff (1964).

alleged to be mentally ill, they would rarely if ever take the responsibility for releasing a mental patient without a medical recommendation to that effect) The question which is crucial, therefore, for the entire screening process is whether or not the court-appointed psychiatric examiners presume illness. The remainder of the paper will consider this question.

Our observations of 116 judicial hearings raised the question of the adequacy of the psychiatric examination. Eighty-six of the hearings failed to establish that the patients were "mentally ill" (according to the criteria stated by the judges in interviews).[4] Indeed, the behavior and responses of 48 of the patients at the hearings seemed completely unexceptionable. Yet the psychiatric examiners had not recommended the release of a single one of these patients. Examining the court records of 80 additional cases, there was still not a single recommendation for release.

Although the recommendation for treatment of 196 out of 196 consecutive cases strongly suggests that the psychiatric examiners were presuming illness, particularly when we observed 48 of these patients to be responding appropriately, it is conceivable that this is not the case. The observer for this study was not a psychiatrist (he was a first year graduate student in social work) and it is possible that he could have missed evidence of disorder which a psychiatrist might have seen. It was therefore arranged for the observer to be present at a series of psychiatric examinations, in order to determine whether the examinations appeared to be merely formalities or whether, on the other hand, through careful examination and interrogation, the psychiatrists were able to establish illness even in patients whose appearance and responses were not obviously disordered(The observer was instructed to note the examiner's procedures, the criteria they appeared to use in arriving at their decision, and their reaction to uncertainty.)

Each of the courts discussed here employs the services of a panel of physicians as medical examiners. The physicians are paid a flat fee of ten dollars per examination, and are usually assigned from three to five patients for each trip to the hospital. In court A, most of the examinations are performed by two psychiatrists, who go to the hospital once a week, seeing from five to ten patients a trip. In court B, C and D, a panel of local physicians is used. These courts seek to arrange the examinations so that one of the examiners is a psychiatrist, the other a general practitioner. Court B has a list of four such pairs, and appoints each pair for a month at a time. Courts C and D have a similar list, apparently with some of the same names as court B.

To obtain physicians who were representative of the panel used in these courts, we arranged to observe the examinations of the two psychiatrists employed by court A, and one of the four pairs of physicians used in court B, one a psychiatrist, the other a general practitioner. We observed 13 examinations in court A and 13 examinations in court B. The judges in courts C and D refused to give us the names of the physicians on their panels, and we were unable to observe examinations in these courts. (The judge in court D stated that he did not want these physicians harassed in their work, since it was difficult to obtain their services even under the best of circumstances.) In addition to observing the examinations by four psychiatrists, three other psychiatrists used by these courts were interviewed.

The medical examiners followed two lines of questioning. One line was to inquire about the circumstances which led to the patient's hospitalization, the other was to ask standard questions to test the patient's orientation and his capacity for abstract thinking by asking him the date, the President, Governor, proverbs, and problems requiring arithmetic calcula-

why + method intervs

---

[4]In interviews with the judges, the following criteria were named: Appropriateness of behavior and speech, understanding of the situation, and orientation.

tion. These questions were often asked very rapidly, and the patient was usually allowed only a very brief time to answer.

It should be noted that the psychiatrists in these courts had access to the patient's record (which usually contained the Application for Judicial Inquiry and the hospital chart notes on the patient's behavior), and that several of the psychiatrists stated that they almost always familiarized themselves with this record before making the examination. To the extent that they were familiar with the patient's circumstances from such outside information, it is possible that the psychiatrists were basing their diagnoses of illness less on the rapid and peremptory examination than on this other information. Although this was true to some extent, the importance of the record can easily be exaggerated, both because of the deficiencies in the typical record, and because of the way it is usually utilized by the examiners.

The deficiencies of the typical record were easily discerned in the approximately one hundred applications and hospital charts which the author read. Both the applications and charts were extremely brief and sometimes garbled. Moreover, in some of the cases where the author and interviewer were familiar with the circumstances involved in the hospitalization, it was not clear that the complainant's testimony was any more accurate than the version presented by the patient. Often the original complaint was so paraphrased and condensed that the application seemed to have little meaning.

The attitude of the examiners toward the record was such that even in those cases where the record was ample, it often did not figure prominently in their decision. Disparaging remarks about the quality and usefulness of the record were made by several of the psychiatrists. One of the examiners was apologetic about his use of the record, giving us the impression that he thought that a good psychiatrist would not need to resort to any information outside his own personal examination of the patient. A casual attitude toward the record was openly displayed in 6 of the 26 examinations we observed. In these 6 examinations, the psychiatrist could not (or in 3 cases, did not bother to) locate the record and conducted the examination without it, with one psychiatrist making it a point of pride that he could easily diagnose most cases "blind".

In his observations of the examinations, the interviewer was instructed to rate how well the patient responded by noting his behavior during the interview, whether he answered the orientation and concept questions correctly, and whether he denied and explained the allegations which resulted in his hospitalization. If the patient's behavior during the interview obviously departed from conventional social standards (e.g., in one case the patient refused to speak), if he answered the orientation questions incorrectly, or if he did not deny and explain the petitioners' allegations, the case was rated as meeting the statutory requirements for hospitalization. Of the 26 examinations observed, eight were rated as Criteria Met.

If, on the other hand, the patient's behavior was appropriate, his answers correct, and he denied and explained the petitioners' allegations, the interviewer rated the case as not meeting the statutory criteria. Of the 26 cases, seven were rated as Criteria Not Met. Finally, if the examination was inconclusive, but the interviewer felt that more extensive investigation might have established that the criteria were met, he rated the cases as Criteria Possibly Met. Of the 26 examined, 11 were rated in this way. The interviewer's instructions were that whenever he was in doubt he should avoid using the rating Criteria Not Met.

Even giving the examiners the benefit of the doubt, the interviewer's ratings were that in a substantial majority of the cases he observed, the examination failed to establish that the

Table 43.1 Observer's Ratings and Examiners' Recommendations.

Observer's ratings		Criteria Met	Criteria Possibly Met	Criteria Not Met	Total
Examiners' recommendations	Commitment	7	9	2	18
	30-day observation	1	2	3	6
	Release	0	0	2	2
	Total	8	11	7	26

statutory criteria were met. The relationship between the examiners' recommendations and the interviewer's ratings are shown in ... Table 43.1.

The interviewer's ratings suggest that the examinations established that the statutory criteria were met in only eight cases, but the examiners recommended that the patient be retained in the hospital in 24 cases, leaving 16 cases which the interviewer rated as uncertain, and in which retention was recommended by the examiners. The observer also rated the patient's expressed desires regarding staying in the hospital, and the time taken by the examination. The ratings of the patient's desire concerning staying or leaving the hospital were: Leave, 14 cases; Indifferent, 1 case; Stay, 9 cases; and Not Ascertained, 2 cases. In only one of the 14 cases in which the patient wished to leave was the interviewer's rating Criteria Met.

The interviews ranged in length from five minutes to 17 minutes, with the mean time being 10.2 minutes. Most of the interviews were hurried, with the questions of the examiners coming so rapidly that the examiner often interrupted the patient, or one examiner interrupted the other. All of the examiners seemed quite hurried. One psychiatrist, after stating in an interview (before we observed his examinations) that he usually took about thirty minutes, stated:

> It's not remunerative. I'm taking a hell of a cut. I can't spend 45 minutes with a patient. I don't have the time, it doesn't pay.

In the examinations that we observed, this physician actually spent 8, 10, 5, 8, 8, 7, 17, and 11 minutes with the patients, or an average of 9.2 minutes.

In these short time periods, it is virtually impossible for the examiner to extend his investigation beyond the standard orientation questions, and a short discussion of the circumstances which brought the patient to the hospital. In those cases where the patient answered the orientation questions correctly, behaved appropriately, and explained his presence at the hospital satisfactorily, the examiners did not attempt to assess the reliability of the petitioner's complaints, or to probe further into the patient's answers. Given the fact that in most of these instances the examiners were faced with borderline cases, that they took little time in the examinations, and that they usually recommended commitment, we can only conclude that their decisions were based largely on a presumption of illness. Supplementary observations reported by the interviewer support this conclusion.]

After each examination, the observer asked the examiner to explain the criteria he used in arriving at his decision. The observer also had access to the examiner's official report, so that he could compare what the examiner said about the case with the record of what actually occurred during the interview. This supplementary information supports the conclusion that the examiner's decisions are based on the presumption of illness, and sheds light on the manner in which these decisions are reached:

1. The "evidence" upon which the examiners based their decision to retain often seemed arbitrary.
2. In some cases, the decision to retain was made even when no evidence could be found.
3. Some of the psychiatrists' remarks suggest prejudgment of the cases.
4. Many of the examinations were characterized by carelessness and haste. The first question, concerning the arbitrariness of the psychiatric evidence, will now be considered.

In the weighing of the patient's responses during the interview, the physician appeared not to give the patient credit for the large number of correct answers he gave. In the typical interview, the examiner might ask the patient fifteen or twenty questions: the date, time, place, who is President, Governor, etc., what is 11×10, 11×11, etc., explain "Don't put all your eggs in one basket," "A rolling stone gathers no moss," etc. The examiners appeared to feel that a wrong answer established lack of orientation, even when it was preceded by a series of correct answers. In other words, the examiners do not establish any standard score on the orientation questions, which would give an objective picture of the degree to which the patient answered the questions correctly, but seem at times to search until they find an incorrect answer.

For those questions which were answered incorrectly, it was not always clear whether the incorrect answers were due to the patient's "mental illness," or to the time pressure in the interview, the patient's lack of education, or other causes. Some of the questions used to establish orientation were sufficiently difficult that persons not mentally ill might have difficulty with them. Thus one of the examiners always asked, in a rapid-fire manner: "What year is it? What year was it seven years ago? Seventeen years before that?" etc. Only two of the five patients who were asked this series of questions were able to answer it correctly. However, it is a moot question whether a higher percentage of persons in a household survey would be able to do any better. To my knowledge, none of the orientation questions that are used have been checked in a normal population.

Finally, the interpretations of some of the evidence as showing mental illness seemed capricious. Thus one of the patients, when asked, "In what way are a banana, an orange, and an apple alike?" answered, "They are all something to eat." This answer was used by the examiner in explaining his recommendation to commit. The observer had noted that the patient's behavior and responses seemed appropriate and asked why the recommendation to commit had been made. The doctor stated that her behavior had been bizarre (possibly referring to her alleged promiscuity), her affect inappropriate ("When she talked about being pregnant, it was without feeling") and with regard to the question above:

> She wasn't able to say a banana and an orange were fruit. She couldn't take it one step further, she had to say it was something to eat.

In other words, this psychiatrist was suggesting that the patient manifested concreteness in her thinking, which is held to be a symptom of mental illness. Yet in her other answers to classification questions, and to proverb interpretations, concreteness was not apparent, suggesting that the examiner's application of this test was arbitrary. In another case, the physician stated that he thought the patient was suspicious and distrustful, because he had asked about the possibility of being represented by counsel at the judicial hearing. The observer felt that these and other similar interpretations might possibly be correct, but that further investigation of the supposedly incorrect responses would be needed to establish that they were manifestations of disorientation.

In several cases where even this type of evidence was not available, the examiners still recommended retention in the hospital. Thus, one examiner, employed by court A stated that he had recommended 30-day observation for a patient whom he had thought *not* to be mentally ill, on the grounds that the patient, a young man, could not get along with his parents, and "might get into trouble." This examiner went on to say:

> We always take the conservative side. [Commitment or observation] Suppose a patient should commit suicide. We always make the conservative decision. I had rather play it safe. There's no harm in doing it that way.

It appeared to the observer that "playing safe" meant that even in those cases where the examination established nothing, the psychiatrists did not consider recommending release. Thus in one case the examination had established that the patient had a very good memory, was oriented and spoke quietly and seriously. The observer recorded his discussion with the physician after the examination as follows:

> When the doctor told me he was recommending commitment for this patient too (he had also recommended commitment in the two examinations held earlier that day) he laughed because he could see what my next question was going to be. He said, "I already recommended the release of two patients this month." This sounded like it was the maximum amount the way he said it.

Apparently this examiner felt that he had a very limited quota on the number of patients he could recommend for release (less than two percent of those examined).

The language used by these physicians tends to intimate that mental illness was found, even when reporting the opposite. Thus in one case the recommendation stated: "No gross evidence of delusions or hallucinations." This statement is misleading, since not only was there no gross evidence, there was not any evidence, not even the slightest suggestion of delusions or hallucinations, brought out by the interview.

These remarks suggest that the examiners prejudge the cases they examine. Several further comments indicate prejudgment. One physician stated that he thought that most crimes of violence were committed by patients released too early from mental hospitals. (This is an erroneous belief.)[5] He went on to say that he thought that all mental patients should be kept in the hospital at least three months, indicating prejudgment concerning his examinations. Another physician, after a very short interview (8 minutes), told the observer:

> On the schizophrenics, I don't bother asking them more questions when I can see they're schizophrenic because *I know what they are going to say.* You could talk to them another half hour and not learn any more.

Another physician, finally, contrasted cases in which the patient's family or others initiated hospitalization ("petition cases," the great majority of cases) with those cases initiated by the court:

> The petition cases are pretty *automatic.* If the patient's own family wants to get rid of him you know there is something wrong.

The lack of care which characterized the examinations is evident in the forms on which the examiners make their recommendations. On most of these forms, whole sections have

---

[5]The rate of crimes of violence, or any crime, appears to be less among ex-mental patients than in the general population (Brill & Maltzberg, n.d.; Cohen & Freeman, 1945; Hastings, 1962).

been left unanswered. Others are answered in a peremptory and uninformative way. For example, in the section entitled Physical Examination, the question is asked: "Have you made a physical examination of the patient? State fully what is the present physical condition." A typical answer is "Yes. Fair" or, "Is apparently in good health." Since in none of the examinations we observed was the patient actually physically examined, these answers appear to be mere guesses. One of the examiners used regularly in court B, to the question "On what subject or in what way is derangement now manifested?" always wrote in "Is mentally ill." The omissions, and the almost flippant brevity of these forms, together with the arbitrariness, lack of evidence, and prejudicial character of the examinations, discussed above, all support the observer's conclusion that, except in very unusual cases, the psychiatric examiner's recommendation to retain the patient is virtually automatic.

Lest it be thought that these results are unique to a particularly backward Midwestern State, it should be pointed out that this state is noted for its progressive psychiatric practices. It will be recalled that a number of the psychiatrists employed by the court as examiners had finished their psychiatric residencies, which is not always the case in many other states. A still common practice in other states is to employ, as members of the "Lunacy Panel," partially retired physicians with no psychiatric training whatever. This was the case in Stockton, California, in 1959, where the author observed hundreds of hearings at which these physicians were present. It may be indicative of some of the larger issues underlying the question of civil commitment that, in these hearings, the physicians played very little part; the judge controlled the questioning of the relatives and patients, and the hearings were often a model of impartial and thorough investigation.

DISCUSSION

Ratings of the qualifications for involuntary confinement of patients newly admitted to the public mental hospitals in a Midwestern state, together with observations of judicial hearings and psychiatric examinations by the observer connected with the present study, both suggest that the decision as to the mental condition of a majority of the patients is an uncertain one. The fact that the courts seldom release patients, and the perfunctory manner in which the legal and medical procedures are carried out, suggest that the judicial decision to retain patients in the hospital for treatment is routine and largely based on the presumption of illness. Three reasons for this presumption will be discussed: financial, ideological, and political.

Our discussions with the examiners indicated that one reason that they perform biased "examinations" is that their rate of pay is determined by the length of time spent with the patient. In recommending retention, the examiners are refraining from interrupting the hospitalization and commitment procedures already in progress, and thereby allowing someone else, usually the hospital, to make the effective decision to release or commit. In order to recommend release, however, they would have to build a case showing why these procedures should be interrupted. Building such a case would take much more time than is presently expended by the examiners, thereby reducing their rate of pay.

A more fundamental reason for the presumption of illness by the examiners, and perhaps the reason why this practice is allowed by the courts, is the interpretation of current psychiatric doctrine by the examiners and court officials. These officials make a number of assumptions, which are now thought to be of doubtful validity:

1. The condition of mentally ill persons deteriorates rapidly without psychiatric assistance.

2. Effective psychiatric treatments exist for most mental illnesses.
3. Unlike surgery, there are no risks involved in involuntary psychiatric treatment: it either helps or is neutral, it can't hurt.
4. Exposing a prospective mental patient to questioning, cross-examination, and other screening procedures exposed him to the unnecessary stigma of trial-like procedures, and may do further damage to his mental condition.
5. There is an element of danger to self or others in most mental illness. It is better to risk unnecessary hospitalization than the harm the patient might do himself or others.

Many psychiatrists and others now argue that none of these assumptions are necessarily correct.

1. The assumption that psychiatric disorders usually get worse without treatment rests on very little other than evidence of an anecdotal character. There is just as much evidence that most acute psychological and emotional upsets are self-terminating.[6]
2. It is still not clear, according to systematic studies evaluating psychotherapy, drugs, etc., that most psychiatric interventions are any more effective, on the average, than no treatment at all.[7]
3. There is very good evidence that involuntary hospitalization and social isolation may affect the patient's life: his job, his family affairs, etc. There is some evidence that too hasty exposure to psychiatric treatment may convince the patient that he is "sick," prolonging what might have been an otherwise transitory episode.[8]
4. This assumption is correct, as far as it goes. But it is misleading because it fails to consider what occurs when the patient who does not wish to be hospitalized is forcibly treated. Such patients often become extremely indignant and angry, particularly in the case, as often happens, when they are deceived into coming to the hospital on some pretext.
5. The element of danger is usually exaggerated both in amount and degree. In the psychiatric survey of new patients in state mental hospitals, danger to self or others was mentioned in about a fourth of the cases. Furthermore, in those cases where danger is mentioned, it is not always clear that the risks involved are greater than those encountered in ordinary social life. This issue has been discussed by Ross (1959), an attorney:

> A truck driver with a mild neurosis who is "accident prone" is probably a greater danger to society than most psychotics; yet, he will not be committed for treatment, even if he would be benefited. The community expects a certain amount of dangerous activity. I suspect that as a class, drinking drivers are a greater danger than the mentally ill, and yet the drivers are tolerated or punished with small fines rather than indeterminate imprisonment [p. 962].

From our observations of the medical examinations and other commitment procedures, we formed a very strong impression that the doctrines of danger to self or others, early treatment, and the avoidance of stigma were invoked partly because the officials believed

---

[6]For a review of epidemiological studies of mental disorder see Plunkett & Gordon (1960). Most of these studies suggest that at any given point in time, psychiatrists find a substantial proportion of persons in normal populations to be "mentally ill." One interpretation of this finding is that much of the deviance detected in these studies is self-limiting.

[7]For an assessment of the evidence regarding the effectiveness of electroshock, drugs, psychotherapy, and other psychiatric treatments, see Eysenck (1961).

[8]For examples from military psychiatry, see Glass (1953) and Bushard (1957). For a discussion of essentially the same problem in the context of a civilian mental hospital, cf. Erikson (1957).

them to be true, and partly because they provided convenient justification for a pre-existing policy of summary action, minimal investigation, avoidance of responsibility and, after the patient is in the hospital, indecisiveness and delay.

The policy of presuming illness is probably both cause and effect of political pressure on the court from the community. The judge, an elected official, runs the risk of being more heavily penalized for erroneously releasing than for erroneously retaining patients. Since the judge personally appoints the panel of psychiatrists to serve as examiners, he can easily transmit the community pressure to them, by failing to reappoint a psychiatrist whose examinations were inconveniently thorough.

Some of the implications of these findings for the sociology of deviant behavior will be briefly summarized. The discussion above, of the reasons that the psychiatrists tend to presume illness, suggests that the motivations of the key decision-makers in the screening process may be significant in determining the extent and direction of the societal reaction. In the case of psychiatric screening of persons alleged to be mentally ill, the social differentiation of the deviant from the non-deviant population appears to be materially affected by the financial, ideological, and political position of the psychiatrists, who are in this instance the key agents of social control.

Under these circumstances, the character of the societal reaction appears to undergo a marked change from the pattern of denial which occurs in the community. The official societal reaction appears to reverse the presumption of normality reported by the Cummings (1957, p. 102) as a characteristic of informal societal reaction, and instead exaggerates both the amount and degree of deviance.[9] Thus, one extremely important contingency influencing the severity of the societal reaction may be whether or not the original deviance comes to official notice. This paper suggests that in the area of mental disorder, perhaps in contrast to other areas of deviant behavior, if the official societal reaction is invoked, for whatever reason, social differentiation of the deviant from the non-deviant population will usually occur.

CONCLUSION

This paper has described the screening of patients who were admitted to public mental hospitals in early June, 1962, in a Midwestern state. The data presented here suggest that the screening is usually perfunctory, and that in the crucial screening examination by the court-appointed psychiatrists, there is a presumption of illness. Since most court decisions appear to hinge on the recommendation of these psychiatrists, there appears to be a large element of status ascription in the official societal reaction to persons alleged to be mentally ill, as exemplified by the court's actions. This finding points to the importance of lay definitions of mental illness in the community, since the "diagnosis" of mental illness by laymen in the community initiates the official societal reaction, and to the necessity of analyzing social processes connected with the recognition and reaction to the deviant behavior that is called mental illness in our society.

REFERENCES

Brown, E. L. *Newer dimensions of patient care.* Part I. New York: Russell Sage, 1961.
Brill, H., & Maltzberg, B. Statistical report based on the arrest record of 5354 ex-patients released

---

[9] For further discussion of the bipolarization of the societal reaction into denial and labeling, see Scheff (1963b).

from New York State mental hospitals during the period 1946–48. Mimeographed. Available from the authors.

Bushard, B. L. The U.S. Army's mental hygiene consultation service. In *Symposium on Preventive and Social Psychiatry*, Washington, D.C., April, 1957, Walter Reed Army Institute of Research, Pp. 431–443.

Cohen, L. H., & Freeman, H. How dangerous to the community are state hospital patients? *Connecticut State Medical Journal*, 1945, **9**, 697–700.

Cumming, E., & Cumming, J. *Closed ranks.* Cambridge, Mass.: Harvard University Press, 1957.

Erikson, K. T. Patient role and social uncertainty — A dilemma of the mentally ill. *Psychiatry*, 1957, **20**, 263–275.

Eysenck, H. J. *Handbook of abnormal psychology.* Part III. New York: Basic Books, 1961.

Glass, A. J. Psychotherapy in the combat zone. In *Symposium on Stress*, Army Medical Service Graduate School, Washington, D.C., 1953.

Goffman, E. *Asylums.* Chicago: Aldine, 1962.

Hastings, D. W. Follow-up results in psychiatric illness. *American Journal of Psychiatry*, 1962, **118**, 1078–1086.

Kitsuse, J. I. Societal reaction to deviant behavior: Problems of theory and method. *Social Problems*, 1962, **9**, 247–257.

Kutner, L. The illusion of due process in commitment proceedings. *Northwestern University Law Review*, 1962, **57**, 383–399.

Lemert, E. M. *Social pathology.* New York: McGraw-Hill, 1951.

Mechanic, D. Some factors in identifying and defining mental illness. *Mental Hygiene*, 1962, **46**, 66–75.

Plunkett, R. J., & Gordon, J. E. *Epidemiology and mental illness.* New York: Basic Books, 1960.

Ross, H. A. Commitment of the mentally ill: Problems of law and policy. *Michigan Law Review*, 1959, **57**, 945–1018.

Scheff, T. J. Decision rules, types of error and their consequences in medical diagnosis. *Behavioral Science*, 1963, **8**, 97–107. (a)

Scheff, T. J. The role of the mentally ill and the dynamics of mental disorder: A research framework. *Sociometry*, 1963, **26**, 436–453. (b)

Scheff, T. J. Social conditions for rationality: How urban and rural courts deal with the mentally ill. *American Behavioral Scientist*, 1964, **7**, 21–24.

44

On Being Sane in Insane Places*

D. L. ROSENHAN

If sanity and insanity exist, how shall we know them?

The question is neither capricious nor itself insane. However much we may be personally convinced that we can tell the normal from the abnormal, the evidence is simply not compelling. It is commonplace, for example, to read about murder trials wherein eminent psychiatrists for the defense are contradicted by equally eminent psychiatrists for the prosecution on the matter of the defendant's sanity. More generally, there are a great deal of conflicting data on the reliability, utility, and meaning of such terms as "sanity," "insanity," "mental illness," and "schizophrenia"[1]. Finally, as early as 1934, Benedict suggested that normality and abnormality are not universal [2]. What is viewed as normal in one culture may be seen as quite aberrant in another. Thus, notions of normality and abnormality may not be quite as accurate as people believe they are.

To raise questions regarding normality and abnormality is in no way to question the fact that some behaviors are deviant or odd. Murder is deviant. So, too, are hallucinations. Nor does raising such questions deny the existence of the personal anguish that is often associated with "mental illness." Anxiety and depression exist. Psychological suffering exists. But normality and abnormality, sanity and insanity, and the diagnoses that flow from them may be less substantive than many believe them to be.

At its heart, the question of whether the sane can be distinguished from the insane (and whether degrees of insanity can be distinguished from each other) is a simple matter: do the salient characteristics that lead to diagnoses reside in the patients themselves or in the environments and contexts in which observers find them? From Bleuler, through Kretchmer, through the formulators of the recently revised *Diagnostic and Statistical Manual* of the American Psychiatric Association, the belief has been strong that patients present symptoms, that those symptoms can be categorized, and, implicitly, that the sane are distinguishable from the insane. More recently, however, this belief has been questioned. Based in part on theoretical and anthropological considerations, but also on philosophical, legal, and therapeutic ones, the view has grown that psychological categorization of mental illness is useless at best and downright harmful, misleading, and pejorative at worst. Psychiatric diagnoses, in this view, are in the minds of the observers and are not valid summaries of characteristics displayed by the observed [3–5].

Gains can be made in deciding which of these is more nearly accurate by getting normal people (that is, people who do not have, and have never suffered, symptoms of serious psychiatric disorders) admitted to psychiatric hospitals and then determining whether they were discovered to be sane and, if so, how. If the sanity of such pseudopatients were always detected, there would be prima facie evidence that a sane individual can be

Uses norms who say they are sane to vouch up argument

distinguished from the insane context in which he is found/ Normality (and presumably abnormality) is distinct enough that it can be recognized wherever it occurs, for it is carried within the person. If, on the other hand, the sanity of the pseudopatients were never discovered, serious difficulties would arise for those who support traditional modes of psychiatric diagnosis. Given that the hospital staff was not incompetent, that the pseudopatient had been behaving as sanely as he had been outside of the hospital, and that it had never been previously suggested that he belonged in a psychiatric hospital, such an unlikely outcome would support the view that psychiatric diagnosis betrays little about the patient but much about the environment in which an observer finds him.

This article describes such an experiment. Eight sane people gained secret admission to 12 different hospitals [6]. Their diagnostic experiences constitute the data of the first part of this article; the remainder is devoted to a description of their experiences in psychiatric institutions. Too few psychiatrists and psychologists, even those who have worked in such hospitals, know what the experience is like. They rarely talk about it with former patients, perhaps because they distrust information coming from the previously insane. Those who have worked in psychiatric hospitals are likely to have adapted so thoroughly to the settings that they are insensitive to the impact of that experience. And while there have been occasional reports of researchers who submitted themselves to psychiatric hospitalization [7], these researchers have commonly remained in the hospitals for short periods of time, often with the knowledge of the hospital staff. It is difficult to know the extent to which they were treated like patients or like research colleagues. Nevertheless, their reports about the inside of the psychiatric hospital have been valuable. This article extends those efforts.

PSEUDOPATIENTS AND THEIR SETTINGS

The eight pseudopatients were a varied group. One was a psychology graduate student in his 20's. The remaining seven were older and "established." Among them were three psychologists, a pediatrician, a psychiatrist, a painter, and a housewife. Three pseudopatients were women, five were men. All of them employed pseudonyms, lest their alleged diagnoses embarrass them later. Those who were in mental health professions alleged another occupation in order to avoid the special attentions that might be accorded by staff, as a matter of courtesy or caution, to ailing colleagues [8]. With the exception of myself (I was the first pseudopatient and my presence was known to the hospital administrator and chief psychologist and, so far as I can tell, to them alone), the presence of pseudopatients and the nature of the research program was not known to the hospital staffs [9].

The settings were similarly varied. In order to generalize the findings, admission into a variety of hospitals was sought. The 12 hospitals in the sample were located in five different states on the East and West coasts. Some were old and shabby, some were quite new. Some were research-oriented, others not. Some had good staff-patient ratios, others were quite understaffed. Only one was a strictly private hospital. All of the others were supported by state or federal funds or, in one instance, by university funds.

After calling the hospital for an appointment, the pseudopatient arrived at the admissions office complaining that he had been hearing voices. Asked what the voices said, he replied that they were often unclear, but as far as he could tell they said "empty," "hollow," and "thud." The voices were unfamiliar and were of the same sex as the pseudopatient. The choice of these symptoms was occasioned by their apparent similarity to existential symptoms. Such symptoms are alleged to arise from painful concerns about the perceived meaninglessness of one's life. It is as if the hallucinating person were saying, "My life is empty and hollow." The choice of these symptoms was also determined by the *absence* of a single report of existential psychoses in the literature.

Beyond alleging the symptoms and falsifying name, vocation, and employment, no further alterations of person, history, or circumstances were made. The significant events of the pseudopatient's life history were presented as they had actually occurred. Relationships with parents and siblings, with spouse and children, with people at work and in school, consistent with the aforementioned exceptions, were described as they were or had been. Frustrations and upsets were described along with joys and satisfactions. These facts are important to remember. If anything, they strongly biased the subsequent results in favor of detecting sanity, since none of their histories or current behaviors were seriously pathological in any way.

Immediately upon admission to the psychiatric ward, the pseudopatient ceased simulating *any* symptoms of abnormality. In some cases, there was a brief period of mild nervousness and anxiety, since none of the pseudopatients really believed that they would be admitted so easily. Indeed, their shared fear was that they would be immediately exposed as frauds and greatly embarrassed. Moreover, many of them had never visited a psychiatric ward; even those who had, nevertheless had some genuine fears about what might happen to them. Their nervousness, then, was quite appropriate to the novelty of the hospital set- ting, and it abated rapidly.

[margin note:] Acted normal

Apart from that short-lived nervousness, the pseudopatient behaved on the ward as he "normally" behaved. The pseudopatient spoke to patients and staff as he might ordinarily. Because there is uncommonly little to do on a psychiatric ward, he attempted to engage others in conversation. When asked by staff how he was feeling, he indicated that he was fine, that he no longer experienced symptoms. He responded to instructions from attendants, to calls for medication (which was not swallowed), and to dining-hall instructions. Beyond such activities as were available to him on the admissions ward, he spent his time writing down his observations about the ward, its patients, and the staff. Initially these notes were written "secretly," but as it soon became clear that no one much cared, they were subsequently written on standard tablets of paper in such public places as the dayroom. No secret was made of these activities.

The pseudopatient, very much as a true psychiatric patient, entered a hospital with no foreknowledge of when he would be discharged. Each was told that he would have to get out by his own devices, essentially by convincing the staff that he was sane. The psychological stresses associated with hospitalization were considerable, and all but one of the pseudopatients desired to be discharged almost immediately after being admitted. They were, therefore, motivated not only to behave sanely, but to be paragons of cooperation. That their behavior was in no way disruptive is confirmed by nursing reports, which have been obtained on most of the patients. These reports uniformly indicate that the patients were "friendly," "cooperative," and "exhibited no abnormal indications."

THE NORMAL ARE NOT DETECTABLY SANE

Despite their public "show" of sanity, the pseudopatients were never detected. Admitted, except in one case, with a diagnosis of schizophrenia[10], each was discharged with a diagnosis of schizophrenia "in remission." The label "in remission" should in no way be dismissed as a formality, for at no time during any hospitalization had any question been raised about any pseudopatient's simulation. Nor are there any indications in the hospital records that the pseudopatient's status was suspect. Rather, the evidence is strong that, once labeled schizophrenic, the pseudopatient was stuck with that label. If the pseudopatient was to be discharged, he must naturally be "in remission"; but he was not sane, nor, in the institution's view, had he ever been sane.

The uniform failure to recognize sanity cannot be attributed to the quality of the hospitals, for, although there were considerable variations among them, several are considered excellent. Nor can it be alleged that there was simply not enough time to observe the pseudopatients. Length of hospitalization ranged from 7 to 52 days, with an average of 19 days. The pseudopatients were not, in fact, carefully observed, but this failure clearly speaks more to traditions within psychiatric hospitals than to lack of opportunity.

Finally, it cannot be said that the failure to recognize the pseudopatients' sanity was due to the fact that they were not behaving sanely. While there was clearly some tension present in all of them, their daily visitors could detect no serious behavioral consequences—nor, indeed, could other patients. It was quite common for the patients to "detect" the pseudopatients' sanity. During the first three hospitalizations, when accurate counts were kept, 35 of a total of 118 patients on the admissions ward voiced their suspicions, some vigorously. "You're not crazy. You're a journalist, or a professor [referring to the continual note-taking]. You're checking up on the hospital." While most of the patients were reassured by the pseudopatient's insistence that he had been sick before he came in but was fine now, some continued to believe that the pseudopatient was sane throughout his hospitalization [11]. The fact that the patients often recognized normality when staff did not raises important questions.

Failure to detect sanity during the course of hospitalization may be due to the fact that physicians operate with a strong bias toward what statisticians call the type 2 error [5]. This is to say that physicians are more inclined to call a healthy person sick (a false positive, type 2) than a sick person healthy (a false negative, type 1). The reasons for this are not hard to find: it is clearly more dangerous to misdiagnose illness than health. Better to err on the side of caution, to suspect illness even among the healthy.

But what holds for medicine does not hold equally well for psychiatry. Medical illnesses, while unfortunate, are not commonly pejorative. Psychiatric diagnoses, on the contrary, carry with them personal, legal, and social stigmas [12]. It was therefore important to see whether the tendency toward diagnosing the sane insane could be reversed. The following experiment was arranged at a research and teaching hospital whose staff had heard these findings but doubted that such an error could occur in their hospital. The staff was informed that at some time during the following 3 months, one or more pseudopatients would attempt to be admitted into the psychiatric hospital. Each staff member was asked to rate each patient who presented himself at admissions or on the ward according to the likelihood that the patient was a pseudopatient. A 10-point scale was used, with a 1 and 2 reflecting high confidence that the patient was a pseudopatient.

Judgments were obtained on 193 patients who were admitted for psychiatric treatment. All staff who had had sustained contact with or primary responsibility for the patient—attendants, nurses, psychiatrists, physicians, and psychologists—were asked to make judgments. Forty-one patients were alleged, with high confidence, to be pseudopatients by at least one member of the staff. Twenty-three were considered suspect by at least one psychiatrist. Nineteen were suspected by one psychiatrist *and* one other staff member. Actually, no genuine pseudopatient (at least from my group) presented himself during this period.

The experiment is instructive. It indicates that the tendency to designate sane people as insane can be reversed when the stakes (in this case, prestige and diagnostic acumen) are high. But what can be said of the 19 people who were suspected of being "sane" by one psychiatrist and another staff member? Were these people truly "sane," or was it rather the case that in the course of avoiding the type 2 error the staff tended to make more errors of the first sort—calling the crazy "sane"? There is no way of knowing. But one thing is certain: any diagnostic process that lends itself so readily to massive errors of this sort cannot be a very reliable one.

THE STICKINESS OF PSYCHODIAGNOSTIC LABELS

Beyond the tendency to call the healthy sick—a tendency that accounts better for diagnostic behavior on admission than it does for such behavior after a lengthy period of exposure—the data speak to the massive role of labeling in psychiatric assessment. Having once been labeled schizophrenic, there is nothing the pseudopatient can do to overcome the tag. The tag profoundly colors others' perceptions of him and his behavior.

From one viewpoint, these data are hardly surprising, for it has long been known that elements are given meaning by the context in which they occur. Gestalt psychology made this point vigorously, and Asch[13] demonstrated that there are "central" personality traits (such as "warm" versus "cold") which are so powerful that they markedly color the meaning of other information in forming an impression of a given personality[14]. "Insane," "schizophrenic," "manic-depressive," and "crazy" are probably among the most powerful of such central traits. Once a person is designated abnormal, all of his other behaviors and characteristics are colored by that label. Indeed, that label is so powerful that many of the pseudopatients' normal behaviors were overlooked entirely or profoundly misinterpreted. Some examples may clarify this issue.

Earlier I indicated that there were no changes in the pseudopatient's personal history and current status beyond those of name, employment, and, where necessary, vocation. Otherwise, a veridical description of personal history and circumstances was offered. Those circumstances were not psychotic. How were they made consonant with the diagnosis of psychosis? Or were those diagnoses modified in such a way as to bring them into accord with the circumstances of the pseudopatient's life, as described by him?

As far as I can determine, diagnoses were in no way affected by the relative health of the circumstances of a pseudopatient's life. Rather, the reverse occurred: the perception of his circumstances was shaped entirely by the diagnosis. A clear example of such translation is found in the case of a pseudopatient who had had a close relationship with his mother but was rather remote from his father during his early childhood. During adolescence and beyond, however, his father became a close friend, while his relationship with his mother cooled. His present relationship with his wife was characteristically close and warm. Apart from occasional angry exchanges, friction was minimal. The children had rarely been spanked. Surely there is nothing especially pathological about such a history. Indeed, many readers may see a similar pattern in their own experiences, with no markedly deleterious consequences. Observe, however, how such a history was translated in the psychopathological context, this from the case summary prepared after the patient was discharged.

> This white 39-year-old male.... manifests a long history of considerable ambivalence in close relationships, which begins in early childhood. A warm relationship with his mother cools during his adolescence. A distant relationship to his father is described as becoming very intense. Affective stability is absent. His attempts to control emotionality with his wife and children are punctuated by angry outbursts and, in the case of the children, spankings. And while he says that

he has several good friends, one senses considerable ambivalence embedded in those relationships also....

The facts of the case were unintentionally distorted by the staff to achieve consistency with a popular theory of the dynamics of a schizophrenic reaction[15]. Nothing of an ambivalent nature had been described in relations with parents, spouse, or friends. To the extent that ambivalence could be inferred, it was probably not greater than is found in all human relationships. It is true the pseudopatient's relationships with his parents changed over time, but in the ordinary context that would hardly be remarkable—indeed, it might very well be expected. Clearly, the meaning ascribed to his verbalizations (that is, ambivalence, affective instability) was determined by the diagnosis: schizophrenia. An entirely different meaning would have been ascribed if it were known that the man was "normal."

All pseudopatients took extensive notes publicly. Under ordinary circumstances, such behavior would have raised questions in the minds of observers, as, in fact, it did among patients. Indeed, it seemed so certain that the notes would elicit suspicion that elaborate precautions were taken to remove them from the ward each day. But the precautions proved needless. The closest any staff member came to questioning these notes occurred when one pseudopatient asked his physician what kind of medication he was receiving and began to write down the response. "You needn't write it," he was told gently. "If you have trouble remembering, just ask me again."

If no questions were asked of the pseudopatients, how was their writing interpreted? Nursing records for three patients indicate that the writing was seen as an aspect of their pathological behavior. "Patient engages in writing behavior" was the daily nursing comment on one of the pseudopatients who was never questioned about his writing. Given that the patient is in the hospital, he must be psychologically disturbed. And given that he is disturbed, continuous writing must be a behavioral manifestation of that disturbance, perhaps a subset of the compulsive behaviors that are sometimes correlated with schizophrenia.

One tacit characteristic of psychiatric diagnosis is that it locates the sources of aberration within the individual and only rarely within the complex of stimuli that surrounds him. Consequently, behaviors that are stimulated by the environment are commonly misattributed to the patient's disorder. For example, one kindly nurse found a pseudopatient pacing the long hospital corridors. "Nervous, Mr. X?" she asked. "No, bored," he said.

The notes kept by pseudopatients are full of patient behaviors that were misinterpreted by well-intentioned staff. Often enough, a patient would go "berserk" because he had, wittingly or unwittingly, been mistreated by, say, an attendant. A nurse coming upon the scene would rarely inquire even cursorily into the environmental stimuli of the patient's behavior. Rather, she assumed that his upset derived from his pathology, not from his present interactions with other staff members. Occasionally, the staff might assume that the patient's family (especially when they had recently visited) or other patients had stimulated the outburst. But never were the staff found to assume that one of themselves or the structure of the hospital had anything to do with a patient's behavior. One psychiatrist pointed to a group of patients who were sitting outside the cafeteria entrance half an hour before lunchtime. To a group of young residents he indicated that such behavior was characteristic of the oral-acquisitive nature of the syndrome. It seemed not to occur to him that there were very few things to anticipate in a psychiatric hospital besides eating.

A psychiatric label has a life and an influence of its own. Once the impression has been formed that the patient is schizophrenic, the expectation is that he will continue to be schizophrenic. When a sufficient amount of time has passed, during which the patient has done nothing bizarre, he is considered to be in remission and available for discharge. But the label endures beyond discharge, with the unconfirmed expectation that he will behave as a schizophrenic again. Such labels, conferred by mental health professionals, are as influential on the patient as they are on his relatives and friends, and it should not surprise anyone that the diagnosis acts on all of them as a self-fulfilling prophecy. Eventually, the patient himself accepts the diagnosis, with all of its surplus meanings and expectations, and behaves accordingly[5].

The inferences to be made from these matters are quite simple. Much as Zigler and Phillips have demonstrated that there is enormous overlap in the symptoms presented by patients who have been variously diagnosed[16], so there is enormous overlap in the behaviors of the sane and the insane. The sane are not "sane" all of the time. We lose our tempers "for no good reason." We are occasionally depressed or anxious, again for no good reason. And we may find it difficult to get along with one or another person—again for no reason that we can specify. Similarly, the insane are not always insane. Indeed, it was the impression of the pseudopatients while living with them that they were sane for long periods of time—that the bizarre behaviors upon which their diagnoses were allegedly predicated constituted only a small fraction of their total behavior. If it makes no sense to label ourselves permanently depressed on the basis of an occasional depression, then it takes better evidence than is presently available to label all patients insane or schizophrenic on the basis of bizarre behaviors or cognitions. It seems more useful, as Mischel[17] has pointed out, to limit our discussions to *behaviors*, the stimuli that provoke them, and their correlates.

It is not known why powerful impressions of personality traits, such as "crazy" or "insane," arise. Conceivably, when the origins of and stimuli that give rise to a behavior are remote or unknown, or when the behavior strikes us as immutable, trait labels regarding the *behaver* arise. When, on the other hand, the origins and stimuli are known and available, discourse is limited to the behavior itself. Thus, I may hallucinate because I am sleeping, or I may hallucinate because I have ingested a peculiar drug. These are termed sleep induced hallucinations, or dreams, and drug-induced hallucinations, respectively. But when the stimuli to my hallucinations are unknown, that is called craziness, or schizophrenia—as if that inference were somehow as illuminating as the others.

THE EXPERIENCE OF PSYCHIATRIC HOSPITALIZATION

The term "mental illness" is of recent origin. It was coined by people who were humane in their inclinations and who wanted very much to raise the station of (and the public's sympathies toward) the psychologically disturbed from that of witches and "crazies" to one that was akin to the physically ill. And they were at least partially successful, for the treatment of the mentally ill *has* improved considerably over the years. But while treatment has improved, it is doubtful that people really regard the mentally ill in the same way that they view the physically ill. A broken leg is something one recovers from, but mental illness allegedly endures forever[18]. A broken leg does not threaten the observer, but a crazy schizophrenic? There is by now a host of evidence that attitudes toward the mentally ill are characterized by fear, hostility, aloofness, suspicion, and dread[19]. The mentally ill are society's lepers.

That such attitudes infect the general population is perhaps not surprising, only upsetting. But that they affect the professionals—attendants, nurses, physicians, psychologists, and social workers—who treat and deal with the mentally ill is more disconcerting, both because such attitudes are self-evidently pernicious and because they are unwitting. Most mental health professionals would insist that they are sympathetic toward the mentally ill, that they are neither avoidant nor hostile. But it is more likely that an exquisite ambivalence characterizes their relations with psychiatric patients, such that their avowed impulses are only part of their entire attitude. Negative attitudes are there too and can easily be detected. Such attitudes should not surprise us. They are the natural offspring of the labels patients wear and the places in which they are found.

Consider the structure of the typical psychiatric hospital. Staff and patients are strictly segregated. Staff have their own living space, including their dining facilities, bathrooms, and assembly places. The glassed quarters that contain the professional staff, which the pseudopatients came to call "the cage," sit out on every dayroom. The staff emerge primarily for caretaking purposes—to give medication, to conduct a therapy or group meeting, to instruct or reprimand a patient. Otherwise, staff keep to themselves, almost as if the disorder that afflicts their charges is somehow catching.

So much is patient-staff segregation the rule that, for four public hospitals in which an attempt was made to measure the degree to which staff and patients mingle, it was necessary to use "time out of the staff cage" as the operational measure. While it was not the case that all time spent out of the cage was spent mingling with patients (attendants, for example, would occasionally emerge to watch television in the dayroom), it was the only way in which one could gather reliable data on time for measuring.

The average amount of time spent by attendants outside of the cage was 11.3 percent (range, 3 to 52 percent). This figure does not represent only time spent mingling with patients, but also includes time spent on such chores as folding laundry, supervising patients while they shave, directing ward cleanup, and sending patients to off-ward activities. It was the relatively rare attendant who spent time talking with patients or playing games with them. It proved impossible to obtain a "percent mingling time" for nurses, since the amount of time they spent out of the cage was too brief. Rather, we counted instances of emergence from the cage. On the average, daytime nurses emerged from the cage 11.5 times per shift, including instances when they left the ward entirely (range, 4 to 39 times). Late afternoon and night nurses were even less available, emerging on the average 9.4 times per shift (range, 4 to 41 times). Data on early morning nurses, who arrived usually after midnight and departed at 8 a.m., are not available because patients were asleep during most of this period.

Physicians, especially psychiatrists, were even less available. They were rarely seen on the wards. Quite commonly, they would be seen only when they arrived and departed, with the remaining time being spent in their offices or in the cage. On the average, physicians emerged on the ward 6.7 times per day (range, 1 to 17 times). It proved difficult to make an accurate estimate in this regard, since physicians often maintained hours that allowed them to come and go at different times.

The hierarchical organization of the psychiatric hospital has been commented on before [20], but the latent meaning of that kind of organization is worth noting again. Those with the most power have least to do with patients, and those with the least power are most involved with them. Recall, however, that the acquisition of role-appropriate behaviors occurs mainly through the observation of others, with the most powerful having the most influence. Consequently, it is understandable that attendants not only spend more time with patients than do any other members of the staff—that is required by their station in the hierarchy—but also, insofar as they learn from their superiors' behavior, spend as little time with patients as they can. Attendants are seen mainly in the cage, which is where the models, the action, and the power are.

I turn now to a different set of studies, these dealing with staff response to patient-initiated contact. It has long been known that the amount of time a person spends with you can be an index of your significance to him. If he initiates and maintains eye contact, there is reason to believe that he is considering your requests and needs. If he pauses to chat or actually stops and talks, there is added reason to infer that he is individuating you. In four hospitals, the pseudopatient approached the staff member with a request which which took the following form: "Pardon me, Mr. [or Dr. or Mrs.] X, could you tell me when I will be eligible for grounds privileges?" (or ". . . . when I will be presented at the staff meeting?" or ". . . . when I am likely to be discharged?"). While the content of the question varied according to the appropriateness of the target and the pseudopatient's (apparent) current needs the form was always a courteous and relevant request for information. Care was taken never to approach a particular member of the staff more than once a day, lest the staff member become suspicious or irritated. In examining these data, remember that the behavior of the pseudopatients was neither bizarre nor disruptive. One could indeed engage in good conversation with them.

The data for these experiments are shown in Table 44.1, separately for physicians (column 1) and for nurses and attendants (column 2). Minor differences between these four institutions were overwhelmed by the degree to which staff avoided continuing contacts that patients had initiated. By far, their most common response consisted of either a brief response to the question, offered while they were "on the move" and with head averted, or no response at all.

The encounter frequently took the following bizarre form: (pseudopatient) "Pardon me, Dr. X. Could you tell me when I am eligible for grounds privileges?" (physician) "Good morning, Dave. How are you today?" (Moves off without waiting for a response.)

It is instructive to compare these data with data recently obtained at Stanford University. It has been alleged that large and eminent universities are characterized by faculty who are so busy that they have no time for students. For this comparison, a young lady approached individual faculty members who seemed to be walking purposefully to some meeting or teaching engagement and asked them the following six questions.

(1) "Pardon me, could you direct me to Encina Hall?" (at the medical school: ". . . to the Clinical Research Center?").
(2) "Do you know where Fish Annex is?" (there is no Fish Annex at Stanford).
(3) "Do you teach here?"
(4) "How does one apply for admission to the college?" (at the medical school: ". . . . to the medical school?").
(5) "Is it difficult to get in?"
(6) "Is there financial aid?"

Without exception, as can be seen in Table 44.1 (column 3), all of the questions were answered. No matter how rushed they were, all respondents not only maintained eye contact, but stopped to talk. Indeed, many of the respondents went out of their way to direct or take the questioner to the office she was seeking, to try to locate "Fish Annex," or to discuss with her the possibilities of being admitted to the university.

Similar data, also shown in Table 44.1 (columns 4, 5, and 6), were obtained in the hospital. Here too, the young lady came prepared with six questions. After the first question, however, she remarked to 18 of her respondents (column 4), "I'm looking for a psychiatrist," and to 15 others (column 5), "I'm looking for an internist." Ten other respondents received no inserted comment (column 6). The general degree of cooperative responses is considerably higher for these university groups than it was for pseudopatients in psychiatric hospitals. Even so, differences are apparent within the medical school setting. Once having indi-

Table 44.1 Self-initiated Contact by Pseudopatients with Psychiatrists and Nurses and Attendants, Compared to Contact with Other Groups.

Contact	Psychiatric Hospitals		University Campus (Nonmedical)	University Medical Center Physicians		
	(1) Psychiatrists	(2) Nurses and Attendants	(3) Faculty	(4) "Looking for a Psychiatrist"	(5) "Looking for an Internist"	(6) No Additional Comment
Responses						
Moves on, head averted (%)	71	88	0	0	0	0
Makes eye contact (%)	23	10	0	11	0	0
Pauses and chats (%)	2	2	0	11	0	10
Stops and talks (%)	4	0.5	100	78	100	90
Mean number of questions answered (out of 6)	*	*	6	3.8	4.8	4.5
Respondents (No.)	13	47	14	18	15	10
Attempts (No.)	185	1283	14	18	15	10

*Not applicable.

cated that she was looking for a psychiatrist, the degree of cooperation elicited was less than when she sought an internist.

POWERLESSNESS AND DEPERSONALIZATION

Eye contact and verbal contact reflect concern and individuation: their absence, avoidance and depersonalization. The data I have presented do not do justice to the rich daily encounters that grew up around matters of depersonalization and avoidance. I have records of patients who were beaten by staff for the sin of having initiated verbal contact. During my own experience, for example, one patient was beaten in the presence of other patients for having approached an attendant and told him, "I like you." Occasionally, punishment meted out to patients for misdemeanors seemed so excessive that it could not be justified by the most radical interpretations of psychiatric canon. Nevertheless, they appeared to go unquestioned. Tempers were often short. A patient who had not heard a call for medication would be roundly excoriated, and the morning attendants would often wake patients with, "Come on, you m-----f-----s, out of bed!"

Neither anecdotal nor "hard" data can convey the overwhelming sense of powerlessness which invades the individual as he is continually exposed to the depersonalization of the psychiatric hospital. It hardly matters *which* psychiatric hospital—the excellent public ones and the very plush private hospital were better than the rural and shabby ones in this regard, but, again, the features that psychiatric hospitals had in common overwhelmed by far their apparent differences.

Powerlessness was evident everywhere. The patient is deprived of many of his legal rights by dint of his psychiatric commitment[21]. He is shorn of credibility by virtue of his psychiatric label. His freedom of movement is restricted. He cannot initiate contact with the staff, but may only respond to such overtures as they make. Personal privacy is minimal. Patient quarters and possessions can be entered and examined by any staff member, for whatever reason. His personal history and anguish is available to any staff member (often including the "grey lady" and "candy striper" volunteer) who chooses to read his folder, regardless of their therapeutic relationship to him. His personal hygiene and waste evacuation are often monitored. The water closets may have no doors.

At times, depersonalization reached such proportions that pseudopatients had the sense that they were invisible, or at least unworthy of account. Upon being admitted, I and other pseudopatients took the initial physical examinations in a semipublic room, where staff members went about their own business as if we were not there.

On the ward, attendants delivered verbal and occasionally serious physical abuse to patients in the presence of other observing patients, some of whom (the pseudopatients) were writing it all down. Abusive behavior, on the other hand, terminated quite abruptly when other staff members were known to be coming. Staff are credible witnesses. Patients are not.

A nurse unbuttoned her uniform to adjust her brassiere in the presence of an entire ward of viewing men. One did not have the sense that she was being seductive. Rather, she didn't notice us. A group of staff persons might point to a patient in the dayroom and discuss him animatedly, as if he were not there.

One illuminating instance of depersonalization and invisibility occurred with regard to medications. All told, the pseudopatients were administered nearly 2100 pills, including Elavil, Stelazine, Compazine, and Thorazine, to name but a few. (That such a variety of medications should have been administered to patients presenting identical symptoms is itself worthy of note.) Only two were swallowed. The rest were either pocketed or deposited in the toilet. The pseudopatients were not alone in this. Although I have no precise records on how many patients rejected their medications, the pseudopatients frequently found the medications of other patients in the toilet before they deposited their own. As long as they were cooperative, their behavior and the pseudopatients' own in this matter, as in other important matters, went unnoticed throughout.

Reactions to such depersonalization among pseudopatients were intense. Although they had come to the hospital as participant observers and were fully aware that they did not "belong," they nevertheless found themselves caught up in and fighting the process of depersonalization. Some examples: a graduate student in psychology asked his wife to bring his textbooks to the hospital so he could "catch up on his homework"—this despite the elaborate precautions taken to conceal his professional association. The same student, who had trained for quite some time to get into the hospital, and who had looked forward to the experience, "remembered" some drag races that he had wanted to see on the weekend and insisted that he be discharged by that time. Another pseudopatient attempted a romance with a nurse. Subsequently, he informed the staff that he was applying for admission to graduate school in psychology and was very likely to be admitted, since a graduate professor was one of his regular hospital visitors. The same person began to engage in psychotherapy with other patients—all of this as a way of becoming a person in an impersonal environment.

THE SOURCES OF DEPERSONALIZATION

What are the origins of depersonalization? I have already mentioned two. First are attitudes held by all of us toward the mentally ill—including those who treat them—attitudes characterized by fear, distrust, and horrible expectations on the one hand, and benevolent intentions on the other. Our ambivalence leads, in this instance as in others, to avoidance.

Second, and not entirely separate, the hierarchical structure of the psychiatric hospital facilitates depersonalization. Those who are at the top have least to do with patients, and their behavior inspires the rest of the staff. Average daily contact with psychiatrists, psychologists, residents, and physicians combined ranged from 3.9 to 25.1 minutes, with an overall mean of 6.8 (six pseudopatients over a total of 129 days of hospitalization). Included in this average are time spent in the admissions interview, ward meetings in the presence of a senior staff member, group and individual psychotherapy contacts, case presentation conferences, and discharge meetings. Clearly, patients do not spend much time in interpersonal contact with doctoral staff. And doctoral staff serve as models for nurses and attendants.

There are probably other sources. Psychiatric installations are presently in serious financial straits. Staff shortages are pervasive, staff time at a premium. Something has to give, and that something is patient contact. Yet, while financial stresses are realities, too much can be made of them. I have the impression that the psychological forces that result in depersonalization are much stronger than the fiscal ones and that the addition of more staff would not correspondingly improve patient care in this regard. The incidence of staff meetings and the enormous amount of record-keeping on patients, for example, have not been as substantially reduced as has patient contact. Priorities exist, even during hard times. Patient contact is not a significant priority in the traditional psychiatric hospital, and fiscal pressures do not account for this. Avoidance and depersonalization may.

Heavy reliance upon psychotropic medication tacitly contributes to depersonalization by convincing staff that treatment is indeed being conducted and that further patient contact may not be necessary. Even here, however, caution needs to be exercised in understanding the role of psychotropic drugs. If patients were powerful rather than powerless, if they were viewed as interesting individuals rather than diagnostic entities, if they were socially significant rather than social lepers, if their anguish truly and wholly compelled our sympathies and concerns, would we not *seek* contact with them, despite the availability of medications? Perhaps for the pleasure of it all?

THE CONSEQUENCES OF LABELING AND DEPERSONALIZATION

Whenever the ratio of what is known to what needs to be known approaches zero, we tend to invent "knowledge" and assume that we understand more than we actually do. We seem unable to acknowledge that we simply don't know. The needs for diagnosis and remediation of behavioral and emotional problems are enormous. But rather than acknowledge that we are just embarking on understanding, we continue to label patients "schizophrenic," "manic-depressive," and "insane," as if in those words we had captured the essence of understanding. The facts of the matter are that we have known for a long time that diagnoses are often not useful or reliable, but we have nevertheless continued to use them. We now know that we cannot distinguish insanity from sanity. It is depressing to consider how that information will be used.

Not merely depressing, but frightening. How many people, one wonders, are sane but not recognized as such in our psychiatric institutions? How many have been needlessly stripped of their privileges of citizenship, from the right to vote and drive to that of handling their own accounts? How many have feigned insanity in order to avoid the criminal consequences of their behavior, and, conversely, how many would rather stand trial than live interminably in a psychiatric hospital—but are wrongly thought to be mentally ill? How many have been stigmatized by well-intentioned, but nevertheless erroneous, diagnoses? On the last point, recall again that a "type 2 error" in psychiatric diagnosis does not have the same consequences it does in medical diagnosis. A diagnosis of cancer that has been found to be in error is cause for celebration. But psychiatric diagnoses are rarely found to be in error. The label sticks, a mark of inadequacy forever.

Finally, how many patients might be "sane" outside the psychiatric hospital but seem insane in it—not because craziness resides in them, as it were, but because they are responding to a bizarre setting, one that may be unique to institutions which harbor nether people? Goffman[4] calls the process of socialization to such institutions "mortification"— an apt metaphor that includes the processes of depersonalization that have been described here. And while it is impossible to know whether the pseudopatients' responses to these processes are characteristic of all inmates—they were, after all, not real patients—it is difficult to believe that these processes of socialization to a psychiatric hospital provide useful attitudes or habits of response for living in the "real world."

SUMMARY AND CONCLUSIONS

It is clear that we cannot distinguish the sane from the insane in psychiatric hospitals. The hospital itself imposes a special environment in which the meanings of behavior can easily be misunderstood. The consequences to patients hospitalized in such an environment—the powerlessness, depersonalization, segregation, mortification, and self-labeling—seem undoubtedly countertherapeutic.

I do not, even now, understand this problem well enough to perceive solutions. But two matters seem to have some promise. The first concerns the proliferation of community mental health facilities, of crisis intervention centers, of the human potential movement, and of behavior therapies that, for all of their own problems, tend to avoid psychiatric labels, to focus on specific problems and behaviors, and to retain the individual in a relatively nonpejorative environment. Clearly, to the extent that we refrain from sending the distressed to insane places, our impressions of them are less likely to be distorted. (The risk of distorted preceptions, it seems to me, is always present, since we are much more sensitive to an individual's behaviors and verbalizations than we are to the subtle contextual stimuli that often promote them. At issue here is a matter of magnitude. And, as I have shown, the magnitude of distortion is exceedingly high in the extreme context that is a psychiatric hospital.)

The second matter that might prove promising speaks to the need to increase the sensitivity of mental health workers and researchers to the *Catch 22* position of psychiatric patients. Simply reading materials in this area will be of help to some such workers and researchers. For others, directly experiencing the impact of psychiatric hospitalization will be of enormous use. Clearly, further research into the social psychology of such total institutions will both facilitate treatment and deepen understanding.

I and the other pseudopatients in the psychiatric setting had distinctly negative reactions. We do not pretend to describe the subjective experiences of true patients. Theirs may be different from ours, particularly with the passage of time and the necessary process of adaptation to one's environment. But we can and do speak to the relatively more objective indices of treatment within the hospital. It could be a mistake, and a very unfortunate one, to consider that what happened to us derived from malice or stupidity on the part of the staff. Quite the contrary, our overwhelming impression of them was of people who really cared, who were committed and who were uncommonly intelligent. Where they failed, as they sometimes did painfully, it would be more accurate to attribute those failures to the environment in which they, too, found themselves than to personal callousness. Their perceptions and behavior were controlled by the situation, rather than being motivated by a malicious disposition. In a more benign environment, one that was less attached to global diagnosis, their behaviors and judgments might have been more benign and effective.

REFERENCES AND NOTES

1. P. Ash, *J. Abnorm. Soc. Psychol*, 1949, **44**, 272; A. T. Beck, *Amer. J. Psychiat.*, 1962, **119**, 210; A. T. Boisen, *Psychiatry*, 1938, **2**, 233; N. Kreitman, *J. Ment Sci.*, 1961, **107**, 876; N. Krietman, P. Sainsbury, J. Morrisey, J. Towers, J. Scrivener, *ibid.*, p. 887; H. O. Schmitt and C. P. Fonda, *J. Abnorm. Soc. Psychol.*, 1956, **52**, 262; W. Seeman, *J. Nerv. Ment. Dis.*, 1953, **118**, 541. For an analysis of these artifacts and summaries of the disputes, see J. Zubin, *Annu. Rev. Psychol.*, 1967, **18**, 373; L. Phillips and J. G. Draguns, *ibid.*., 1971, **22**, 447.
2. R. Benedict, *J. Gen Psychol.*, 1934, **10**, 59.
3. See in this regard H. Becker, *Outsiders: Studies in the Sociology of Deviance* (Free Press, New York, 1963); B. M. Braginsky, D. D. Braginsky, K. Ring, *Methods of Madness: The Mental Hospital as a Last Resort* (Holt, Rinehart & Winston, New York, 1969); G. M. Crocetti and P. V. Lemkau, *Amer. Sociol. Rev.*, 1965 **30**, 577; E. Goffman, *Behavior in Public Places* (Free Press, New York, 1964); R. D. Laing, *The Divided Self: A Study of Sanity and Madness* (Quadrangle, Chicago, 1960); D. L. Phillips, *Amer. Sociol. Rev.*, 1963, **28**, 963; T. R. Sarbin, *Psychol. Today*, 1972, **6**, 18; E. Schur, *Amer. J. Sociol.*, 1969, **75**, 309; T. Szasz, *Law, Liberty and Psychiatry* (Macmillan, New York, 1963); *The Myth of Mental Illness: Foundations of a Theory of Mental Illness*

(Hoeber-Harper, New York, 1963). For a critique of some of these views, see W. R. Gove, *Amer. Sociol. Rev.*, 1970, **35**, 873.

4. E. Goffman, *Asylums* (Doubleday, Garden City, N.Y., 1961).

5. T. J. Scheff, *Being Mentally Ill: A Sociological Theory* (Aldine, Chicago, 1966).

6. Data from a ninth pseudopatient are not incorporated in this report because, although his sanity went undetected, he falsified aspects of his personal history, including his marital status and parental relationships. His experimental behaviors therefore were not identical to those of the other pseudopatients.

7. A. Barry, *Bellevue Is a State of Mind* (Harcourt Brace Jovanovich, New York, 1971); I. Belknap, *Human Problems of a State Mental Hospital* (McGraw-Hill, New York, 1956); W. Caudill, F. C. Redlich, H. R. Gilmore, E. B. Brody, *Amer. J. Orthopsychiat.*, 1952, **22**, 314; A. R. Goldman, R. H. Bohr, T. A. Steinberg, *Prof. Psychol.*, 1970, **1**, 427; unauthored, *Roche Report*, 1971, **1** (No. 13), 8.

8. Beyond the personal difficulties that the pseudopatient is likely to experience in the hospital, there are legal and social ones that, combined, require considerable attention before entry. For example, once admitted to a psychiatric institution, it is difficult, if not impossible, to be discharged on short notice, state law to the contrary notwithstanding. I was not sensitive to these difficulties at the outset of the project, nor to the personal and situational emergencies that can arise, but later a writ of habeas corpus was prepared for each of the entering pseudopatients and an attorney was kept "on call" during every hospitalization. I am grateful to John Kaplan and Robert Bartels for legal advice and assistance in these matters.

9. However distasteful such concealment is, it was a necessary first step to examining these questions. Without concealment, there would have been no way to know how valid these experiences were; nor was there any way of knowing whether whatever detections occurred were a tribute to the diagnostic acumen of the staff or to the hospital's rumor network. Obviously, since my concerns are general ones that cut across individual hospitals and staffs, I have respected their anonymity and have eliminated clues that might lead to their identification.

10. Interestingly, of the 12 admissions, 11 were diagnosed as schizophrenic and one, with the identical symptomatology, as manic-depressive psychosis. This diagnosis has a more favourable prognosis, and it was given by the only private hospital in our sample. On the relations between social class and psychiatric diagnosis, see A. deB. Hollingshead and F. C. Redlich, *Social Class and Mental Illness: A Community Study* (Wiley, New York, 1958).

11. It is possible, of course, that patients have quite broad latitudes in diagnosis and therefore are inclined to call many people sane, even those whose behavior is patently aberrant. However, although we have no hard data on this matter, it was our distinct impression that this was not the case. In many instances, patients not only singled us out for attention, but came to imitate our behaviors and styles.

12. J. Cumming and E. Cumming, *Community Ment. Health*, 1965, **1**, 135; A. Farina and K. Ring, *J. Abnorm. Psychol.*, 1965, **70**, 47; H. E. Freeman and O. G. Simmons, *The Mental Patient Comes Home* (Wiley, New York, 1963); W. J. Johannsen, *Ment. Hygiene*, 1969, **53**, 218; A. S. Linsky, *Soc. Psychiat.*, 1970, **53**, 166.

13. S. E. Asch, *J. Abnorm. Soc. Psychol.*, 1946, **41**, 258. *Social Psychology* (Prentice-Hall, New York, 1952).

14. See also I. N. Mensh and J. Wishner, *J. Personality*, 1947, **16**, 188; J. Wishner, *Psychol. Rev.*, 1960, **67**, 96; J. S. Bruner and R. Tagiuri, in *Handbook of Social Psychology*, G. Lindzey, Ed. (Addison-Wesley, Cambridge, Mass., 1954), vol. 2, pp. 634–654; J. S. Bruner, D. Shapiro, R. Tagiuri, in *Person Perception and Interpersonal Behavior*, R. Tagiuri and L. Petrullo, Eds. (Stanford Univ. Press, Stanford, Calif., 1958), pp. 277–288.

15. For an example of a similar self-fulfilling prophecy, in this instance dealing with the "central" trait of intelligence, see R. Rosenthal and L. Jacobson, *Pygmalion in the Classroom* (Holt, Rinehart & Winston, New York, 1968).

16. E. Zigler and L. Phillips, *J. Abnorm. Soc. Psychol.*, 1961, **63**, 69. See also R. K. Freudenberg and J. P. Robertson, *A.M.A. Arch. Neurol. Psychiatr.*, 1956, **76**, 14.

17. W. Mischel, *Personality and Assessment* (Wiley, New York, 1968).

18. The most recent and unfortunate instance of this tenet is that of Senator Thomas Eagleton.

19. T. R. Sarbin and J. C. Mancuso, *J. Clin. Consult. Psychol.* 1970, **35**, 159; T. R. Sarbin, *ibid.*, 1967, **31**, 447; J. C. Nunnally, Jr., *Popular Conceptions of Mental Health* (Holt, Rinehart & Winston, New York, 1961).
20. A. H. Stanton and M. S. Schwartz, *The Mental Hospital: A Study of Institutional Participation in Psychiatric Illness and Treatment* (Basic, New York, 1954).
21. D. B. Wexler and S. E. Scoville, *Ariz. Law Rev.*, 1971, **13**, 1.
22. I thank W. Mischel, E. Orne, and M. S. Rosenhan for comments on an earlier draft of this manuscript.

Contrary to indep (handwritten)

45

Science and Public Policy:
The Crime of Involuntary Mental
Hospitalization*

THOMAS S. SZASZ

For some time I have maintained that commitment—that is, the detention of persons in mental institutions against their will—is a form of imprisonment; that such deprivation of liberty is contrary to the moral principles embodied in the Declaration of Independence and the Constitution of the United States; and that it is a crass violation of contemporary concepts of fundamental human rights. The practice of "sane" men incarcerating their "insane" fellowmen in "mental hospitals" can be compared to that of white men enslaving black men. In short, I consider commitment a crime against humanity.

Existing social institutions and practices, especially if honored by prolonged usage, are generally experienced and accepted as good and valuable. For thousands of years slavery was considered a "natural" social arrangement for the securing of human labor; it was sanctioned by public opinion, religious dogma, church, and state; it was abolished a mere one hundred years ago in the United States, and is still practiced in some parts of the world, notably Africa. Commitment of the insane has enjoyed equally widespread support since its origin, approximately three centuries ago. Physicians, lawyers, and the laity have asserted as if with a single voice, the therapeutic desirability and social necessity of institutional psychiatry.

My claim that commitment is a crime against humanity may thus be countered—as indeed it has been—by maintaining, first, that the practice is beneficial for the mentally ill, *(unintelligible handwritten note)* and second, that it is necessary for the protection of the mentally healthy members of society. This conventional explanation is but a culturally accepted justification for certain quasimedical but extralegal forms of social control exercised against both individuals and groups whose behavior does not violate criminal laws but threatens established social values.

Mental illness is a metaphor. If by *disease* we mean a disorder of the physicochemical machinery of the body, then we can assert that what we call functional mental diseases are not diseases at all. Persons said to be suffering from such disorders are socially deviant or inept, or in conflict with individuals, groups, or institutions. Since they do not suffer from disease, it is impossible to "treat" them for any sickness.

Although the term *mentally ill* is customarily applied to persons who have no disease, it is sometimes also applied to persons who do. However, when patients with demonstrable diseases of the brain are involuntarily hospitalized, the primary purpose is to exercise social control over their behavior; treatment of the disease is, at best, a secondary consideration. Frequently, therapy is nonexistent, and custodial care is dubbed "treatment."

---

*From *Medical Opinion and Review*, 1968, May 25–35. Copyright © 1968 by *Medical Opinion and Review*. Reprinted by permission of *Medical Opinion and Review*, and Dr. Szasz. (Photographs have been omitted.)

Even if, as a result of future research, certain conditions now believed to be "functional" mental illness were shown to be "organic," my argument against involuntary mental hospitalization would remain unaffected.

In free societies, the relationship between physician and patient is predicated on the legal presumption that a person "owns" his body and his personality. The physician can examine and treat a patient only with his consent; the latter is free to reject treatment (for example, an operation for cancer). After death, "ownership" of the person's body is transferred to his heirs; the physician must obtain permission from them for a postmortem examination. John Stuart Mill explicitly affirmed that "each person is the proper guardian of his own health, whether bodily, or mental and spiritual." Commitment is incompatible with this moral principle.

Commitment practices flourished long before there were any mental or psychiatric "treatments" of "mental diseases." Indeed, madness or mental illness was not always a necessary condition for commitment. (See "Medical Ethics: A Historical Perspective," by Dr. Szasz, *MO & R*, February 1968.)

The claim that commitment of the "mentally ill" is necessary for the protection of the "mentally healthy" is more difficult to refute, not because it is valid, but because the danger that "mental patients" supposedly pose is of such an extremely vague nature.

However, in the absence of disease there is no medical justification for isolating patients with mental illness as there is for isolating patients with leprosy or tuberculosis.

If the so-called mental patient threatens others by virtue of his beliefs or actions, he could be dealt with by methods other than "medical." If his conduct is ethically offensive, moral sanctions might be appropriate; if forbidden by law, legal sanctions might be appropriate. In my opinion, both informal sanctions such as social ostracism or divorce and formal judicial sanctions such as fines and imprisonment are more dignified and less injurious to the human spirit than involuntary hospitalization.

To be sure, confinement does protect the community from certain problems. However, the question we ought to ask is not *whether* commitment protects the community from "dangerous mental patients," but rather, from precisely *what danger* it protects and by *what means?*

Slavery, too, protected the community: it freed the owners from manual labor. Commitment likewise shields the nonhospitalized members of society: first, from having to accommodate themselves to the annoying or idiosyncratic demands of persons who have not violated any criminal statutes; and, second, from having to apprehend and prosecute community members who have broken the law but who either cannot be convicted in court, or, if convicted, might not be restrained as effectively or as long in prison as in a mental hospital.

I have stated that commitment constitutes a social arrangement whereby one part of society secures certain advantages for itself at the expense of another part. To do so, the oppressors must possess an ideology to justify their actions; and they must be able to use the police power of the state. It may be argued that such use of state power is legitimate when law-abiding citizens punish lawbreakers. What is the difference between this use of state power and its use in enforcing slavery or involuntary commitment?

"Criminals" are subjected to such controls because they have violated laws applicable equally to all; "psychotics" and "slaves" are subjected to coercive controls of the state because they are members of a special class of inferior beings.

The principal purpose of imprisoning criminals is to protect the liberties of the law-abiding members of society. Since the individual subject to commitment is not considered a threat to these liberties in the same way as the accused criminal is (if he were, he would be

Compares slavery w/ commitment

prosecuted), his removal from society cannot be justified on the same grounds. Justification for commitment must thus rest on its therapeutic promise and potential: it will help restore the "patient" to "mental health." But if this can be accomplished only at the cost of robbing him of liberty, this goal is no more compatible with the moral principles of a free society than is the drafting (in the absence of a national emergency) of young men to serve as doctors or farmers; or of women, as nurses or maids.

Critical examination of the practice of involuntary mental hospitalization compels one to confront the basic moral dilemma of contemporary psychiatry: in a conflict between the values of liberty and mental health (no matter how defined), which should rank higher? The architects of the Open Society chose liberty; I want to reecho their choice. The architects of the Therapeutic Society chose mental health; the present-day supporters of commitment procedures reecho their choice.

The fundamental parallel between master and slave on the one hand, and institutional psychiatrist and involuntarily hospitalized patient on the other, lies in this: in each instance, the former member of the pair *defines* the social role of the latter, and *casts* him in that role by force.

Wherever there is slavery, there must be criteria for who may and who may not be enslaved. In ancient times, any people could be enslaved; bondage was the usual consequence of military defeat. After the advent of Christianity, although the people of Europe continued to make war on each other, they ceased enslaving prisoners who were Christians. By the time of the colonization of America, the peoples of the Western world considered only black men appropriate subjects for slave trade.

The criteria for distinguishing between those who may be incarcerated in mental hospitals and those who may not be are similar: poor and socially unimportant persons may be, and Very Important Persons may not be. This rule is manifested in two ways: first, through our mental hospital statistics, which show that the majority of institutionalized patients belong in the lowest socioeconomic classes; second, through the rarity and difficulty with which VIPs are committed. Yet even the sophisticated social scientists often misunderstand or misinterpret these correlations by attributing the low incidence of committed upper-class persons to a denial of the "medical fact" that "mental illness" can "strike" anyone. To be sure, powerful people may feel anxious or depressed, or behave in an excited or paranoid manner; but that, of course, is not the point at all.

Let us suppose that a person wishes to study slavery. How would he go about doing so? First, he might study slaves. He would then find that such persons are, in general, brutish, poor, and uneducated, and he might accordingly conclude that slavery is their "natural" or appropriate social state. Such, indeed, have been the methods and conclusions of innumerable men throughout the ages. Even the great Aristotle held slaves were "naturally" inferior and hence justly subdued. "From the hour of their birth," he asserted, "some are marked for subjection, others for rule." This view is similar to the modern concept of schizophrenia as a genetically caused disease.

Another student, "biased" by contempt for the institution of slavery, might proceed differently. He would maintain that there can be no slave without a master holding him in bondage; and he would accordingly consider slavery a type of human relationship and, more generally, a social institution supported by custom, law, religion, and force, From this point of view, the study of masters is at least as relevant to the study of slavery as is the study of slaves.

The latter point of view is generally accepted today with regard to slavery, but not with regard to institutional psychiatry. "Mental illness" of the type found in psychiatric hospitals has been investigated for centuries, and continues to be investigated today, in much the same way as slaves were studied in the antebellum South and before. The "existence" of slaves was taken for granted; their biological and social characterisics were noted and classified. Similarly, the "existence" of "mental patients" is now taken for granted; indeed, it is widely believed that their number is steadily increasing. The psychiatrist's task is to observe and classify their biological, psychological, and social characteristics.

This perspective is a manifestation, in part, of what I have called "the myth of mental illness"—that is, of the notion that mental illnesses are similar to diseases of the body; and in part, of the psychiatrist's intense need to deny the fundamental complementarity of his relationship to the involuntary mental patient. The same complementarity obtains in all situations where one person or party assumes a superior or dominant role and ascribes an inferior or submissive role to another; for example, master and slave, accuser and accused, inquisitior and witch. (Sometimes people willingly assume a submissive role and cast their partners in a dominant role. I am not concerned with this aspect of the problem here.)

A basic assumption of American slavery was that the Negro slave was racially inferior. "There is no malice toward the Negro in Ulrich Phillips' work," wrote S. M. Elkins about that author's book, *American Negro Slavery*, a work sympathetic to the Southern position. "Phillips was deeply fond of the Negroes as a people; it was just that he could not take them seriously as men and women; they were children."

Similarly, the basic assumption of institutional psychiatry is that the "mentally ill" person is psychologically and socially inferior. He is like a child: he does not know what is in his best interests and therefore needs others to control and protect him. Psychiatrists often care deeply for their involuntary patients, whom they consider—in contrast with the merely "neurotic" persons—"psychotic," which is to say, "very sick." Hence, such patients must be cared for as the "irresponsible children" they are considered to be.

The perspective of paternalism has played an exceedingly important role in justifying both slavery and involuntary mental hospitalization. Aristotle defined slavery as "an essentially domestic relationship"; in so doing, wrote D. B. Davis, in *The Problem of Slavery in Western Culture*, he "endowed it with the sanction of paternal authority, and helped to establish a precedent that would govern discussions of political philosophers as late as the eighteenth century." The relationship between psychiatrists and mental patients has been and continues to be viewed in the same way. The fact that, as in the case of slavery, the physician needs the police power of the State to maintain his relationship with his so-called patient does not alter this self-serving image of the oppressive institution.

Paternalism is the crucial explanation for the stubborn conflict about whether the practices employed by slaveholders and institutional psychiatrists are "therapeutic" or "noxious." Masters and psychiatrists profess their benevolence; their slaves and involuntary patients protest against their malevolence. As S. L. Halleck, a defender of contemporary mental health practices, put it in *Psychiatry and the Dilemmas of Crime*: "... the psychiatrist experiences himself as a helping person, but his patient may see him as a jailer. Both views are partially correct." Not so. Both views are completely correct. Each is a proposition about a different subject: the former, about the psychiatrist's self-image; the latter, about the involuntary mental patient's image of his captor. In Ward 7, Valeriy Tarsis presents the following dialogue between his protagonist-patient and the mental hospital physician: "This is the position. I don't regard you as a doctor. You call this a hospital, I call it a prison.... So now, let's get everything straight. I am your prisoner, you are my jailer, and there isn't going to be any nonsense about my health...or treatment."

This is the characteristic dialogue of oppression and liberation. The ruler looks in the mirror and sees a liberator; the ruled looks at the ruler and sees a tyrant. If the physician has the power to incarcerate the patient and uses it, the relationship between the two will inevitably fit into this mold, If one cannot ask the subject whether he likes being enslaved or commited, whipped or electroshocked—because he is not a fit judge of his own "best interests"—then one is left with the contending opinions of the practitioners and their critics.

The defenders of slavery claimed that the Negro was happier as a slave than he could have been as a free man because of the "peculiarities of his character." The defenders of involuntary mental hospitalization claim that the mental patient is healthier—the twentieth-century synonym for *happier*—as a psychiatric prisoner than he would be as a free citizen because of the nature of his illness. It requires no great feat of imagination to see how comforting—indeed, how absolutely necessary—these views are, even when contradicted by fact.

For example, although it was held that the Negro slave was happy, there was an ever-lurking fear of Negro violence and revolt. As S. M. Elkins (*Slavery: A Problem in American Institutional and Intellectual Life*) put it: "The failure of any free workers to present themselves for enslavement can serve as one test of how much the analysis of the 'happy slave' may have added to Americans' understanding of themselves."

The same views and the same inconsistencies apply to involuntary psychiatric hospitalization. (Defenders of the system maintain that the committed patient is better off in the hospital; at the same time, the patients are feared for their potential violence, their escapes from captivity occasion intense manhunts, and their crimes are prominently featured in the newspapers.) Moreover, as with slavery, the failure of free citizens to present themselves for involuntary psychiatric hospitalization can serve as a test of how much the currently popular analysis of mental health problems may have added to Americans' understanding of themselves.

The social necessity, and hence the basic value, of involuntary mental hospitalization, at least for some people, is not seriously questioned today. (It is thus possible to debate *who* should be hospitalized, or *how*, or for *how long*—but not whether *anyone* should be.) I submit, however, that just as it is improper to enslave anyone—black or white, Moslem or Christian—so it is improper to hospitalize anyone without his consent, whether he is depressed or paranoid, hysterical or schizophrenic.

Our unwillingness to look at this problem searchingly may be compared to the unwillingness of the South to look at slavery. "…a democratic people," writes Elkins, "no longer 'reasons' with itself when it is all of the same mind. Men will then only warn and exhort each other, that their solidarity may be yet more perfect. The South's intellectuals, after the 1830s, did really little more than this. And when the enemy's reality disappears, when his concreteness recedes, then intellect itself, with nothing more to resist it and give it resonance, merges with the mass and stultifies, and shadows become monsters."

Our growing preoccupation with the menace of mental illness may be a manifestation of just such a process. A democratic nation, as we have been warned by Tocqueville, is especially vulnerable to the hazards of a surfeit of agreement: "The authority of a king is physical, and controls the actions of men without subduing their will. But the majority possesses a power that is physical and moral at the same time, which acts upon the will as much as upon the actions, and represses not only all contests, but all controversy."

(There are essential similarities in relationships between masters and subjects—no matter whether owners and slaves or psychiatrists and confined patients.)

To maintain a relationship of personal or class superiority, it is necessary, as a rule, that the oppressor keep the oppressed uninformed, especially about matters pertinent to their relationship. In America the history of the systematic efforts by the whites to keep the Negro ignorant is well known. A dramatic example is the law, passed in 1824 by the

Virginia Assembly, that provided a fifty-dollar fine and two months' imprisonment for teaching *free Negroes* to read and write. Nor was the situation very different in the North. In January 1833, Prudence Crandall admitted to her private school, in Canterbury, Connecticut, a young lady of seventeen, the daughter of a highly respected Negro family. Miss Crandall was thereupon ostracized and persecuted by her neighbors. She was formally tried for breaking a law that forbade the harboring, boarding, or instruction in any manner of any person of color and was convicted. Finally, her school was set on fire.

A similar effort to educationally degrade and psychologically impoverish their charges characterizes the acts of the managers of mad houses. In most prisons in the United States, it is possible for a convict to obtain a high school diploma, to learn a trade, to become an amateur lawyer, or to write a book. None of these is possible in a mental hospital. Moreover the principal requirement for an inmate of such an institution is that he accept the psychiatric ideology about his "illness," and the things he must do to "recover" from it. The committed patient must thus accept the view that he is "sick," and that his captors are "well"; that his own view of himself is false, and that of his captors true; and that to effect any change in his social situation he must relinquish his "sick" views and adopt the "healthy" views of those who have power over him. By accepting himself as "sick", and his institutional environment and the various manipulations imposed on him by the staff as "treatment," the mental patient is compelled to authenticate the psychiatrist's role as that of a benevolent physician curing mental illness. The mental patient who maintains the forbidden image of reality, i.e., that the institutional psychiatrist is a jailer, is considered paranoid. Moreover, since most patients—as do oppressed people generally—sooner or later accept the ideas imposed on them by their superiors, hospital psychiatrists are constantly immersed in an environment in which their identity as "doctors" is affirmed. The moral superiority of white men over black was similarly authenticated and affirmed.

In both situations, the oppressor first subjugates his adversary, and then cites his status as proof of his inferiority. Once this process is set in motion, it develops its own momentum and psychological logic.

Looking at the relationship, the oppressor will see his superiority and hence his well-deserved dominance; the oppressed will see his inferiority and hence his well-deserved submission. In race relations in the United States, we continue to reap the bitter results of this philosophy, and in psychiatry, we are even now sowing seeds of this poisonous fruit, whose eventual harvest may be equally bitter and long.

Convicts are entitled to fight for their "legal rights"; but not involuntary mental patients. Like slaves, such patients have no rights except those granted them by their medical masters. According to Benjamin Apfelberg, Clinical Professor of Psychiatry and Medical Director of the Law-Psychiatry Project at New York University: "Our students come to realize that by fighting for a patient's *legal* rights they may actually be doing him a great disservice. They learn that there is such a thing as a person's *medical* rights, the right to get treatment, to become well," (*SK & F Psychiatric Reporter, July-August* 1965.)

The 'medical right' to which Apfelberg refers is a euphemism for the *obligation* to remain confined in a mental institution, not the *opportunity* to choose between hospitalization and no hospitalization. But calling involuntary mental hospitalization a "medical right" is like calling involuntary servitude in antebellum Georgia a "right to work."

Oppression and degradation are unpleasant to behold and are, therefore, frequently disguised or concealed. One method for doing so is to segregate—in special areas, such as camps or "hospitals"—the degraded human beings. Another is to conceal the social realities behind the fictional facade of what we call, after Wittgenstein, "language games."

While psychiatric language games may seem fanciful, the psychiatric idiom is actually only a dialect of the common language of oppressors. Thus slaveholders called the slaves live-stock, mothers *breeders* their children *increase*, and gave the term *drivers* to the men set over them at work. The defenders of psychiatric imprisonment call their institutions *hospitals*, the inmates *patients*, and the keepers *doctors*; they refer to the sentence as *treatment*, and to the deprivation of liberty as *protection of the patient's best interests*.

In both cases, the semantic devices are supplemented by appeals to tradition, morality, and social necessity. The proslavery factions in America argued that the abolitionists were wrong because they were seeking to overthrow an ancient institution recognized by the Scriptures and the Constitution.

The contemporary reader may find it difficult to believe how unquestioningly slavery was accepted as a natural and beneficial social arrangement. Even as great a liberal thinker as John Locke did not advocate its abolition. Moreover, protests against the slave trade would have provoked the hostility of powerful religious and economic groups.

Similar considerations apply to challenging the institution of involuntary mental hospitalization.

In Western nations and the Soviet Bloc alike, there are two views on commitment. According to the one, involuntary mental hospitalization is an indispensable method of medical healing and a humane type of social control; according to the other, it is a contemptible abuse of the medical relationship and a type of imprisonment without trial. We adopt the former view and consider commitment "proper" if we use it on victims of our choosing whom we despise; we adopt the latter view and consider commitment "improper" if our enemies use it on victims of their choosing whom we esteem.

The change in perspective— from seeing slavery occasioned by the "inferiority" of the Negro and commitment by the "insanity" of the patient, to seeing each occasioned by the interplay of, and especially the power relation between, the participants— has far-reaching practical implications. In the case of slavery, it meant not only that the slaves had an obligation to revolt and emancipate themselves, but also that the masters had an even greater obligation to renounce their roles as slaveholders. Naturally, a slaveholder with such ideas felt compelled to set his slaves free, at whatever cost to himself. This is precisely what some slaveowners did.

Their action had profound consequences in a social system based on slavery. For the act led almost invariably to the former master's expulsion from the community—through economic pressure or personal harassment or both. Such persons usually emigrated to the North. For the nation as a whole, these acts and the abolitionist sentiments behind them symbolized a fundamental moral rift between those who regarded the Negroes as objects or slaves, and those who regarded them as persons or citizens. The former could persist in regarding the slave as existing in nature; whereas the latter could not deny his own moral responsibility for creating man in the image, not of God, but of the slave-animal.

The implications of this perspective for institutional psychiatry are equally clear. A psychiatrist who accepts as his "client" a person who does not wish to be his client, defines him as a "mentally ill" person, then incarcerates him in an institution, bars his escape from the institution and from the role of mental patient and proceeds to "treat" him against his will—such a psychiatrist, I maintain, creates "mental illness" and "mental patients." He does so in exactly the same way as the white man who sailed for Africa, captured the black man, brought him to America in shackles, and then sold him as if he were an animal, created slavery and slaves. To be sure, in both cases, the process is carried out in accordance with the law of the land. The assertion that only the "insane" are committed to mental hospitals is, in this view, comparable to the claim that only the black man is enslaved. It is the most damaging evidence, for it signifies that the oppressor recognizes the "special " condition of his adversary.

The parallel may be carried one step further. The renouncing of slaveholding by some slaveowners led to certain social problems, such as Negro unemployment and a gradual splitting of the country into pro- and anti-slavery factions. The renouncing by some psychiatrists of relationships with involuntary mental patients has led to certain professional problems in the past and is likely to do so in the future. Psychiatrists restricting their work to psychoanalysis and psychotherapy have been accused of not being "real doctors"—as if depriving a person of his liberty required medical skills; of "shirking their responsibilities" to their colleagues and to society by accepting only the "easier cases" and refusing to treat the "seriously mentally ill" patient—as if practicing self-control and eschewing violence were newly discovered forms of immorality.

The psychiatric profession has, of course, a huge stake, both existential and economic, in being socially authorized to rule over mental patients, just as the slave-owning classes did in ruling over slaves. In contemporary psychiatry, indeed, the expert gains superiority not only over members of a specific class of victims, but over nearly the whole of the population, whom he may "psychiatrically evaluate."

The economic similarities between chattel slavery and institutional psychiatry are equally evident. The economic strength of the slaveowner was determined by the number of slaves he owned. The economic strength of the institutional psychiatrist lies, similarly, in his involuntary mental patients, who are not free to move about, work, marry, divorce, or make contracts, but are, instead under the control of the hospital director. The income and power of the psychiatric bureaucrat rises with the size of the institution he controls and the number of patients he commands. Moreover, just as the slaveholder could use the police power of the state to help him recruit and maintain his slave labor force, so can the institutional psychiatrist rely on the state to help him recruit and maintain a population of hospital inmates.

Finally, since the various governments have vast economic stakes in the operation of psychiatric hospitals and clinics, the interests of the state and of institutional psychiatry tend to be the same. Formerly the state and federal governments had a vast economic stake in the operation of plantations worked by slaves, and hence the interests of the state and of the slaveowning classes tended to be the same. The wholly predictable consequence of such an arrangement is that the oppressive institution is invincible; its defects, no matter how glaring, cannot be much improved. On the other hand, once such an institution loses the support of the state, it rapidly disintegrates; there can be no oppression without power.

If this argument is valid, pressing the view that psychiatrists now create mentally sick clients just as slaveholders used to create slaves is likely to lead to a cleavage in the psychiatric profession, and perhaps in society generally, between those who condone and advocate the relationship between psychiatrist and involuntary mental patient and those who condemn and oppose it.

It is not clear whether, or on what terms, these two psychiatric factions could coexist. The practices of coercive psychiatry and of paternalistic psychiatrists do not, in themselves, threaten the practices of noncoercive psychiatry and of contracting psychiatrists. Economic relations based on slavery coexisted over long periods with relations based on contract. But the moral conflict poses a more difficult problem. For just as the abolitionists tended to undermine the social justifications of slavery and the psychological bonds of the slave, so the abolitionists of psychiatric slavery tend to undermine the justifications of commitment and the psychological bonds of the committed patient.

Ultimately, the forces of society will probably be enlisted on one side or the other. If so, we may, on the one hand, be ushering in the abolition of involuntary mental hospitalization and treatment; on the other, we may be witnessing the fruitless struggles of an individualism bereft of popular support against a collectivism proferred as medical treatment.

We know that man's domination over his fellowman is as old as history; and we may safely assume that it is traceable to prehistoric times and to prehuman ancestors. Perennially, men have oppressed women; white men, colored men; Christians, Jews. However, traditional reasons and justifications for discrimination have lost much of their plausibility. What justification is there for man's age-old desire for domination of his fellowman? Modern liberalism (in reality, a type of statism), allied with scientism, has met the need for a fresh defense of oppression and has supplied a new battle cry: Health!

In this therapeutic-meliorist view of society, the ill form a special class of "victims" who must, both for their own good and for the interests of the community, be "helped"—coercively and against their will, if necessary—by the healthy; and among the healthy, especially by physicians, who are "scientifically" qualified to be their masters. This perspective developed first and has advanced farthest in psychiatry, where the oppression of "insane patients" by "sane physicians" is by now a social custom hallowed by medical and legal tradition. At present, the medical profession as a whole seems to be emulating this model. In the Therapeutic State toward which we appear to be moving, the principal requisite for the role of Big Brother may be an MD degree.

Suggested Additional Readings

Farina, A., & Ring, K. The influence of perceived mental illness on interpersonal relations. *Journal of Abnormal Psychology*, 1965, **70,** 47–51.

Goffman, E. *Stigma.* Englewood Cliffs, N. J.: Prentice-Hall, 1963.

Honey, C. A., & Miller, K. S. Definitional factors in mental incompetency. *Sociology and Social Research*, 1970, **54,** 520–532.

Hugh, A. P. Commitment of the mentally ill: Problems of law and policy. *Michigan Law Review*, 1959, **57,** 945–1018.

Kesey, K. *One flew over the cuckoo's nest.* New York: Viking, 1962.

Lindman, F. T., & McIntyre, D. M., Jr. *The mentally disabled and the law.* Chicago: University of Chicago Press, 1961.

Maisel, R. Decision making in a commitment court. *Psychiatry*, 1970, **33,** 352–361.

Miller, D., & Dawson, W. H. Effects of stigma on re-employment of ex-mental patients. *Mental Hygiene*, 1965, **49,** 281–287.

Nunnally, J. C., Jr. *Popular conceptions of mental health.* New York: Holt, Rhinehart & Winston, 1961.

Nunnally, J. C., Jr., & Kittross, J. M. Public attitudes toward mental health professions. *American Psychologist*, 1958, **13,** 589–594.

Phillips, D. Rejection: A possible consequence of seeking help for mental disorders. *American Sociological Review*, 1963, **28,** 963–972.

Phillips, D. L. Rejection of the mentally ill: The influence of behavior and sex. *American Sociological Review*, 1964, **29,** 679–689.

Rabkin, J. G. Opinions about mental illness: A review of the literature. *Psychological Bulletin*, 1972, **77,** 153–171.

Rosen, A. C. Changes in the perception of mental illness and mental health. *Perceptual and Motor Skills*, 1971, **31,** 203–208.

Rosenhan, D. L. On being sane in insane places. *Science*, 1973, **179,** 250–258.

Simon, R. J., & Shackelford, W. The defenses of insanity: A survey of legal and psychiatric opinion. *Public Opinion Quarterly*, 1965, **29,** 411–424.

Stone, A. D. Psychiatry and the law. *Psychiatric Annals*, 1971, **1,** 19–43.

Swanson, R. M., & Spitzer, S. P. Stigma and the psychiatric patient career. *Journal of Health and Social Behavior*, 1970, **11,** 44–51.

Szasz, T. *The myth of mental illness.* New York: Harper & Row, 1961.

Szasz, T. *Ideology and insanity,* New York: Anchor Books, 1970.

Topp, J. L. Psychology and the law: The dilemma. *Psychology Today*, 1969, **2,** 16–22.

Whatley, C. D. Social attitudes toward discharged mental patients. *Social Problems*, 1959, **6,** 313–330.

Name Index

(References are noted by numerals in italics)

Subject Index

TITLES IN THE PERGAMON GENERAL PSYCHOLOGY SERIES (Continued)